Clinical Pediatric Physical Therapy

A GUIDE FOR THE PHYSICAL THERAPY TEAM

Clinical Pediatric Physical Therapy

A GUIDE FOR THE PHYSICAL THERAPY TEAM

KATHERINE T. RATLIFFE, MA, PT

Project Coordinator
Hawai'i University Affiliated Program
University of Hawai'i

Physical Therapist
Rehabilitation Services Department
Kapiolani Medical Center for Women and Children

Lecturer
Physical Therapist Assistant Program
Kapiolani Community College
Honolulu, Hawai'i

Photographs by Clark E. Ratliffe, RN, MS
Illustrations by Jeanne Robertson

with 364 illustrations

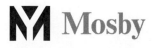 Mosby

St. Louis Baltimore Boston Carlsbad Chicago Minneapolis New York Philadelphia Portland
London Milan Sydney Tokyo Toronto

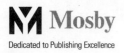

Printed in the United States of America

Mosby, Inc.
11830 Westline Industrial Drive
St. Louis, Missouri 63146

Library of Congress Cataloging in Publication Data

Ratliffe, Katherine T.
    Clinical pediatric physical therapy : a guide for the physical
therapy team / Katherine T. Ratliffe.
        p.   cm.
    Includes bibliographical references and index.
    ISBN 0-8151-7088-2
    1. Physical therapy for children.   I. Title.
    [DNLM: 1. Physical Therapy—infancy & childhood.   WB 460 R236c
1998]
RJ53.P5R38   1998
615.8′2′083—dc21
DNLM/DLC
                                                              97-29089

  99 00 01 / 9 8 7 6 5 4 3 2

Contributors

LINDA McCORMICK, PhD

Professor
Department of Special Education
College of Education
University of Hawaiʻi
Honolulu, Hawaiʻi

IRENE R. McEWEN, PhD, PT, PCS

Associate Professor
Department of Physical Therapy
University of Oklahoma
Oklahoma City, Oklahoma

MARILYN E. MILLER, PhD, PT, GCS

Associate Professor and Director
Physical Therapist Assistant Program
Department of Health Sciences
University of Hawaiʻi–Kapiolani Community College
Honolulu, Hawaiʻi

GAY M. NAGANUMA, MS, PT

Therapy Department Coordinator
Boyer Children's Clinic
Seattle, Washington

KATHERINE A. O'REILLY, PT, MPH

Director
Rehabilitation Services Department
Kapiolani Medical Center for Women and Children
Honolulu, Hawaiʻi

CLARK E. RATLIFFE, RN, MS

Instructor of Pediatrics
School of Nursing
University of Hawaiʻi
Honolulu, Hawaiʻi

KATHERINE T. RATLIFFE, MA, PT

Project Coordinator
Hawaiʻi University Affiliated Program
University of Hawaiʻi
Physical Therapist
Rehabilitation Services Department
Kapiolani Medical Center for Women and Children
Lecturer
Physical Therapist Assistant Program
Kapiolani Community College
Honolulu, Hawaiʻi

NANCY B. ROBINSON, PhD, CCC-SLP

Assistant Professor
Associate Director and Interdisciplinary Training Director
University Affiliated Program
University of Hawaiʻi
Honolulu, Hawaiʻi

JAMES R. SKOUGE, EdD

Assistant Professor
Director, Media, Computing and Assistive Technology Center
Hawaiʻi University Affiliated Program
Honolulu, Hawaiʻi

LORRAINE SYLVESTER, MS, PT

Physical Therapist
Kamuela, Hawaiʻi

KAREN J. TESSIER, MS, RN

Pediatric Faculty
School of Nursing
University of Hawaiʻi
Honolulu, Hawaiʻi

This book is dedicated to the children and their families
who have opened their hearts and their homes to help us all understand,
especially Andrew, Camila, Clinton, Coreen, Cyril, Ian, Kal,
Kawailani, Luke, Matthew, Noelani, Shelly, and Tyler

Foreword

Throughout the history of our profession, pediatric physical therapists have been at the forefront in developing and implementing innovative models of practice (Stuberg & Harbourne, 1994), in conducting and disseminating leading-edge clinical research (Campbell, 1990; Harris & Mulero Portela, 1994), and in facilitating the learning of current and future pediatric therapy practitioners through creative teaching tools and educational curricula (Campbell & Carter, 1990; Spake, 1994). Katherine Ratliffe's outstanding text on clinical pediatric physical therapy, written as a guide for physical therapists (PTs) and physical therapist assistants (PTAs) working together as a team, maintains the tradition of excellence set forth by her predecessors in pediatric physical therapy. I applaud her creativity in conceiving this extremely worthwhile book and her diligence in completing it, as well as her commitment to such important principles as people-first language, family-centered therapy, functionally and ecologically based interventions, and a life span continuum of service provision.

Written in a well-organized, straightforward, and family-sensitive manner, this text will appeal to both entry-level physical therapy students and PTAs who plan to work with children who have special needs. A comprehensive Case Study of a child with a particular illness or disability provides a focal point for each chapter and serves as an excellent learning tool. Rather than using a medically oriented, problem-based approach to each case example, Ms. Ratliffe has chosen to emphasize the child's everyday activities within the context of home, family, and school. The children and their families come from a variety of ethnic and cultural backgrounds, and each child literally "comes alive" as you learn about how he or she interacts with parents, siblings, teachers, peers, and health care providers. Each Case Study includes a physical therapy evaluation summary and a home-based or school-based therapy program with sample individualized educational plan (IEP) or individualized family support plan (IFSP) goals. In addition, special Applications sections, written by a variety of well-known contributing authors, are imbedded within each disability-focused chapter. These sections include important topics such as the multicultural aspects of physical therapy intervention; the role of school-based therapy; the use of splints, orthoses, and assistive technology; seating, positioning, and mobility; and the use of positive behavioral strategies. The final chapter, focusing on medical disorders of childhood, includes a Case Study of a teenager recovering from cancer. It presents an Applications section on death and dying with sensitive, pragmatic strategies for providing practical support, empathetic listening, and helpful things to say.

Having supervised PTA students while I worked as a public school PT, I have long believed that the role of the PTA in working with children with special needs is extremely important. The PTA's potential for contributing as an integral member of the interdisciplinary team has not been well acknowledged or well understood by many of my own professional peers. The publication of this exciting text, which not only acknowledges but also defines the complementary roles of the pediatric PT and the pediatric PTA, is a much-needed addition to the field. Not only will our two professions benefit from this book, but, more important, it will enhance our ability to serve these special children and their families better.

It is, indeed, a great honor to have been invited to write the foreword for this unique, compelling, and well-written guide to the education of pediatric PTs and PTAs. Hats off to Katherine Ratliffe and the other contributing authors for a landmark achievement in sensitively and creatively enhancing the knowledge base of those of us who are privileged to work with children with special needs and their families!

SUSAN R. HARRIS, PhD, PT, FAPTA
Professor, School of Rehabilitation Sciences
University of British Columbia
Vancouver, British Columbia, Canada

References

Campbell, S.K. (Guest Ed.) (1990). Proceedings of the consensus conference on the efficacy of physical therapy in the management of cerebral palsy. *Pediatric Physical Therapy,* 2(3), 123-176.

Campbell, S.K., & Carter, R.E. (1990). *Topics in pediatrics* (*In Touch* Continuing Education Series). Alexandria, VA: American Physical Therapy Association.

Harris, S.R., & Mulero Portela, A.L. (1994). Research in pediatric physical therapy: Past, present, and future. *Pediatric Physical Therapy,* 6(3), 133-138.

Spake, E.F. (1994). Reflections and visions: The state of pediatric curricula. *Pediatric Physical Therapy,* 6(3), 128-132.

Stuberg, W., & Harbourne, R. (1994). Theoretical practice in pediatric physical therapy: Past, present, and future considerations. *Pediatric Physical Therapy,* 6(3), 119-125.

Preface

Physical therapists (PTs) and physical therapist assistants (PTAs), especially those working with children, generally enter the profession because they want to help. Helping is an admirable goal; however, we must make sure that we do not overestimate the contributions of our own knowledge and expertise. It is only through partnerships with children and families, as well as with other team members, that we can truly make a difference.

Several years ago I attended a keynote lecture by Norman Kunc, a family therapist from British Columbia who has cerebral palsy, at the Pacific Rim conference in Honolulu (Kunc, 1995). Mr. Kunc discussed the insensitivity he experienced at the hands of PTs during his childhood, but he spiced his talk with enough humor to keep therapists in their seats. He recounted feeling violated when his clothes were removed and he was touched without his consent. He perceived the interventions as separating him from his peers rather than helping him fit in with them. Instead of going swimming like his peers, he had aquatherapy; instead of playing in the dirt, he had garden therapy; instead of eating lunch, he had feeding therapy. He never felt as if he belonged, and he blamed therapists for much of this isolation. Listening to him from the audience, I cringed as I recognized myself in his portrayal of the "evil" PT. His voice echoed that of others who have described feelings of intrusion, isolation, and alienation during childhood that were aided and abetted by PTs. These voices are being heard and are changing many of our attitudes and practices as pediatric PTs.

When we meet someone with a disability, the disability itself seems prominent. The medical appliances, deformities, and deficits stand out as being different. This is especially true for students and others who have not known many individuals with disabilities. The differences draw the attention. The personality, character, and capabilities of the child remain in the background. Therapy providers need to see the child before the disease, the personality and strengths before the disability. By presenting case studies of children as whole beings—with families, dreams, and fears—this book attempts to avoid the tendency of many textbooks to focus on the disease or the disability first. It is in the context of a child's life—the classroom, playground, bus, or grocery store—where individual needs for children emerge. We may note that Bobby needs to learn to walk, but we need to know that he specifically wants to walk between his classroom and the cafeteria at the same speed as his classmates, walk between his bedroom and bathroom at night without help, or walk in the mall while shopping with his mother. Teaching Bobby to take steps independently may or may not help him walk while being jostled by other children, walk down a dimly lit hall at night, or negotiate the varied levels and surfaces of the mall with visual and auditory distractions. Teaching skills in isolation does not always lead to generalization of the skills to functional contexts. Providing therapy in varied environments is much more difficult than the old "pull-out" model in which children are removed from their classrooms for therapy. Professional peers may not be available for consultation, tools may not be available when we need them, and old routines may not work in new situations. Creativity, ingenuity, and self-reliance are necessary tools of the trade.

Many children can benefit from physical therapy services provided by PTAs in hospitals, schools, clinics, and homes. However, what became very apparent while I was writing this book was that the PTA does not work in isolation. The PT is always working with the PTA to provide initial and continued assessment of the child, as well as guidance about the provision of physical therapy services. The PT has an important role in this team, yet many PTs, especially those in pediatric settings, have no idea of the scope of practice of the PTA or how to use or supervise the PTA effectively. In addition to teaching PTAs and others about pediatric physical therapy practices, this book attempts to educate physical therapy providers about the roles of the PT and the PTA in pediatrics and how they can work together to serve children and their families optimally. The concept of a physical therapy team that provides a coordinated approach to meet the child's physical therapy needs appropriately describes the relationship between the different individuals attending to the physical therapy needs of a child. The physical therapy team includes primarily the PT and the PTA but also others who may provide physical therapy supports to children, for example, teachers, educational assistants, parents, and other therapists. The advent of this physical therapy team and the specific role of the PTA in pediatrics may change and expand the role previously played by the PT, but the needs of children still dictate the services provided. The PT is the leader of the physical therapy team. He or she conducts initial and ongoing assessment of the child and—with team input—develops goals and objectives as well as an intervention plan for the child. The PTA's role on the team is to assist in carrying out the interventions with some autonomy as to what activities are used to meet the established goals. Other team members may also perform activities with children to meet their physical therapy goals. As in any team, all the members must communicate regularly to ensure that the child's needs are being met.

This book was originally intended to be primarily for the PTA. It grew out of a pediatrics course for PTAs that I teach collaboratively with Wendy Tada, PhD, PT, at Kapiolani Community College in Honolulu. Emphasis is on the day-to-day intervention with the child who has physical therapy needs rather than on assessment procedures. It is hoped that the information offered here will be of practical help to physical therapy providers in many settings. Students can learn from specific suggestions of techniques, strategies, and approaches, as well as the generous numbers of photographs and drawings illustrating many of the points discussed. Special features of the text include an outline of the chapter contents and a list of Key Terms. Study aides include Exercises for readers to learn about resources in their own communities and to explore more personal feelings related to the topics presented. Questions to Ponder are posed to initiate discussions or personal reflection on the part of the reader. An Annotated Bibliography at the end of each chapter introduces the reader to further resources. Although specific techniques and strategies for working with children and families are embedded in the text, several have also been highlighted in special boxes throughout the chapters. Applications sections in each chapter discuss in depth specific topics that are applicable to children with the disorders discussed.

The text is organized in four parts. Part One discusses the context of physical therapy intervention with children. Social, legal, and practice issues related to pediatric practice in general are presented in Chapter 1. Issues such as laws mandating services to children, approaches to the child and family, and current and future practice issues related to pediatric physical therapy, including health care reform and genetic testing, are discussed. The development of the PTA job category, issues related to supervision of the PTA, and specific skills that the PTA possesses to work with children are discussed in Chapter 2. Chapter 3 considers the typical development of children as they grow from birth to adolescence. Part Two addresses orthopedic disorders of children, including hip disorders, developmental orthopedic disorders, and other orthopedic disorders. Part Three discusses neurological disorders—including cerebral palsy, genetic disorders, and traumatic disorders—and cognitive, sensory, and processing disorders. Part Four focuses on medical disorders of childhood, including prematurity. Parts Two, Three, and Four all consist of two to four chapters organized around groups of disorders. Each chapter begins with a Case Study to illustrate the school, community, and home environments of a child with one of the disorders being discussed.

This book can be used in several ways for teaching in entry-level PT or PTA programs. In traditional teaching models based on didactic methods, the text can be used as reference material to support classroom discussions and lectures. Alternatively, the case studies can be used as focal points in a problem- or inquiry-based approach to teaching. In this method students reading the cases identify issues they want to learn more about and use other resources, including the Background and Theory sections of the chapters, the Applications sections, the resources highlighted in the annotated bibliographies, and other references, to research identified learning issues. This method of teaching encourages problem solving and independent learning.

Physical therapy for children is evolving as financial and social pressures bring changes to service delivery systems. Increasingly, many practitioners are working in isolation from professional peers as service delivery occurs in homes, neighborhood schools, and community settings. This text is an effort to bring the practice of pediatric physical therapy to life for both practicing PTs and PTAs, as well as for students aspiring to work with children. Information is presented in ways that can be useful and practical. My own biases are readily apparent, and I apologize in advance to those I may offend. I simply hope that the book is useful and that it benefits children who can learn and grow with help from physical therapy services.

References

Kunc, N. (Jan. 9, 1995). *Inclusive education: Disability to diversity.* Keynote presentation at the Pacific Rim Conference, Honolulu, HI.

Acknowledgments

I consider it an honor to have worked with the many children and their families who have come into my life. The experience of getting to know each child and his or her world is exciting and broadening for me personally, and these relationships continue to be enriching for me and my family. The children presented in this book are all real children. Some names and situations have been changed to safeguard privacy or to emphasize certain points. All the stories have been read and approved by the children and their families. I sincerely appreciate their valuable and very personal contributions.

My family supported me through long months of writing and researching. This was a family project as well as an individual one. Most of the photographs were taken by my husband, Clark Ratliffe, during the many hours we spent with children in the daily contexts of their lives. Our daughter Meghan accompanied us during most of these excursions and appears in some of the photographs. I am deeply appreciative of my husband's skill and insight, which have made the photographs in the book so powerful. He also reviewed many sections and gave me useful advice throughout the writing process.

This project has also been a community effort. My colleagues wrote sections of this book, critiqued many sections that I wrote, and helped identify resources. I particularly want to thank all the contributing authors whose rich sections give the project depth and energy. I also want to thank the following individuals who gave of their time and expertise to read portions of the text and give me feedback: Anna Ah Sam, Nancy Bloomfield, Andrea Ceppi, Marion Coste, Lyda Hodgins, Lucille Lew, Adrienne Mark, Lisa Miyamoto, Karol Richardson, Cindy Sanekane, Cheryl Stoa, Alice Teruya, Gerda Turner, Sandra Wood, and Margo Wray. Wendy Tada not only read sections and gave me advice but was a sounding board for ideas and provided helpful comments, professional support, and friendship. Dana Meitz helped immeasurably with essential tasks of organizing photographs and text. Dr. Kent Reinker gave freely of his expert advice and encouragement, as well as the use of his photographs (Figures 6-8 and 6-16). Jeanne Robertson got most of it right the first time and was never hesitant to revise her beautiful drawings. She continually offered positive perspectives and encouragement.

Although I cannot name them all, many other children, parents, teachers, educational assistants, PTA students at Kapiolani Community College, and other peers and colleagues throughout Hawai'i all helped in many different ways. The challenge of working together to teach skills and adapt activities and equipment to help a child be successful has great rewards for all of us.

KATHERINE T. RATLIFFE

Contents

PART IV

Medical Disorders of Childhood

PART ONE

The Context of Pediatric Physical Therapy

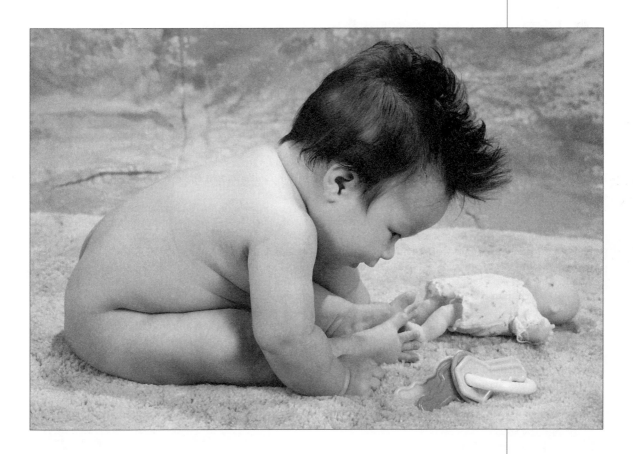

Legal, Social, and Practice Issues Related to Pediatric Physical Therapy

1

History of Physical Therapy Services for Children in the United States
Current Trends in the Provision of Physical Therapy Services to Children
People-first language
Family-centered therapy
Services across the life span
Functional/ecological approach
Integrated therapy
Practice Issues for Pediatric Physical Therapy
Laws regulating the practice of physical therapy
Approaches to physical therapy
Working in teams
Ethics and values relating to providing physical therapy to children
Future Trends in Pediatric Physical Therapy
Health care and legislative reform
National Human Genome Research Institute
Evolution of physical therapy as a profession

Physical therapy, especially as provided to children, has evolved and changed over the past century because of the influence of new laws, evolving "best practices," changing community needs and perceptions, fiscal constraints, and increasing recognition of the rights and roles of individuals with disabilities. This chapter focuses on the evolution and current practice of physical therapy in the provision of services to children. This evolution cannot be seen out of the context of social, fiscal, and legislative events of the times.

History of Physical Therapy Services for Children in the United States

The provision of rehabilitation services to individuals with disabilities, especially children, has changed significantly over the past century. The types of disability seen during the past hundred years, in addition to public opinion, have shaped federal legislation directing services to children and adults. Reviewing the evolution of these services can provide insight into influences that may affect the coming century.

In the early days of the physical therapy profession, services were given primarily to those with musculoskeletal disorders. Individuals with injuries to the head or spinal cord did not usually survive to participate in rehabilitation. World War I produced many injured soldiers. Rehabilitation was provided by "reconstruction aides," a category of personnel produced by the Reconstruction Aid Programs, which were started by the surgeon general to address the needs from World War I. A significant growth in physical therapy occurred in the 1920s, when an epidemic of polio affected many adults and children throughout the United States. In 1921 the American Physical Therapy Association (APTA) was formed to regulate and facilitate the growth of the profession. From 1916 through 1955, until the advent of the polio vaccine, physical therapists (PTs) were involved primarily in the treatment of flaccid limbs and weakness. Dorothy Voss (1982) characterizes this period as the "era of flaccidity." The "era of spasticity" began in the early 1940s as more individuals with cerebral palsy, spinal cord injuries, strokes, and head injuries began to survive their initial trauma and progress to rehabilitation (Voss, 1982). During the 1940s and 1950s an interest in treating children and adults with neurological problems led to the development of neurophysiological and developmental approaches to treatment, including neurodevelopmental treatment (NDT), proprioceptive neuromuscular facilitation (PNF), and other methods. PTs developed skills to prevent secondary disabilities and enhance life skills in children and adults with cerebral palsy and other neurological disabilities. They practiced only with physician referrals during these early years.

In the 1950s and 1960s the profession of physical therapy defined itself as distinct from medicine and from other professions that provided rehabilitation services. The era of civil rights laws and liberal policies generated federal legislation that benefited older adults, children, and individuals with disabilities. This legislation allowed physical therapy services to be covered under

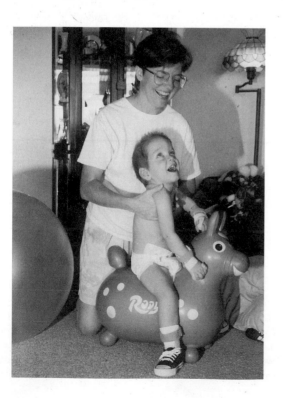

Medicare and Medicaid health plans, increasing the population base for physical therapy services. In the late 1960s the first physical therapist assistant (PTA) program was started.

The 1970s brought greater efforts from legislators to provide federal assistance for those who were disabled or poor. Landmark legislation mandating education for children with disabilities (Education for All Handicapped Children Act [EHA]) was passed in 1975 (Public Law 94-142). Aspects of this legislation are described more fully in the Applications section in Chapter 5. The EHA not only mandated a free and appropriate public education for all children in the least restrictive environment, but it also stated that children were entitled to receive related services to benefit from their education. Physical therapy is one of these related services.

Other influences during this decade included an awareness of the high costs of health care. Although health care reform measures were not undertaken formally, health care dollars became tighter; and efforts were made to modify service delivery systems. PTs began to advocate for practice without referral, but in many states third-party payers would not pay for services unless a physician prescribed them.

The APTA took an active role in physical therapy education, sharing the accreditation for schools that trained physical therapists with the American Medical Association. In 1983 the APTA became the sole accrediting agency for PT and PTA educational programs. Seeing the burgeoning amount of knowledge needed to treat the general population and recognizing the need for advanced education to support the profession through research and teaching, the APTA developed a policy statement that entry-level education for PTs should be at the postbaccalaureate level by 1990. The APTA also began to develop specializations, allowing therapists with advanced skills to become certified as specialists in certain areas including geriatrics, pediatrics, and orthopedics. The pediatric section of the APTA was formed in 1974, and a pediatric specialization certification program was begun in 1978 with the first specialists certified in 1985.

The number of PTA programs grew as physical therapists began to open private businesses and needed help to maintain therapy programs with their clients. Because more individuals were mandated to receive services, a shortage of PTs prompted some to redefine their roles to include consulting and to rely on PTAs to perform some of the day-to-day interventions with children and adults with chronic disabilities.

Awareness of the high costs of institutions to care for individuals with developmental disabilities and mental illness prompted the move toward deinstitutionalization during the 1970s. A further consideration was recognition that an institutional life did little to prepare an individual to live productively and independently. Efforts were made to develop community supports for adults and children with mental retardation and other disabilities. This movement, in addition to the mandate to provide physical therapy to children in schools, opened up new venues for physical therapy practice. Besides hospitals and large institutions, physical therapy was beginning to flourish in community settings such as schools, day treatment programs, and homes. The need to work closely with other professions to provide optimal services necessitated the development of different models of teamwork, such as interdisciplinary and transdisciplinary care.

Court cases testing the limits of PL 94-142 emerged in the 1980s, and individual court decisions helped to define further what supports schools needed to provide to children. The law stated that children should be served in the "least restrictive environment (LRE)," and the debate over the definition of LRE produced advocates for fully including children with disabilities in regular education environments. Services were initially provided to most children with severe disabilities in self-contained classrooms, but the idea of supporting them in regular classrooms gained momentum as the benefits to the children were realized. The difficulties of this approach in terms of cost, level of support services, and ethics continue to be debated today as school districts develop an array of options for children with disabilities. In 1986 the EHA was amended to provide for early intervention services for infants, toddlers, and preschool children. This amendment expanded the pediatric settings where physical therapy was provided. The needs of very young children included even more family involvement, and new models of service delivery were necessary.

Progress in other areas, including the further development of practice specializations in the APTA and the advent of practice without referral in some states, gave hope to those who had a vision of PTs as independent practitioners. Practice acts in many states were rewritten between 1985 and 1990 to include practice without referral. Many PT educational programs converted to entry-level masters programs from the baccalaureate level during the 1980s.

In 1990 the Individuals with Disabilities Education Amendments (IDEA) (PL 101-476) was passed, reauthorizing EHA. It expanded the earlier legislation, including the definition of related services. This legislation continues to be the primary influence in the implementation of educational services to children with disabilities. IDEA was scheduled to be reauthorized in 1995, but the debate over a few areas of the law was so pronounced that it was not reauthorized until 1997. Areas of debate in the reauthorization include aspects of discipline relating to children with behavioral challenges.

Another landmark legislation, the Americans with Disabilities Act (ADA), was passed in 1990. This legislation not only addresses civil rights for all Americans with disabilities but also has applications to children. Areas applicable to children include employment, public and private accommodations, transportation, and telecommunications (Lowes & Effgen, 1996). Being aware of the rights of individuals with disabilities can help PTs work with educational teams to support children to participate as fully as possible in school and community activities and make the transition to productive lives after graduation.

An important influence on therapy in the 1990s is health care reform. Managed care has become common, with restrictions on the amount of time therapists can see individuals who need help recovering from an injury or learning new skills. Therapists in private practice have had to join group practices and make other concessions to maintain a referral base of patients. Services in schools and infant programs have suffered because of significantly lower pay than the private sector, resulting in a critical shortage of pediatric therapists.

As we live and work in our evolving field, we should all make an effort to be aware of changes taking place in the environments in which we work and to carefully reflect on the issues and work actively to influence the direction of political and social change, according to our conscience, to benefit the children and families we serve.

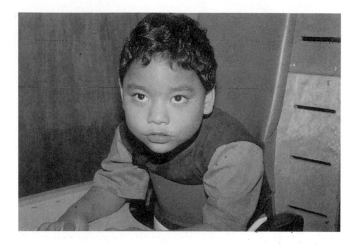

Current Trends in the Provision of Physical Therapy Services to Children

Changing attitudes are shaping both the language that we use and the way we think about children and their families. The awareness that we are preparing children for a full and productive life dictates that we look at what skills they will need over time and expand our vision to include the future. This vision of children as multifaceted individuals has changed the way therapy goals are written. Rather than isolating skills, such as strength or range of motion, goals now must be functional in nature. For example, a functional goal would read that a child will learn to walk from the classroom to the cafeteria. A nonfunctional goal would have the child increase stance time on the right leg during ambulation.

People-First Language

Categorizing people has become a way of life. We come in contact with so many individuals in our daily lives that some categorization is helpful; however, categorization can lead to stereotypes if attention is not paid to the effect of language on our perceptions. The move toward "politically correct" language is an attempt to decrease stereotypes that can be perpetuated through language. Language and perception are intimately connected. Change language, and perceptions will also change. Change perceptions, and language will change.

With individual and community awareness that those affected with disabilities have rights, personalities, and strengths come changes in language to reflect changes in attitude. A profound change in language reflecting changes in perception has been that of speaking of a person *before* the disability. Rather than referring to a "wheelchair-bound, crippled man," it is both more respectful and more accepting to refer to the "man with a disability who uses a wheelchair." Instead of saying "the CP kid" or "the Down's kid," "the child with cerebral palsy" or "the child with Down syndrome" could be substituted. The child can also be described by using other attributes than the disability; for instance, "the girl with red hair who sits at the first table in the cafeteria" provides sufficient information.

In people-first language, the term *handicap* does not refer to an individual. This term is applied to a barrier that results in an individual being excluded. For example, an individual using a wheelchair is presented with a handicap when the elevator is broken and he or she needs to go upstairs. In another example classmates' perception of a child as stupid is a handicap to being included in the peer group. Attention to language and putting the individual before the disability can lead to new understandings and perceptions.

Family-Centered Therapy

The realization that families provide the context of life for children has opened up new ways of relating to families and of providing services to children. The roles that families play in the eyes of service providers have shifted significantly over the past 20 years. Traditional medical intervention has been professionally centered, with families viewed as needing the help of expert professionals who planned and implemented interventions that they considered appropriate. Family-allied models allowed family members to assist in implementing interventions such as carrying out a home exercise program for their child. Family-focused models of intervention demonstrate increased collaboration between families and professionals but continue to view families as having less knowledge and power than the professionals. Child-centered models view the intervention as being directed solely by the child's needs, and they do not consider the family's needs. In the family-centered model the family directs the services and supports, which are set up to last even after the professionals are no longer involved (Shelton & Stepanek, 1994).

So the continuum has shifted from the professional at the center to the family at the center. Different models may be encountered in different programs or environments. The family-centered model is more frequently seen in early childhood programs for infants and toddlers. Child-centered models may be seen in the schools, and professionally centered models may be seen in hospitals. The concept of putting the family and the child first when assessing or planning therapy intervention, however, is an important shift in perception and attitude that can extend for the entire life span in any environment.

The concept of "professional distance" that has traditionally been taught to protect medical service providers from the emotional pain of getting too close to their patients is characterized by maintaining an emotional distance through power differential and authoritarianism. Professional distance is more commonly seen in the professionally centered models of intervention and is incompatible with the family-centered model. The experience of having a child who is acutely ill or chronically ill or who has a disability can be overwhelming and isolating for a family. If medical and other service providers maintain an emotional distance, important information may not be communicated and essential needs of the child and family may be missed. Taking the extra step of visiting the home, providing services in the home, assessing the environments and functions of daily life, and incorporating the family's needs and preferences into therapy plans and strategies are ways to include the family in all aspects of the child's care.

Parents as problem or solution. Parents used to be viewed as part of the child's problem. Emotional frigidity, poor parent-child relationships, and poor caregiving were assumed to have caused or played a role in causing some disabilities in children. Now it is recognized that many of the theories of causation for autism and other disorders were erroneous. Parents have been blamed for something over which they had no control.

Although a few parents have had a role in the causation of some disorders, including fetal alcohol syndrome, traumatic brain injury from abuse, and some genetic disabilities, the influence of the parent in the life of a child with disabilities is usually positive. These parents can move beyond the role of causation and become part of the solution if they and service providers will make the leap in perception. Most parents, however, find themselves in the situation of parenting a child with a disability through no causative action of their own.

Parents are with the child more than any other caregivers are, and most take active roles in their child's development and health. They may need significant support to shift their own dreams and perceptions from the child they expected to the child they have. Their efforts to help their child achieve all that is possible should be encouraged and supported. The development of services and programs around parent and family needs has become more prevalent as a result of the medical and educational professional's shift in perceptions.

Parents in passive or active roles. Parents used to be merely the recipients of professional evaluations of their child, with accompanying recommendations of what the parent should do. They were expected to follow through, or they were labeled "noncompliant." Most parents are now encouraged and expected to take an active role in planning a program for their child. Service providers more often recognize that family needs may be varied and complex. Parent needs, considerations, and feelings are part of the discussion. As an example, Rik, the boy featured in the Case Study in Chapter 8, has trouble sleeping at night. His parents are up with him six to eight times throughout the night, and both work demanding full-time professional jobs during the day. Rik's brother Sean is still an infant and has his own needs. The stresses on this family are enormous. Expecting Rik's parents to perform daily therapy exercises with him is unrealistic. To expect them to give up their careers to care for Rik demonstrates a lack of respect for them and their own dreams. Identifying the problem and working with the family to help find a solution to Rik's nighttime sleeplessness is a more practical approach to providing Rik services. Building a rapport with the family and with Rik is necessary to identify and address the relevant issues.

Expanding definition of family. Families traditionally viewed as primarily the mother and child dyad are now perceived to include the father and other members, including nontraditional family members such as neighbors, babysitters, or stepfamilies. This perspective can be broadened to include grandparents, bus drivers, and others who regularly engage and interact with children who have disabilities. Recognition of the support from this extended group can make a great difference in a child's life.

Addressing needs of individuals in the family. Although family needs were previously recognized in a general way, recognizing and allowing for individual needs for each family member related to the child with a disability can provide a greater amount of understanding and support. A broad example is the growth in programs to support siblings of children with disabilities. For a specific example, we can look at Cyril Rivera (see Case Study, Chapter 7). His mother is now unable to transfer him into or out of his wheelchair by herself because of his size. Yet she is alone with him all afternoon, when he may need to use the toilet. Rather than expecting her to find some way to transfer Cyril to the toilet, therapy providers can work with her to find some equipment, respite, or other assistance in meeting Cyril's needs in the afternoons. Mrs. Rivera is housebound when Cyril is home because she must use the city bus for transportation and cannot take Cyril with her. Finding her respite care for one afternoon per week will allow her to do the family shopping, visit with her friends, and improve her self-esteem.

Legal mandates to include families. Legislation has mirrored these shifts in perception. The Individuals with Disabilities Education Act (IDEA) of 1990 mandates that families be included on the educational team as an equal member for infants and school-aged children. Parents with more formal education and more experience may participate actively; however, many family members may refrain from contributing to the team because of feelings of inadequacy. Sensitivity to these issues can help team members include parents more effectively. Parents can be supported and encouraged to participate by team members who are sensitive to their needs. Team members can form individual alliances with family members to include them in designing the overall program for their child and in implementing therapy services.

The Individual Family Support Plan (IFSP) that is mandated for children less than 3 years old includes family needs in the plan itself. This recognizes that families are the most important context of life for small children. Family members are included in all aspects of service provision, and goals are written for families as well as for the individual child. Implicit in family-centered intervention is the assumption that family functioning interacts with the environment and influences child development (Kolobe, 1992). Therefore supporting family needs directly impacts the child.

Cultural sensitivity. Sensitivity to cultural issues may help team members understand some parent concerns. For example, Cyril's (see Case Study, Chapter 7) Filipino parents felt very strongly that they could not ask the landlord to modify their apartment to make it more accessible for Cyril. The Filipino culture discourages direct confrontation, and the parents were afraid that they might lose their inexpensive apartment if they advocated for themselves. Yet the situation seemed untenable; 13-year-old Cyril could only take a bath with his father, who lifted him into the tub and bathed with him in the early mornings. Privacy was also an issue for this teenager. When his father had back pain, Cyril made do with sponge baths. Cyril missed a

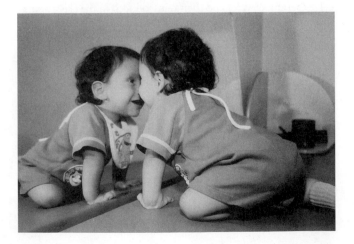

year of summer school to relieve the stress on the family associated with getting up early to bathe. Helping the family cope within the constraints of their own beliefs and ethics is important. Finding equipment to help—without structurally modifying the apartment and without judging the parents—is the only way to help Cyril's bathing situation. The Applications section in Chapter 4 addresses cultural issues more fully.

Challenges and stresses to families. Different families have different stresses related to demanding jobs, precarious socioeconomic situations, family dynamics or dysfunction, or lack of social resources. Identifying stress factors can help teams work more effectively with families and address issues that may impact on their ability to care for their child.

Coping skills vary among families and are based on extended family support systems, availability of social resources, and perception of their child's disability. Teaching family members methods to cope by relying more on extended family, developing a broader, informed perspective of their child's disability, and developing new social resources for support can help the family function better overall.

Relationships between parents and support for siblings of a child with a disability can all take a "back seat" under the daily stresses of caring for a child with multiple needs. Encouraging both parents to take an active role in caring for the child and including siblings both in supporting the child during therapy sessions and in separate groups designed to enhance their own feelings of self-worth are examples of strategies for addressing potential conflicts. Parents may or may not disclose marital problems to the therapy provider. If it is clear that a parent is asking for help or needs help in dealing with marital issues, the therapy provider should refer him or her to an appropriate resource such as the social worker or psychologist or a family support group. Simply providing the parent with the telephone number of a support group is not the solution to the problem; the team and relevant team members should be involved in following up with any identified needs.

Therapists can facilitate interactions between parents and their child with a disability by highlighting the child's abilities. Parents may focus on the activities their child cannot do and may not be fully aware of his or her capabilities. This negative focus may lead to negative methods of interacting, including rigidity, frequent disapproval, or overprotectiveness. The child's awareness of environmental stimuli, social responses, and early motor skills can all be emphasized during a therapy session. The parent can be taught to enhance these skills, as well as skills directly related to "therapy." Modeling and encouraging behaviors such as turn taking, allowing the child extra time to accomplish a task, modifying a task so that a child can be successful, and praising a child for successes can all help parents learn appropriate and rewarding ways of interacting.

Services Across the Life Span

When working with a child, therapists may find it easy to concentrate on the immediate task of helping the child learn a particular skill. The mechanics of therapy, the anatomy and physiology of the disorder, the immediate interactions of the family, and volatile health issues of the child take on immediate importance. Sometimes focusing on the present is easier for families and therapists than looking forward 20 years to when the child is an adult.

This looking forward is essential. Therapy providers are in a unique situation to help support family members to think ahead and plan for the future. Therapy goals should be related to an overall vision for the child.

Mapping the future. Several methods exist to help teams develop a life span perspective. The McGill Action Planning System (MAPS) (Vandercook, York, & Forest, 1989) is a semistructured method for eliciting broad-thinking dreams and visions from a group of individuals gathered for the benefit of a child. The child and family are an integral part of the group. Seven questions are posed:

- What is the individual's history?
- What are your dreams for the individual?
- What is your nightmare?
- Who is the individual?
- What are the individual's strengths, gifts, and abilities?
- What are the individual's needs?
- What would the individual's ideal day at school look like, and what must be done to make it happen? (pp. 3-4)

In a traditional format, large poster paper would be placed on a wall so that team members could draw or map their visions. This method allows for broad thinking, not constrained by what is known to be possible. MAPS may be used in a school Integrated Education Program (IEP) conference. Because of the length of time the MAPS process requires, performing the MAPS before the IEP is sometimes helpful. The MAPS process should involve individuals from all parts of a child's life, including friends, neighbors, babysitters, and relatives.

Futures planning. Another form of visioning is to create a personal futures plan for the child. A personal futures plan involves:

- Creating a personal profile of the child, including background, positive and negative experiences, critical events, and current dynamics that affect the individual's immediate future, family issues, general health, and ethnic and community ties
- Documenting the child's accomplishments in all areas of life
- Documenting the child's preferences and desires (Field & Haring, 1994)

The personal futures plan is especially helpful for an older child who is getting ready to make the transition from high school to a job, sheltered workplace, day program, or other environment. It can be an uplifting experience to focus on the positive accomplishments and dream about what could be possible for the child without constraints or limitations such as finances, services, or programs. Often the team realizes that more is possible for the child than they had originally thought.

The process of envisioning the future has an impact on the present. By having in mind a vision of the individual in the future, choices can be made about what to focus on today. No longer will we get to the point where a 30-year-old man with mental retardation can sort shapes and insert them in the correct slots of a child's toy but cannot sort coins and put the correct ones in a vending machine to buy himself a softdrink.

Functional/Ecological Approach

A recent emphasis in service provision is to consider the child's needs in the context of the environment and activities where he or she will need to use the skills. Needs are expressed functionally, meaning that they are related to a particular activity or use. The functional approach includes assessment of functional skills (not merely strength and range of motion unless they directly affect function) and establishing of goals that are functionally based. A functional goal for Cyril (see Case Study, Chapter 7) is to be able to stand with assistance for transfers to and from his wheelchair. In comparison, a traditional goal is to have at least good strength in his right quadriceps and gluteal muscles. Although strength in these muscle groups is essential to master the skill of standing with support, the goal is not expressed in a functional context. The emphasis on functional goals is similar in most settings where physical therapy is practiced. Third-party payers, for example, are requiring functional goals for patients with acute or rehabilitation needs.

Related to the functional approach is the ecological approach. In this perspective a child's world is looked at as a series of environments, for instance, the bathroom, the kitchen, the classroom, or the beach. In assessing a child's ecological needs, the question is posed, "What skills does the child possess, and what skills does he or she need to function in this environment?" Activities that occur in the environment are assessed to determine the child's needs to participate more fully. If the school bathroom is taken as an example of an environment for Cyril and if brushing his teeth after lunch were the activity, he might need to learn skills involving choosing between two toothbrushes, opening the toothpaste tube, turning on the water, balancing while standing at the sink, applying toothpaste to the brush, getting his hand to his mouth, making brushing movements with the brush, rinsing the brush, putting it away, and wiping his face and hands on a towel. Physical therapy might be involved with helping him learn to stand at the sink or reach for objects while standing at the sink. A team approach to develop a plan to learn these skills is needed because most are broader than any one discipline.

Integrated Therapy

Physical therapy has traditionally been provided as a direct hands-on method of service delivery. The professionally centered model of therapy provision was translated to schools when therapy services began to be offered to children in school. Therapists evaluate children, decide what their needs are, and work with them individually to gain particular skills to remedy an identified deficiency. Children have been pulled out of classrooms to receive therapy services and then reintroduced to the classroom at the end of the therapy session. If a child needed to learn specific skills related to classroom activities, those skills were taught individually outside the classroom; then the skills were expected to be generalized to the classroom setting. This method of service provision may not always provide optimal outcomes for children in educational environments.

McWilliam (1995) has identified six different methods of providing school-based physical therapy services:

- Individual pull-out: The child is removed from the class and returned after the therapy session. Therapy addresses concerns related to the individual child.
- Small group pull-out: The child with a small number of peers is removed from the rest of the class and returned after the therapy session. Therapy addresses individual concerns related to the specific child and/or others in the group.

- One-on-one in the classroom: The child is treated in the corner of the classroom, possibly working on skills unrelated to the class routine.
- Group activity: The child and classmates are engaged in a group activity addressing physical therapy needs of one or more of the children in the context of class activities.
- Individual therapy during classroom routine: The child is supported during a class routine to develop specific skills related to class activities.
- Consultation: The therapy provider consults with the teacher to exchange information and expertise regarding a particular child's needs in the context of class activities.

The last three methods deliver physical therapy in an integrated manner, with educational and physical therapy interventions accomplished during the same activities. Integration of services helps to promote greater team collaboration, improved outcomes for children because skills are learned in the context of normal routines, and opportunities to address problems as they arise. Teachers and therapists have greater opportunity to work with and learn from each other, and classroom teaching is not fragmented by children constantly being pulled out of class (McWilliam, 1996).

McWilliam's continuum of service delivery contains methods that may each be appropriate for different circumstances. Efforts to provide integrated services depend on the entire team and the commitment of the administration to allow flexible scheduling and adequate time for collaboration. The Applications section in Chapter 5 explores methods of service delivery in the schools in more depth.

Practice Issues for Pediatric Physical Therapy

The mechanics of carrying out physical therapy with children are dictated by current laws regulating physical therapy practice, varying approaches to therapy between different sites where services may be provided, and mechanics of team organization in the various settings. Issues such as provision of community service, research to validate the techniques that are used, and ethics

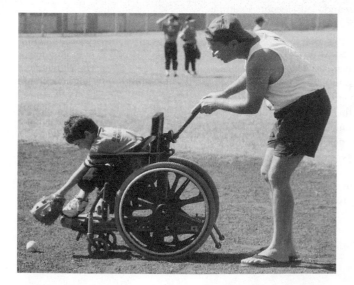

and values relating to the provision of physical therapy services to children usually are secondary to the day-to-day needs of scheduling and providing services, but they are issues that every physical therapy provider should consider and self-evaluate regularly.

The American Physical Therapy Association (APTA), especially the pediatric section of the APTA, works with members of the profession to develop materials to support pediatric PTs and PTAs. These materials include brochures and instructional materials for specific content areas, journals to present current research and to discuss current issues, and formulations of policy regarding the practice of pediatric physical therapy. Each of us makes a choice to support this professional organization, both through monetary dues and volunteer participation.

Laws Regulating the Practice of Physical Therapy

Each state defines what is meant by physical therapy and who can provide these services through the state professional practice act and administrative rules governing the practice act. The state legislature passes legislation defined as a practice act, which is reviewed periodically by the legislature in what is called a "sunset review." Each time the practice act is considered for review, others have an opportunity to give input. For instance, chiropractors may think that PTs should not do spinal manipulations and may try to change the language of the physical therapy practice act to prohibit them from providing this service. Unless the physical therapy community in the state is active and diligent, changes may be made that detract from the scope of practice of physical therapy. On the other hand, changes also may be made to expand the scope of service. For instance, changes in the requirements for physician referrals can be made to allow PTs to practice without referrals. Practice acts differ significantly between states, and each practitioner should be familiar with his or her own state laws governing physical therapy practice.

Administrative rules govern the implementation of the practice act. Requirements for supervision of ancillary personnel such as PTAs and aides are usually well defined in the administrative rules. Other aspects include requirements for licensing and procedures to follow if a therapist is practicing in conflict with professional ethics or with the administrative rules.

In states where PTAs are licensed they may have their own administrative rules and licensing boards to oversee the implementation of these rules. In most cases the physical therapy licensing board addresses the needs of the PTAs as well. In states where PTAs are not yet licensed the rules governing supervision of ancillary personnel for PTs direct what the PTA and other support staff are able to do.

Approaches to Physical Therapy

As documented throughout this book, physical therapy services provided to children vary according to the needs of the child. These needs dictate where the services are provided. For instance, a child in an acute care hospital will usually have acute medical needs. The goals of physical therapy will be to avoid problems related to the illness, such as contracture or weakness, and to help the child gain the functional skills needed to return home. The child in a school setting will generally be healthy but may need help in developing skills to benefit from the educational services offered at school. A child in a rehabilitation setting will need intensive physical therapy to learn or relearn basic functional skills such as moving in bed, standing, walking, and playing. The setting and needs of the child determine the types of intervention and the intensity that is provided. The same child may receive physical therapy services concurrently at school and in an outpatient setting, with different goals in each setting. In school the physical therapy provider may teach the classroom aide proper methods of transfer and develop a positioning program for the child in the classroom. In the outpatient setting the program for the same child may be exercises to improve strength and motor control of the lower extremities and trunk, with emphasis on improving balance in sitting. Different therapists working with the same child should coordinate and support each other's interventions.

Working in Teams

Physical therapy is usually provided to children as part of a coordinated team of individuals, no matter what setting the child may be in; however, the composition and mechanics of the teams may differ between settings. A discussion of different team models can help to define varying roles. Table 1-1 outlines different types of teams, typical settings in which they practice, and how interactions may differ between them. Usually the younger the child, the greater the coordination between team members. Smaller intervention settings located in community settings, such as infant development programs, usually have more integration of services than the more institutionalized settings like hospitals. Legal mandates dictate that services be provided in an integrated manner in the least restrictive setting for all children (Rainforth, York, & Macdonald, 1992).

Members of teams may differ according to the setting, but most teams that include physical therapy also include the child and parents, occupational therapy, speech-language pathology, medicine, and nursing. Other members may include audiology, nutrition, psychology, recreation, education, and social work. Parent advocates, friends of the child, neighbors, or bus drivers may also participate on the team. Key team members and their roles are described in the following sections.

Child and family. The child and family are the most important members of the team; the degree of their inclusion depends on the setting and type of team. The family is likely to take a more active role in teams that use a more interdisciplinary, transdisciplinary, or collaborative model of working together. In practice, teams that have a medical base, such as those in hospitals or rehabilitation facilities, may include families less than teams that work in education settings like schools or infant development programs. Families should be included in all settings as much as possible.

Occupational therapy. The role of occupational therapy and physical therapy are closely intertwined, especially when working with very young children. Occupational therapy is usually overtly responsible for functional areas that include activities of daily living, such as dressing, bathing, and toileting, and fine motor skills involved in handwriting and manipulating small objects such as buttons or beads. Roles vary between the occupational therapist (OT) and PT in different settings. For instance, in some settings it is the OT who is responsible for seating and positioning; in others it is the PT. These roles may be interchangeable be-

TABLE 1-1	Team Models		
Team model	**Characteristics**		**Common settings**
Intradisciplinary	The PT conducts an evaluation of the child, plans a treatment intervention, and carries it out. The PTA may help collect data for the evaluation and carry out the intervention.		Private practice setting Some outpatient facilities
Multidisciplinary	The PT will conduct an evaluation of the child, then make the written report available in a central location so that other team members are aware of each other's assessments and plans. Meetings may be held to present each member's findings. Therapy is conducted without direct input from other disciplines.		Acute care hospital Some outpatient facilities
Interdisciplinary	Different team members make their assessments individually, including recommendations and plan of intervention. Meetings are held to plan interventions jointly and discuss the child's needs and progress toward agreed on objectives. Team members may incorporate some aspects of each other's care plans in their own interventions.		School settings Some acute care hospitals Rehabilitation facilities
Transdisciplinary	Team members work closely with one another in the evaluation process, designing an intervention program and carrying out interventions. Roles cross boundaries of typical disciplines.		Infant development programs Some acute care settings, especially neonatal intensive care unit (NICU)
Collaborative (Rainforth, York, & Macdonald, 1992)	Team members work closely together in a combination of a transdisciplinary and integrated therapy approach to service provision. The therapist may not provide the majority of motor instruction during the day, teaching the teacher and classroom aide to carry out programs that are collaboratively designed.		School settings Adult day health programs

tween OT and PT for very young children because both address developmental activities. Working closely with the OT or certified occupational therapy assistant (COTA) can be a great learning experience. Co-treating children offers many benefits to the therapy providers as well as to the child, including an extra pair of hands, the consolidation of knowledge and observation skills, and more efficient joint planning.

Speech-language pathology. Sometimes called a speech therapist, the speech-language pathologist (SLP) is responsible for working with the child's expressive and receptive language skills. Expressive language is what the child can communicate to others, and receptive language is what the child understands of others' attempts to communicate with him or her. Language pervades daily life, whether orally in speech, manually in gestures or signs, or nonverbally in facial expressions or actions. Language skills can easily be incorporated into physical therapy treatment sessions and goals if the therapy provider is aware of the language goals. The PTA working with a child with a language impairment should make the effort to learn the signs and communication methods that the child uses and reinforce them regularly during therapy sessions.

Audiology. The audiologist tests the child's hearing and recommends and fits hearing aids or other listening devices. The audiologist works closely with the SLP regarding assessing the child's hearing capability and developing strategies to help the child use hearing aids and communicate most effectively.

Medicine. The physician is frequently an active member of the team, especially on medically based teams in a hospital or rehabilitation setting. In some communities the physician may feel responsible for being aware of the spectrum of services available and ensuring that a child has access to and is receiving appropriate services. In many community settings, such as schools or infant development programs, however, the physician is responsible for signing prescriptions for therapy services or durable medical equipment but may not take a more active role.

Nursing. Nursing is involved with any child who has medical issues, such as an acute or chronic illness. In a medical setting the nurse is an active part of the team. Nursing is also active in schools and community settings through school health services or public health nursing. Nurses or nurses aides may provide respite services for children who are medically fragile. Children who have medical appliances, such as feeding tubes or endotrachial tubes, those who need suctioning, and those who have frequent seizures need regular nursing care. Nurses are a valuable resource to therapy providers, giving insight into the child's medical limitations and restrictions, as well as capabilities.

Nutrition. The nutritionist is responsible for monitoring the child's food and nutrition intake, as well as physical growth. Many nutritionists are trained as dietitians to give specific dietary advice, but they also address larger issues affecting nutrition, including community awareness and policies regarding health and nutrition. Children with medical problems related to diet include those with obesity, multiple food allergies, and diabetes; those who have a feeding tube; children with nutritional uptake problems such as short bowel syndrome; medical/ behavioral disorders such as bulimia or anorexia; and those with psychological or behavioral issues about feeding related to medical interventions or other causes. Recommendations regarding ideal weight for a child are usually based on the child's height and body type. Diets may need to be adjusted to accommodate medical needs, such as phenylketonuria or diabetes, and feeding practices may need to be changed to provide the most conducive environment to facilitate optimal nutrition.

Psychology. The psychologist is an important team member when a child has psychological needs. A child in a stressful home situation, one with behavioral problems related or unrelated to the disability, and a child who is having difficulty coping with the effects of a disease or disability can all benefit from the intervention of a child psychologist. The psychologist can give valuable insight to team members regarding effective strategies for working with a child and can help develop intervention plans to accommodate or work with challenging behaviors. The psychologist is also responsible for psychometric testing resulting in diagnosis of mental retardation, autism, or other disorders with a behavioral component.

Recreation. The recreation therapist works with individuals to promote maximal participation in recreation and leisure activities. For children this almost always involves play. Recreation for children can range from helping an acutely ill child access a video player to watch a favorite movie, to assisting a child with a lower extremity amputation learn to ski. The child-life specialist is an individual trained to work with children in acute care settings to promote age-appropriate play and allow exploration of feelings through play. In some communities the child-life specialist may also work outside a hospital doing developmental assessments such as the Denver Developmental Screening Test (DDST).

Education. School is a pervasive part of childhood. Teachers play key roles in promoting learning in children. Special education teachers are trained to adapt curriculum for children and may support them in the regular education setting or in a self-contained classroom. Children may be enrolled in regular education classes and have the services of both a regular and a special education teacher. Older children may have several teachers. Educational assistants may work closely with a child with a physical or behavioral disability in the classroom. Teachers may provide tutoring to a child with medical problems that keep the student out of school. Because each of these individuals has insight into the child's needs, each should participate on the team to make decisions about the child's educational plan.

Social work. Social workers have multiple roles, including providing social support and counseling, making referrals to appropriate service agencies, and explaining programs and resources to families. They may provide practical assistance by transporting family members to appointments with community agencies, making telephone calls, and visiting the family regularly to ensure that their needs are met.

Ethics and Values Relating to Providing Physical Therapy to Children

Teaching skills to others. As a profession, physical therapy is governed by provisions that are written into the practice acts for each state and guided by a code of ethical standards that was written by the American Physical Therapy Association (APTA, 1991). Although the ethical standards only bind those physical therapy providers who are members of the professional association, they represent careful thought about the profession by PTs.

Newer methods of providing services to children, which include teaching others to perform some of the techniques and practices that a PT traditionally performed, have been challenged as not being under legal or ethical guidelines for practice. Rainforth and Roberts (1996) have examined the legal and ethical implications of this method of practice and have concluded that "role release" is not only allowed in legal and ethical guidelines but also encouraged if it benefits the children who are served.

Controversies regarding "role release" have been generated by members of the profession who feel that, by teaching others skills and techniques, we are giving away our profession and decreasing our share of the service provision pie. Others feel that the skills learned through years of training and practice cannot be adequately taught to teachers, aides, or even PTAs who have not undergone the same training. Teaching skills to others is viewed as making the skills themselves less effective and perhaps even dangerous.

When seen from the perspective of the benefit to the child, there is no question as to the best method of service provision. For example, a child whose teacher can apply some principles of myofacial release to loosen cervical musculature and encourage an aligned head and neck position before eating is receiving more consistent intervention than the child who gets the treatment during two direct physical therapy sessions each week that may or may not coincide with mealtime. Although the teacher can learn the skills to apply the technique to one child for a particular situation, he or she will not have the underlying knowledge to generalize the skill to other children for other purposes. The PT still has an important role in determining appropriate intervention strategies and deciding on the correct time and personnel for implementation.

The PTA may want to teach a classroom teacher or aide specific strategies to help a child walk during the day at school or to adjust positioning equipment to accommodate different functions. Sometimes these skills are taught to support the therapy provider who cannot be available to every child or every classroom at all times. A confident practitioner can easily determine which skills are appropriate to teach others.

Community service and research. Just as it is important to be aware of the child's entire life span when providing therapy services, it is also important to grow in professional practice beyond the daily routines of therapy provision. The unique skills that each pediatric PT and PTA develop over the years of practicing can be helpful to larger numbers of children and their families and in shaping the direction of the profession. Community service can include coaching challenged sports teams, talking about the profession to high school students, participating in events to promote disability awareness in the community, writing and giving testimony to state legislatures regarding bills that affect children in the community, and participating in the local chapter of the APTA.

Research to validate specific techniques used in physical therapy and to assess outcomes for children can add to the existing body of knowledge and shape the directions that physical therapy services to children take in coming decades. PTAs who are not trained in research methods can participate in research projects by collecting data, participating in focus groups, enlisting the help of families and children, and advocating for research in educational environments. Reading professional journals to stay abreast of current directions in research regarding pediatric physical therapy is important to review existing treatment philosophies and treatments, as well as learn about new strategies in the provision of services to children.

Future Trends in Pediatric Physical Therapy

Health Care and Legislative Reform

Health care reform may change the ability of individuals to access and pay for health care. It may also change the environments and circumstances under which physical therapy for children is provided in the future. Skyrocketing costs for health care have prompted tightening of health care dollars. This has resulted in increasing productivity requirements for therapists working in hospitals (Tolley, 1993) and has prompted insurance companies to require prior approval for outpatient therapy sessions and to limit the number of sessions.

The underlying intent of health care reform is to halt or slow the increase in health care spending rather than to improve the quality and quantity of care for Americans. Managed care is private industry's method of containing health care costs (Budetti, 1997; Solomon, Collins, Silverberg, & Glass, 1996). Controversy exists about the quality of care and whether children will receive necessary services. Future unknown factors include what health care reforms may be passed or what policies may be instituted to further limit or restrict health care access including physical therapy. Health care reform may affect the status, or at least the reimbursement potential, of PTs who practice without physician referral, which is now allowed in 28 states (Rainforth & Roberts, 1996).

Current laws mandating the education of children with disabilities may be weakened or dismantled in the future. Support for related services in education including physical therapy may decrease as budget constraints become more forceful.

Each of us can become involved in the legislative process to maintain and improve the level of services for children. Decreases are not inevitable, and our own efforts can affect future outcomes. The APTA keeps us abreast of current legislative issues. Writing letters to legislators, testifying at state legislative hearings, and becoming involved in activities to promote community awareness can make a difference.

National Human Genome Research Institute

Formerly known as the Human Genome Project, the National Human Genome Research Institute (NHGRI) is a 15-year project coordinated by the Department of Energy and the National Institutes of Health to find and map all the genes on every chromosome in the human body and to determine their biochemical nature. The project is ahead of schedule because of international cooperation and the development of new technologies allowing for faster processing of information. The success of the project is exciting to individuals who have diseases of genetic origin that might be identified and treated through information derived from the research. Although treatments for most genetic diseases are still years away, scientists are hopeful that by identifying specific genes and the resulting deficient proteins, treatments can be developed that will be effective at either curing diseases or ameliorating their effects. Children with genetic diseases such as Duchenne muscular dystrophy, cystic fibrosis, or spinal muscular atrophy have much to gain from this research.

Ethical concerns regarding confidentiality of testing results and personal choice about undergoing genetic testing are being considered by the NHGRI. In 1995 the Equal Employment Opportunity Commission (EEOC) passed guidelines to extend the Americans with Disabilities Act (ADA) employment protection to individuals being discriminated against based on genetic information related to disease, illness, or other conditions. Employment is only the tip of the iceberg, however. Confidentiality related to genetic testing may affect health insurance coverage and other rights and privileges related to living in our complex society. These issues have yet to be fully discussed and will continue to emerge in the coming decade.

Evolution of Physical Therapy as a Profession

Just as social, legal, and political issues affected the direction of physical therapy as provided to children through the twentieth century, these issues will continue to affect the evolution of the profession into the twenty-first century. Current directions of practice, including integration of therapy in educational settings, collaborative relationships with other service providers, and therapy directed toward functional outcomes for children in all settings, will evolve according to new or changing events and ideas. Students today are in the best position to watch and direct the changing landscape.

EXERCISES

1. Attend a meeting of your state board of physical therapy (or the equivalent) to understand the legal and practice issues this body addresses. Before the meeting, obtain a copy of the agenda and research the topics that will be discussed by talking with informed individuals in the profession.
2. Hold a MAPS session or a futures planning meeting around someone you know. This could be yourself, a classmate, or someone you know with a disability. It is important to include family members and other key persons in the individual's life, especially if the individual has a significant disability. To have an effective meeting, you may need to research the method you choose by using references in this chapter.
3. Read a few pages of an old textbook, promotional material, or a local news article about those with disabilities; identify examples where people-first language is not used. Rewrite the offending sections to reflect the individual before the disability. This exercise can be done individually or in a group. Begin now to use people-first language with your classmates.

QUESTIONS TO PONDER

1. Should physical therapy for children always be provided in an integrated format? Why or why not?
2. What are some values that you would ascribe to an excellent pediatric PT or PTA? Why did you choose these values? What do your choices reflect about your own values?
3. What are the roles of the PT and the PTA in community service and research? How do you see your role in these activities in the coming years?

References

American Physical Therapy Association. (1991). *Code of ethics and guide for professional conduct.* Alexandria, VA: Author.

Budetti, P. P. (1997). Health reform for the 21st century? It may have to wait until the 21st century. *Journal of the American Medical Association, 277,* 193-198.

Field, S., & Haring, N. G. (1994). Transition to work and community living. In N. G. Haring, L. M. McCormick, & T. G. Haring (Eds.), *Exceptional children and youth* (6th Ed.). New York: Macmillan.

Kolobe, T. H. A. (1992). Working with families of children with disabilities. *Pediatric Physical Therapy, 4(2),* 57-63.

Lowes, L. P., & Effgen, S. (1996). The Americans with Disabilities Act of 1990: Implications for pediatric physical therapists. *Pediatric Physical Therapy, 8,* 111-116.

McWilliam, R. A. (1995). Integration of therapy and consultative special education, A continuum in early intervention. *Infants and Young Children, 7(4),* 29-38.

McWilliam, R. A. (1996). How to provide integrated therapy. In R. A. McWilliam (Ed.), *Rethinking pull-out services in early intervention* (pp. 147-184). Baltimore: Brookes.

Rainforth, B., & Roberts, P. (1996). Physical therapy. In R. A. McWilliam (Ed.), *Rethinking pull-out services in early intervention* (pp. 243-265). Baltimore: Brookes.

Rainforth, B., York, J., & Macdonald, C. (1992). *Collaborative teams for students with severe disabilities.* Baltimore: Brookes.

Shelton, T. L., & Stepanek, J. S. (1994). *Family-centered care for children needing specialized health and developmental services* (3rd ed.). Bethesda, MD: Association for the Care of Children's Health.

Solomon, B. A., Collins, R., Silverberg, N. B., & Glass, A. T. (1996). Quality of care: Issue or oversight in health care reform? *Journal of the American Academy of Dermatology, 34,* 601-607.

Tolley, B. (1993). Productivity expectations for hospital-based pediatric physical therapists. *Pediatric Physical Therapy, (5)1,* 16-21.

Vandercook, T., York, J. & Forest, M. (1989). MAPS: A strategy for building the vision. *Journal of the Association for Persons with Severe Handicaps, 14(3),* 205-215.

Voss, D. E. (1982). Seventeenth Mary Macmillan lecture. "Everything is there before you discover it." *Physical Therapy, 62,* 1617-1624.

The Emerging Role of the Physical Therapist Assistant in Pediatrics

2

Marilyn E. Miller
Katherine T. Ratliffe

Pediatric Education for the PTA
Growth of PTA educational programs
Supervision of the PTA
Utilization of the PTA
Utilization of the PTA in pediatric settings

Delegation of Tasks in Pediatrics
Identify the tasks
Outline the process of the tasks
Assess the purpose of the task
Assess the locale of the task
Competence

KEY TERMS

physical therapist assistant (PTA)
American Physical Therapy
 Association (APTA)
pediatric education
pediatric curriculum
supervision
legal guidelines
PTA licensure
utilization of the PTA
delegation of tasks
competence

The definition of the physical therapist assistant (PTA) is "an educated health care provider who assists the physical therapist in the provision of physical therapy" (APTA, 1993). The American Physical Therapy Association (APTA) specifies that "the physical therapist assistant is a graduate of a physical therapist assistant associate degree program accredited by an agency recognized by the Secretary of the United States Department of Education or the Council on Post Secondary Accreditation (APTA, 1993). The PTA practices under the supervision of a physical therapist (PT).

One could argue that the PTA role evolved from the professional history of teaching caregivers to implement a plan of care. This delegation of responsibilities has been documented as early as the 1920s, barely after the introduction of physical therapy in the United States and before the formation of the APTA. The APTA, the professional organization formed to unite PTs in defining practice issues and looking toward the future, is the principal force in the development of the PTA.

Much has changed for the PTA since 1967, when the APTA first accepted the development of this category of personnel. Milestones in the development of the PTA are listed in Table 2-1 and provide a context for the difficulties PTAs have had in defining their role in the provision of physical therapy and in gaining a voice in the professional organization. Much work has been done by many individuals to define practice issues for the PTA. Box 2-1 lists relevant documents available from the APTA that outline roles and responsibilities of the PTA.

The introduction of the PTA job classification in the last 25 years has prepared a new category of personnel to provide physical therapy services to children. The PTA can work in schools, clinics, and hospitals and can provide home care to children who are medically stable. If used effectively, the PTA may help alleviate critical shortages in pediatric physical therapy practice and extend the capability of PTs to provide services to more children (Zaslow & Benedetto, 1994).

Many PTs resisted using the PTA during the early years, and many continue to resist today. Some may have concerns of being replaced in providing direct service to children or being forced to take primarily administrative or decision-making roles. Further concern may include questions regarding the PTA's level of skill and capabilities to work with children.

Although all PTAs receive a comprehensive education in the basic principles of anatomy, physiology, kinesiology, and therapeutic exercise, as well as therapeutic techniques and modalities, preparation in the fundamentals of pediatric practice may vary. This chapter outlines the educational background of the PTA related to pediatrics, the legal and practice issues shaping the practice of the PTA, and the definition of some of the concepts that the PTA must understand to work effectively with children. The purpose is to give PTAs working in pediatrics concrete information to share about their abilities to work with this population. In the past 30 years much work has been done to define the knowledge base needed by the PTA to work alongside the PT in pediatrics as well as in other areas of practice.

PTAs are currently working in many pediatric settings, and fiscal realities will ensure that the PTA will take on more responsibilities in providing services to children over the next decade. To be effective in the workplace, PTA students and new graduates must educate PTs and other team members about their skills and capabilities. PTAs who want to work in pediatrics must be ready to identify and learn essential skills related to working with children that they may not learn in their educational curriculum.

Pediatric Education for the PTA

PTA educational programs have been in existence since 1967. Content in pediatrics is a criterion for accreditation for both PT

TABLE 2-1	Milestones for the PTA
Year	**Milestones and implications**
1949	The APTA House of Delegates (HOD) adopted a statement that officially recognized the need and value of utilizing nonprofessional assistants in physical therapy.
1964	APTA ad hoc committee was formed to study the title, responsibilities, education, training, supervision, and regulation of nonprofessional assistants.
1967	Ad hoc committee presented a policy statement, "Training and Utilization of the Physical Therapy Assistant," to HOD and it was accepted. Two PTA education programs accepted their first students.
1969	The first 15 PTA students graduated.
1970	PTAs were accepted as temporary members in the APTA as "Affiliates."
	• PTs were having a difficult time accepting the new category of the PTA.
1973	The "affiliate" designation was made permanent.
	• PTs recognized that PTAs were here to stay. However, no mechanism existed for affiliates to meet or develop and discuss practice issues that pertained to them.
1975	The HOD approved the "Essentials of an Accredited Educational Program for Physical Therapist Assistants."
1983	The Affiliate Special Interest Group (ASIG) was formed.
	• The ASIG provided some cohesiveness to the group and a voice for concerns although still did not allow PTAs input in the policy-making house of delegates.
1989	A new type of APTA component that has a voice in the HOD was instituted and called an assembly; the ASIG formed the affiliate assembly.
	• Finally PTAs had a voice in APTA policy.
1992	The HOD voted to allow affiliate members to hold office at the component level (state chapters or sections united by practice such as pediatrics or orthopedics) with the exception of president.
	• PTAs were permitted to take leadership roles in local and regional APTA organizations.

Documents Related to the PTA*

| BOX 2-1 | |

1. Standards of Ethical Conduct of Physical Therapist Assistants (order no. P-135)
2. Guidelines for Conduct of Affiliate Members (order no. P-135)
3. A Future in Physical Therapy (order no. PR-23A)
4. Physical Therapist and Physical Therapist Assistant Educational Programs (order no. PR-23B)
5. Position Statement on the Utilization of Physical Therapist Assistants in the Provision of Pediatric Physical Therapy (available through the pediatric section)

*These documents are available from the American Physical Therapy Association. To order, call the APTA at 800-999-2782 during business hours on the East Coast, and ask to be transferred to the service center.

and PTA educational programs; however, the specific requirements are not defined (Commission for Accreditation of Physical Therapy Education, 1995). To be more specific, several groups have identified what they feel is appropriate content for pediatric education of the PTA.

The Commission for Accreditation of Physical Therapy Education (CAPTE) solicited input from PTA educators and other interested individuals in the field to evaluate and make general recommendations for the content of pediatric education for the PTA (Commission for Accreditation of Physical Therapy Education, 1995). This information is available to PTA programs and other interested individuals.

A series of PTA educator colloquia entitled "Defining the Outer Limits of Subject Matter in PTA Curricula" was held from 1992 through 1994 in various locations across the country. The outcomes provide one perspective on what should be included in pediatric education for the PTA. The participants thought that the development of the body across the life span, including motor milestones, motor control, recognition of abnormal muscle tone, reflex activity, a basic introduction to interventions for neurological diagnoses, positioning strategies, use of adaptive equipment, and exposure to developmental testing were all appropriate to include in pediatric curricula. The participants felt that it was not appropriate to include selection of adaptive equipment, therapeutic exercise for the neurologically involved child, and independence in developmental testing. The psychosocial aspects of interacting with families were also considered to be beyond the scope of entry-level PTA curriculum (Personal notes, M. Miller, 1992-1994).

Pediatric curriculum is taught in many ways. It may be included as part of a larger course covering the life span of an individual or may be taught separately in a designated course. The content of pediatric curriculum varies considerably between different programs. Although all PTAs receive education about child development and certain disease entities, most do not receive direct instruction related to working with families, handling and interaction skills with children, or the specific needs of children receiving services through an infant/toddler development program or school system. These aspects of care provide a context for working with children and cannot be omitted from an integrated curriculum; therefore this book provides some introduction to these matters. Most PTAs entering the pediatric work force will need additional training that addresses these important concepts in working with children (Figure 2-1).

Growth of PTA Educational Programs

In 1970 there were nine PTA programs. This number grew to 67 programs in 1985; in 1996 there were 226 programs that were either accredited or waiting to become accredited. The numbers of graduates have increased proportionately. In 1969, 15 graduates entered the work force; in 1995, 3,396 PTA graduates joined their peers in providing physical therapy services to individuals with rehabilitation needs in the United States (APTA, 1996).

In 1996 more than 10% of students enrolling in an associate degree PTA program held either a bachelor's degree or a graduate degree (APTA, 1996). Although statistics are not available, anecdotal evidence indicates that at least some of these numbers reflect students who have tried unsuccessfully or who want to be

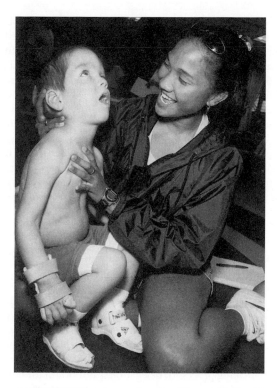

Figure 2-1 This PTA student enjoys handling and interacting with Ian after a demonstration in class.

accepted by physical therapy schools in the future. They hope that a PTA degree will give them a greater competitive advantage when applying or reapplying to a PT education program.

Supervision of the PTA

In a discussion of support personnel, the definition of required supervision is an important focus. A PT must supervise all phases of the provision of physical therapy. The PT assumes ultimate responsibility for the provision of physical therapy services.

Supervision may have different meanings in various practice situations and geographical jurisdictions. Primary forces defining the supervision of the PTA include (1) APTA standards; (2) individual state and federal laws regulating practice acts, including administrative rules for practice; and (3) specifications of entitlement programs such as Medicare. In state practice acts or administrative rules, supervision of the PTA may be spelled out separately from other support personnel, or the PTA may be included in language that defines supervision for all support personnel. How this supervision is delineated may restrict or expand the role of the PTA in any particular jurisdiction. In fact, a PTA who lives near the border of another state and whose practice crosses state lines may need to contend with different rules regarding supervision.

The APTA policy statement "Direction, Delegation and Supervision in Physical Therapy Services" (1993) provides basic guidelines with four requirements for off-premises supervision of the PTA. These are as follows:

1. A qualified PT must be accessible by telecommunications to the PTA at all times while the PTA is treating patients.
2. The initial visit must be made by a qualified PT for every evaluation of the patient and establishment of a plan of care.
3. There must be regularly scheduled and documented conferences with the PTA regarding patients, the frequency of which is determined by the needs of the patient and the needs of the PTA.
4. In those situations in which a PTA is involved in the care of a patient, a supervisory visit by the PT will be made:
   a. Upon the PTA's request for reevaluation, when a change in treatment plan of care is needed, prior to any planned discharge, and in response to a change in the patient's medical status
   b. At least once a month or at a higher frequency when established by the PT in accordance with the needs of the patient
   c. A supervisory visit should include:
      (1) On-site reassessment of the patient
      (2) On-site review of the plan of care with appropriate revision or termination
      (3) Assessment and recommendation for utilization of outside resources.

When the state laws do not delineate supervision requirements, PTs should rely on the APTA guidelines. Some state laws and rules closely follow the APTA guidelines; however, in those states where the rules are stricter than those defined by the APTA, state regulations must be followed. Each PT and each PTA should be familiar with his or her own state or jurisdiction regulations regarding supervision of the PTA and other support personnel. Laws and administrative rules are dynamic and may be revised; therefore vigilance regarding the content of current laws and rules regarding practice issues is very important.

Supervision of the PTA in pediatrics also varies according to the needs of the child, the level of education or experience of the PTA, the comfort level of the supervising PT, and the type of setting. For instance, the PTA working in a pediatric hospital setting may need more direct supervision from the PT because the children's needs are changing more quickly than in other settings. The PTA working in school health may need significantly less direct supervision because most children have chronic needs that change slowly. The PTA who has significant experience working with children and who has attended continuing education programs that address working with children may need less direct supervision than a new graduate. The supervising PT must determine the correct amount and type of supervision for the PTA based on multiple factors. Supervision needs may change over time.

The PTA, especially someone working for the first time in a pediatric setting, must let the supervising PT know about the level of supervision with which he or she is comfortable. Other personnel such as nurses, teachers, other PTAs, or program staff may be able to help the PTA learn about the mechanics of the organization or system in which the therapy is provided. The PT, however, should be available to direct and assist with the actual provision of therapy services. Specific information should be available to the PTA regarding indications and contraindications for therapeutic procedures, length and frequency of intervention, a current plan of care, and therapy goals and objectives.

Utilization of the PTA

Utilization of PTAs is not usually taught in PT education programs, and many therapists continue to think that the use of PTAs will dilute and further fragment physical therapy services. Lack of experience in working with the PTA, lack of knowledge about the capabilities of the PTA, and fears of losing control over categories of practice have led many PTs to reject or limit their use of PTAs. In spite of this resistance from some PTs, significantly greater numbers of PTAs are graduating from accredited programs in every state. The PTA is practicing in many different settings, including geriatrics, home care, orthopedics, acute care, rehabilitation, and pediatrics (Figure 2-2).

Legal variation in PTA practice between different states can lead to different patterns of utilization of PTAs in different jurisdictions. In some states PTAs are licensed, but in others their practice is dictated by rules governing the supervision of ancillary personnel by PTs; yet in others various aspects of the PTA's job are not specified in any legal document. Currently 41 states have PTA licensure. Thus PTAs may find themselves in ambiguous legal territory, possibly restricted from practicing certain skills in one state, when they may have developed those skills and practiced under the supervision of PTs in another state. Some state chapters of the APTA are addressing ambiguities in practice law.

Utilization of the PTA in Pediatric Settings

Discussion of the PTA's role in pediatrics prompted the pediatric section of the APTA to issue a draft document outlining appropriate utilization of the PTA in pediatric physical therapy ("Draft Position Statement," 1995). The position statement on the utilization of PTAs in the provision of pediatric physical therapy states that, "physical therapist assistants can be appropriately utilized in pediatric practice settings with the exception of the medically unstable, such as neonates in the NICU" (p. 14). This document has undergone several changes based on feedback from members of the pediatric section of the APTA; the latest document addresses issues of background, education, delegation and supervision, and exceptions for pediatric intervention by the PTA.

The exceptions to PTA practice in pediatrics, as noted by the pediatric section, are notable in their brevity. The authors considered situations in which "the need for rapid interpretation of physiologic data and behavioral responses to treatment would require multiple adjustment of sequence and procedures during treatment would not be appropriate to be delegated to a physical therapist assistant" ("Draft Position Statement," 1995, p. 16). Situations that fit this criteria include any child with medical needs necessitating intensive care including neonatal intensive care and pediatric intensive care. Care for children who are medically fragile and may be in the hospital, at home or at school may also fall into this category.

Delegation of Tasks in Pediatrics

Delegating tasks to support personnel is not usually taught in physical therapy educational programs. The PT must decide which responsibilities to delegate to the PTA, as well as to other personnel such as an aide or a teacher. The PTA needs to evaluate the delegation of responsibilities to him or her and decide which of those tasks can be taught to others. Understanding the decision-making process of delegation is important for both the individual doing the delegating and the one receiving the delegation.

In 1971, just as the first graduates of PTA programs were entering the work force, Dr. Nancy Watts wrote an article defining decision making around delegating responsibilities in physical therapy. These strategies can help those of us who continue to struggle with issues surrounding delegation more than 25 years later.

Let us take the example of Andrew (see Case Study, Chapter 7) to identify and apply the steps delineated by Dr. Watts in making decisions regarding delegation. Andrew is a 5-year-old boy with severe cerebral palsy. He attends his neighborhood school and is in a segregated special education classroom for most of the day. A special education teacher and an educational aide work in the classroom, and specialists, including a PT, an occupational therapist (OT), and a speech-language pathologist, visit the classroom regularly for consultation and to work directly with Andrew. Andrew's PT is trying to decide whether to turn over all or some of his physical therapy intervention to a PTA and to determine how much the classroom staff should be expected to do.

Identify the Tasks

The first step is to identify the tasks involved. Andrew receives direct therapy once every other week to work on trunk and head control in sitting and standing, gait training in his walker, and consultation with the teacher and aide regarding positioning and handling for Andrew in the classroom and other school environments. The PT also attends and contributes to Integrated Education Program (IEP) meetings, communicates with Andrew's family regarding his needs and his progress, and identifies appropriate equipment for Andrew to access his educational environment. A current goal is to teach Andrew to be more independent when moving from a lying position to sitting on the

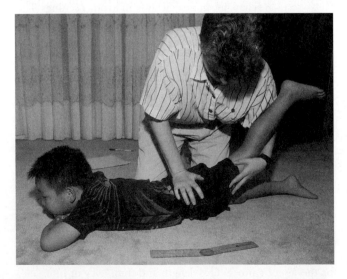

Figure 2-2 The PTA student learns basic skills with children by practicing them.

floor for circle time (see Applications, Chapter 5). Rather than address all the preceding physical therapy tasks, in this example we will focus on teaching Andrew to move from lying down to sitting on the floor.

Outline the Process of the Tasks

The next step is to outline the process of the tasks. This includes deciding whether the tasks involve decision making or doing, or both. The PT is trained to assess change continually while administering a treatment method or modality. Continual assessment involves both deciding and doing, frequently at the same time. The PTA has been trained to administer a treatment method or modality under the supervision of a therapist. This involves primarily doing with some deciding, such as when to change or adapt activities or when to call in the PT for consultation. It is the PT who makes most of the major decisions regarding changing objectives or introducing new treatment modalities or strategies. Determining situations that are appropriate for a PTA and those that are not is the job of a supervising PT. According to Watts (1971), five major factors determine the degree to which deciding and doing can be performed effectively by different individuals (e.g., PT, PTA, teacher, aide). These factors are as follows:

1. Predictability of consequences—How uncertain is the situation? How confident can the decision maker be in predictions about the consequences of action?
2. Stability of the situation—How much and how quickly is change likely to occur in the factors on which decisions are based?
3. Observability of basic indicators—How difficult is it to elicit the phenomena on which decisions are based? How easy are these phenomena to perceive?
4. Ambiguity of basic indicators—How difficult are the key phenomena to interpret? How easily might they be confused with other phenomena?
5. Criticality of results—How serious are the consequences of a poor choice of goals or method? (p. 27).

To apply these principles to the example of teaching Andrew to be more independent in moving from lying down to sitting on the floor, a task analysis of the process is important.

A simplified task analysis might include:

1. Assess Andrew's ability to move from lying down to sitting on the floor.
2. Determine what intervention must be done to help him learn the needed skills.
3. Provide intervention to Andrew to help him learn the skills.
4. Assess his capabilities and adjust the intervention as needed.

If we apply Watts's principles to this example, we can see that (1) the initial assessment of Andrew's skill is unknown, and therefore consequences of the strategies used are unpredictable. Regarding (2) the stability of the situation, Andrew will not likely learn new skills very quickly because of his severe motor impairments. Therefore changes to the program will likely take some time based on his learning new skills. Basic indicators (3) will be fairly easy to observe. Andrew will either be able to hold his head and trunk upright when moving through space or not. The PTA will be able to assess his progress in the skills taught.

Some indicators may be ambiguous (4). For instance, Andrew's inability to bear weight through his arms may be a function of his persistent symmetrical tonic neck reflex (STNR) and his head position. The PTA may not have the skills to assess this factor. The results (5), although important to his integration in the classroom, are not critical to Andrew's health or safety.

Based on this analysis, the PT will need to assess Andrew's current level of skill and design an intervention plan from which the PTA will work. This decision-making role cannot be accomplished by someone without the necessary skills. The assessment could be done with the PTA as an initial training opportunity. The PTA can come to the classroom daily to work with Andrew on the skill during circle time. The PTA could perform the doing portion of the training because the PTA has knowledge of the structure and function of the human body, as well as motor differences related to cerebral palsy. As Andrew's skills change or problems arise, the PTA can consult with the PT to adapt the program, the goal, or the strategies used. In this way the individual executing the intervention consults with the decision maker. This person also makes some important decisions such as assessing whether PT input is necessary. As Andrew's capabilities become stable, the decision-making hierarchy can shift one level. The PTA can instruct the teacher or classroom aide in how to support Andrew in his skills of moving from a lying-down position to sitting on the floor and can act as a consultant.

Assess the Purpose of the Task

Watts's next principle, that of assessing the purpose or function of the task, can be categorized as instrumental or expressive. Instrumental means that which has a practical purpose, such as teaching Andrew new skills, adjusting his wheelchair, or adjusting his head position to decrease the influence of the STNR. Expressive tasks, on the other hand, involve communication and interaction. Some examples include communicating with the family and classroom staff about the program and helping Andrew feel comfortable with moving from lying down to sitting on the floor. The task of helping Andrew has both instrumental and expressive components, and the individual providing support needs to have skills in both areas. The PT must assess not only his or her own skills in the two areas but also that of any supportive personnel. This assessment will determine what components to delegate.

Assess the Locale of the Task

Watts's final principle, that of the locale of a task performance, means assessing how much physical proximity exists between the service provider and the child or family. Some tasks, such as writing a program, do not need direct proximity; others, such as handling a child, require close proximity. The delegation of responsibilities to the PTA may cause the PT to have less contact with children, focusing on paperwork or decision making rather than direct hands-on services. This issue may affect job satisfaction for the PT and may, in fact, be a major reason for resisting the use of PTAs in practice settings.

Awareness of both the PT's and the PTA's needs regarding balancing the two categories of locale can help a PT determine what aspects of intervention to delegate and what aspects to retain. For instance, the PTA may work with Andrew daily during the initiation of the program, with the PT coming in once per week to assess his progress and adjust the tasks as needed. The PTA may eventually provide most of the direct services to Andrew, with the PT coming in as needed. This schedule frees the PT to take on another child for direct intervention. In this way the needs for direct contact with children are met for both the PT and the PTA, and more children receive services.

Competence

Competence is defined as "a significant behavior, performed in a specific setting, to a specified standard (Davis, Anderson, & Jag-

ger, 1979)." Competence is the essence of physical therapy education. It is the professional accountability to the consumer. Because the standard educational curriculum cannot include all aspects important for pediatric practice, PTA graduates entering the pediatric field may need to develop skills not taught in school to practice effectively in educational settings. Student affiliations in pediatric settings can be a starting point for becoming aware of needed skills. Some examples of general competencies for students expecting to work in a pediatric setting after graduation are listed in Box 2-2, along with examples of practical experiences that may help them gain the relevant competencies (Ratliffe & Tada, 1997). These competencies may help the PTA appreciate what skills and strategies are needed to work in a pediatric setting.

BOX 2-2   Competencies for PTA Students in Educational Settings*

1. Students will appropriately handle and position a child with a severe motor disability to facilitate motor skills, socialization, functional skills, and participation in school activities.
   Examples of practical experiences to gain competency:
   a. Facilitate and inhibit movement in a child with severe disabilities during a therapy session.
   b. Work with a specific child with severe disabilities in a group setting such as circle time.
   c. Adapt positioning equipment to better meet the needs of a particular child.
   d. Develop ideas regarding how to better include a student with severe disabilities in daily activities.
   e. Adapt a game or activity to include a student with severe disabilities.
2. Students will assist the PT in taking measurements, observing children's capabilities and needs, and screening children with motor disabilities.
   Examples of practical experiences to gain competency:
   a. Take goniometric measurements of a child with contractures.
   b. Observe limitation in range of motion.
   c. Help fill out a developmental assessment on a child with a disability.
   d. Observe a physical therapy evaluation.
   e. Estimate strength of a child with motor disabilities.
3. Students will design and administer age-appropriate treatment activities based on the results of the PT's assessment results and planned intervention goals that foster integration of a student into a classroom, school, or community setting.
   Examples of practical experiences to gain competency:
   a. Plan a treatment session based on PT goals.
   b. Organize the treatment area or equipment to prepare for a treatment session.
   c. Implement an individual treatment session with supervision, guided by PT goals and objectives.
   d. Carry out a treatment session in the context of a group, with supervision.
   e. Adapt activities based on a child's changing needs or circumstances.

4. Students will have adequate written communication skills for gathering relevant information and providing documentation of services.
   Examples of practical experiences to gain competency:
   a. Write a progress note, summary statement, or SOAP (subjective, objective, assessment, and plan) note documenting the child's current level of performance or documenting a treatment session.
   b. Communicate in a written form with other team members, including occupational therapist, speech-language pathologist, program manager, social worker, physician, or parent regarding the child's needs, including letters, notes in a child's communication book, and memos.
   c. Review a medical, physical therapy, or educational record.
   d. Complete required paperwork for billing or documenting provided services to third-party payers or administrators.
   e. Communicate to supervising therapist regarding a child's needs.
5. Students will be creative in using available resources, including space, equipment, toys, peers, and learning materials to assist in therapy activities.
   Examples of practical experiences to gain competency:
   a. Adapt existing positioning equipment for improved access or position for a child.
   b. Create a new piece of equipment to help the child with positioning or mobility skills.
   c. Adapt a toy with switch access.
   d. Plan for or rearrange furniture or equipment to promote improved access to classroom, recess, physical education, or therapy services.
   e. Adapt learning materials such as pencils, worksheets, or computer for improved access for a child.
6. Students will demonstrate understanding of family support principles through encouraging family advocacy, facilitating family involvement in the team process, and respecting family rights and perspectives.
   Examples of practical experiences to gain competency:

*Developed with the support of U.S. Department of Education, Office of Special Education and Rehabilitation Services, Grant #H029A60099.

BOX 2-2 Competencies for PTA Students in Educational Settings—cont'd

a. Interact with individuals from different agencies involved with a child.
b. Research community support to help a family solve a particular problem. (Example: Find the address for the local Down syndrome support group, and give it to the family if they are interested.)
c. Adapt activities and teach family members to carry out therapy activities at home.
d. Give family members information about agencies, programs, and services that may be available to them after discussing the information with the PT and the team.

7. Students will understand the various types of team relationships and interact collaboratively with team members to implement therapy activities, participate in planning meetings, and assist in developing goals and strategies for integrated inclusive education.
Examples of practical experiences to gain competency:
a. Actively participate in a team meeting.
b. Collaborate with another team member to plan an integrated therapy session. (Example: Collaborate with the occupational therapist, teacher, or speech-language pathologist to conduct a group session with children, which integrates goals of several different disciplines.)
c. Write Integrated Education Program/Individual Family Service Plan (IEP/IFSP) goals and objectives, either as an exercise or draft for an actual IEP/IFSP.
d. Sit in on and participate in planning meetings for the agency, school, or program.
e. Schedule therapy sessions for children and therapy activities based on the needs of the child and of other team members.

8. Students will have adequate oral communication skills to foster relationships with and work collaboratively with other team members.
Examples of practical experiences to gain competency:
a. Observe and interact with other team members during the day (e.g., occupational therapist, speech-language pathologist, teacher, and registered nurse).
b. Plan collaborative activities with other team members.
c. Express opinions, plans, or ideas during team meetings or during collaborative sessions.

9. Students will understand cultural influences on attitudes, family adaptation, and program development for children with disabilities.
Examples of practical experiences to gain competency:
a. Research a cultural perspective different from the student's own.

b. Present an inservice to staff regarding cultural issues.
c. Suggest program alterations based on cultural needs of a family and child.
d. Have opportunity to work with children and families of varying cultural backgrounds.

10. Students will understand how special education teachers interact with children in various educational environments such as self-contained classrooms, mainstreamed situations, and inclusive classrooms.
Examples of practical experiences to gain competency:
a. Work with children in different types of classrooms or settings.
b. Collaborate with a special education teacher to address needs of a child in school.
c. Research an issue, such as inclusion either to present to the staff or to document in written form for staff information.
d. Visit and observe different educational settings (e.g., self-contained and inclusive).

11. Students will explain how PTAs might interact with special educators in the various environments described above in order to provide integrated services to students.
Examples of practical experiences to gain competency:
a. Discuss issues of collaboration with special educators with the PT supervisor.
b. Plan intervention that is directly related to the educational goals of a student.
c. Collaborate with a special education teacher to plan an integrated group or individual therapy session.
d. Consult with a special education teacher regarding one or more students with motor needs.

12. Students will know and act according to professional ethical standards and in accordance with local laws governing the provision of physical therapy services to children in educational settings.
Examples of practical experiences to gain competency:
a. Make a presentation to the staff regarding the supervision of PTAs by PTs, administrative rules governing physical therapy in your state, or ethical considerations as to PTA practice (refer to APTA ethical guidelines).
b. Create a handout for parents that documents the legal issues regarding physical therapy provision to children (e.g., specific legislation such as IDEA, or case law).
c. Discuss ethical issues that arise with a PT supervisor when providing treatment to children.

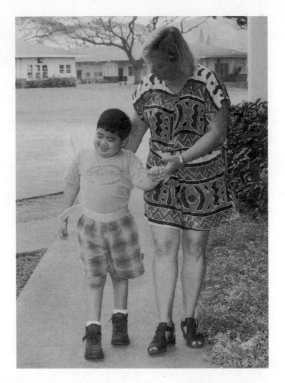

Figure 2-3 This PTA helps Clinton walk between classes.

Summary

The role of the PTA in pediatrics is not easy to delineate because of the complex nature of the tasks involved with working with children (Figure 2-3). Skills of the PTA are varied; but with adequate support, most PTAs are able to handle challenging situations. Care should be taken that specific tasks or children with certain problems are not always assigned to either a PT or a PTA. Watts (1971) states that:

It is impractical and potentially dangerous to classify specific treatment and evaluation procedures as routinely belonging in the domain of a specific level of worker.... Tasks can vary immensely depending upon the stage of evolution of treatment planning and the stability of the patient's condition. Very few procedures are truly simple or complex under all circumstances (p. 32).

Appropriate decision-making skills of the PT are needed to work with supportive personnel such as PTAs and aides. These skills should be taught in physical therapy education programs. However, it is also the responsibility of the PTA to ensure that his or her time is used efficiently and appropriately. All PTAs should be familiar with local rules and regulations governing PTA practice and should take an active role in educating PTs and other service provision personnel about the PTA's role.

Regardless of the initial difficulty in acceptance of PTAs by the PT community, the PTA job category is one of the fastest growing in the country, with expected growth of 83% in the next 10 years ("Physical Therapist Assistant," 1997). As PTs and PTAs continually struggle to redefine their own roles through the changing social and political climate of the turn of the century, they need to learn to work effectively together.

PTAs have a significant role in pediatrics and can help extend physical therapy services by providing skilled intervention to children in schools, home, clinics, and hospitals, under the supervision of PTs. The role of the PTA in pediatrics will continue to evolve as more PTAs enter this area of practice.

● ━━ EXERCISES ━━

1. Obtain a copy of the practice act and administrative rules for PTAs in your state or jurisdiction. Read it and prepare a summary including any specific criteria for pediatric practice. How do the criteria for practice in your practice act compare with the APTA guidelines?
2. Choose a case study provided in this text. Based on the practice act governing PTA practice in your jurisdiction, what parts of the therapeutic intervention are appropriate for the PTA to implement?
3. Choose a case study provided in this text. Create a task analysis of the physical therapy intervention. Decide which tasks you think should be delegated to the PTA and which tasks should be delegated to other support personnel. Hold a dialogue with your peers to see if everyone agrees.

● ━━ QUESTIONS TO PONDER ━━

1. Should policy statements governing PTA practice be explicit? What are the advantages? Disadvantages?
2. Should all PTA programs present the same curriculum content in pediatrics? Why or why not?
3. How should a PTA address a situation where he or she feels either undersupervised or oversupervised?

References

American Physical Therapy Association. (1993). *Direction, delegation and supervision in physical therapy services. HOD 06-93-08-09 (Program 32).* Alexandria, VA: Author.

American Physical Therapy Association. (1996). *1996 Physical Therapist Assistant Education Program fact sheet.* Alexandria, VA: Author.

Commission for Accreditation of Physical Therapy Education. (1995). *Criteria for accreditation.* Alexandria, VA: Author.

Davis, C. M., Anderson, M. J., & Jagger, D. (1979). Competency: The what, why, and how of it. *Physical Therapy, 59,* 1088-1094.

Draft position statement on the utilization of physical therapist assistants in the provision of pediatric physical therapy. (1995, March). *Section on Pediatrics Newsletter, 5,* 14-17.

Fowles, B. H., & Young, J. E. (1965). On-the-job training. *Physical Therapy, 45,* 124-126.

Physical therapist assistant classified by BLS as one of fastest-growing careers. (1997, February 28). *PT Bulletin.*

Ratliffe, K. T., & Tada, W. L. (1997). *Competencies for physical therapist assistant students in educational settings.* Unpublished manuscript.

Watts, N. (1971). Task analysis and division of responsibility in physical therapy. *Physical Therapy, 51(01),* 23-35.

Zaslow, L., & Benedetto, M. (1994). Is the PTA an untapped resource in pediatric PT? *PT Magazine of Physical Therapy, 2(3),* 52-54.

The Typically Developing Child

typical development
gross motor development
fine motor development
cognitive development
social development
language development
adaptive skills development
infant
toddler
preschool-aged child
early school-aged child
older school-aged child
adolescent
play
Piaget
Vygotsky
motivation
evaluation
interdisciplinary
multidisciplinary
transdisciplinary

Background and Theory
Influences of genetics and the environment
  Temperament
Prenatal growth and development
  Patterns of growth and development
  Embryonic stage
  Fetal stage
Infant reflexes
  Asymmetrical tonic neck reflex
  Galant reflex
  Palmar and plantar grasp reflexes
  Tonic labyrinthine reflex
  Rooting and sucking reflexes
  Moro reflex
  Positive supporting reflex
  Walking or stepping reflex
Postural reactions
  Righting and equilibrium responses
  Protective responses
Domains of development
A typically developing child
  The newborn period
  The 2- to 3-month-old infant
  The 4- to 5-month-old infant
  The 6- to 7-month-old infant
  The 8- to 9-month-old infant
  The 10- to 11-month-old infant
  The young child of 12 to 15 months
  The 15- to 24-month-old child
  The 2-year-old and a preschool-aged child
  The early school-aged child
  The older school-aged child
  The adolescent

Applications: Pediatric Evaluation for the PTA
Purpose of evaluation
  Information gathering
  Treatment planning
  Eligibility determination
  Outcome measurement
  Screening
Types of evaluation
  Interdisciplinary or multidisciplinary evaluation
  Transdisciplinary evaluation
  Play-based evaluation
Process of evaluation
  Location
  Timing
  Participants
Components of the evaluation
  History
  Observations
  Specific tests
Use of evaluation tools
  Tyler
  Rik
  Cyril
  Andrew
  Luke
Applications: The Role of Play in Therapy for Children
The importance of play
  Play as developmental learning
  Children's development and play
  Strategies for incorporating play in treatment sessions
  Addressing a child's abilities and interests
  Adaptive toys and play
  Motivational strategies

Healthy children are born every day. Most children are born without developmental problems and grow and change like their peers. Individual differences between children abound, including physical characteristics, temperament, and personality; but the sequence of development is fairly predictable. Most children sit up by themselves before they walk, speak in single words before they learn sentences, and grow larger as they get older. Many first-time parents turn to books or experienced friends and rel-atives to help them predict and celebrate their child's accomplishments as the child grows and changes. Milestones that include taking the first step, speaking the first word, going to school for the first time, having the first date, and graduating from high school are recorded and cherished by parents.

Children with developmental disabilities such as cerebral palsy or myelomeningocele also develop on a fairly predictable, although perhaps a different, timetable than children without these disabilities. When working with children who develop atypically, it is important to be aware of typical development. This is not to compare those who are different with a "standard" but to have a vision of what is possible, so we do not sell our children short. By knowing what skills or strengths are important for children of different ages, and by helping them work toward these, we can help promote peer relationships among differently abled children, improve school success, and ensure vocational success for children with different needs. Being aware of what is possible, or what is expected of most children, can help us to be creative in making adaptations and accommodations for children with special needs to help them succeed. Appropriate early intervention for children with special needs can help them live, play, learn, and work with their peers throughout their lives. Understanding the interrelationships between different domains of development and seeing a child as a whole person can make a significant difference in the life of a child with a disability.

In this chapter we discuss some universal aspects of child development, including the effects of environment and genetics, neonatal reflexes, and the development of balance and motor control. The major focus of the chapter, however, is on following one child through childhood and watching the emergence and change of gross motor skills and how these skills interact with the development of fine motor, language, cognition, and adaptive skills. To discuss the domains of childhood skills, it is sometimes easier to separate them, but in reality the development of these skills is inextricably intertwined. Tables are presented for ease in seeing the progression of specific domains of behavior over time, but the emphasis is on movement and gross motor skills with which physical therapy is particularly interested. The Applications sections on the importance of play in therapy and on physical therapy evaluation of children explore these topics from the perspective of the physical therapist assistant (PTA).

Influences of Genetics and the Environment

Theories of the pervasiveness of environmental influences on children have given rise to blaming parents of troubled children for not providing enough structure, not giving them enough love, or not doing something "right." Parents of children with physical and cognitive disabilities have been blamed for abusing their children prenatally, taking drugs, arguing, or thinking impure thoughts during the pregnancy, and thus causing their child's disability. Others, who attribute childhood problems primarily to genetics, may absolve parents of all responsibility for the rearing of their children but blame them for the genetic problems. These people believe that it is the child's genes, not the influence of the parents, which have the most effect. Parents get blamed in a "double whammy" for their physically or cognitively challenged offspring who inherit defective genes. The debate between the effects of "nature" versus "nurture" is continuing, and compromises are being made as researchers and theorists realize that there is a complex interweaving of genetic predispositions with environmental influences on all children. Most parents care deeply about their children's well-being and future. It is hoped that the emphasis is fading from placing blame for a disability or problem and is moving toward optimizing the future for all children, both through genetic research and creating optimal environments in which children can grow and thrive.

Temperament

Children clearly have different personalities and temperaments that they bring to the events in their lives. Recent research is identifying specific genes that correlate with different temperamental attributes. Some research has focused on the resilient child, who, even under very difficult life circumstances, perseveres and succeeds, as opposed to the child in similar circumstances who becomes oppressed by what life has dealt and is not able to rise above it. Identifying and sorting out the effects of the myriad inborn and environmental influences on a child is a quest that will probably engage researchers for many years.

Researchers have identified and categorized temperamental attributes (Chess & Thomas, 1986). On the basis of the patterns of these attributes, many children can be classified into one of three temperamental categories: (a) the easy child, (b) the difficult child, and (c) the slow-to-warm-up child. The easy child is defined as having predictable habits, an easygoing personality, and a positive approach to changes. The difficult child is usually very active, has irregular habits, and has difficulty adjusting to change. The slow-to-warm-up child is usually inactive and moody and adapts slowly to changes in routine. Although children with each of these temperaments have their own challenges growing up, the risk resulting from having a specific temperament is not the temperament itself but the fit between the specific child and the environment. Therefore an "easy child" in an active household full of stress and uncertainty can have more trouble than a "difficult child" who may have better coping skills in the same environment. The child who is very shy and passive and the child who "bounces off the walls" may need different kinds of help in coping with life events such as beginning school, having an accident, or attending a physical therapy appointment. Parents and health professionals may need to interact in different ways with children of similar ages and development who have varying temperaments. It is important to recognize the strengths of children's personalities and temperaments during interactions with them.

Prenatal Growth and Development

The phenomenal growth of the tiny embryo that develops from one undifferentiated cell to millions of cells in a well-organized living being in the space of 9 months is one of the wonders of life. The growth of the fetus is directed by inborn genetic material and modified by environmental influences. Understanding the patterns of growth and development of the fetus can lead to greater understanding of the continued growth and development of the infant, as well as the effects of disturbances in the prenatal time period.

Patterns of Growth and Development

Some general patterns of growth are consistent in the fetus and continue in the infant and child. The first pattern is that growth occurs in a *cephalocaudal* direction, or from head to tail. The head of the fetus initially forms more completely than the body and limbs. Then the trunk and limbs of the fetus develop. In following this pattern after birth, the infant develops beginning head control before learning to control the trunk or limbs functionally. Development moves downward, with the child learning to control the upper trunk before the lower and using the eyes to engage the environment before learning the skills to use the hands to grasp and manipulate.

Another pattern of development is from the center outward, or *proximal to distal.* The fetus develops the spinal cord and trunk, as limb buds are barely formed. As the fetus develops, the limb buds continue to grow into fully formed limbs and the peripheral nerves form to provide sensory data to the central nervous system, the brain. The infant follows the same pattern of proximal to distal development, with brain growth fastest in the first few years of life when the development of more fine control of limbs is still emerging. As the child grows, the movements of the limbs become more refined and the child develops specific skills, such as throwing, writing, and dancing.

The third major pattern of growth is from the *general to the specific,* or from the simple to more complex. As the fetus grows, undifferentiated cells migrate to specific locations in the fetus and take on specific roles (brain cells, skin, blood). In the developing child, this pattern is also strong. The child learns general skills first; for example, the child will cry to communicate. General communication strategies are refined to specific language over time. Limb movements start out as gross patterns that are directed by reflexes, and mature into skilled movements that are functional for life and safety such as running, jumping, and climbing.

Embryonic Stage

Growth during the prenatal period is predictable and sequential. During the first few weeks of gestation, the early blastocyst implants into the uterine wall and the cells differentiate into embryonic cells, which will develop into the infant, and trophoblastic cells, which will become the placenta and other supporting structures. Early in the embryonic period, from 2 to 8 weeks of gestation, the embryonic cells differentiate further into layers of *ectodermal* cells, which will mature into skin, hair, teeth, nails, and nerves of the infant; *mesodermal* cells, which will develop into muscles, bones, heart, and blood vessels of the infant; and *endodermal* cells, which will form the major organs of the developing infant. It is during the embryonic period that the developing organs go through their most critical growth period and the embryo is the most susceptible to environmental disruptions, such as teratogens (Eckert, 1987; Sadler, 1985). During this period many women do not yet know they are pregnant.

Fetal Stage

After 8 weeks of gestation, the developing infant is called a fetus. Growth and maturation of all the structures that were formed in the embryonic stage occurs. The fetus is about 4 cm long at 9 weeks of gestation. By 12 weeks, it is 10 cm in length. By the end of the first trimester of pregnancy, the fetus is making sucking motions with the mouth and the external genitalia are mature. The tiny heart is beating, and respiratory movements can be seen on ultrasound.

By 16 weeks, the fetus is 18 cm long, and 8 weeks later at the end of the second trimester of pregnancy, it is 28 cm long. By this time it is also ingesting and absorbing amniotic fluid through the gastrointestinal tract and the kidneys are excreting urine. Most of the peripheral neurological reflexes are present in the fetus during this trimester. The fetus weighs a little more than 1 pound (Sadler, 1985).

By 28 weeks of gestation, the fetus is 30 cm long and weighs about 2½ pounds. The eyes open and close, and the fetus has regular breathing movements. With aggressive medical intervention, a fetus would usually survive a premature birth at this stage, although the risk of developmental problems is high (Eckert, 1987). By 32 weeks, subcutaneous fat is present and fingernails and toenails have developed. The fetus weighs about 3½ pounds and may actually look chubby. At 36 weeks the fetus weighs 4½ pounds, and at birth the average weight is 7 to 7½ pounds. The average length of a newborn is 53 cm. During this last trimester of pregnancy the fetus gains the most weight, and the fatty tissue myelin is laid down in the central nervous system to help speed messages through the nervous system. The myelinization of the central nervous system is not complete until 1 year after birth.

Infants born before the completion of 37 weeks of gestation are called *premature.* Chapter 11 addresses physical therapy problems related to prematurity.

Infant Reflexes

The newborn's movements are dominated by innate reflexes. Many of these reflexes are active during the prenatal period and are thought to help the infant learn to organize motor behavior. Some of the reflexes have recognizable roots to our primate ancestors and may have once been functional for safety and social bonding. Each reflex has a stimulus and an automatic response (Barnes, Crutchfield, & Heriza, 1978). Commonly observed reflexes are summarized in Table 3-1 with the ages at which they are active. Also included in the table are possible negative effects on developmental skills if the reflexes persist. Abnormally persistent reflexes may interfere with the development of more advanced motor skills for some children with early brain injuries.

Asymmetrical Tonic Neck Reflex (Figure 3-1)

When an infant who is younger than 6 months old turns the head to the side, the arm and the leg on the scalp side tend to move into flexion, and the arm and the leg on the face side tend to move into extension. The trunk may also curve with the concave side toward the flexed extremities. A typically developing child will move in and out of this pattern, even with the head turned. If a child cannot move out of this pattern, a developmental problem may be suspected.

Galant Reflex

When a finger or other solid object is drawn down the side of an infant's spine from the shoulder to the hip, lateral flexion of the trunk will occur with the concavity toward the side of the stimulus. The reflex is easily elicited when the infant is held in prone suspension. This is a fun reflex to show parents because the re-

TABLE 3-1   Infant Reflexes and Possible Effects If Reflex Persists Abnormally

Primitive reflex	Possible negative effect on movement with abnormal persistence of reflex
Asymmetrical Tonic Neck Reflex (ATNR) Stimulus: Head position, turned to one side Response: Arm and leg on face side are extended, arm and leg on scalp side are flexed, spine curved with convexity toward face side Normal age of response: Birth to 6 months	Interferes with: • Feeding • Visual Tracking • Midline use of hands • Bilateral hand use • Rolling • Development of crawling Can lead to skeletal deformities (e.g., scoliosis, hip subluxation, hip dislocation)
Symmetrical Tonic Neck Reflex (STNR) Stimulus: Head position, flexion or extension Response: When head is in flexion, arms are flexed, legs extended. When head is in extension, arms are extended, legs are flexed Normal age of response: 6 to 8 months	Interferes with: • Ability to prop on arms in prone position • Attaining and maintaining hands-and-knees position • Crawling reciprocally • Sitting balance when looking around • Use of hands when looking at object in hands in sitting position
Tonic Labyrinthine Reflex (TLR) Stimulus: Position of labyrinth in inner ear—reflected in head position Response: In the supine position, body and extremities are held in extension; in the prone position, body and extremities are held in flexion Normal age of response: Birth to 6 months	Interferes with: • Ability to initiate rolling • Ability to prop on elbows with extended hips when prone • Ability to flex trunk and hips to come to sitting position from supine position Often causes full body extension, which interferes with balance in sitting or standing
Galant Reflex Stimulus: Touch to skin along spine from shoulder to hip Response: Lateral flexion of trunk to side of stimulus Normal age of response: 30 weeks of gestation to 2 months	Interferes with: • Development of sitting balance Can lead to scoliosis
Palmar Grasp Reflex Stimulus: Pressure in palm on ulnar side of hand Response: Flexion of fingers causing strong grip Normal age of response: Birth to 4 months	Interferes with: • Ability to grasp and release objects voluntarily • Weight bearing on open hand for propping, crawling, protective responses
Plantar Grasp Reflex Stimulus: Pressure to base of toes Response: Toe flexion Normal age of response: 28 weeks of gestation to 9 months	Interferes with: • Ability to stand with feet flat on surface • Balance reactions and weight shifting in standing
Rooting Reflex Stimulus: Touch on cheek Response: Turning head to same side with mouth open 28 weeks of gestation to 3 months	Interferes with: • Oral-motor development • Development of midline control of head • Optical righting, visual tracking, and social interaction
Moro Reflex Stimulus: Head dropping into extension suddenly for a few inches Response: Arms abduct with fingers open, then cross trunk into adduction; cry Normal age of response: 28 weeks of gestation to 5 months	Interferes with: • Balance reactions in sitting • Protective responses in sitting • Eye-hand coordination, visual tracking

TABLE 3-1	Infant Reflexes and Possible Effects If Reflex Persists Abnormally—cont'd
Primitive reflex	**Possible negative effect on movement with abnormal persistence of reflex**

Startle Reflex

Stimulus: Loud, sudden noise

Response: Similar to Moro response but elbows remain flexed and hands closed

Normal age of response: 28 weeks of gestation to 5 months

Interferes with:
- Sitting balance
- Protective responses in sitting
- Eye-hand coordination, visual tracking
- Social interaction, attention

Positive Support Reflex

Stimulus: Weight placed on balls of feet when upright

Response: Stiffening of legs and trunk into extension

Normal age of response: 35 weeks of gestation to 2 months

Interferes with:
- Standing and walking
- Balance reactions and weight shift in standing
- Can lead to contractures of ankles into plantar flexion

Walking (Stepping) Reflex

Stimulus: Supported upright position with soles of feet on firm surface

Response: Reciprocal flexion/extension of legs

Normal age of response: 38 weeks of gestation to 2 months

Interferes with:
- Standing and walking
- Balance reactions and weight shifting in standing
- Development of smooth, coordinated reciprocal movements of lower extremities

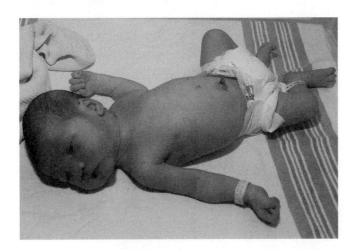

Figure 3-1   The asymmetrical tonic neck reflex (ATNR) dictates a typical neonatal resting posture.

sponse to the stimulus is usually very strong. This reflex is sometimes called the trunk incurvation reflex.

Palmar and Plantar Grasp Reflexes (Figure 3-2)

The palmar grasp is elicited when pressure is placed in the palm of an infant's hand. An adult's finger, or a toy pressed into the hand, works well to demonstrate this response. The infant will grasp an object strongly enough to lift his or her entire body weight briefly. Parents often mistakenly assume that the infant is grasping Daddy or Mommy's finger purposefully, and may be disappointed to learn that the infant has no choice! The plantar grasp reflex is similar, but the pressure stimulus is placed at the base of the toes and the response is a curling of the toes around the object.

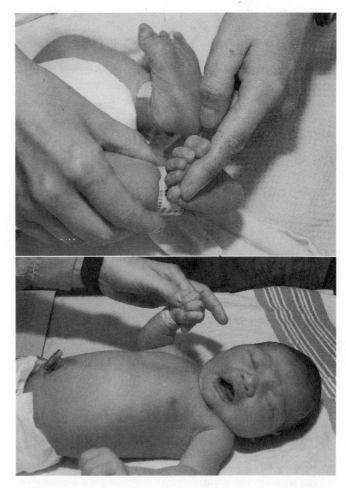

Figure 3-2   All infants will demonstrate the plantar (**A**) and palmar (**B**) grasp reflexes.

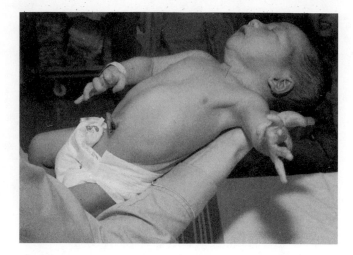

Figure 3-3   When an infant's head drops backward, the Moro reflex can be elicited.

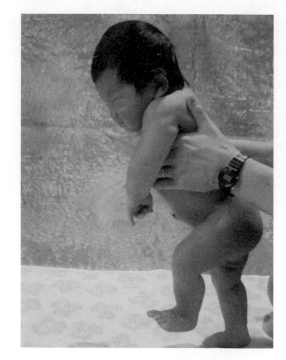

Figure 3-4   The walking or stepping reflex is strongest a few weeks after birth.

Tonic Labyrinthine Reflex

The stimulus for this reflex is the position of the infant's head, or actually of the labyrinths inside the infant's ears, which informs the infant of position in space. When the infant is supine or the neck is extended in an upright position, the infant's legs tend to move into extension and the shoulders retract. When the opposite is true, either the infant is in a prone position or the head is dropped forward in an upright position, the infant's legs tend to pull into flexion, and the shoulders protract pulling the arms into flexion as well.

Rooting and Sucking Reflexes

When the infant's cheek is touched or stroked, he or she will turn the head to that side and open pursed lips. If a nipple, fist, or other object is encountered, the infant will latch on and suck. These reflexes are obviously essential for survival and have been helpful to many new mothers learning to breastfeed their infants.

Moro Reflex (Figure 3-3)

When the infant's head drops back a few degrees abruptly, the arms will abduct and fingers splay. The arms will then adduct across the infant's body and cries may be elicited. This reflex probably helped primate infants grab hold of their caregivers if they started to fall and now are useful for alerting a parent of distress or the danger of falling.

Positive Supporting Reflex

The stimulus for this reflex is weight placed on the balls of the feet when in an upright position. A newborn will stiffen both legs into extension, looking as if he or she is standing. This reflex fades by 2 months of age and returns in a more mature form when the infant is 6 months old. Therefore a 2- to 6-month-old infant will not usually bear sustained weight through the legs.

Walking or Stepping Reflex (Figure 3-4)

When an infant is held upright and leaning forward slightly with a solid surface beneath the feet, the legs will reciprocally flex and extend in a stiff "walking" pattern. This reflex is sometimes heralded by new parents as evidence that their child is advanced, but it occurs in all children.

Postural Reactions

As neonatal reflexes give way to more mature voluntary movements, postural and equilibrium responses develop. These responses help the infant to develop strength and balance for upright activities. Postural and equilibrium reactions can be organized into three major categories. Righting responses help the infant learn to keep the head oriented in relation to the body, or to gravity. Equilibrium reactions adjust for changes of the body's orientation in space. These reactions include righting the head and trunk against gravity when tilted. Protective responses help the infant to learn protection from falls as well as bearing weight through the arms and legs in preparation for more upright positions and mobility. Table 3-2 summarizes the development of these reactions, including the general ages at which they develop.

Righting and Equilibrium Responses

Head righting.   The earliest equilibrium responses to develop are the head-righting responses. The infant tries to keep the head in a vertical position to gravity. Even a tiny infant will try to lift

TABLE 3-2   Reflexes and Developmental Reactions of Childhood

Developmental reaction	Effect on development of motor skills
Birth to 1 Month	
Reflexes	
Sucking and swallowing	Infant learns vertical orientation to world
Palmar grasp	Infant beginning to strengthen postural muscles
Plantar grasp	Infant can lift head in prone position to clear airway
Asymmetrical tonic neck	
Tonic labyrinthine	
Galant	
Moro	
Startle	
Positive support	
Developmental reactions	
Head righting	
2 to 3 Months	
Reflexes	
Traction response of arms in pull to sit stronger	Able to hold head up when held at shoulder
Sucking and swallowing reflexes weaker	Holds head up to 90 degrees briefly in prone position
Galant reflex inhibited	Head bobbing upright in supported sitting position
Positive supporting reflex inhibited	Chest up in prone position with some weight through forearms
Stepping reflex inhibited	
Developmental reactions	
Optical and labyrinthine head righting develops	
4 to 5 Months	
Reflexes	
Integration of asymmetrical tonic neck reflex (ATNR)	Infant rolls from prone to supine position
Integration of palmar grasp reflex	Pivots in prone position
Developmental reactions	Bears weight through extended arms in prone position
Equilibrium reactions in prone position develop	Forward propping beginning in sitting position
Protective extension forward in sitting position develops	Sits alone briefly
Landau response getting stronger	Grasps and releases toys
6 to 7 Months	
Reflexes	
Symmetrical tonic neck reflex develops	Rolls from supine to prone position
Moro reflex inhibited	Holds weight on one hand to reach for toy
Developmental reactions	Gets to sitting position without assistance
Protective extension sideward in sitting position	Stands holding on
Equilibrium reactions in supine position	
8 to 9 Months	
Reflexes	
Inhibition of plantar grasp	Gets into hands-and-knees position
STNR is inhibited	Moves from sitting to prone position
Developmental reactions	Sits without hand support
Protective extension backward develops in sitting position	Creeps on hands and knees
	Cruises along furniture
10 to 11 Months	
Developmental reactions	
Equilibrium responses emerge in quadruped position	Stands briefly without support
	Pulls to stand using half-kneel intermediate position

Continued

TABLE 3-2 **Reflexes and Developmental Reactions of Childhood—cont'd**

Developmental reaction	Effect on development of motor skills
12 to 15 Months	
Developmental reactions	
Equilibrium reactions emerging in standing position	Walks without support
Protective extension forward in standing position	Walks backward
	Walks sideways
16 to 24 Months	
Developmental reactions	
Protective extension sideways and backward in standing position	Squats in play
	Kicks ball
	Propels ride-on toys

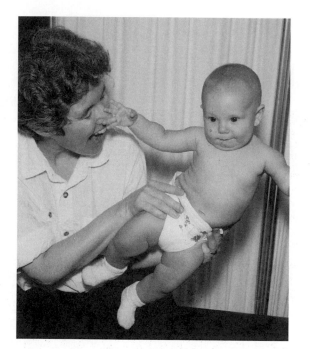

Figure 3-5 Head righting in vertical suspension.

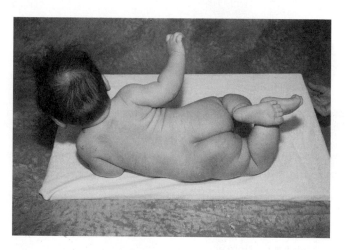

Figure 3-6 The 4-month-old infant demonstrates equilibrium responses in the prone position.

the head upright when at a parent's shoulder. When an older infant or a child is held in vertical suspension and tilted to the side, the head, and eventually the trunk, will accommodate by moving laterally so the head is vertical to the floor (Figure 3-5). There are two mechanisms working to help the child adjust the position in space. In optical head righting the child accommodates visually; in labyrinthine head righting the inner ear balance mechanisms help adjust the head position in space.

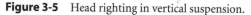

☀ Get down to a child's eye level. This means squat, sit, or kneel on the floor when talking to or interacting with a child.

Prone and supine equilibrium responses (Figure 3-6). When an infant is placed on a firm surface in the prone position, and

the surface is tilted, the infant will adjust to the tilt by raising the arm and leg on the higher side for balance. Soon, the infant will develop this response in the supine position. The mature response can be seen in all neurologically intact children and adults.

Sitting and quadruped equilibrium responses (Figure 3-7). The older infant develops accommodations to equilibrium shifts in sitting and in quadruped, where the trunk and extremities move to accommodate the change in position. Try sitting on a chair and have someone tilt the chair backward. Your arms and legs will accommodate to the change in position in an equilibrium response, usually moving forward. These early infant responses develop into more mature responses that accommodate movement and weight shift. Soon self-initiated weight shifts lead to independent transitions between positions and to mobility skills such as rolling, creeping, and walking.

The *Landau response,* in which the head and lower extremities are extended in line with or above the plane of the body when a child is held in prone suspension, demonstrates many of the righting and equilibrium responses. Children begin exhibiting the Landau response at 3 months, and it is not integrated until the second year of life.

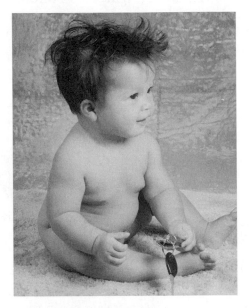

Figure 3-7 The 6-month-old infant demonstrates equilibrium responses in sitting.

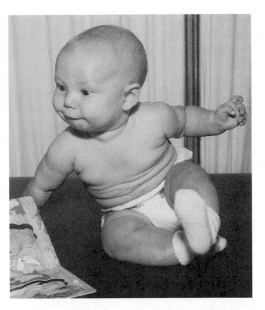

Figure 3-9 The 6-month-old infant demonstrates protective extension sideways in sitting.

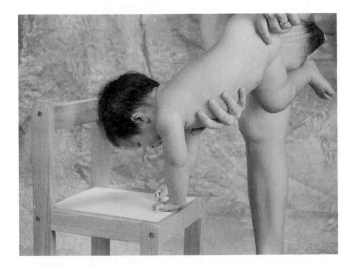

Figure 3-8 An infant will put hands out to protect from a fall, demonstrating protective extension.

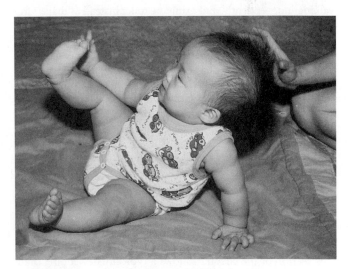

Figure 3-10 The 8-month-old is just beginning to demonstrate protective extension backward in sitting.

Protective Responses

Protective responses downward and forward are the first to develop. When a child is lifted up vertically and brought downward quickly, the legs will extend to catch the child. Likewise, when a child is brought downward head first, the arms will extend to catch the child (Figure 3-8). Next, the child learns to protect from a sideways displacement of balance (Figure 3-9). When sitting, the child can move the arms sideways to stop a fall. The last direction to develop protective responses is backward. By the time the child is 9 to 11 months old, backward protective extension in sitting should have developed (Figure 3-10). Protective responses in standing emerge later than those in sitting, during the second year, but follow the same pattern of development: forward, side, and then backward.

Domains of Development

When assessing or measuring a child's development, professionals usually divide the child's behaviors and skills into specific domains. Different professionals may take responsibility for assessing and treating various areas, perform their assessments and treatments, and write their reports separately. Some of the key areas addressed in a child's development include gross motor, fine motor, receptive language, expressive language, social, emotional, and cognitive domains.

In reality these areas do not develop in isolation. Each is dependent on all the others. The interrelatedness of domains of development is particularly important for children because they are changing a great deal over relatively short periods. Methods of assessment, including play-based assessment, arena assessment, and transdisciplinary assessment, allow professionals to work together to assess more than one domain (see the Applications section in this chapter). Collaborative and integrated treatments of children encourage all therapy providers to consider multiple domains of development when working with children. This method of treatment is now considered to be "best practice," especially in educational environments.

Unless a pediatric therapy provider understands how the domains of development interrelate, understanding how one component of a child's developmental changes can affect all areas may be difficult. However, this approach is fundamental when working with children.

The skilled therapist must look beyond the surface of observable developmental skills in a child. Many tables and references on child development address specific skills as milestones of achievement for the child. Thus speaking in single words, walking independently, and using the toilet instead of diapers for elimination are seen as independent skills that can be celebrated. The development of these skills is dependent on a variety of underlying mechanisms. Underlying gains in motor control; increase in variety of independent movements; and improved control of intrinsic muscles such as tongue, sphincter, and intrinsic skeletal muscles are key to the development of many skills for the child. Improved balance and greater coordination of opposing muscle groups also provide a foundation for the development of skills.

It is these underlying changes that the therapy provider must be aware of to facilitate optimal developmental skills in a young child.

A Typically Developing Child

This section of the chapter follows a typically developing child through infancy, childhood, and adolescence. Observing this child's activities, capabilities, and struggles through selected vignettes of her life will demonstrate key changes in social, language, cognitive, and adaptive skills, as well as gross and fine motor skills.

These skills are summarized in Tables 3-3 and 3-4 at the end of this section for reference (see pp. 45-50).

It is important to keep in mind that each child is an individual person with a slightly different pattern and pace of skill development. The vignettes and the tables are only a guide, and individual children may develop skills before or after the tables predict (Frieberg, 1992; Furuno, O'Reilly, Inatsuka, Hosaka, & Falbey, 1993).

The Newborn Period (Figures 3-11 through 3-15)

Lani and Joe looked down at their beautiful daughter. After three boys it was time to have a girl! Karrie was alert with her eyes open, resting in her 23-year-old mother's arms, only 1 hour after her birth. Her parents had unwrapped her from the warm cotton blanket to count all her toes and fingers. Her

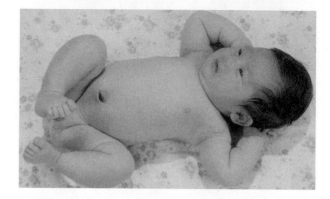

Figure 3-11 The posture of a neonate is one of physiological flexion. In the supine position a neonate is able to turn the head to both directions. Gravity acts upon the limbs to allow the infant to extend them briefly, but they always move back into flexion. Newborns are able to kick reciprocally.

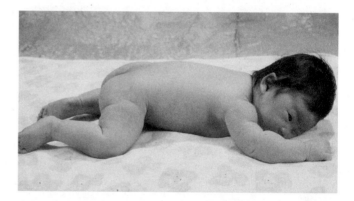

Figure 3-12 In prone the pelvis of a newborn is held up off the support surface because of flexion of the hips and knees. The infant is able to extend the legs reciprocally in prone, and turn the head to clear the airway.

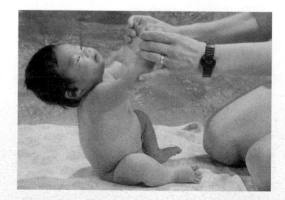

Figure 3-13 The newborn's head falls back completely when pulled to a sitting position.

knees and hips were bent and her legs were kicking in the air. Her arms were moving in strong jerky motions. She turned her head from side to side. Joe sat next to the bed in an armchair with his hand on the infant's abdomen to help her keep calm and settled. The boys—2-year-old Kevin, 3-year-old David, and 5-year-old Joey—would come to visit this evening with their grandparents. Joe and Lani were enjoying these few hours with each other and their newborn. "She's so beautiful." Lani looked at Joe smiling. The infant turned toward her mother's voice, and the blanket brushed gently against her cheek. She turned her head further, opening her mouth, and searched for a nipple. She was not successful. A monotone cry erupted from the infant's lungs and her face turned red. Lani and Joe laughed and watched her for a few minutes. Karrie turned her head toward her father, fists waving. A fist came into brief contact with her mouth, and she sucked vigorously on it, her cries slowing down. Then her head turned farther to the side, and the fist dropped away. Her entire face, neck, and arms turned red as she cried louder. Lani lifted the infant to her breast. Karrie felt her mother's nipple on her cheek, turned her head, and latched on immediately. As she sucked, her attentive eyes watched her mother's face. Lani spoke gently to her infant as she nursed. After a few minutes of sucking, Karrie's eyes closed and she fell asleep.

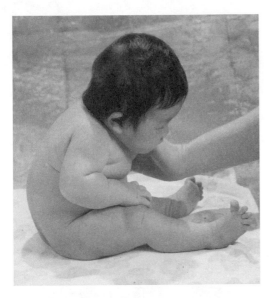

Figure 3-14   Once in the sitting position, the newborn falls completely forward if not supported. The spine is curved forward into flexion.

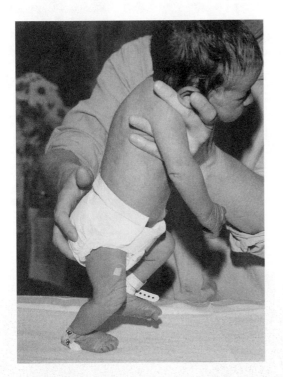

Figure 3-15   In the supported standing position, the newborn takes weight through the legs. Holding the head up briefly is possible, especially when paired with activation of the positive supporting reflex.

The 2- to 3-Month-Old Infant
(Figures 3-16 through 3-22)

Karrie lay upright against her mother's chest, tucked inside a protective arm, and resting her head on her mother's shoulder with her eyes wide open. Her brothers were playing on the floor around them. Lani bustled around the kitchen making dinner with her free hand, and the scene was constantly changing in front of Karrie's eyes. When 5-year-old Joey climbed onto a chair to put his face right next to Karrie's, she picked her head up, laughed out loud, and waved her arms jerkily at him. Joey grinned at his infant sister and leaned over his mother's shoulder to talk to the infant. Karrie listened attentively and smiled when Joey smiled. When Joey stepped off the chair onto his 2-year-old brother, Kevin cried loudly. Karrie jerked her head and arms and widened her eyes, in a startle

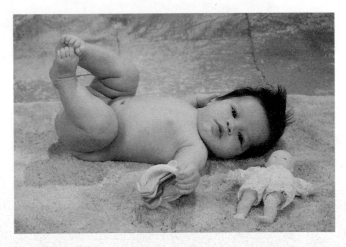

Figure 3-16   At 2 to 3 months of age, an infant will turn the head side to side full range in the supine position and prefers to keep the head to the side. The legs will generally be tucked into a flexed position, although the infant will be able to kick reciprocally and move both legs into extension. The ATNR is still a strong influence.

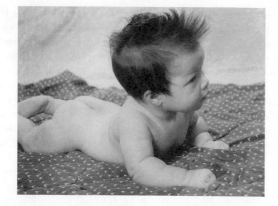

Figure 3-17 The infant has more possible movements in the prone position. As opposed to the younger infant, who still has strong physiological flexion, the 2- to 3-month-old infant's weight will be further back toward the pelvis to allow the lifting of the head and chest. In the prone position the infant will be able to lift the head up briefly to 90 degrees to look around, the chest will be off the support surface, and some weight will be taken through the fore-arms. From the prone position the infant may inadvertently roll into a side-lying or supine position by turning the head with the body following.

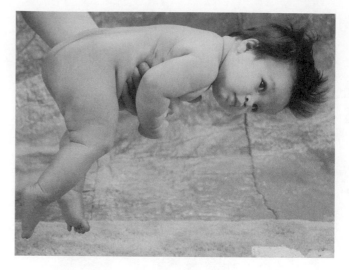

Figure 3-18 When a 2- to 3-month-old infant is held in ventral suspension, the head may be in line or beyond the line of the body as more voluntary trunk extension is observed.

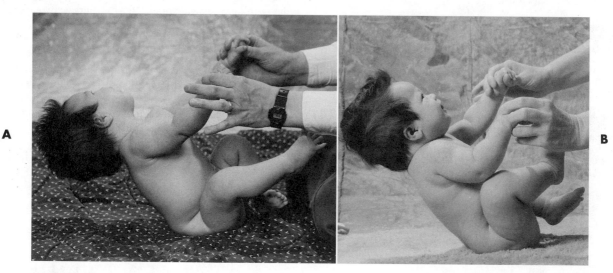

A

B

Figure 3-19 When being pulled to sit, the 2-month-old infant will still have a full head lag (**A**), whereas the 3-month-old infant has a lesser head lag or may be able to hold the head in line with the body (**B**). The older infant will also demonstrate a stronger traction response of the arms, pulling them into some flexion to help when being pulled into a sitting position.

Figure 3-20 The trunk is still rounded with poor extension through the thoracic and lumber spine. The 3-month-old infant may be able to take some weight through the arms and hold the head up close to the line of the shoulders. Once in a supported sitting position, the head can be held upright briefly, although bobbing movements demonstrate fragile control.

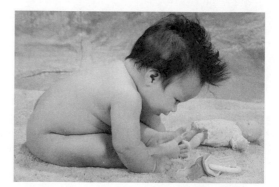

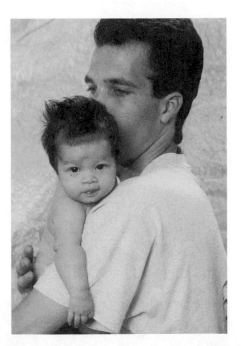

Figure 3-21   When held at a parent's shoulder, a 2- to 3-month-old infant will be able to hold the head up briefly and turn the head to visually track at least 45 degrees.

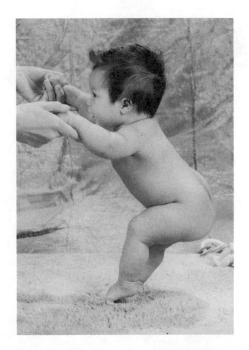

Figure 3-22   In a supported standing position, the 2- to 3-month-old infant is not able to extend the hips and has lost the ability to bear significant weight through the legs. The hips are held behind the shoulders, and the ankles may be plantar flexed with the toes curled as the infant tries to bear weight.

response, her head bobbing. Lani put Karrie down onto a blanket on the floor so she could console Kevin. Karrie lay quietly on her back, turning her head to the side and looking at the activity around her. She closed her fist around a rattle that Joey put in her hand but did not notice when the rattle moved with her hand. She brought her hands together in front of her but kept her head to the side watching Joey. When he approached her with another toy, Joey had to pry Karrie's hand open to take the rattle out of her hand. Joey soon lost interest, and Karrie cried loudly when left on her own for a few minutes. Her cries were rhythmic and louder than the cry she used to tell her mother she was hungry. Lani picked the infant up again and continued working on dinner preparations. The new toy dropped out of Karrie's hand as she forgot it and snuggled into her mother's arms.

The 4- to 5-Month-Old Infant
(Figures 3-23 through 3-27)

Karrie lay on her stomach on the bed, where her mother had put her, watching her brothers get ready for bed. Her eye caught a blue and red plastic airplane on the edge of the bed, and she arched her back, trying to reach for it. Wiggling and squirming to get herself closer to the toy, her knee came up beside her trunk, and she pushed off with her foot. Her left arm collapsed underneath her, and all of a sudden she rolled over, very near the edge of the bed. She was so surprised that she burst into tears. Joey ran to her and pulled her further into the middle of the bed. He patted her stomach and talked to her until she stopped crying. He saw her looking at the airplane and picked it up, holding it out to her. Karrie reached out and grasped the toy with her right hand. She brought it to her mouth with both hands and happily mouthed it while gazing at her brother. When she turned her head and smiled as Lani approached, the toy ended up in Karrie's

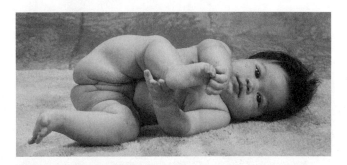

Figure 3-23   In the supine position the 4- to 5-month-old will move all extremities actively through space, explore knees and then feet with the hands, and may at first inadvertently, and then purposefully, roll to the side.

left hand. Lani helped Joey pile pillows around Karrie so that she would not roll off the bed. Then she picked Karrie up and put her on her feet while she held onto her hands. Karrie stood firmly on fully extended knees, bent forward at her hips. She moved her head in jerky motions to look around the room. When Lani sat her down in front of the pillows, she held the baby's hands and talked to her. Karrie was able to actively explore her environment visually and held her head and trunk up. She cooed "aah" and "ee" in response to her mother's voice. When her mother let go of her hands, however, Karrie drooped continually forward as she sat alone for a few seconds. When she became stuck leaning forward, she started to cry and fell over sideways. Lani untangled her from the pillows and let her play on her stomach with the airplane while she helped the boys finish getting dressed in their pajamas.

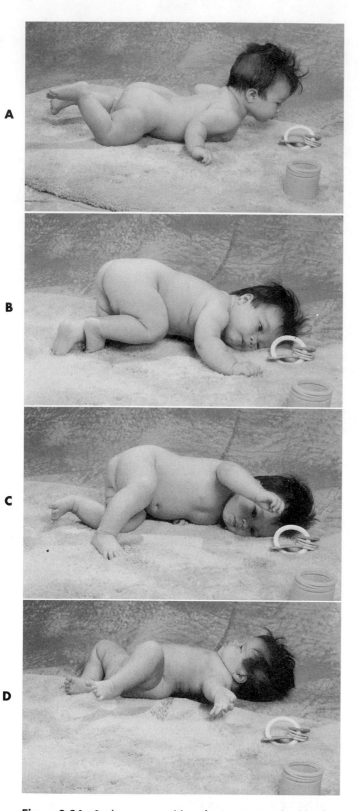

Figure 3-24 In the prone position, the 4- to 5-month-old infant can lift all extremities off the surface and may accidentally, and then purposefully, roll to supine from prone.

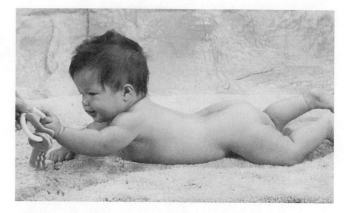

Figure 3-25 In the prone position the 4- to 5-month-old infant can lift the head upright to 90 degrees, can reach for toys, and by 5 months is successful at grasping toys in a wider range.

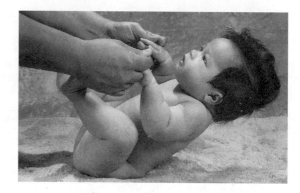

Figure 3-26 The 4- to 5-month-old infant tucks the chin and helps when pulled to a sitting position. In supported sitting the infant can prop briefly and sit for several minutes with minimal support at the trunk or hands.

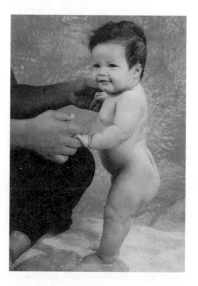

Figure 3-27 In a supported standing position, a 4- to 5-month-old infant can take full weight through wide-based legs, but the hips remain in flexion so that the pelvis is behind the plane of the shoulders. A 5-month-old infant may begin to flex and extend the knees.

The 6- to 7-Month-Old Infant
(Figures 3-28 through 3-33)

Karrie stood on her mother's lap protected by a bright-yellow infant life jacket and her mother's arms as the wind whistled through her hair. She held her legs stiffly against the bouncing of the boat, and her hands fidgeted with the buckles on the life jacket. She squinted into the sunset as the boat headed west toward the reef. Lani and Joe were headed out to collect edible reef fish, sunset being the best time to catch certain varieties. When they anchored, Lani put Karrie down on a towel on the floor of the boat and told Joey to watch her while she went up to the bow to help Joe who was in the water with a mask, a net, and a fishing spear. The two younger boys were home with their grandparents.

Karrie sat independently, her hands firmly on the deck, watching her mother. Joey brought over three brightly colored fishing lures with the hooks removed for her to play with. She

was able to grasp two of them, one with each hand, but could not figure out how to get the third one. She brought them both to her mouth and mouthed them, grimacing and sticking her tongue out when she tasted the salt. She played in a sitting position without hand support for several minutes. Her mother called out, "Hi, Karrie!" Karrie looked up and found Lani with her eyes, smiling at her. She babbled to Joey who was sitting near her playing with some newspaper, "bababa." When Joey covered up the fishing lures with the newspaper, Karrie pushed it aside to find the toy. She discovered that the newspaper was fun, too. She leaned over until she fell onto her side. Then she grabbed the newspaper. It crinkled and made noise. Joey laughed when she put it in her mouth, munching up and down. When her mother came near, she made Karrie spit out the wet gobs of paper. Karrie rolled onto her stomach and pushed up onto her hands and knees by pushing back with her arms. She seemed stuck, so Joey lifted her up to stand at the cooler. She bounced a little by bending and straightening her knees and leaned to the right to get the lures, which were just out of her reach on the top of the cooler.

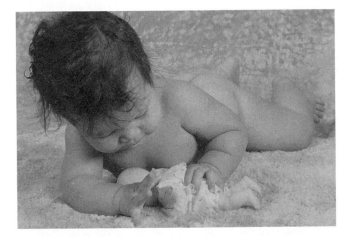

Figure 3-28   In a prone position the 6- to 7-month-old infant can reach forward or to the side for toys, use lateral trunk flexion with hip and knee flexion on that side to shift weight, and lift one arm up to reach. In a supine position the infant can roll to the side and to a prone position. Sidelying is a common play position because the infant can more easily manipulate toys.

Carry something in your pocket that a child may find intriguing. Depending on the age of the child, this could be a set of keys, a small squeaky toy (the ones from pet stores are great), a pen, or a tape measure. Make sure the object is clean if the child is likely to mouth it. Use the object or toy as an intermediary to make friends with the child.

When she started to lose her balance, her foot moved over to catch her. The next time she leaned over, her foot did not catch her, and she fell to the side, rolling and bouncing on the deck as she landed. She did not put out her hands to catch herself, but the life jacket provided some cushioning. Karrie was surprised and scared. She ended up on her back, crying. Lani came back, laughing, and picked her up. Soon Joe had caught all the fish he needed, and Karrie was seated back on her mother's lap as the boat headed away from the sunset, back home.

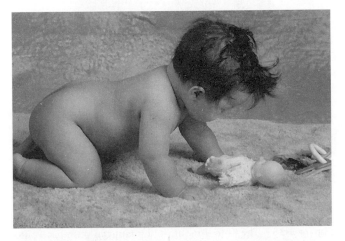

Figure 3-29   The 6- to 7-month-old infant can push back into the quadruped position from prone and rock on all fours.

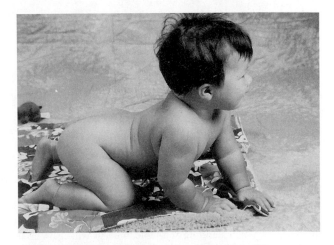

Figure 3-30   Eventually the 7-month-old infant will learn to move one knee forward to begin the creeping motion, but disassociation will be poor between the lower extremities.

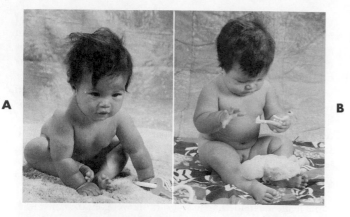

Figure 3-31   In a sitting position the 6- to 7-month-old infant will prop initially (**A**) but will gradually spend more and more time with both hands engaged with a toy (**B**).

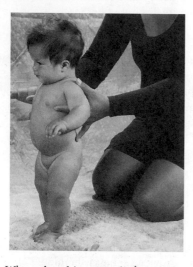

Figure 3-32   When placed in a standing position, the 6- to 7-month-old infant will have the hips in greater extension with the legs closer together than in earlier months.

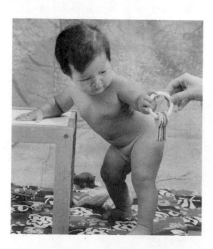

Figure 3-33   When standing at a table, the legs will again be abducted and the 6- to 7-month-old infant will have difficulty keeping the base of support underneath the body. When reaching forward or to the side, the infant may fall.

The 8- to 9-Month-Old Infant
(Figures 3-34 through 3-39)

Karrie clung to her mother, tears streaking her cheeks, and both fists grasping her mother's shirt. She buried her face in her mother's chest, crying loudly. Kevin, her 3-year-old brother, started crying too. Lani, looking worried, handed the infant to her mother. "I'm sorry, Mom, she only started this recently."

Karrie's grandmother took the infant, making soothing sounds. "Say bye-bye to Mommy." Karrie weakly raised her hand through her tears and opened and closed her fingers in a bye-bye gesture. Lani leaned over and kissed her, then with Joe and Joey left to go fishing. Karrie was now too active to be safe on the boat, so she stayed with the younger two boys and her grandmother.

Grandma put her into the high chair and gave her a bottle filled with juice. She also gave her some cereal pieces on the tray of her high chair. Karrie quieted down as soon as her mother left.

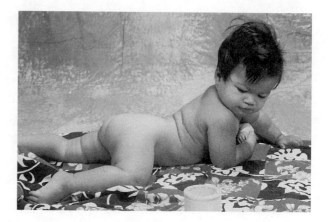

Figure 3-34   The 8- to 9-month-old infant rarely stays in a supine position, rolling immediately into prone. Moving between positions is fairly easy, and in prone the infant can use lateral flexion and beginning rotation to pivot to reach toys.

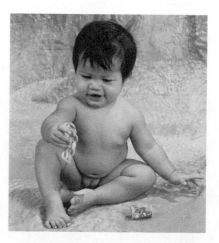

Figure 3-35   The 8- to 9-month-old infant can push back onto the hands-and-knees position and push up into a sitting position.

She drank from her bottle, then dropped it carefully over the side of the high chair, watching it fall. She ate a few of the cereal pieces, picking them up carefully between her thumb and the side of her index finger. Then she started dropping cereal off her tray onto the floor. Her grandmother put her down on the floor and cleaned up the cereal.

Karrie sat for a few minutes playing with the bottle that she had retrieved. Then she moved forward over her knees into a quadruped position and crawled over to her brothers, who were peacefully coloring at the coffee table. She crawled over the top of the bottle that had been in her hand, pulled herself up to standing at the coffee table by getting into a half-kneel position, and then pulled up with her arms. She watched the boys for a few seconds, babbling "dadadada," and banged on the table top. When she moved sideways over to where the crayons were kept in a plastic container, her voice rose in pitch and volume. When

she grasped the container, the boys shouted at her to stop, but she leaned on it and the container slid off the table onto the floor, along with Karrie. Crayons were everywhere. As Grandma helped the boys pick them up, Karrie lay on her back, grasping a few crayons in each hand and looking at them. She brought one crayon to her mouth and turned it over. Then she put it in her mouth and sucked on it until her brother grabbed it from her and put it back into the container. Karrie immediately turned back over onto her stomach and crawled back over to the table. She pulled herself to stand again and looked at the boys. She let go of the table with one hand and then the other to reach for two crayons that Kevin handed her. Her legs were wide apart and externally rotated with her belly protruding. She balanced just a few seconds before she leaned against the table again. Her grandmother gave her a piece of paper to color on, but Karrie picked it up and tried to eat it instead.

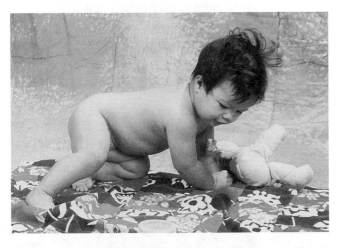

Figure 3-36 Moving back and forth between sitting and hands and knees is a frequent transition, and the 8- to 9-month-old infant can actively explore the environment.

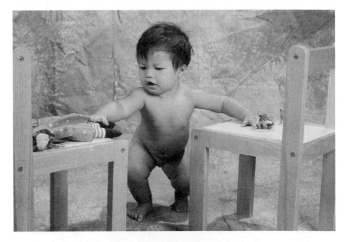

Figure 3-38 Cruising sideways at the furniture and walking with one or two hands held provide beginning upright mobility for the 8- to 9-month-old child.

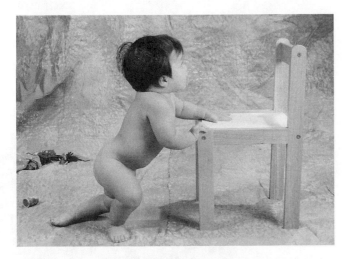

Figure 3-37 The 8- to 9-month-old infant has many more options for mobility, including creeping efficiently on hands and knees and pulling to standing through a half-kneel position.

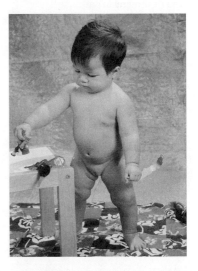

Figure 3-39 Stability is improving in the upright position, with some 8- to 9-month-old infants being able to stand briefly without upper extremity support. In this case the legs are widely based in abduction and external rotation.

The 10- to 11-Month-Old Infant
(Figures 3-40 through 3-46)

The children were pouring out of the walkway that led to the classrooms. Karrie stood next to her mother and brothers and watched them walk by. When Joey came out, her face brightened and she walked toward him. Her legs were abducted and her arms held out to the side for balance in a high guard position. A child brushed by her, and Karrie fell down by sitting. She carefully got onto her hands and knees, pushed up onto extended legs and arms, squatted, and stood again. Six-year-old Joey ran over to her and took her hand to lead her back to their mother.

Kevin, 3 years old, and David, 4 years old, were running on the school playground, and Joey begged to stay for a while and play. Lani agreed and sat on a bench. She pulled three toy cars out of her bag for Karrie to play with while the older boys played on the playground equipment. When David fell off the slide, Lani ran to him. Karrie rolled a car along the bench until it rolled out of her reach. She climbed onto the bench to get it. When Lani turned back, Karrie was leaning off the bench looking for the car that she had dropped over the edge. Before Lani could get to her, Karrie tumbled off the bench and landed on her back in the grass. Tears gave way to smiles when Lani distracted her by piling the cars on top of each other. Then she hid them under her bag. Karrie moved the bag aside and found them again. Lani then hid the cars inside the bag. Karrie pulled objects out of the bag until she found the cars. Karrie held a car out to show to David who came over for some more comfort. When he tried to take it, she shrieked and pulled her hand back. Then she turned her back to him and clutching the car, toddled over to a nearby water fountain.

"Mama, mama," she called, gesturing up at the water fountain. Lani had held her up to the fountain to get a drink the previous day, and Karrie wanted to do it again. When Lani did not come, Karrie squatted down to play in the mud at the base of the fountain. She sat down in the mud and squeezed it between her fingers. She reached all around her, leaning on her hands and

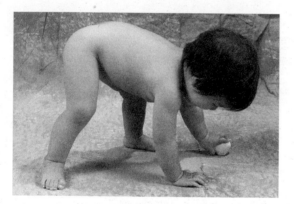

Figure 3-40   The infant of 10 to 11 months is highly mobile. Creeping on hands and knees or hands and feet (bear walk) can be an efficient method of moving around.

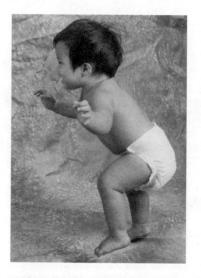

Figure 3-42   Early walking is characterized by arms held in high guard, abducted and externally rotated lower extremities, and leaning forward to shift the center of gravity to take steps.

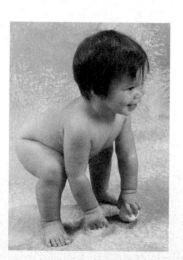

Figure 3-41   Many children by 10 to 11 months can come to a standing position by using a squatting intermediate position.

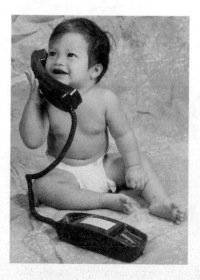

Figure 3-43   Children at 10 to 11 months old have dynamic sitting posture and can assume varied positions in sitting.

shifting her weight to gather some colorful pebbles. She was able to grasp the pebbles by using her thumb and finger and put some of them in her mouth. Telltale signs of mud streaked her face and shirt. When Lani saw her, she hurried over and swept Karrie's mouth with her finger. Three pebbles came out. She rinsed Karrie off using water from the fountain and gathered up the boys to go home.

The Young Child of 12 to 15 Months
(Figures 3-47 through 3-51)

Karrie dragged a large plastic bag that her mother had given her across the yard to her father to fill with yard clippings. "Dada, ba." Joe thanked her and started to take the bag. "No no." Joe tried to take the bag again, but Karrie protested by grabbing it back and screaming. When Joe insisted, Karrie ran back to her mother, empty handed and screaming. Little sympathy came from her mother, and Karrie lay down on the ground and

screamed louder. Her red face was tear streaked. Lani gave her another bag, but this did not assuage her feelings. Finally, when Lani offered her a cracker, Karrie lay on the ground munching, sniffing, and watching the boys. Joey, 6 years old, and David, 5 years old, were raking over by the corner of the house, and 4-year-old Kevin was helping his father stuff the raked clippings into the bags. A cat walked through the yard. Karrie rolled over and stood up. She walked fast across the yard, her arms out, following the cat that disappeared through the hedge. "Ca," she said, pointing after it.

Joey looked up from his raking. "Yes, cat," he said, smiling. Karrie stuffed the rest of the cracker back into her mouth, moving it to the side of her mouth with her tongue. She fiddled with her diaper and finally pulled off the sticky tabs that held it closed. The diaper came undone, and she carefully pulled it off, throwing it on the grass. Joey laughed at her, then put down his rake to go and pick up her diaper and throw it away. Karrie wandered over to the rake and picked it up. She pushed and pulled at it to

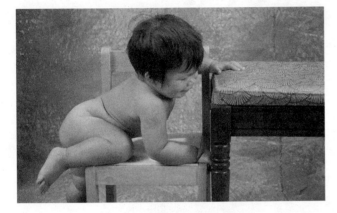

Figure 3-44 Climbing is becoming an option for vigorous environmental exploration. Children initially keep their body close to the supporting surface when climbing to provide stability and use their arms to pull themselves up. Safeguards are important to prevent injury.

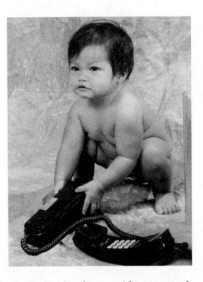

Figure 3-46 Squatting in play provides a more dynamic base of support from which to move.

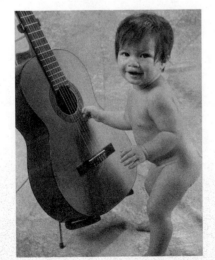

Figure 3-45 Play in standing is easier as stability has improved in upright positions.

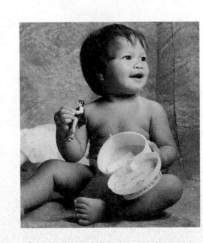

Figure 3-47 The child of 12 to 15 months can sit and play with a toy for 5 to 10 minutes. The improved fine motor skills of being able to put things into and out of containers allows greater variety in play.

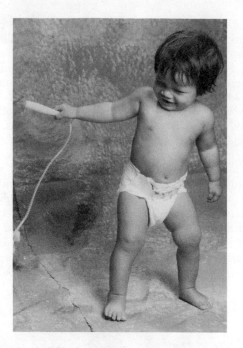

Figure 3-48   Stability has improved in standing so the child can combine locomotion with playing, pull toys attached to strings, or drag toys while walking.

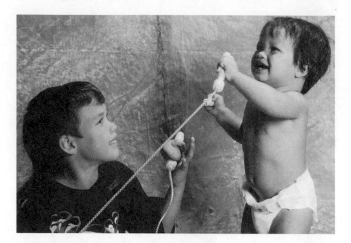

Figure 3-49   The child is becoming more independent in actions and movement and can use the improved stability in standing for physical resistance when arguing with a sibling.

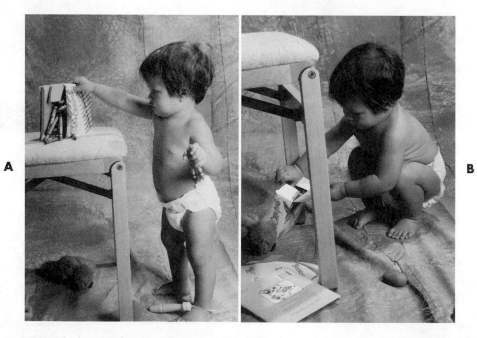

Figure 3-50   The legs are closer together in standing (**A**) and squatting (**B**), allowing the child more variety of movements and reflecting greater balance skills.

get it to move across the lawn, but it would not move. When her older brother returned, Karrie looked at her naked bottom and then at Joey. "Uh-oh." She watched urine run down her legs onto the grass. When Joey tried to take back his rake, she held it close to her and said, "No!" She then started walking toward her mother pulling the rake after her. Lani watched the interchange between the two children, laughing, and sent Joey to get another diaper for his little sister. After rediapering Karrie, Lani helped Karrie start playing with some other toys so Joey could take the rake back to finish his job.

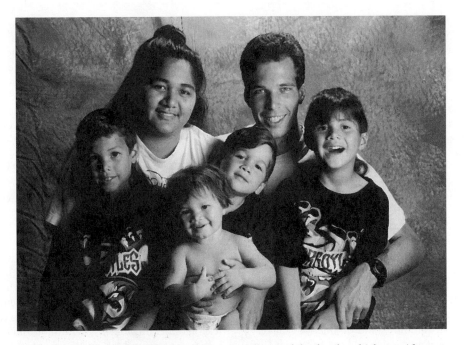

Figure 3-51 The child cannot be separated from the context of the family, which provides support and nurturing.

The 15- to 24-Month-Old Child

Karrie shrieked as she ran through the house. Four-year-old Kevin was chasing her. They both came to an abrupt stop when Karrie slipped on a shirt left on the floor and fell. Kevin landed on top of her, and they both started crying. Lani untangled the children and sat them down to play more quiet games. She gave each a coloring book, and they shared a basketful of crayons. Karrie sat with her book on the floor. She watched Kevin to see what he did with his book and turned some pages, copying him. She then chose a crayon and colored in ever-widening scribbles over the page she had chosen. Kevin was trying to color inside the lines and asked his mother for help. After Lani had sat with Kevin for a few minutes, Karrie abandoned her coloring book and climbed onto her mother's lap, "Me, too."

"Not now Karrie, I'm helping Kevin." Lani put Karrie down on the floor. Karrie put her arms around her mother, leaning against her and looking forlornly up at her mother's face. When Lani did not respond, she wandered away and got on her ride-on-toy, a rolling dog. "Woof, woof," she said loudly as she propelled herself through the kitchen, glancing at her mother and Kevin to see if she could get their attention this way. When they did not respond, she began to talk loudly to herself as she propelled her dog across the room with her feet. Her voice rose and fell, but few words were recognizable. When she reached the kitchen counter, she got off her dog and climbed on a chair to reach something on the counter.

"Karrie, what are you doing?" Lani smiled at her young daughter.

"Karrie cookie?"

Lani laughed and got up to get cookies for both her children. Karrie sat on the floor with her cookie and broke it into small pieces. She put several into her mouth at once and chewed carefully, enjoying the taste of her cookie. She reached up to take the small cup her mother offered and drank a large sip of juice be-

fore swallowing her cookie. She choked and spewed cookie and juice all around her as she coughed and sputtered.

"Oh Karrie!" Lani cleaned up the mess with a cloth. "Look, it went as far as your foot!" Karrie reached out and touched her foot. "And it's on your nose." Karrie touched her nose. "And your chin." She touched her chin. Lani laughed as she grasped Karrie's hands with the damp cloth. "And even on your fingers!" Karrie looked carefully at her fingers as her mother wiped her face.

The 2-Year-Old and a Preschool-Aged Child

Lani and her mother walked along the beach, watching the two children run along the ocean's edge. Kevin was 4 years old, and Karrie was 2. "Kevin, hold her hand," Lani called to her son. Although he tried, Kevin couldn't persuade Karrie to let him hold her hand. She grabbed it back from him and shouted, "NO!" Lani shrugged when Kevin glanced back at her, and then she settled down on a warm sandy area to keep an eye on the children and to enjoy the day.

> Talk with the parent first, making small overtures to the child at the same time. This is sometimes a less threatening method of developing a relationship with a small child.

Karrie collected rocks and shells in a pile. Kevin added his own treasures to the pile as he found them. When he wanted to take one to show his mother, Karrie objected. "No, my pile!" Kevin insisted on taking the shell, and a grabbing fight ensued. Lani finally had to come and admire the treasures where they were.

Later in the morning, the children were playing on a picnic table at the edge of the beach. Kevin climbed on the bench and jumped off. Karrie did the same, although she crouched down on the bench before stepping off and was not always able to stay on her feet. They both crawled under the table and began to play house. Karrie lay down as if asleep at one end of their "house," and Kevin collected sticks for firewood. He laid a "fire," and they cooked lunch using shells and rocks. Kevin carefully separated the shells and rocks into categories for different foods. Later the sticks for the fire turned into fences that they had to jump over. Kevin was able to easily jump over them, but Karrie had a little more trouble. She was able to clear the ground with both feet but did not always clear the stick!

"Mommy, I have to pee." Karrie clutched at her crotch. It turned out that Kevin had to go, too, so all of them went to the public restroom at the far end of the park together. The children ran on ahead and climbed the few stairs to the bathroom. When Lani and her mother arrived, Kevin had already used the toilet and was helping Karrie to pull down her pants.

"Karrie, lift your foot up like this so I can get your pants off." Kevin stood on one foot for a few seconds. He hopped a few steps as he tried to stay upright and laughed as he fell onto his other foot.

Karrie said "No," although she tried to follow Kevin's directions. Unfortunately, she could not stand on one foot for very long. She also could not wait any longer and wet her pants. Lani had extra underpants and shorts in her bag and cleaned Karrie up quickly. She helped Karrie wash her hands. Kevin washed his hands by himself. Then everyone scampered down the stairs again. Kevin alternated his feet on the steps, but Karrie stepped with both feet on each step to go down.

The Early School-Aged Child

Seven-year-old Karrie walked out of her classroom in a group of other second graders. The children spread out over the playground, mingling with the third graders who streamed out of their classrooms. Karrie moved over to the hopscotch squares with her friends Emily and Sarah. They collected their rock markers from behind a bush and began their game of hopscotch. Karrie threw her rock onto the first square. She jumped over it, landing on one foot in the second square. She successfully hopped on one foot through all nine squares, turned around, and hopped back to the beginning again. When she reached the second square, she squatted down on one leg and picked up her marker. Then she leaped over the first square to land on two feet at her starting off place. She carefully threw her marker toward the second square, but it rolled out, and it was Emily's turn.

While Emily was playing, Karrie looked around the playground. Children were over by the basketball nets arguing over who could use the space. The boys wanted to shoot baskets, and the girls wanted to jump rope. Finally, a teacher divided the space in half so both groups could play. The boys were using a rubber playground ball rather than a regulation basketball, and it bounced very high, causing them to lose it frequently. They called loudly to each other as they ran after it when it rolled out into the grassy part of the playground. The girls were playing with long ropes, swinging for each other and taking turns jumping in. The rhythms of their chants drifted across the playground, mixed with the yells and laughter of the boys. Other children played tether ball. There was such a variety of sizes of children that sometimes tearful arguments occurred. Playground monitors had to intervene frequently.

The kindergartners and first graders were on the lower playground where there was more playground equipment. Karrie could see them swinging, playing on the slide, and swarming over the climbing equipment. She remembered how she had loved to play shipwreck and pirates, using the climbing equipment as a ship with her friends last year. She watched a group of girls holding hands and skipping together as they sang. Sometimes she missed being on the lower playground.

Karrie and her friends played through the entire recess but did not yet finish their game. When the bell rang, they marked where their stones were and carefully hid them behind the bush again. The groundskeepers would not see the stones behind the bush, and they would be safe until the next recess period.

The Older School-Aged Child

Karrie, aged 10, listened carefully to her hula teacher. The music started. She swayed her hips and moved her feet, and her arms and body moved to tell the story of Pelé, the goddess of fire. This was a dance she had done many times before, but this time her teacher was preparing the group for a hula competition. The precision of her movements, her timing and coordination with the other dancers, and the quality of expression of her movements were very important.

This dance was an old one, reinterpreted through the years by different hula teachers. Step-together-step, Karrie coordinated her steps and arm movements, her mouth forming the ancient Hawaiian words of the chant as her teacher chanted them. She remembered struggling though this dance when she was first learning hula, but now the steps and movements were relatively easy. It was the subtle aspects of the dance, reaching higher, smiling, feeling the movements so she could make them real that consumed her attention as she danced.

Because she was one of the older girls in the children's hula group and therefore one of the tallest, she was in the back row. Altogether there were 20 girls ranging in age from 7 to 11 years old. Karrie was tall for her age, and her arms and legs sometimes felt as if they were growing faster than the rest of her. She was able to learn fast, though, faster than some of the younger girls who still struggled to learn sequences of steps. She was also stronger and able to do longer dances before getting tired than when she first started learning hula when she was 7 years old.

Although this hula competition was only among children, Karrie's teacher had told them that, if they did well, some of the more proficient children might be able to join the adults for the Merrie Monarch competition in the spring. Karrie was excited at the idea of traveling to the competition and competing among the best hula schools in the world. She turned her attention again to the music and the chant.

The Adolescent

Fifteen-year-old Karrie waited, the bat poised above her shoulder, her eyes on the pitcher. When the pitch came, she swung and hit the ball solidly. Dropping the bat, she took off for first base. She pumped her arms and legs as she ran full out, stamping on the base just before the ball reached the glove of the first base player. Trotting back to first base after her overrun and breathing heavily, she grinned. Her running and hitting had both improved since last year. She might even make the first team this year. She tagged the base and led out toward second, eyes on the pitcher, who could try to get her out by throwing the ball to first base again. She kept her legs about shoulder width apart, and she shifted her weight from right to left foot constantly so she could easily run back to the base or off toward second if the ball was hit.

"Crack!" What a hit! Karrie took off for second base. The third base coach was gesturing to her to keep coming, so she tagged second and kept going for third. Her team members were yelling. The crowd was wild with excitement. She rounded third and kept her eye on the catcher, who was waiting on home plate. Although she was running as fast as she had ever run, she felt as though she were in slow motion. When she saw the catcher raise her arm to catch the ball, Karrie dove for the plate. She ploughed right through the catcher and was consumed in a pile of moving dust, arms, legs, and sound. The umpire yelled "Safe!," and she saw the ball rolling away from her. The catcher was untangling herself, and Karrie's team was going crazy.

As she dusted herself off, Karrie caught a glimpse of her family in the stands. Her gaze passed over them, however, to a group of teenagers lower down. Yes, he was there. Luckily, the dust hid her blush as she tried not to look at Nathan. Karrie was glad he had seen her slide, and she hoped he would be at the party that night. She walked over to the bench to greet her enthusiastic teammates.

TABLE 3-3   Developmental Gross and Fine Motor Skills

Gross motor skills	Fine motor skills
Newborn to 1 Month	
Prone	
Physiological flexion	Regards objects in direct line of vision
Lifts head briefly	Follows moving object to midline
Head to side	Hands fisted
Supine	Arm movements jerky
Physiological flexion	Movements may be purposeful or random
Rolls partly to side	
Sitting	
Head lag in pull to sit	
Standing	
Reflex standing and walking	
2 to 3 Months	
Prone	
Lifts head 90 degrees briefly	Can see further distances
Chest up in prone position with some weight through forearms	Hands open more
Rolls prone to supine	Visually follows through 180 degrees
Supine	Grasp is reflexive
Asymmetrical tonic neck reflex (ATNR) influence strong	Uses palmar grasp
Legs kick reciprocally	
Prefers head to side	
Sitting	
Variable head lag in pull to sitting position	
Needs full support to sit	
Head upright but bobbing	
Standing	
Poor weight bearing	
Hips in flexion, behind shoulders	
4 to 5 Months	
Prone	
Bears weight on extended arms	Grasps and releases toys
Pivots in prone to reach toys	Uses ulnar-palmar grasp
Supine	
Rolls from supine to side position	
Plays with feet to mouth	
Sitting	
Head steady in supported sitting position	
Turns head in sitting position	
Sits alone for brief periods	
Standing	
Bears all weight through legs in supported stand	

Continued

TABLE 3-3   Developmental Gross and Fine Motor Skills—cont'd

Gross motor skills	Fine motor skills
6 to 7 Months	
Prone	
Rolls from supine to prone position	
Holds weight on one hand to reach for toy	
Supine	
Lifts head	Approaches objects with one hand
Sitting	Arm in neutral when approaching toy
Lifts head and helps when pulled to sitting position	Radial-palmar grasp
Gets to sitting position without assistance	"Rakes" with fingers to pick up small objects
Sits independently	Voluntary release to transfer objects between hands
Standing	
Stands holding on when placed	
Bounces in standing	
Mobility	
May crawl backward	
8 to 9 Months	
Prone	
Gets into hands-and-knees position	
Supine	
Does not tolerate supine position	
Sitting	Develops active supination
Moves from sitting to prone position	Radial-digital grasp develops
Sits without hand support for longer periods	Uses inferior pincer grasp
Pivots in sitting position	Extends wrist actively
	Points with index finger
	Pokes with index finger
	Release of objects is more refined
Standing	
Stands at furniture	Takes objects out of container
Pulls to stand at furniture	
Lowers to sitting position from supported stand	
Mobility	
Crawls forward	
Walks along furniture (cruising)	
10 to 11 Months	
Standing	
Stands without support briefly	Fine pincer grasp developed
Pulls to stand using half-kneel intermediate position	Puts objects into container
Picks up object from floor from standing with support	Grasps crayon adaptively
Mobility	
Walks with both hands held	
Walks with one hand held	
Creeps on hands and feet (bear walk)	
12 to 15 Months	
Mobility	
Walks without support	Marks paper with crayon
Fast walking	Builds tower using two cubes
Walks backward	Turns over small container to obtain contents
Walks sideways	
Bends over to look between legs	
Creeps or hitches upstairs	
Throws ball in sitting position	

TABLE 3-3 Developmental Gross and Fine Motor Skills—cont'd	
Gross motor skills	**Fine motor skills**

16 to 24 Months

Squats in play
Walks upstairs and downstairs with one hand held—both feet
   on step
Propels ride-on toys
Kicks ball
Throws ball forward
Picks up toy from floor without falling

Folds paper
Strings beads
Stacks six cubes
Imitates vertical and horizontal strokes with crayon on paper
Holds crayon with thumb and fingers

2 Years

Rides tricycle
Walks backward
Walks on tiptoe
Runs on toes
Walks downstairs alternating feet
Catches large ball
Hops on one foot

Turns knob
Opens and closes jar
Buttons large buttons
Uses child-size scissors with help
Does 12- to 15-piece puzzles
Folds paper or clothes

Preschool Age (3-4 Years)

Throws ball 10 feet
Walks on a line 10 feet
Hops 2-10 times on one foot
Jumps distances of up to 2 feet
Jumps over obstacles up to 12 inches
Throws and catches small ball
Runs fast and avoids obstacles

Controls crayons more effectively
Copies a circle or cross
Matches colors
Cuts with scissors
Draws recognizable human figure with head and two extremities
Draws squares
May demonstrate hand preference

Early School Age (5-8 Years)

Skips on alternate feet
Gallops
Can play hopscotch, balance on one foot, controlled hopping,
   and squatting on one leg
Jumps with rhythm, control (jump rope)
Bounces large ball
Kicks ball with greater control
Limbs growing faster than trunk allowing greater speed, leverage

Hand preference is evident
Prints well, starting to learn cursive writing
Able to button small buttons

Later School Age (9-12 Years)

Mature patterns of movement in throwing, jumping, running
Competitiveness increases, enjoys competitive games
Improved balance, coordination, endurance, attention span
Boys may develop preadolescent fat spurt
Girls may develop prepubescent and pubescent changes in
   body shape (hips, breasts)

Develops greater control in hand usage
Learns to draw
Handwriting is developed

Adolescence (13 Years+)

Rapid growth in size and strength, boys more than girls
Puberty leads to changes in body proportions: center of gravity
   rises toward shoulders for boys, lowers to hips for girls
Balance skills, coordination, eye-hand coordination, endurance
   may plateau during growth spurt

Develops greater dexterity in fingers for fine tasks (knitting,
   sewing, art, crafts)

TABLE 3-4   Social, Language, Cognitive, and Adaptive Skills of Childhood

Age	Social	Language
Newborn to 1 month	Eye contact Molds body when held Relaxes when held Regards face	Crying to indicate needs Monotonous nasal cry Makes comfort sounds
2 to 3 months	Watches speaker's eyes and mouth Responds with smile when socially approached Enjoys physical contact Vocalizes in response to conversation	Coos open vowel sounds Cries vary in pitch and volume to indicate different needs Laughs Squeals
4 to 5 months	Socializes with strangers/anyone Lifts arms to mother Enjoys social play Vocalizes pleasure/displeasure	Reacts to music Reacts to own name Babbles consonant chains "bababa" Babbles to people
6 to 7 months	Smiles at self in mirror Does not like to be separated from mother Recognizes mother visually Anxious about strangers Yells to get attention Loves vigorous play	Babbles double consonants "baba" Waves bye-bye Produces more consonant sounds when babbling
8 to 9 months	Lets only mother meet needs Explores environment enthusiastically Enjoys social games	Babbles single consonant "ba" Adult pattern of inflection in babbling Says "dada" or "mama" nonspecifically
10 to 11 months	Tests parental reactions Extends toy to show, not give	Babbles monologue when alone Says "dada" or "mama" specifically Repeats sounds or gestures if laughed at Unable to talk while walking
12 to 15 months	Displays tantrum behaviors Acts impulsively Enjoys imitating adult behaviors Says "no"—resists adult control Distractible	Uses exclamatory sentences ("uh-oh", "no-no") Uses words or word approximations to express self Has one-to three-word vocabulary Says "no" meaningfully Speech may plateau as child learns to walk
16 to 24 months	Expresses affection Plays alone for short times Gets frustrated easily Displays wide range of emotions, including jealousy of a family member Parallel play Interacts with peers using gestures, vocalizations	Imitates environmental sounds Uses two-word sentences Attempts to sing songs Expressive vocabulary up to 50 words Uses own name to refer to self Uses jargon mixed with intelligible words
2 years	Talks loudly Becomes bossy and demanding Obeys simple rules Has trouble with changes Separates easily from mother in familiar surroundings May have tantrums May develop fears of unfamiliar things such as animals or clowns	Child gains language quickly, up to four words per day Uses three-word sentences Frustrated when not understood Tells full name Recites simple nursery rhymes Sings phrases of songs
Preschool-aged child (3-4 years)	Enjoys making friends Plays cooperatively Needs praise and guidance from adults Enjoy helping with adult activities (shopping, setting table) Enjoys imitating adult behavior Fears may continue	Child talks to self at play and rest Uses rhythmic language Uses language actively Has expressive vocabulary of up to 1000 words Learns entire songs and nursery rhymes Loves to talk

Cognitive	Adaptive/self-help
Quiets when picked up	Opens and closes mouth in response to food
Responds to voice	Beginning coordination of sucking, swallowing, and breathing
Consoles self by sucking	
Searches with eyes for sound	Brings hand to mouth
Shows active interest in person or object for 1 minute	Better coordination of sucking, swallowing, and breathing
Inspects and plays with own hands	Stays awake longer periods during day
	Sleeps for longer periods at night
Looks for hidden voice	Holds bottle
Plays for 2 to 3 minutes with one toy	Eats pureed or strained foods
Finds partially hidden object	Drinks from cup
Works to obtain object out of reach	Naps 2 to 3 times per day
	Sleeps up to 12 hours at night
Looks for family members when named	Mouths solid food
Shakes toys to hear sound	Feeds self cracker
Plays peek-a-boo	Bites and chews toys
Plays with paper	
Imitates simple gestures	
Responds to simple verbal requests ("come here," "give mommy")	Finger-feeds self
Throws and drops objects	Chews using munching pattern
Looks at pictures when named	Sleeps up to 14 hours at night
Enjoys looking at pictures in books	Holds spoon
Stacks and unstacks rings	Extends arm or leg for dressing
Guides action toy manually	
Dances	
Enjoys messy activities such as finger-painting, feeding self	Brings spoon to mouth
Recognizes individuals outside family	Holds cup and drinks with some spilling
Helps turn pages	Indicates discomfort over dirty diaper
	Shows pattern of elimination behavior
Can put things away	Feeds self with spoon, some spilling
Names six body parts	Uses rotary jaw movements to chew food
Matches sounds to pictures of animals	Removes shoes
Sorts objects	Plays with food
	Helps with washing hands
	Turns knob to open doors
	Begins toilet training
Matches shapes	Undresses/dresses with help
Completes a 3- to 4-piece puzzle	Uses spoon and fork
Understands concept of one	Uses napkin
Understands concept of two	Washes and dries hands
Plays house	Uses toilet consistently
Loves being read to	Hangs clothes up on hook
Sorts colors, matches some colors	Blows nose with help
	Insists on doing things without help
Identifies colors and shapes	Dresses/undresses independently except back buttons
Able to do a 30-piece puzzle or more	Uses toilet without help
Identifies money, coins	Uses utensils (fork, spoon) independently
Enjoys books	Brushes teeth with supervision
Has vivid imagination	May be very modest with dressing, toileting, bathing
May confuse fantasy with reality	

Continued

TABLE 3-4   Social, Language, Cognitive, and Adaptive Skills of Childhood—cont'd

Age	Social	Language
Early school-aged child (5 to 8 years)	Prefers to play with peers rather than adults Refines social skills of giving, sharing, receiving Cares deeply what others think of them Likes to impress peers	Uses plurals, pronouns, tenses correctly Recites or sings rhymes, TV commercials, songs Interested in new words Vocabulary of 2000 to 4000 words
Late school-aged child (9 to 12 years)	Increased interest in group activities Spirit of adventure high Interested in organized sports—athletes as heroes Interested in practicing skills to gain social approval and develop skills	Increasing vocabulary and maturity of language skills
Adolescent (13 to 18 years)	Peer-oriented Self-conscious Interest in opposite sex Increase in social maturity	Expressive writing skills improve

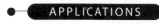

APPLICATIONS   Pediatric Evaluation for the PTA

KATHERINE A. O'REILLY

Evaluation of a child's physical and developmental status is performed by the physical therapist (PT). The terms *evaluation* and *assessment* are used differently by different authors. Evaluation is defined here as the total process of measuring a child's abilities and drawing conclusions that result in a final report. Assessments are the ministeps included in the evaluation process, such as the use of a specific measurement tool and its interpretation. The role of the physical therapist assistant (PTA) is defined by the pediatric section of the APTA as a "clinician who can implement a plan of care designed by a physical therapist" (Chapman, 1995). However, to fully and appropriately implement a pediatric plan of care, it is important that the PTA have an understanding of the purpose and process of evaluation that the PT is likely to use in developing the plan of care. An awareness of commonly used evaluation tools can also help the PTA participate more fully in the collaborative team working with a child. An understanding of how the PT makes decisions about developing the plan of care is important because the PTA participates by (a) assisting in parts of the evaluation process, (b) observing the results of treatment strategies, and (c) communicating observations and ideas with the PT.

Purpose of Evaluation

Physical therapy evaluations of children are performed for many reasons: information gathering, treatment planning, eligibility determination, outcome measurement, and screening (Goodwin & Driscoll, 1980).

Information Gathering

Information on an individual child's development is needed to compare that development with established norms for other children of the same age or to plot where a child's development falls on a continuum. Information about the child's movement abilities can be valuable to the physician in the diagnostic process. Families benefit from information about their child's functional abilities and needs, both to put their child's needs into perspective and to plan for the future. Early identification of deviations from normal development can help the family access early intervention programs that offer services, support, and education.

Treatment Planning

The plan of care for a child is based on an analysis of the strengths and areas of need identified during an evaluation. The areas of need are the obvious areas that will be targeted for support, correction, or improvement, but it is also important to note and build on strengths to develop the child's functional skills, as well as a sense of competence and self-esteem.

In pediatrics the treatment plan will become part of an Individualized Family Support Plan (IFSP) for infants from birth to 3 years of age. For older children in the school system there will be an Individualized Educational Program (IEP) that includes those aspects of physical therapy that assist a child in optimizing his/her education. Physical therapy treatment goals should be integrated with other goals—such as social, educational, recreational, language, or fine motor—in the comprehensive plan.

Eligibility Determination

Programs provided by public or private agencies typically need information about the functional level of disability a child exhibits to justify placement in classes or to receive special services. Likewise, eligibility for funds through medical insurance payments and Supplemental Security Income (SSI) may be partially based on the functional level of disability that a child exhibits

Cognitive	Adaptive/self-help
Learns to read	May have stomach aches related to school attendance
Learns basic math skills of addition and subtraction	Definite likes and dislikes with food
Learns concept of conservation	Learns to use knife for spreading, cutting
Learns to write (printing)	Learns to tie shoes
Enjoys table games	Can bathe independently, wash hair with supervision
Able to think more abstractly	Independent in daily care activities
Increased attention span	Learns to cook
Intellectually curious	Takes role in household tasks
Reads greater variety of materials including nonfiction	
Can develop hypotheses, theories	Takes on greater household roles (laundry, cooking, cleaning)
Increased attention span	Learns to drive
Interests expand beyond self to environment, those less fortunate, etc.	

(Mental Health, 1991). Level of disability can be documented by test scores and descriptive statements. For example, some infant programs have entry requirements of significant delays in two areas of development, such as cognitive and gross motor domains. To receive SSI assistance, a child must have a physical or mental impairment that limits the ability to function independently, appropriately, effectively, and in an age-appropriate manner. For determination of eligibility, the child may have a diagnosis that presumes eligibility or the agency may request an individualized functional assessment (Mental Health, 1991).

Outcome Measurement

Initial evaluations of children provide the baseline against which change can be measured. It is essential to measure progress or skill loss over time to document the effectiveness of treatment (or lack of treatment). In developing specific goals and objectives for each child as part of the care plan, a clinician is predicting future function for that child. Subsequent evaluations determine the success of the predicted target outcomes.

Many programs use outcome data from large groups of children to evaluate the success of their programs. These more global evaluations are important in justifying their efforts to program administrators and to funding sources. Group data also become useful in conducting research. A study may hypothesize that certain intervention strategies are more effective than others. Appropriate group evaluation data can confirm or refute the hypothesis.

Screening

A screening test is one in which only a few significant items are given and measured against standard norms. A screen is intended to be fast (15 to 30 minutes) and is usually given to large numbers of apparently normal children in an effort to identify any children who have suspicious signs of delays. Pediatricians,

for example, regularly screen children at well-child checkups. A child who failed a screen would then be referred for a more in-depth evaluation.

Screening tests for young children are commonly called developmental tests because they assess what behavior, skills, or characteristics are typical for children at different age levels. For example, the Denver Developmental Screening Test (DDST) (Frankenburg & Dodds, 1990) is used by many pediatricians across the country. A neurological screen is another type of test that looks at expected reflexes and reactions based on a child's age. These are often used in hospital nurseries or outpatient clinics. Scoliosis screening is sometimes offered to school-age children to identify early signs of spine deviations. Fitness screening may also be provided for children who are involved in sports programs.

Types of Evaluation

Interdisciplinary or Multidisciplinary Evaluation

This traditional type of evaluation would be conducted by an individual therapist with the child in a quiet, private room with or without a parent present. The interdisciplinary or multidisciplinary evaluation tends to be a structured, formal evaluation. It is usually conducted in a clinic or hospital setting. Separate evaluations of the child are conducted by each discipline who may subsequently share information for treatment planning.

Transdisciplinary Evaluation

A transdisciplinary evaluation is conducted by members of different disciplines who are all present at the same time. It is sometimes called *arena assessment*. The child and family are usually engaged in activities by one team member while the others observe. Many test items can be scored by observation rather than direct interaction. This evaluation format provides the advantage of reducing the number of different people with whom a child and family must interact and also reduces the time needed for evaluation. It also ensures that team members observe the child under similar circumstances. A major advantage to families is a reduced need to answer the same questions repeatedly by different professionals. Family members are frequently included in the subsequent discussion, which promotes good communication and mutual respect. Program planning is done as a team.

Play-Based Evaluation

The child is involved in a play situation, either individually or with a parent, sibling, or team member, while being observed by members of various disciplines. Team members may periodically interact with the child to get optimum results. The setting is usually relaxed and informal (Linder, 1990).

Process of Evaluation

Location

Physical therapy evaluations can occur in many different locations. Traditional medical settings include hospitals, outpatient clinics, and rehabilitation centers. Community-based programs such as schools, infant development programs, and daycare centers are also typical now as a result of laws requiring therapy services in educational settings. The home environment is also an option that is usually reserved for those children who are medically fragile or dependent on technology for survival. Others who might be served in the home are those in rural communities who are unable to find transportation to a center-based program.

Where the evaluation takes place can have an effect on the outcome. Typically, a child is more relaxed in the home environment. This may provide a more realistic picture of his or her abilities. A disadvantage to evaluating a child in the home, however, can be the lack of peers to stimulate interaction and the absence of certain types of testing equipment, such as large balls, vestibular boards, or balance beams. A community-based program such as a school or daycare center is ideal for evaluation because the child can be observed participating in normal routines. Difficulties in mobility, strength, coordination, and range of motion can be seen functionally, and the key individuals in the child's life can be included in goal setting and program planning to create an optimal environment for the child.

Timing

The timing of an initial assessment depends on the first occurrence or suspicion of a problem in the child. Subsequent evaluation is determined on the basis of the child's age, the nature of the condition, how rapidly progress is being made, and requirements of agencies or third-party payers. For example, in infancy where change is rapid, reevaluations every 3 months are typical. An older child in a school setting may only require annual reevaluations. A child who is admitted to a hospital with a head injury may have reevaluations on a weekly basis until discharged from the hospital. In chronic conditions, when a child has received maximum benefit from therapy services, there may only be a need for reevaluation at significant periods, such as during

growth spurts or when entering or leaving school or day programs.

Participants

The team exists to meet child and family needs, so it is critical that the evaluation process focus on family wishes and the understanding of their child's problems. The initial request for an assessment usually comes from the child's physician. Some states and some insurance companies require a physician's referral as an entrance to services. Some states permit an evaluation without a physician order but require the physician to approve treatment recommendations. A few states have no physician referral requirements for physical therapy. It is important to determine what is true for your state.

In addition to physicians, there are frequently other team members participating in the care of a child with a disability. Pediatric programs will frequently involve occupational therapists (OTs) and speech language pathologists (SLPs) as a regular part of the team. The OT's role is to assess fine motor skills such as ability to use the hands and the eyes in a coordinated manner. For children this usually involves play activities. In addition, the OT attends to areas of self-care as a child is learning feeding, dressing, bathing, and grooming skills. The SLP assesses a child's receptive and expressive speech and language skills and often cognitive development. Because of particular expertise in oral-motor structures, the SLP is also very involved with the feeding process, particularly related to swallowing ability. The child's ability to hear is closely related to speech development. Usually there will be a request for an audiological evaluation whenever there is a speech-language delay. Educators also play an important role on the team of any school-aged child. The teacher assesses the child's learning style and is also an important resource for incorporating therapy activities into a child's daily routine at school.

The psychologist is an occasional team member who assesses a child's intellectual, behavioral, and social abilities. Recommendations from the psychologist are frequently important to all team members as they implement treatment programs for children and their families. A social worker can provide valuable information to a team about the families resources and support systems. Other team members can include educational assistants, aides, nutritionists, and bus drivers. Finally, the most important team members are the family members themselves. The family may include parents, siblings, grandparents, aunts, and uncles. Family support members of the team could include a babysitter or neighbors.

Components of the Evaluation

Evaluations typically require a history, observations, and specific tests appropriate for the age of the child.

History

A parent interview is a good way to obtain information about history and current problems related to the child's medical conditions, behaviors, and skills. A medical history from the child's physician is also important with information related to the mother's prenatal care, labor, and delivery. Information about hospitalizations, medications, diagnoses, and current health status all may be important for a complete physical therapy evaluation.

Observations

Observation of the child at play or during an unstructured activity can furnish information about the child's general social, language, and cognitive abilities. Decisions can be made about how to approach the evaluation, based on the information learned. Developmentally and age-appropriate toys, activities, and communication styles need to be selected for the interactive part of the evaluation. Styles of parent-child interaction also give clues regarding strategies that can be used in the evaluation and/or treatment process. For example, a child who is clinging to the parent needs to be approached more gradually than one who easily separates and shows interest in toys.

Specific Tests

Evaluations include a series of tests that, when combined, are interpreted by the PT, who will then make appropriate recommendations. A formal evaluation would typically take longer than a screening test, 1 hour or more. Evaluation of children includes components similar to those of adult testing. Range of motion, flexibility, sensation, muscle strength, muscle tone, neurological status, posture, mobility, and function all should be considered. However, evaluation of children requires adaptation of adult techniques. Games and toys replace traditional methods. For example, a game of "Simon Says," in which the child copies your movements, can be a good way to check active range of motion. When a child is unable to follow complex directions, such as those required in manual muscle tests, estimates are made through observation. Results from observation typically reflect whether the child can move against gravity or take some resistance. For instance, if a child can push up from a side-lying to a sitting position with the arms, one could infer that the upper extremity strength is probably in the good range.

Motor tests. Testing of motor skills could include joint range of motion, manual muscle testing, and functional and developmental tests. Functional abilities include how a child moves (rolling, crawling, walking); transitions (getting to sitting, standing, or into a chair or bed); the quality of movements, (speed, smoothness, coordination); how much assistance is required; and use of assistive devices such as walker or wheelchair. Some examples of motor tests include the Bayley Scales of Infant Development (Bayley, 1993), the Tufts Assessment of Motor Performance (Haley, Inacio, & Mann, 1992), and the Bruininks and Oseretsky Test of Motor Performance (Bruininks, 1978) (Figure 3-52).

Neurological tests. Measurements of central nervous system function are a routine part of the physical therapy evaluation. Examples of tests that might be incorporated in this are The Neurological Evaluation of the Newborn and Infant (Amiel-Tison, 1976) and the Milani-Comparetti Motor Development Screening Test (Tremblath, Kliewer, & Brauce, 1977). These tests identify normal developmental reflexes, as well as righting and equilibrium reactions, which would be expected to develop in the first few years of life.

Sensory tests. A child's response to sensory input provides important information to the PT. One would evaluate response to touch including: light versus firm pressure, pinprick, and responses to different temperatures and textures. Responses to auditory, visual, and vestibular input are also evaluated. Tests of sensory integration assess the child's ability to use the information received through the senses in a functional way as well as the child's ability to understand the information. (Figure 3-53)

Developmental tests. Developmental testing is a critical component of a complete child evaluation that is not necessary in adults who have completed the growth process. During the first 6 years of a child's life there are dramatic changes in abilities. The dependent infant gradually becomes competent in motor skills, which include mobility, posture, and coordination. Developmental assessments, such as the Bayley Scales of Infant Development (Bayley, 1993), are usually comprehensive in testing many domains of development, such as motor, cognitive, speech-language, and social skills. Many are designed to give a score that compares the child's developmental age with chronological age. The purpose is to demonstrate how the child compares with others of the same age. Other evaluation tools are used for purposes of program planning rather than a developmental score such as the Hawaii Developmental Charts (Furuno, O'Reilly, Inatsuka, Hosaka, & Falbey, 1993). Therapists will determine where the child currently functions, make estimates of future functioning, and then use the tool to plot the skills that need to be achieved to reach the goal. These tools frequently are accompanied by suggestions of activities to promote attainment of the new skills, which can be used by parents or therapist.

Understanding what is normal for children at different age levels is critical in interpreting the results of the evaluation. As children grow and mature, we have different expectations. For ex-

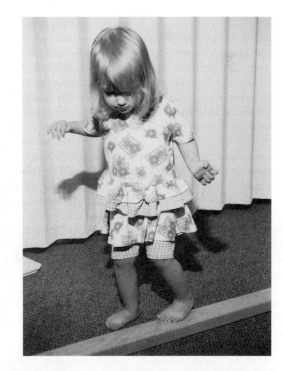

Figure 3-52 Ability to walk on a 2 x 4–inch board is tested in several motor and developmental scales. As skills improve, children can walk with two feet on the board: sideways, forward, and backward.

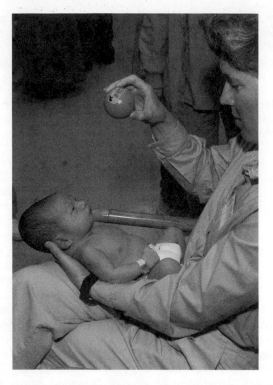

Figure 3-53 The Neonatal Behavioral Assessment Scale includes sensory, reflex, and adaptive behaviors exhibited by newborns.

ample, an infant of 6 weeks would be expected to have hip extension of − 20°, whereas this would be considered abnormal in a child 6 years of age. Likewise, there would be different expectations of muscle strength, reflex activity, and functional skills according to the child's age. Proper interpretation of test results is obviously important when making decisions about what is normal or abnormal and how to intervene with a therapy program.

The PTA's training in measuring and recording joint range of motion, muscle strength, and gross motor development provides an important contribution to the total physical therapy evaluation. The PT will incorporate the information from the PTA in the total written evaluation. The PT's additional responsibility is to interpret the results and to determine an intervention plan.

Evaluation report. The format for a typical assessment uses the following headings: Subjective, Objective, Assessment, and Plan (SOAP). Subjective findings include the history and observation sections. Objective findings include the details of any testing conducted. Assessment includes the PT's interpretation of the results and identification of normal and abnormal findings and functional strengths and weaknesses. The plan includes the recommended plan of care and suggestions for therapy, adaptive equipment, parent and teacher education, and perhaps suggested referrals to other community resources. When therapy is recommended, there must be specific functional outcomes that are projected and a time frame in which they should be achieved. Therapy recommendations should also include the frequency and type of intervention (direct or consult) and an anticipated reevaluation date. The parents (and child when appropriate) should be included in development of the treatment plan. Agreement about each aspect of the plan can help to achieve optimum outcome.

Use of Evaluation Tools

Examples of how different evaluation instruments may be used are illustrated through the case studies that are presented in various chapters throughout the book.

Tyler

Tyler is an infant with congenital torticollis and Erb's palsy. He spent his first week of life in the hospital, followed by outpatient physical therapy for 2 months to help his tight neck and weak arm. Tyler received the Neonatal Behavioral Assessment Scale (Brazelton, 1973) before discharge from the hospital after his birth. This scale helped his parents to see some of Tyler's abilities. He was able to visually track his mother's face and turn to the sound of his father's voice. His parents were pleased to know that there were many positive, age-appropriate things that Tyler could do because otherwise there was a lot of focus on his problems.

At the first outpatient PT visit, the Movement Assessment of Infants (Chandler, Swanson, & Andrews, 1980) was completed to serve as a baseline against which Tyler's progress could be measured. It also helped the therapist to identify specific treatment objectives. For example, Tyler's reflex responses were deficient in his left arm. This led to formation of an objective to have his left arm responding the same way as the right arm in automatic as well as voluntary movements. Active turning of the head was noted to be asymmetrical, and a goal was formulated to have equal range in active rotation. The treatment plan of regular therapy with his parents providing exercises at home addressed these goals. Tyler's objective evaluation and the goals developed from it were used by Medicaid to determine whether or not they would pay for PT services.

After Tyler's discharge from therapy his pediatrician or nurse can follow Tyler's progress every 6 months through the Denver Developmental Screening Test (Frankenburg & Dodds, 1990). This will help to ensure that his skills are maintained as he grows. If not, the pediatrician could refer him to the PT for further intervention.

Rik

Rik is a boy with spinal muscular atrophy who attends public school with other children his age. During infancy and the preschool years, Rik and his family received help from infant development programs and Shriner's Hospital. As part of the comprehensive assessment for his IFSP in the infant development program, the team completed the Hawaii Developmental Charts (Furuno et al., 1993). The charts, which included gross motor, fine motor, self care, social, language and cognitive skills, gave the family a good look at many areas of Rik's development and helped them to choose what were the most important skills to target as part of Rik's therapy. It was important to them that they could also see Rik's strengths on the charts; his cognitive skills were advanced for his age and were good resources to use in planning therapy strategies. For example, his enjoyment of looking at pictures in books helped to entertain him while the therapist was working to improve sitting balance. The school therapists found the Pediatric Evaluation of Disability Inventory (Haley, Faas, Coster, Webster, & Gans, 1992) to be a helpful evaluation tool because it could measure Rik's function in practical terms, even in a wheelchair. It helped them to determine goals

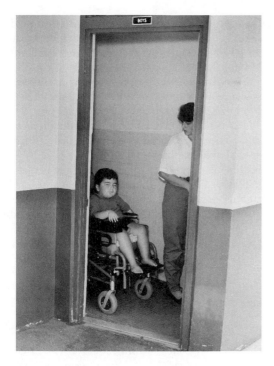

Figure 3-54 Independent wheelchair mobility allows a level of independence in other skills as well as socialization at school.

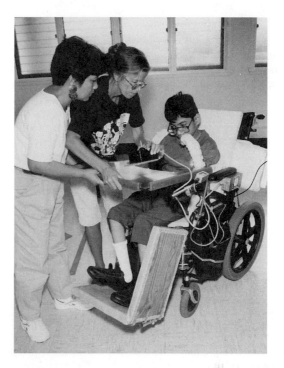

Figure 3-55 Therapists provide appropriate equipment and positioning supports to promote maximum independence.

for Rik, including the ability to use the wheelchair outdoors on uneven surfaces and ramps, so that he could be included in recess activities (Figure 3-54).

Cyril

Cyril is a teenager with cerebral palsy. He has been enrolled in special education classes in his community school since grade three. The school PT initially used the Milani-Comparetti Motor Development Screening Test (Tremblath et al., 1977) to assess his reflexes and their relationship to his gross motor abilities. Although the Milani-Comparetti Test is normed for children from birth to 2 years of age, it was appropriate to use with Cyril at age 8 years because his gross motor abilities were significantly delayed. The Tufts Assessment of Motor Performance (Haley et al., 1992) was used to determine Cyril's functional skills in moving about his environment, how much assistance he required, and how long he would need to accomplish an activity. This information was helpful in working with his team as they planned his IEP (Figure 3-55).

Andrew

Andrew is a 5-year-old boy with cerebral palsy. He is currently in kindergarten but has been followed by a healthcare team since birth, when he was in a hospital neonatal intensive care unit (NICU). The PT in the NICU follow-up clinic used the Gesell and Amatruda Developmental Neurological Exam (Knobloch & Pasamanick, 1974) and the Neurological Evaluation of the Newborn Infant (Amiel-Tison, 1976) as tools to track his development at each 6-month visit. By comparing his skills to the norms on the tests, they were able to let the parents and the pediatri-

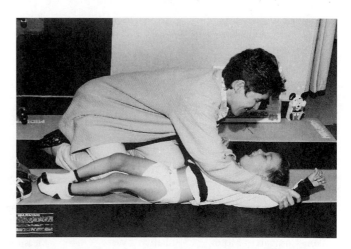

Figure 3-56 Range of motion testing can be fun when the PTA and the child interact visually, vocally, and through synchonous movement.

cian know how he compared with other infants of the same age. Each check-up demonstrated the progress he was making as a result of early intervention. The NICU clinic team was also using the data from all the infants they observed as part of an evaluation study by their hospital to measure the long-term outcome for premature infants who received intensive care. At 5 years of age, when Andrew started kindergarten, his PT used the Peabody Developmental Motor Scale (Folio, Fewell, & Allen, 1983) because it provided both a standard score and an age-equivalent score that could provide a baseline measure for Andrew over his years in the school system (Figure 3-56).

Luke

Luke is a boy with autism who is currently in the sixth grade. During infancy Luke's development was unusual, showing some delays in motor skills, but some advances in cognitive skills. His physician reassured the parents by saying that boys were slow. However, after a move that required finding a new pediatrician, Luke was referred to an infant development program at 2 years of age.

The Bayley Scales of Infant Development (Bayley, 1993) were used as part of a comprehensive evaluation of his motor, mental, and behavioral abilities. The developmental score helped the parents to understand Luke's strengths as well as areas where he needed more help.

When Luke started kindergarten at age 5 years, the PT used the Bruininks & Oseretsky Scale (Bruininks, 1978) to document his gross and fine motor functions. With this baseline the thera-pist could make recommendations for the therapy needed to enhance Luke's education in his IEP. In the sixth grade another assessment was conducted. This time the PT used the Purdue Perceptual Motor Survey (Roach & Kephart, 1966) to determine whether there were more subtle problems that needed attention, such as balance, body image, and perceptual motor skills. The Test of Motor Impairment (Stott, Moyes, Henderson, 1972) was also included to gain information about coordination and manual dexterity. The information gained helped Luke's teacher plan how to teach Luke computer skills.

A variety of evaluation tools are part of the pediatric PT's practice because of the many different ages, diagnoses, and functions that must be assessed. Table 3-5 lists commonly used evaluation tools. The PTA should have a basic understanding of these tools and their use to fully participate as part of the intervention team.

TABLE 3-5 Commonly Used Evaluation Tools

Evaluation tool	Age range	Key features	Reference
Neonatal Behavioral Assessment Scale	3 days to 4 weeks	Assesses interactive behavior, infant competence, and neurological status. An effective predictor of future neurological problems. A good tool for teaching parents about infant behaviors.	Brazelton, T. B. (1973). *Clinics in developmental medicine* (No. 50). Philadelphia: J.B. Lippincott.
Neurological Evaluation of the Newborn and Infant	Birth to 12 months	Measures reflexes and muscle tone and provides range of motion expectations.	Amiel-Tison, C., & Grenier, A. (1976). *Current problems in pediatrics* (Vol. III, No. 1). Chicago: Year Book Medical.
Movement Assessment of Infants	Birth to 12 months	Assesses muscle tone, reflexes, automatic reactions, and purposeful movement.	Chandler, L. S., Swanson, M. W., & Andrews, M. S. (1980). *Movement assessment of infants*. Rolling Bay, WI: Infant Movement Research.
Alberta Infant Motor Scale	Birth to age of walking	An observational tool that identifies the components of motor development. Differentiates what is atypical development and small increments that may be attributed to maturation or intervention.	Piper, M. C., Darrah, J., Pinnell, L., Maguire, T., & Byrne, P. (1993). *Motor assessment of the developing infant*. Philadelphia: W.B. Saunders.
Milani-Comparetti Motor Development Screening Test	Birth to 2 years	Measures functional movement and related reflex and automatic responses. A profile demonstrates age-appropriate responses.	Tremblath, J., Kliewer, D., & Brauce, W. (1977). Omaha: Nebraska Medical Center.
Hawaii Developmental Charts (formerly Hawaii Early Learning Profile)	Birth to 3 years	Used to graphically demonstrate approximate age ranges in motor, cognitive, language, self-help and social skills. Intended for use in planning intervention programs, documenting progress, and monitoring achievement of individual objectives.	Furuno, S., O'Reilly, K., Inatsuka, T., Hosaka, C., & Falbey, B. Z. (1993). *Hawaii developmental charts*. Tucson, AZ: Therapy Skill Builders.

TABLE 3-5	Commonly Used Evaluation Tools—cont'd		
Evaluation tool	**Age range**	**Key features**	**Reference**
Revised Gesell and Amatruda Developmental Neurological Exam	1 month to 5 years	Gives a developmental quotient in four areas: motor, adaptive, language, personal-social.	Knobloch, H., & Pasamanick, B. (1974). *Developmental diagnosis* (3rd ed.). Philadelphia: J.B. Lippincott.
Bayley Scales of Infant Development II	Birth to 42 months	Includes a mental scale, motor scale, and behavioral record. Scored as a developmental index. Includes data on special populations (e.g. prematurity, Down syndrome, HIV, developmental delays).	Bayley, N. (1993). *Bayley scales of infant development.* San Antonio, TX: Harcourt Brace.
Denver Developmental Screening Test	2 weeks to 6 years	Measures four domains: personal-social, fine motor adaptive, language, and gross motor. Screens children for delays and determines need for further evaluation.	Frankenburg, W. K., & Dodds, J. (1990). *Denver developmental screening test.* Denver, CO: Archer Petal.
Peabody Developmental Motor Scales	Birth to 83 months	Includes gross and fine motor scales. Gives standard scores and age-equivalent scores. Identifies emerging skills. Child does not need to understand verbal language to be scored on test.	Folio, M., & Fewell, R. (1983). *Peabody developmental motor scales.* Allen, TX: DLM Teaching Resources.
The Pediatric Evaluation of Disability Inventory	6 months to 7.5 years	Assesses functional skills; designed for rehabilitation use. Includes self care, mobility, and social skills. Scores based on function, amount of assistance required, and need for equipment or modification.	Haley, S. M., Faas, R. M., Coster, W. J., Webster, H., & Gans, B. M. (1989). Boston: New England Medical Center.
Miller Assessment for Preschoolers	2 years, 9 months to 5 years, 8 months	Identifies children with mild to moderate delays. Combines sensory-motor and cognitive domains. Uses developmental approach. No age-equivalent scores.	Miller, L. J. (1982). *The foundation of knowledge in development.* San Antonio, TX: The Psychological Corporation.
Tufts Assessment of Motor Performance-Pediatric Clinical Version	3 years and above	Measures functional and motor performance skills to monitor child's response to treatment and to determine if treatment goals were met. Measurements include proficiency of skill and time to complete skill.	Haley, S. M., Inacio, C. A., & Mann, N. R. (1989). *Tufts assessment of motor performance–Pediatric clinical version.* Boston: Tufts New England Medical Center.
Bruininks-Oseretsky Test of Motor Performance	4.5 to 14.5 years	Assesses gross and fine motor function in order to make educational and therapeutic placement decisions. Scores given as age equivalents.	Bruininks, R. H. (1978). *Bruininks-Oseretsky test of motor performance.* Circle Pines, MN: American Guidance Service.
Purdue Perceptual Motor Survey	6 to 10 years	Identifies children lacking perceptual motor abilities needed to acquire academic skills. Includes balance and postural flexibility, body image and differentiation, perceptual-motor match, ocular control, and visual achievement forms.	Roach, E. G., & Kephart, N. C. (1966). *The Purdue perceptual motor survey.* Columbus, OH: Merrill.
Test of Motor Impairment	5 to 13 years	Detects motor dysfunction problems indicative of possible neurological dysfunction. Divided into five areas: balance, upper limb coordination, whole body coordination, manual dexterity, and simultaneous movement.	Stott, D. H., Moyes, F. A., & Henderson, F. A. (1972). *Test of motor impairment.* Guelph, Ontario: Brook Educational.

● **APPLICATIONS**   The Role of Play in Therapy for Children

A 5-year-old child pumps his legs vigorously to get the swing to go higher. Wind blows his hair back and forth as the swing reaches the top of the arc. The child grins as he watches his playmates running on the playground far below.

A 3-year-old girl splashes her mother with water from the small plastic wading pool. She shrieks as her mother splashes her back. When her mother's attention wanders, the child splashes her again.

Three 8-year-old boys race across the playground chasing a ball. The first one to reach it throws himself down and clutches the ball to his chest. The others pile on top of him, wrestling it away. The boy who ends up with the ball kicks it and all three race across the grassy area, following it again.

Two 6-year-old girls plant leaves stem down in the loose dirt. One girl places rocks next to the leaves, and the other draws roads in the dirt between them. Between silent periods of constructive activity, they relate ideas about the world they are creating.

The Importance of Play

All of us would recognize the preceding scenes as children playing, but we may have difficulty in defining exactly what we mean by play. There is magic when children enter the world of play (Figure 3-57). Have you seen the intense concentration on a child's face when absorbed in play? Have you connected with the sparkle in a child's eye when he or she includes you in play? When we enter the realm of play with a child, we can enter the magic too. This section presents some definitions of play but focuses on the developmental aspects of play, the use of toys and games in therapy, and the cultivating of our flexible and adaptive playful personalities.

Researchers and academics have suggested many different and sometimes conflicting definitions of play (Spodek & Saracho, 1988). Some definitions juxtapose play and work. Others define play by the reasons it is engaged in; for example, play for elaboration on an experience, for exploration, for social development, or for development of coordination skills. Smith and Vollstedt (1985) found that most observers characterized play as

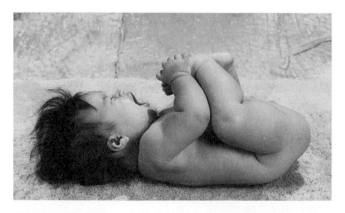

Figure 3-57   This 5-month-old infant enjoys sensorimotor exploration. The body is one of the first playthings.

enjoyable, flexible, and "pretend." Bronfenbrenner (1979) defines three themes to play; it is performed for its own sake, it is undertaken by choice, and it is enjoyable.

Donaldson (1993) characterizes play on a more fundamental level. He discusses "original play" as separate from "cultural play," which is taught by adults to "make" children fit better into their cultures.

Original play is not a mere vacation from life; it is life. Both you and a child are always growing and changing. Accepting this and playing without answers requires a great deal of openness. Original play is based not on fear, but on a trust relationship with life. As a playmate you join the child in such a way that both of you feel loved, respected and eager to explore. The skills required of you in play—curiosity, trust, resilience, awareness- are those of a healthy child (p. 31).

Donaldson points out that the quality of true play towers in importance beside the specific activities and "things" of play. This quality of true play is fundamental to connecting with a child in a therapy session. It is a quality that is essential in working/playing with children that we must all cultivate in ourselves.

Because we have specific agendas when we play with children, we must also pay attention to the activities of play. For the purposes of this chapter, play activities are defined as a child-directed interaction with and manipulation of objects, individuals, environment, and thoughts for enjoyment and stimulation. Play activities must have some meaning for the child and therefore can be seen in the context of previous experiences and learning. The types of play activities that interest a child are dependent on the developmental experiences of that child and change in a predictable pattern as the child gains experience.

To therapists who work with children, play activities are a medium to achieve therapeutic goals. Toys and play can be therapeutic tools, motivating forces, and behavioral rewards. Understanding play in the context of child development and cultivating our own playfulness and adaptability can help make therapy more fun for us and the children, as well as more effective and productive.

Play as Developmental Learning

Piaget. Jean Piaget, the Swiss researcher who has had such a profound effect on the field of child development, identified several cognitive stages that children pass through from infancy to adulthood. He was the first theorist to look at children's development as a progression of developmental cognitive skills that build on each other to culminate in the highest form of thinking. His theories, although useful in characterizing what is observed in children's behavior, have been substantially criticized for their rigidity.

More recent research has shown that children's logical processes do not fit as neatly into the stages of development that Piaget would have liked but that skills can bridge different stages and can occur at different ages than Piaget suggested. His theory, however, continues to be useful in a broad sense to see children's learning on a continuum and to recognize that children of different ages, or levels of experience or ability, have different developmental tasks, skills, and strategies for play.

Piaget identified four developmental stages that children pass through as they develop. The *sensorimotor stage* is characterized by exploring through the senses. Children younger than 2 years old generally experience their environment through their eyes, ears, touch, smell, and taste. They grasp and manipulate objects, shake them, and feel them with their mouth, feet, and body. The *preoperational stage* is characterized by interpreting their environment literally and from an egocentric point of view. Young children are not able to take alternate perspectives from their own and will interpret, for example, Mommy's irritability as meanness or anger rather than fatigue from a long day at work. The development and use of language is an important component of the preoperational stage. When children reach 6 or 7 years old, they develop the ability to use logic. The *concrete operational stage* is characterized by the development of logical skills that address the here and now. A child can tell you that a tall, skinny glass has the same amount of water as a fat glass, even though the water heights are not the same. When a child can abstract logical skills to create hypotheses, he or she has reached the *formal operational stage*. An adolescent at this stage is able to manage complex mathematical problems. Although Piaget's developmental stages have been shown to be more flexible than he envisioned, they are useful for understanding the cognitive development of children, including their use of play materials.

Vygotsky. Vygotsky, a Soviet psychologist who lived during the early part of the 1900s, developed theories of child development and learning that are gaining popularity in Europe and the United States. His theory of development encompasses socialization, enculturation, and learning. Children and other less competent members of society are assisted by adults and other more competent members of society to move from their current level of development to a more complex level (Figure 3-58). Vygotsky's concept of the "zone of proximal development" is that area where a child, with assistance, can move beyond his or her actual level of development to a higher level of potential development. For example, a child who is learning to talk may regularly use only one or two words clearly. A parent will converse with the child, allowing approximations of words and modeling a more complex vocabulary. In this way the child is assisted to move from the current level of development to a more advanced level. The "zone of proximal development" changes as the child gains more skills. A key point in Vygotsky's theory is that a child's development is not static; there is always a "zone of proximal development" where the child's skills have potential to grow and be refined.

Vygotsky believed that play was practice to separate thought from the surrounding world and to rely on ideas to guide behavior. Infants cannot separate the thought of an infant from an actual infant, whereas older children can use their imagination to create an infant from a folded blanket. An imaginary infant therefore can be thought of separately from an actual infant. In this way play helps children learn to abstract their thoughts. Vygotsky believed that this abstraction is the foundation for adult thought. Children also develop rules during play and learn to subvert their own desires to the rules they have constructed (Figure 3-59). For example, a child will not go into the kitchen because a monster is in there, even if a snack is waiting on the kitchen table. In this way children learn to develop self-restraint and to follow social rules.

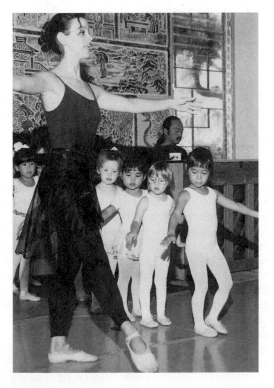

Figure 3-58 Alice, a 4-year-old girl with Down syndrome, participates in an organized community dance class.

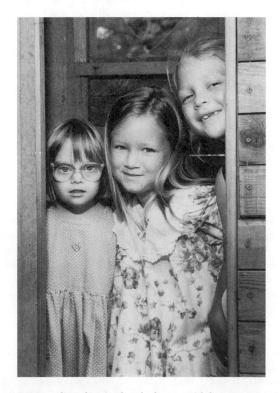

Figure 3-59 Alice plays in the playhouse with her sister Sarah and a friend. Peer relationships and the development of imaginative play are important for both boys and girls.

Children's Development and Play

Infants. Children younger than 1 year old change almost visibly day to day in their physical capabilities, cognitive development, and social skills. Piaget characterizes this stage of development as the "early sensorimotor stage." Infants are using their own senses to explore their environment. Others describe this stage as "exploratory play" (Musselwhite, 1985). Children in the exploratory stage of play grasp, squeeze, throw, and mouth toys. They also watch events around them.

Infants initially are dominated by their own reflexes and reflexive responses to external stimuli. However, they can interact with the world and choose to respond to some things more than others. When in an awake, alert state, newborns respond more to a face presented to them than to other configurations of shapes. They look longer at objects with contrasting colors, such as black and white, and they look at the edges of shapes. They enjoy social stimulation with a face presented 8 to 12 inches away. They like to watch smiling, open mouths and eyes and will track or visually follow a moving face or object. Infants start to smile socially at 2 to 3 months of age.

By 3 months of age, infants are swiping at toys and learning to grasp. Toys should be big enough not to go down their throat when mouthed, should be easily cleaned, and should be a bold color to stimulate visual regard. Toys that younger infants enjoy are things they can easily grasp and see, such as a red ring, a busy box, a rattle that makes noise when they move it, and soft dolls or stuffed animals that may have a rattle inside for auditory stimulation. Mobiles and hanging toys are fun to swipe at and make move, but they should be fastened securely so they will not fall, and any string should be short and securely fastened for safety.

When they are 4 to 5 months old, children learn to roll and can more easily grasp toys. Social stimulation is very important, and they love to look at faces. Beware of your hair or jewelry when you are around children of this age. The mouthing of toys, fingers, and toes is a way for children to explore their bodies and their environment. Toys should be bright colors, make noise or change colors, be easy to grasp, and be safe to put in their mouth. Mobiles, hanging toys, and infant gyms are enjoyed at this age.

At 6 to 8 months old infants are learning to sit up and to reach for toys that are near. They are also learning to release toys, and they enjoy throwing toys and having others retrieve them. Toys that make noise and move when touched are enjoyed.

By 9 to 10 months an infant is creeping on hands and knees, exploring the environment, and pulling up to stand at the furniture. Cabinets should be locked, and breakable items should be removed from low shelves and tables. At this age infants enjoy playing with paper and will eat it with glee. They also enjoy playing with balls that are weighted so they will not roll too far and ride-on or sturdy push toys that the child can hold onto for support when walking. Stacking and nesting toys are enjoyed at this age when they are learning how to manipulate smaller objects more precisely. They enjoy banging toys together and taking things out of containers. Food is great fun and can be smeared all over with some going in the mouth.

By 1 year of age a child will be cruising along the furniture or perhaps walking independently. Large climbing toys such as cube chairs, plastic slides, and cardboard boxes are fun to climb on, in, under, and through. At this age children are learning to pick up smaller objects and should be supervised to prevent choking. They enjoy putting things into containers.

In summary, during this early part of the sensorimotor period, infants change rapidly. Initially they are dependent on caregivers and are passive recipients of external stimuli, but they gradually gain skills and experience to start manipulating their environment and actively explore through their senses. Therapists need to take cues for interaction from the infants and parents and have available a variety of toys that are boldly colored and visually and auditorily interesting. The toys should be easily grasped by little hands and should be safe for infants to put in their mouths. Infants are intrinsically motivated to explore and interact with their environment, and therapists need only direct and shape the behavior with appropriate activities and toys.

Toddlers. During the second year of life, the child refines the mobility skills of walking and climbing and can carry a large toy while walking. Stairs are tackled with help, and a child may start to climb on the furniture. Smaller toys are interesting and can be stacked. Crayons can be grasped and marks made on paper. The development of language may be a priority for a child during this period. This year is the second half of what Piaget called the "sensory-motor period." Young children are still exploring their environment through their senses.

For the toddler, toys are fairly concrete. The 2-year-old child is in Piaget's second stage of preoperations. Piaget defines this stage as being ruled by perception rather than logic. Therefore a child make inferences based on what is seen, rather than what makes logical sense. A child usually plays independently—manipulating blocks, books, stacking toys, and other objects—but plays alone. Older toddlers may play next to peers, demonstrating parallel play.

Older toddlers are very interested in exploring and increasing their own independence, as long as a safe adult is there to return to when they need reassurance. They are generally willing to participate in activities that are set up for them, especially if participation is at their own initiation. Children of this age love to direct others to follow them and love to follow others. They love to help sweep and do other household tasks but may need assistance. Two-year-old children are becoming more assertive and say "no" frequently. Therefore the selection of activities/toys is important in an individual therapy session, as well as being creative in how to use the activities/toys presented. Depending on the therapy goal, the balance beam could be used in a variety of ways during a therapy session. For instance, it may be a piece of wood to practice walking across, a place to set up small toys in a row, something to jump over, something to lift up (with help), a ramp to walk up or roll a ball down, a bridge to go under, or a support for a sheet tent.

Toddlers love obstacle courses and enjoy ball play with adults. They enjoy athletic pursuits such as toddler tennis, golf, and baseball with plastic equipment. Stairs, tunnels, and slides are challenging and fun for a toddler.

Preschoolers. Preschoolers from 3 to 5 years old are developing imaginative skills, but they need guidance. They can use their imagination with help to create simple scenes, such as pirate ships, shark infested waters, or cloud ships moving across the sky. The images should be specific and defined because some preschoolers may be confused between this imaginative reality and the concrete reality of the world. This confusion might lead to nightmares of pirates under the bed.

Preschoolers move between associative play, where they may approach a peer with a toy and have brief physical contact, to cooperative play where they are interacting with a peer during play. A preschooler may, for example, pull a peer in a wagon or help stack blocks in the same tower. Later, preschoolers may be able to play symbolically without direct guidance. These imaginative games may include dress up or house.

School-aged children. Early school-aged children from 6 to 9 years old are fully involved in symbolic play. Imaginative games are the rule with guns, soldiers, and action figures for boys, dolls and house for girls, and store and school for mixed groups. Gender differences are apparent in the choices of toys and activities from age 2 years, with boys enjoying more physically aggressive play than girls (Figure 3-60). Although gender roles are culturally influenced, research shows that there are also biological differences between boys and girls related to prenatal exposure to different hormones that influence patterns and preferences of play (Berenbaum & Hines, 1992; Meyer-Bahlburg, Feldman, Cohen, & Ehrhardt, 1988). Toy guns, adventure fantasy play, and video games (which frequently have aggressive content) are typical of boys' play. Girls tend to choose dolls, household objects, and fantasy games with familiar roles (Goldstein, 1994). Children at this age love stories, books, and board games. They are also gaining some athletic skills and frequently play after-school sports, as well as follow organized sports with older family members (Figure 3-61).

The older school-aged child (10 to 12 years) is generally willing to engage in imaginative play, but not so anyone else can see them! Toys and activities that are likely to engage these children include video games, model building, and computer games. They may be more interested in educational types of games or activities. More sophisticated board games such as Monopoly or Risk may hold their attention. Girls and boys will be interested in participating with peer support in a group exercise class or in a community program such as a swimming or aerobics class.

Children at these ages can follow directions and comply with a therapeutic program, but they can get easily bored with repetition and routine. Even if they are motivated to reach their therapeutic goals, they will resist therapy if it is not fun. It is important that motivational strategies be tailored to the child's interests. For example, stationary bicycle riding can be done in front of a TV while watching a tape of the latest football game. A group exercise program can be helpful to motivate both girls and boys. Other motivational strategies for older school-aged children include the use of interesting equipment such as a kinetic exercise machine, therapy balls, or a pool. Listening to music or creating music through singing or playing instruments can be very motivating for children of any age. Competition can also be useful to motivate an older child. The competition can be against the self or against a parent, peers, or the therapy provider. Charts can be effective motivational tools, with progress in therapy clearly documented by using stickers or colored graphs. Periodic change in routine can keep a child interested. Integration and support in community exercise and activity programs can benefit a child with a chronic disability socially and emotionally and help the child progress toward specific therapeutic goals (Figure 3-62).

Adolescents. The adolescent receiving therapy can provide an interesting challenge to a therapist. The teenager may be consumed by the need to increase autonomy and independent thought and influenced by an increasing social awareness. This, coupled with the hormonal changes of physical maturation, is sometimes overwhelming. Piaget's formal operational stage is reached by many children during this time, although researchers have found that not everyone attains the ability to think abstractly or formulate and test hypotheses while an adolescent. These skills may develop as late as college age in some individuals—or not at all.

Play takes on a greater social context for the adolescent. Children of this age are exploring their own values separate from their family and developing their own sense of who they are. Adolescents may be interested in athletics, academics, job, or

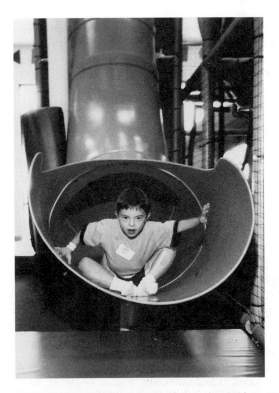

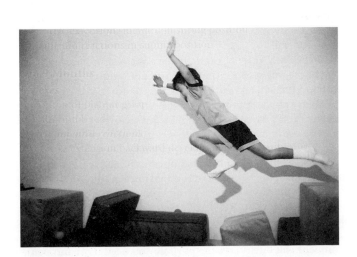

Figure 3-60 This padded play area allows Ryan, a 6-year-old boy with Down syndrome, to push the limits of his gross motor skills.

Figure 3-61 Ryan loves this indoor play area for children. He can run, jump, slide, tumble, and stay safe.

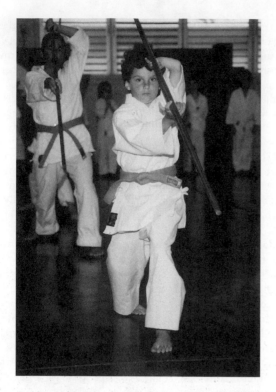

Figure 3-62   Robert, an 8-year-old boy with radial aplasia syndrome, enjoys karate after school. He also plays soccer and baseball.

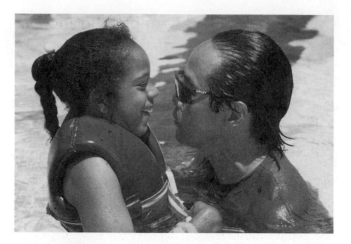

Figure 3-63   Cheryl, a 12-year-old girl with cerebral palsy, shares a moment with her school principal after her swimming event at the Special Olympics.

recreation, with friends being the common thread that weaves their interests together. Play may include athletic practices or games, computer or video games, skill-building activities, or social activities.

Motivational strategies are important when working with an adolescent. Discovering a child's priorities is necessary to create a treatment plan that is relevant for the child. Sometimes this is very difficult. For example, a 16-year-old boy with an above-the-knee amputation secondary to osteosarcoma refused to attend any therapy sessions. Life as an amputee was not in his self-concept, and he refused to accept anything related to it, especially therapy. This boy ultimately chose not to participate in therapy during his teen years. On the other hand, athletes are usually very motivated to return to their sport after an injury and will generally be disciplined in their home programs. Most adolescents fall between these two extremes.

Strategies for Incorporating Play in Treatment Sessions

Plan well.   Before the child arrives, or before you arrive at the child's classroom or home, you should plan how you will use the environment and toys to work toward developmental goals for the child. For a very young child, infant toys should be set out, ready at hand. You should know how you will use the toys to help the child learn to roll, prop on forearms, or shift the center of gravity in sitting to reach.

An older child who is learning mobility skills needs a different environment and different toys than an infant. Because the older child is actively exploring the environment, different "stations" could be set up, close enough so the child could cruise be-

tween them. Toys that the child would enjoy manipulating could be placed on tables—for example, a farm with animals, a gas station with attendants, toys with doors that open, chutes to put objects down, and swings to swing objects on. Different-height tables could be used to facilitate play in standing and kneeling and transitions between them. Cube chairs make an excellent tool for setting up different "stations."

A preschooler who is learning more advanced mobility skills may enjoy an obstacle course. Mat tables, portable therapy mats, balance beams, flexible spring tunnels, sheets, plastic footprints, and step stools can be used to create varied obstacle courses. Skills such as climbing, jumping, creeping, and balancing can be addressed in this type of environment. Toys such as cars, farm sets, and school buses with figures inside can complement an obstacle course and can be used in a variety of ways.

An older child who is learning more precise control of movement may enjoy throwing bean bags at a target, strengthening or balance activities with a therapy ball, or hopscotch on a masking tape hopscotch square. The child may have ideas about what he or she wants to learn to do, such as swing a bat, dive into a pool, or climb onto a horse (Figure 3-63). Equipment that is available can be used to approximate the desired activity to develop the skill.

Be flexible.   It is important to have at least one back-up plan for the therapy session. The child may not want to do the activity you initially planned. The skill may be too hard, the equipment may not be appropriate for the activity, or the child may be more or less active than during the last treatment session. The creative use of equipment and toys is an important skill for anyone working and/or playing with children.

Use the environment.   An adjunct to the above is to learn to use the ambient environment as a tool for therapy. When seeing a child in the home, you may find it impossible to carry a mat, cube chairs, and large toys with you. Kitchen chairs, sofa cushions, walls, coffee tables, and the child's own toys often work just as well. If the child does not have toys, items found in the environment will often serve the purpose you need. Pots and pans, wooden spoons, furniture, clothing or sheets, sticks and rocks found outside, and siblings, pets, and parents work as wonderful playthings. A benefit to using items around the house is that the family will be able to recreate the environments after you leave and can support the therapy sessions when you are not there.

Let the child take the lead. Allowing the child to take the lead is important for children who are learning about independent skills. If you create a therapy environment that can be flexible in addressing therapy goals, you can let the child decide how the toys and equipment should be used. Your role, then, is to follow the child's lead until joint activity routines are developed, then begin to teach the child to follow your lead. You need to shape the child's activity so that goals you believe are important are addressed. For example, for a 2-year-old girl, the goal of therapy is weight bearing through her right upper extremity to promote proximal stability in her shoulder girdle. You have set up a therapy ball in front of the mirror and plan to have the child prone on the ball, pushing up with both arms to see her reflection in the mirror. But the child is afraid of being on top of the ball. You follow her lead by allowing her to sit and to roll the ball back and forth to a parent. You help the child to use both arms to push the ball and, eventually, to prop on her right arm and kick the ball across the room. Soon she is propped backward on both arms while kicking the ball with both feet, laughing gleefully.

Incorporate family members into therapy. Some of the best motivators for young children include siblings, parents, and grandparents. The young child may feel more comfortable interacting with people who are familiar. Family members can frequently get a child to do something that an unfamiliar person cannot. Family members also know what kinds of play the child enjoys and can incorporate familiar games into therapy sessions. Observing family play and interacting to shape play toward therapeutic goals can be a very productive activity for both family members and therapy providers. Therapy providers can learn key motivators for the child, and family members can observe and practice activities that can assist the child toward meeting therapy goals.

Use music. Music is a wonderful therapy tool that can cut across age ranges. Small children enjoy singing with each other and with adults. Familiar tunes can teach rhythm, facilitate movement, and develop social skills for young children. Music can also be an ice breaker and can encourage a young child to enjoy activity with therapy personnel. Older children may enjoy songs from popular movies. These can be incorporated into activity/exercise routines. School-aged children may enjoy helping to develop routines to music, playing instruments, doing child aerobics, or having music as a background to therapy activities. Adolescents and preadolescents enjoy popular music, such as rap and rock and roll. Music can be a significant motivator for them, both as a means for reaching therapy goals and as a reward for successfully reaching goals. Music can be played in the background to set the atmosphere of the therapy session, used as a medium for therapy routines or exercises, played on a tape recorder activated by a switch to encourage specific movements, or played with musical instruments that need certain fine and gross motor skills to play. An adolescent who likes music may be motivated by rewards of listening to favorite tapes, purchasing CDs or tapes, or going to a concert with friends or family.

Integrate the goals of other disciplines. Play is an excellent way to integrate the goals of other disciplines into the physical therapy session. Goals such as improving communication skills,

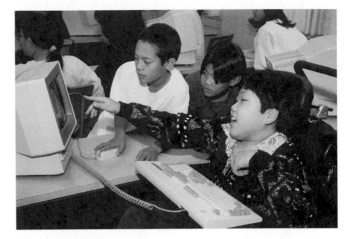

Figure 3-64 Joshua, a 13-year-old boy with spina bifida, finds that computers help make peer relationships possible for him.

developing fine motor skills, or developing social and cognitive skills can be integrated with working on gross motor skills. For example, as a child is practicing balance skills in half-kneeling, fine motor skills will be enhanced by putting small toys in and out of a container on the low table, communication skills will be addressed by using gestures, signs, and oral language with the child during the activity, and social skills will be improved by interacting with the therapy provider and other children in the therapy group.

Addressing a Child's Abilities and Interests

It is important to be aware of a child's chronological age, as well as abilities and interests. In a child with a disability the chronological age frequently does not match abilities and interests. Developmental age can be calculated based on developmental tests of cognitive, gross motor, fine motor, self-help, or language ability. The child's performance is compared with that of children without disabilities to assign a developmental age. The difference between the calculated developmental age and the chronological age is frequently used as a measure of developmental delay to justify therapeutic intervention.

Although tests are useful to justify therapeutic intervention to third-party payers, it is important to caution anyone against interacting with a child based on a developmental age calculated in this manner. Each child is an individual and should be seen as a multifaceted person with individual strengths and needs (Figure 3-64). Personality, emotional strengths, nonverbal communication, interests, and other qualities that make a person unique are not measured well with standardized tests. Toys and activities used in a therapy session should be chronologically age appropriate to respect the dignity of the child and family, and should also reflect the interests and capabilities of the child.

For example, an 18-year-old young man who is nonverbal and has severe mental retardation and multiple physical handicaps will hardly respond to a rousing game of Monopoly or a conversation about his girlfriend. It is just as inappropriate to give this young man a rattle to grasp. He would be able to grasp a microphone, however, and may enjoy listening to popular music during the therapy session. The microphone could be linked by a switch to a tape recorder that will play the music when he lifts his hand to his face. Conversation should be in an adult pitch and cadence and can concern events occurring in the immediate environment.

Adaptive Toys and Play

If therapists, family members, and teachers are aware of the developmental tasks of a child, they can modify the home, classroom, or therapy environment to allow the child access to appropriate toys and experiences. Examples of specific adaptations

TABLE 3-6 Adaptations: Suggestions for Play

Children who may need adaptations	Adaptations (not age specific)
Children with sensory impairments	
Auditory	Colorful toys
	Large facial expressions (smiles)
	Tactile toys such as terrycloth, velour
	Water play
	Gestures and sign
	Toys with light, vibrating switches
	Use FM amplifier, hearing aids
	Speakers for extra volume on computers
	Position child so he or she can see activity
Visual	Toys with sound (rattles)
	Singing
	Music boxes
	Enlarged pictures/print
	Tactile toys such as terrycloth, velour
	Vibrating switches
	Computer programs with large print
	Computer voice output
	Scanner to read to data to computer
	Braille
Children with motor impairments	Hang toys near child's hand/feet (use overhead bar, chair)
	Wrist or ankle fasteners for rattles
	Use squeaky toys from pet store that are easier to squeak (NOTE: these toys may not be safe to mouth)
	Adapt toys so they can be grasped (sew on fabric flap or use bottle with divided trunk that can be grasped by smaller hands)
	Use large crayons, puzzles with large pieces
	Position child so hands or feet can be used optimally (head and trunk supported in midline)
	Positioning devices (corner seat, infant seat, adapted stroller, custom molded seat, stander, mobile stander)
	Adapt toys to give auditory feedback if touched or swiped, even if they are not grasped
	Adapt toys for switch use
	Clamp or glue toys so they will not move away (to lap tray, table, chair, high chair, stroller, floor)
	Build up seat, back, handlebars on ride-on toys/tricycle
	Switch access for computers
	Weight base of toys
	Electric toys or equipment adapted for switch operation (electric car, electric train, battery-operated toys, bubble generator, toy house with lights, tape recorder, fan, blender)
	Use equipment to facilitate movement that child has difficulty with (wedge for rolling, scooter board or floor cart for moving on floor, special seat for swing)
	Use equipment to facilitate access to playground equipment (positioning device for sandbox, seat for swing, seat or cart for playhouse, vest for slide)
Children with cognitive impairments	Simplify rules for games
	Use peer buddy for support
	Give simple instructions clearly
	Create role that child could perform to participate in activity

include attaching a playhouse to a child's lap tray with a C-clamp, adapting a mechanical dog toy to be activated with a switch, and using a puzzle with large pieces. Squeaky rubber toys from a pet store can be easier to squeeze than squeaky toys made for infants. (Be sure to monitor the child continuously because a toy from the pet store may not be safe to mouth.) The bases of dolls or action figures can be weighted so they stand up more easily. Rules of board games can be adapted to make them simpler. Switches can facilitate access to tape recorders, lights, or toy trains for older children. Other environmental adaptations to allow children to play could include hanging toys from an overhead bar, laying a child on a wedge so rolling can be achieved more easily, or using a mobile stander so a child can keep up with peers in the classroom or playground.

Creative adaptations for play evolve from observing a child and assessing the child's needs. What are other children the same age doing? What toys are peers playing with? Adaptations can range from the placement of toys (hanging, gluing to a surface,

moving it closer) to building or buying electronic switches. Do not limit yourself to what you see—be creative! Use family members and other team members to help generate ideas. See Table 3-6 for further suggestions for adapting toys for children with different needs.

Motivational Strategies

Although play is a strong motivational strategy to get children to participate in therapy, sometimes other strategies need to be used, especially for older children. It is important to assess each child for individual strengths, interests, and goals, and to develop an individualized plan for implementing therapy. The child, family members, teachers, medical personnel, and friends can all help with designing and implementing a plan for therapy. Although each child is an individual, there are common strategies grouped to different ages that can help to motivate children. Many of these have been referred to in the preceding paragraphs. See Table 3-7

TABLE 3-7	Appropriate Toys and Motivational Strategies for Working With Children
Age range	**Appropriate toys**	**Motivational strategies**
Young infants (newborn to 6 months)	Rattles Plastic keys Stuffed animals Mobiles Busy boxes Bubbles Pinwheels Black/white or color pictures	Smiling Cooing Tickling Playing pat-a-cake This little piggy went to market Holding toys for infant to reach for; If infant is tired, talk to caregiver and/or demonstrate using doll rather than stressing infant
Older infants (6-12 months)	Music boxes Busy boxes Stackable or nesting toys, blocks Push toys Ride-on toys Infant books (cloth/cardboard) Puzzles with large pieces Stuffed animals Teethers Mirror	Work through caregiver (teach caregiver how to do activity with child) Use interesting toys Follow child's lead until relationship is established; then shape child's behavior toward desired therapy goals
Toddlers (1-3 years)	Balls Dolls Toy animals Ride-on toys/tricycle Toddler slide Plastic baseball/golf/basketball Farm set Playhouse with furniture Pretend food Grocery cart Push or pull toys Shape-sorter toys Simple puzzles Books/crayons Toy telephone Computer Age-appropriate software	Present interesting toys Set up interesting environments Include family members in therapy Allow child to explore beyond boundaries of therapy room Use your body as therapy tool to climb on, under, across Read books Use familiar routines

Continued

Appropriate Toys and Motivational Strategies for Working With Children—cont'd

TABLE 3-7

Age range	Appropriate toys	Motivational strategies
Preschoolers (3-5 years)	Crayons Books Puzzles Play-dough Music tapes/tape recorders Building toys such as blocks Dress-up clothes Legos Groups of related toy figures Puppets Dolls Rocks, sticks, boards Pillows, blankets Action figures Doctor's kits Art supplies Children's athletic equipment (plastic bats, light-weight balls, portable nets, etc.) Marbles Computer with software	Gross motor play Rough-housing Allow child to explore environment Use peer support through closely planned group activities Use simple, imaginative games Create art projects child can take home; follow child's lead Involve family members or classmates in therapy session
Young school-aged children (5 to 8 years)	Same as for preschoolers plus board games Playground equipment Bicycles Athletic equipment (balls, nets, bats, goals, etc) Dolls and action figures Beads to string Knitting Pasting, tracing, and drawing Magic sets Trading cards Checkers Dominoes Make-up Water play	Imaginative games (pirates, ballet dancers, gymnastics, baseball, etc.) Draw family members into therapy session Give child sense of accomplishment (help child complete project to take home or learn specific skill that he or she can demonstrate to family members) Incorporate child's goals into therapy goals Use chart to document progress Use small toys/objects as rewards
Older school-aged children (8-12 years)	Art supplies Board games Tape recorders (music) Exercise equipment (stationary bike, rowing machine, kinetic exercise equipment, pulleys, weights, etc.) Athletic equipment Model kits Puzzles Collections (stamps, marbles, dolls, cars, angels, etc) Computer with software	Competition between child and self, therapy provider, family member or peers Document progress on chart using stars or stickers Find out child's goals and incorporate them into therapy Give child sense of success (make goals small enough that immediate progress can be seen) Find out what motivates child (ask child, family members, and peers)
Adolescents (12-18 years)	Same as above	Develop system of rewards and consequences for doing home programs or making progress that is attainable and meaningful Use chart to document goals and progress

for a synthesis of toys and motivational strategies that may be helpful to consider for different age groups of children.

Most of this section has focused on play activities as tools to reach therapy goals. The toys and games used in therapy and the environment where therapy takes place are essential components of a therapy session, and the appropriate use of these tools can facilitate an effective session. Developing the relationship between a therapist and a child, however, is more central in creating an environment where therapeutic goals are meaningful. Fred Donaldson sums up his argument for original play by saying;

Observing isn't sufficient. You must feel play yourself. Infants are already experts. Get down. Let go. Pay attention. Be in touch. You'll learn more than you can imagine. I'm not just talking about "normal" infants. There is no question of competence in play, as if people with disabilities play less well than those without. I do not play with categories of disease or illness, but individual children (p. 30).

It is this ability to "feel" play that must occur for therapy providers to develop the flexibility and creativity to address the real needs of individual children.

EXERCISES

1. Spend some time observing at a preschool, school, or daycare center for young children. Keep a journal documenting how you see children playing alone or together at different ages. Think of how you could use several of the play activities you observe in therapy with a child for strengthening, increasing range of motion, or improving balance. How could you incorporate physical therapy into the group setting you are observing?

2. Interview at least five parents of typically developing children to find out when their children first rolled, sat up alone, crawled, walked, spoke single words, and spoke in sentences. Does early or late skill acquisition make a difference in their overall development?

3. Choose one typically developing child. Through observing the child and interviewing the parent, fill out a developmental test such as the Denver Developmental Screening Test (DDST) or the Hawaii Developmental Charts.

QUESTIONS TO PONDER

1. How do you feel about developmental tests? Do they stigmatize children who are not developing typically by labeling them, or do they help teachers, parents, and medical personnel identify and address problems related to delays in development?

2. Should children with atypical development be placed in daycare centers, preschools, and school classrooms with children who are developing typically? Why or why not?

Annotated Bibliography

Bly, L. (1994). *Motor skills acquisition in the first year: An illustrated guide to normal development.* Tucson, AZ: Therapy Skill Builders.

Lois Bly has for many years studied the kinesiology of the typically developing child as well as children who have neuromuscular problems. This book has evolved out of her years of study as a physical therapist and a teacher of the Neurodevelopmental Treatment (NDT) approach for children. Her view of motor development is much broader than motor milestones. By looking at the postural reflexes; cognition; the development of problem-solving skills; and the effects of sensory input, reflexes, and behavior on the development of motor skills, the bases for motor development can be addressed. In her preface, Ms. Bly addresses some of the most recent theories of motor development in a brief, straightforward manner. Throughout the text, she addresses indications of possible disturbances in motor development that can be helpful to the clinician. The photographs are descriptive and enhance the detailed text. This book should be in the library of any therapist working with infants.

Alexander, R., Boehme, R., & Cupps, B. (1993). *Normal development of functional motor skills: The first year of life.* Tucson AZ: Therapy Skill Builders.

This team of a speech-language pathologist, occupational therapist, and physical therapist address the development of the infant during the first year of life. They discuss postural control, gross motor development, fine motor development, and oral-motor and respiratory development for infants in a very detailed manner. Unfortunately, the information is presented as fractured components without addressing integration of the skills, cognitive development, effects of the environment, or behavior and temperament on the developing child. The text is a valuable resource, nonetheless, because of the thorough handling of the material, the clear line drawings, and the helpful summary charts.

References

Barnes, M. R., Crutchfield, C. A., & Heriza, C. B. (1978). *The neurophysiological basis of patient treatment: Reflexes in motor development (Vol 2).* Atlanta, GA: Stokesville Publishing Co.

Berenbaum, S. A., & Hines, M. (1992). Early androgens are related to childhood sex-typed toy preferences. *Psychological Science, 3,* 203-206.

Bronfenbrenner, U. (1979). *The ecology of human development.* Cambridge, MA: Harvard University Press.

Chapman, S., Box, O. J., Benedetto, M., Lindsey, D., Babiak, C., Walker, A., Norton, E., Scott, E., & Kuczynski, K. (1995). Report from the task force on physical therapy assistants in pediatrics. *Section on Pediatrics Newsletter,* Vol. 5, No. 1, APTA.

Chess, S., & Thomas, A. (1986). *Temperament in clinical practice.* New York: Guilford Press.

Donaldson, O. F. (1993). *Playing by heart: The vision and practice of belonging.* Deerfield Beach, FL: Health Communications, Inc.

Eckert, H. M. (1987). *Motor development* (3rd ed.). Indianapolis: Benchmark.

Frieberg, K. L. (1992). *Human development: A life-span approach* (4th ed.). Boston: Jones and Bartlett.

Furuno, S., O'Reilly, K., Inatsuka, T., Hosaka, C., & Falbey, B. Z. (1993). *Hawaii developmental charts.* Tucson, AZ: Therapy Skill Builders.

Goldstein, J. H. (1994). Sex differences in toy play. In J. Goldstein (Ed.), *Toys, play and child development* (pp. 110-129). New York: Cambridge University Press.

Goodwin, W. L., & Driscoll, L. A. (1980). *Handbook for measurement and evaluation in early childhood education.* San Francisco: Jossey-Bass.

Mental Health Law Project (1990). *SSI new opportunities for children with disabilities.* [Brochure], Washington D.C.

Meyer-Bahlburg, H. F. L., Feldman, J. F., Cohen, P., & Ehrhardt, A. A. (1988). Perinatal factors in the development of gender-related play behavior: Sex hormones versus pregnancy complications. *Psychiatry, 51,* 260-271.

Musselwhite, C. R. (1986). *Adaptive play for special needs children: Strategies to enhance communication and learning.* San Diego: College-Hill Press.

Sadler, T. W. (1985). *Longman's medical embryology* (5th ed.). Baltimore: Williams & Wilkins.

Smith, P. K., & Vollstedt, R. (1985). On defining play: An empirical study of the relationship between play and various play criteria. *Child development, 56,* 1042-1050.

Spodek, B., & Saracho, O. N. (1988). The challenge of educational play. In D. Bergen (Ed.), *Play as a medium for learning and development: A handbook of theory and practice.* (pp. 9-22) Portsmouth, NH: Heinemann.

PART TWO

Orthopedic Disorders
of Childhood

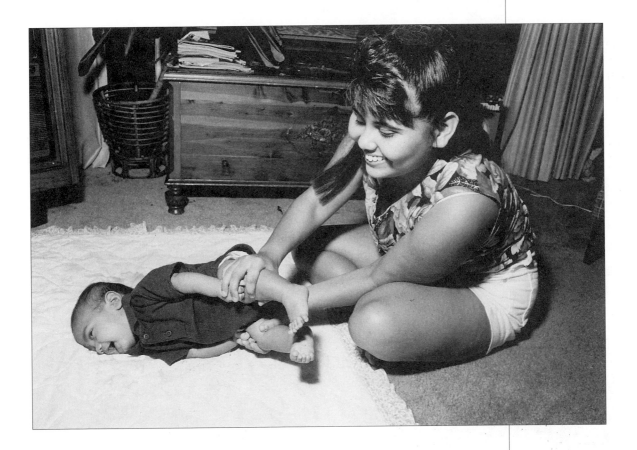

Disorders of the Developing Hip

Shelly, A Girl With Legg-Calvé-Perthes Disease

Shelly dropped her heavy backpack on the grass, then she grasped her crutches firmly and said, "Look, you guys!" Prancing from one crutch to the other, she danced across the sidewalk, neither foot touching the ground at all (Figure 4-1). Other teenagers moving between classes stopped to watch. Her friends were appropriately impressed. "Wait, there's more!" She pushed down on both crutches at the same time, lifting herself up, then jumped, feet and crutches off the ground at the same time. She was able to jump seven or eight times on the crutches without ever touching her feet to the ground. When her arms got too tired, she finally put her left foot down and sprawled back on the grass laughing.

"Wow, Shelly, that was great!"

"How do you do that?"

"Can I try?"

Shelly lay on the grass while her friends tried to copy her antics using her crutches. Most were unable and fell on the ground laughing. She glanced over at the gym where gymnastics practice was being held. She could see through the open double doors and watched as girls and a few boys tumbled across the doorway on mats. On the far side of the gym, she could see part of the uneven bars. Those had been her specialty. Her upper body strength had helped her win a few competitions on that apparatus. She glanced back at her friends. Now her upper body strength helped her show off using crutches. She sighed.

Shelly was the oldest child; her only brother, Russell, was four years younger. Her mother, Tammy, was a teacher who worked full time and was back in school several evenings per week expanding her skills to include teaching special education. Her father, Jack, was self-employed as a landscape artist, creating wa-

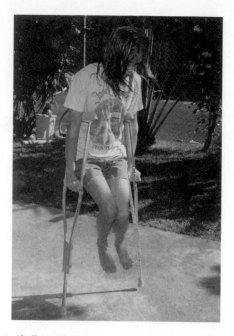

Figure 4-1 Shelly can hop on her crutches for several minutes without putting either foot down.

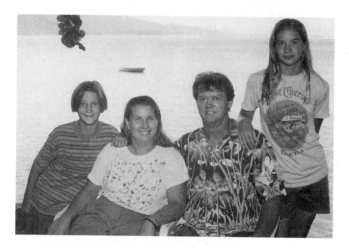

Figure 4-2 Family portrait.

terfalls and handmade replicas of rocks for homes and businesses (Figure 4-2).

Shelly started gymnastics at the end of third grade. She loved it because she enjoyed competing. She also liked being able to fly through the air doing a flip by herself. By sixth grade she was competing on a team. She had to work harder at it than many girls, because she was not naturally flexible. In the summer between fifth and sixth grades, she worked very hard at stretching and was proud to finally be able to perform a full split.

At the end of sixth grade, she started hearing a clicking sound in her right hip; she had pain at night in her right hip, knee, and ankle. She developed a limp that her friends at school noticed before she did. During this time gymnastics became more difficult, and she found she was losing some skills. Her coaches told her to work through it, it was just a slump.

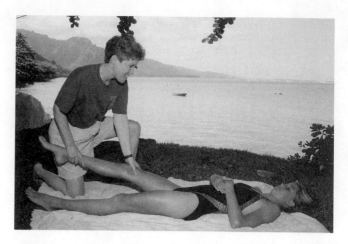

Figure 4-3 Shelly's hip flexor strength is only "fair plus" in her right hip.

Her mother started seriously worrying when she saw Shelly hit her feet on the uneven bars one day during practice. Shelly had never made that mistake before. When she mentioned her concern to Shelly's coach, she was told that Shelly needed to work a little harder to develop her strength and flexibility. Tammy was told that the pains Shelly was experiencing were "growing pains."

Shelly was accepted into a prestigious private school for seventh grade and was thrilled because they had a very good gymnastics team. Team tryouts were held about a month after school began, and Shelly eagerly attended.

One day during tryouts, Shelly tried to do a kip and then straddle on the mat; she found that she could not do it, even though she had done it hundreds of times before. It hurt too much. Her new coach realized that something was seriously wrong and informed Shelly's mother that she should take Shelly to a doctor right away. It was Shelly's last day in gymnastics.

A seemingly endless procession of doctors and medical tests followed (Figure 4-3). Shelly's family doctor referred them to an orthopedic surgeon in town. The orthopedist performed an x-ray examination, and told them immediately that she had Legg-Calvé Perthes disease (LCPD). He recommended a magnetic resonance imaging test (MRI) and an immediate varus osteotomy surgery. He explained that this surgery would help contain the femoral head in the acetabulum as it went through its inevitable disease process of destruction and rebuilding. After considering the x-ray film, he felt that Shelly's hip had started the LCPD process at least 8 months previously. The family, overwhelmed, felt that they needed a second opinion; a friend referred them to Shriners Hospital for Children. Shriners provided orthopedic care free of charge to children who met their criteria. Shelly met the criteria.

The doctors at Shriners could not tell Shelly the reason she had the disease, but they felt that trauma from her gymnastics might have contributed to its development. The orthopedic surgeon at Shriners felt that Shelly's LCPD could be treated by conservative measures for now and suggested several alternatives. One option he suggested was a brace that would hold her leg into abduction with a bar, not allowing her to bear weight through her right leg. Another suggestion was using crutches until the femoral head started remodeling, and using traction at night to

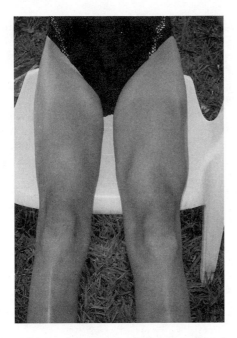

Figure 4-4 The muscle atrophy in Shelly's right thigh is apparent.

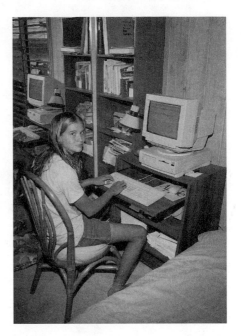

Figure 4-5 Shelly's mother is concerned about her posture when she does her schoolwork. Shelly has a beginning scoliosis from asymmetrical weight bearing.

relieve pressure through the femoral head. Most of the doctors did not feel that the outcome using the brace would be any better than simple non–weight-bearing crutches, so this is what the family decided to do.

Shelly's father installed a pulley system on her bunk bed so that a weight could be applied to a sleeve on her leg pulling it down toward her feet while she slept. Shelly tried this for about a week, but she had such a hard time sleeping that they discontinued it. She used crutches for 7 months, and had x-ray examinations every 6 weeks to monitor the progress of her disease.

In the meantime Shelly struggled with the increased volume of homework from her new school. She missed gymnastics, but she was glad that she had the extra time to apply to her studies. Because the family lived in a rural area, Shelly's commute to and from school was almost 2 hours each way. Although she was able to finish some homework on the bus, leaving the house every day at 6 AM and returning home at 5 PM made for long days. She was also exhausted from using crutches all day. Her new school had a hilly campus and made no accommodations for Shelly's need to use crutches. She was forced to hike up and down the hills between classes. She had a sturdy backpack to carry her books, and friends sometimes helped, but it was still physically draining.

When on crutches, Shelly had to forego some of the recreational activities she loved so much such as surfing, horseback riding, and running. She especially missed being able to run spontaneously if she was late for a class. She was encouraged to keep swimming, though, and frequented the pool near their house. She continued to have pain in her hip for the entire 7 months, but she made efforts to keep herself in shape through swimming.

When she was allowed to walk on two legs again, Shelly found that she had a huge discrepancy in girth between her right and left thighs and calves (Figure 4-4). Her muscles had wasted away

because of disuse. She measured and found that there was a two-inch difference between her thighs and an inch difference between her calves. Her right leg was also shorter than her left, and she had a major limp. Shelly worked hard to strengthen her right leg using exercises the physical therapist (PT) from Shriners had given her, as well as swimming and playing. Although she was able to surf again, she could not sit straddling the surfboard, so she accommodated by kneeling on the board or lying down when she paddled out to meet the waves. Shelly was not able to straddle a horse easily, so she did not go horseback riding any more. Her upper body strength, which had been even further developed as she used crutches, was very helpful in dealing with ocean currents while she was surfing and swimming.

During the years of Shelly's treatment, her parents researched LCPD, and consulted other doctors whom they hoped could offer advice. Tammy was especially concerned about the long-term effect the disease would have on her daughter's health and mobility. She had met a man in his 40s who had LCPD as a child and had experienced back pain and a limp ever since. This man felt that the limp had caused most of his problems over the years. Tammy was therefore very concerned about Shelly's limp.

During the summer after seventh grade, she took Shelly for a consultation in another major city with a larger medical center. The orthopedic surgeon there recommended surgery and felt it would help correct Shelly's limp. Tammy brought the written report back to the doctors at Shriners. Later Tammy consulted an osteopathic doctor who gave Shelly vitamins and examined her x-ray films. This doctor believed that Shelly's spine was becoming unbalanced and that she may be developing a scoliosis. None of the orthopedic physicians had even looked at Shelly's back, and Tammy was concerned (Figure 4-5). A massage therapist treated Shelly for several months during seventh grade. Shelly enjoyed these treatments, commenting that the therapist's hands were like "cat's paws" helping her to relax. Tammy felt that although she trusted the doctors at

BOX 4-1   Physical Therapy Evaluation Summary: Shelly

Social and Medical History

Addressed in the Case Study.

Range of Motion

All within normal limits except for limitations in the following:

	Right	Left
Hip flexion	110	120
Hip internal rotation	20	35
Hip external rotation	20	50
Straight leg raise	40	50
Hip abduction in flexion	25	50
Hip abduction in extension	25	40
Ankle dorsiflexion	10	20

Muscle Strength and Bulk

Muscle strength is within normal limits in her trunk and upper extremities with the following limitations in her lower extremities:

	Right	Left
Hip abduction	F+	Normal
Hip adduction	F+	Normal
Straight leg raise	F+	Good
Knee extension	F+	Normal
Knee flexion	G	Normal
Ankle plantar flexion	Fair (pain in hip)	Normal

Muscle bulk is lean throughout. Girth measurements in inches are as follows:

	Right	Left
Thigh (4 inches above patella)	13	14½
Calf (3 inches below tibial tubercle)	11	11¾

Reflexes and Developmental Reactions

Appropriate for age.

Functional Skills

Shelly put aside her crutches only 1 week before the evaluation, after using them for 3 months after surgery. She walks with a distinct limp. She has decreased weight bearing through her right leg; she unweights it when standing still and has decreased stance time during gait. She walks with internal rotation at the hip, a hip hike, and slight circumduction of her right hip. She was not able or willing to run, jump, or hop pushing off through her right leg. Shelly is able to ascend and descend stairs using a railing with decreased stance time on her right leg. She cannot put her right leg forward to ascend or descend without upper extremity support.

Adaptive Equipment

None.

Activities of Daily Living

Age appropriate.

Summary

Shelly is an active young woman with limitations in her right hip range of motion because of a recent varus osteotomy. She has decreased strength in her hip secondary to disuse. She has gait deviations and limitations in some functional skills secondary to weakness.

BOX 4-2   Home Exercises

1. General exercise, including swimming or walking for 30 minutes, should be done every day.
2. Do the following exercises every day. Try doing them at the same time and place so that they will become routine; for example, carry them out in front of the television during the same show every evening. Another example would be to always listen to the same music in your room while you do your exercises. Make a chart for yourself that you check off or place a sticker on each day to record your exercises. Mark on the chart when you progress to a higher weight or more repetitions.
   a. Lie on your left side. Keep your right leg straight and lift it at least 24 inches off the ground. Hold it for a count of 5. Do this 10 times. Rest. Repeat 10 times. Rest. Repeat 10 times.
   b. Lie on your right side. If it is painful to lie on your right hip, roll slightly back so you are half on your side and half on your back. A pillow behind your back can help you stay partially on your side. Bend your left leg with your foot flat on the ground. Keeping your right leg straight, lift it up off the ground as far as you can. Hold it for a count of 5. Do this 10 times. Rest. Repeat 10 times. Rest. Repeat 10 times.
   c. Lie on your back with your left knee bent and your right leg straight. Lift your right leg off the ground 6 to 12 inches and hold for a count of 5. Lower it gently back to the ground. Repeat, building up to 20 repetitions.
   d. Sitting in a firm chair, straighten your right leg 10 times. Repeat the sequence 2 to 4 times. When this becomes easy for you, place a 4-ounce can in a small plastic bag over your right foot for resistance. When this becomes easy, use an 8-ounce can, and progress to a 12-ounce and 16-ounce can.
   e. Stand with your feet about 12 inches apart. Keep your weight evenly distributed between your legs and your arms out to the side for balance. Have a chair near you that you can easily reach for balance if you need. Gently squat 1 to 2 inches. Hold this position for a count of 5, and come up again. Repeat 20 times. As this becomes easier for you, lower yourself 3 to 4 inches each time.

Shriners to treat her daughter's hip, they were not looking at her daughter's needs as a whole. She was very concerned about Shelly's posture, her limp, and the possible curve in her back.

By the time eighth grade started, Shelly's limp had gotten much better. She continued to go quarterly to Shriners for x-ray examinations so the doctors could monitor the disease process in her hip. They were generally satisfied until March of her eighth grade year. She was told that the surgery that had originally been proposed when her disease was first diagnosed would now be required. Three quarters of her femoral head had collapsed, and it had started to flatten and protrude out of her joint space. A varus osteotomy with derotation would angle the femoral head so that it was maximally contained within the acetabulum.

Shelly was able to take a trip to Europe with her class after school ended in June. By this time she was walking with only a slight limp, and the strength in her right leg had caught up to her left leg.

The surgery was scheduled immediately after her return from Europe. The surgery and the days surrounding it are remembered only vaguely by Shelly, but her mother reports that Shelly was in considerable pain and stayed in the hospital for 3 days. She was on crutches again for 3 months, non–weight bearing through her right leg again. For the first few weeks she was not able to swim because of the healing incision on her hip. As soon as she received permission to swim, Shelly headed for the pool. The doctors, concerned about trauma to her hip from buffeting waves, would not yet allow her to swim in the ocean. Tammy was surprised at and impressed by the amount of hardware she saw in the x-ray film of Shelly's hip. The hardware was scheduled to be removed after 1 year, when the bone had remodeled well enough.

Shelly is now 14 years old and in the ninth grade. She started the school year using crutches again while recovering from her surgery, but recently was able to put them aside. Her most recent physical therapy evaluation is summarized in Box 4-1. Shelly has again developed a terrible limp, and muscle atrophy throughout her right leg is very apparent. The PT gave Shelly exercises to do at home to improve her strength (Box 4-2), but she rarely does

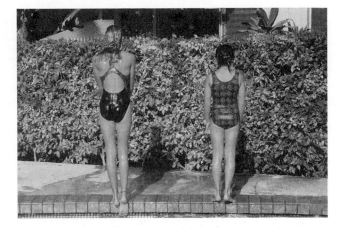

Figure 4-6 Although Shelly stays very athletic, she continues to bear weight asymmetrically. She has taken up diving to replace the gymnastics she was forced to discontinue.

them. She prefers to surf, swim and play actively with her family and her friends. Her mother does not force her to do the exercises, feeling that because Shelly is very active, her strength and flexibility will improve naturally.

Shelly is looking forward to participating in activities with her peers including physical education classes at school. Water polo and diving are on the agenda for this year. The surfing season is just starting, and she is looking forward to getting onto her board and back into the ocean (Figure 4-6). She also looks forward to running spontaneously. She is active and happy; however, sometimes she limps past the gym at school and looks in at the students practicing gymnastic skills. She wonders what her life would be like had she not gotten LCPD? Her parents watch her and wonder what will happen in the future. What will the repercussions of this disease be for their active, athletic daughter?

BACKGROUND AND THEORY

A child is different from an adult in more ways than size. The child is in the process of development, not only of skills and knowledge, but also of tissues and joints that form important anatomical structures. This development begins in utero, but it does not end at birth. The childhood years from birth to skeletal maturity bring physiological and anatomical changes to bones and joints, which produce a mature skeleton by the time a child has completed the first two decades of life. The growing child is vulnerable to influences such as disease, trauma, and environmental effects on the development of tissues and joints.

The hip is the largest joint in the body. Although movement is available in three planes, the hip can carry large amounts of weight and is one of the most stable joints in the body. Stability with remarkable mobility is available because of the unique anatomy of this joint.

The hip is important for postural stability, as well as mobility. A child needs two functioning hips to lie, sit, and stand comfortably, as well as to crawl, walk, and run. Disorders of the developing hip can cause delays or deficiencies in gross motor development

with resultant developmental lag in other areas. Temporary or lifelong pain and deformity can result from disorders that affect the developing hip. Understanding the hip is essential in providing optimal therapy services to children with neurological or musculoskeletal disorders, which affect musculoskeletal development.

This chapter discusses the functional development of the hip and several disorders of hip development, including developmental dysplasia of the hip (DDH), Legg-Calvé-Perthes disease (LCPD), slipped capital femoral epiphysis (SCFE), and infections of the hip. Incidence and causes of the disorders are addressed, as well as their clinical features and the role of physical therapy in their management. Children with these disorders are commonly treated with physical therapy, especially during acute phases of the disease process. Also considered in this chapter is how developmental disorders, such as cerebral palsy, spina bifida, and arthrogryposis, affect the developing hip.

A case study of Shelly, a girl with Legg-Calvé-Perthes disease, demonstrates the effects of significant hip disease on the life of a growing child. Her experiences with the medical profession and physical therapy through the various phases of her disease illustrate the long-term nature of treatment of a child with a hip disorder.

The Applications section of this chapter, which focuses on the multicultural aspects of physical therapy intervention, brings attention to the fact that our colleagues, as well as the children and families we work with, may have different ethnic backgrounds, religious orientations, and cultural practices from our own. Our skills and abilities in working together in a diverse world can affect how we work with children and families with many different types of disabilities.

Normal Hip Development

Anatomy

The hip joint is formed by the junction of the femoral head and the acetabulum of the pelvis (Figure 4-7). The joint is strengthened by ligamentous structures, which anchor the femoral head in the acetabulum and allow movement in three planes: flexion and extension, abduction and adduction, and rotation. Muscles cross the joint and provide extra stability, as well as mobility. The influences of gravity through weight bearing and the stresses of muscle pull contribute pressures to the joint, which cause it to evolve in structure and function throughout childhood.

In a study of hip development, anatomy plays an important role. The anatomy of children differs from that of adults. To understand the evolution of the anatomy of the hip, one should start with the earliest phases of embryonic development. Connective tissue, including bone, cartilage, ligaments, muscles, and tendons develop from embryonic mesenchymal tissue. Early in fetal development (8 to 10 weeks) the acetabulum begins to form and initially almost surrounds the femoral head completely (Ralis & McKibbin, 1973). By the time of birth the acetabulum surrounds about one third of the femoral head, and both the femur and acetabulum are still completely cartilaginous. Ossification centers in the femoral head, greater trochanter, and acetab-

ulum form by 4 to 19 months of age, with ossification becoming complete by 13 to 16 years of age (Chung, 1981).

Several anatomical features of the developing bony hip are remarkable in that they provide a very stable joint. The bony acetabulum is made even deeper by a fibrocartilage labrum around the edge. The acetabulum gets its strength not only from the thickness of the bone, but from reinforcing structures such as ridges in the surrounding bone. Ligaments that cross the joint anteriorly and posteriorly from the pubis, ilium, and ischium also stabilize the joint while allowing mobility.

The junction of the epiphysis, or growth plate, and the developing bone in the femoral head is relatively smooth only until about 1 year of age. After 1 year the bone and cartilage begin to interlock, giving the growth plate extra stability during skeletal growth. This amount of engagement between the bone and the cartilage reaches a peak between 6 and 13 years of age when the child is growing the fastest (Figure 4-8). The interlocking pegs provide extra stability to resist the shear forces of weight-bearing in the adolescent.

Muscle strength, muscle position, and neuromuscular control of muscle can also affect the stability of the developing hip joint. Muscles stabilize the joint and maintain joint position. They also allow for normal weight bearing and movement, which helps the joint further develop stability. However, abnormal muscle pull, can promote joint instability, especially during a growth spurt when stresses on the bones and joints are maximized. An example is the imbalance between adductor and abductor pull in a child with cerebral palsy. The strong adductor pull can exacerbate other structural problems, causing a subluxation or dislocation of the hip even in a young child.

Geometry

The geometry of the hip joint changes as a child matures; bones grow and stresses on the joint change. Some angles that undergo changes include that between the femoral neck and shaft (Figure 4-9) and that of the torsion or rotation of the shaft of the femur in relationship to the head and neck of the femur, also called the angle of anteversion or retroversion (Figure 4-10).

In typically developing children the angle between the neck and the shaft of the femur decreases as the child ages. The functional result of this decrease in angle is that the head of the femur

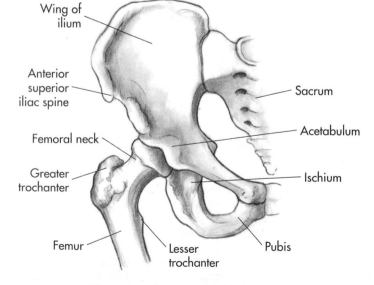

Figure 4-7   The anatomy of the hip joint.

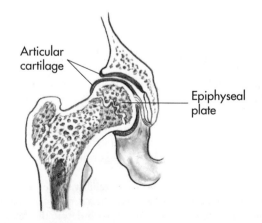

Figure 4-8   The junction of the epiphysis in the femoral head resists shear forces in growing children.

points more directly into the acetabulum, causing it to be more firmly seated in the socket. The decrease in the angle is frequently attributed to weight-bearing or muscle pulls in the growing child. Therefore the child who does not bear weight through the lower extremities or who has abnormal muscle pull on the joint may be more at risk of developing an unstable joint. Walmsley (1915) demonstrated that in individuals with amputation, polio, cerebral palsy, or myelomeningocele, the femoral neck to shaft angle is increased compared to those who have more typical weight-bearing influences on the joint.

In typically developing young children, the femoral head points toward the front of the shaft, toward the same side as the patella. This is called femoral anteversion because the femoral neck points to the front, or anterior of the shaft. The angle of torsion or twist varies at birth between 15 and 50 degrees of anteversion, with a mean of close to 30 degrees (Chung, 1981). As the child grows, the anteversion decreases to a mean of 15 to 20 degrees by adolescence. In a typically developing child whose an-

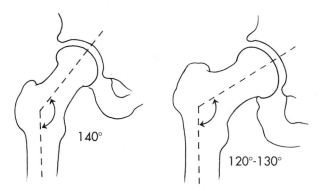

Figure 4-9 The neck to shaft angle of the femur decreases as a child grows.

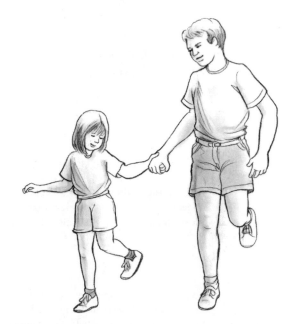

Figure 4-10 The rotation of the femoral neck and head on the shaft of the femur changes as the child grows. Femoral anteversion in young children causes a flailing outward of the lower leg during gait.

teversion decreases as growth occurs, the patella points somewhat inward at birth and rotates with the shaft of the femur until it is pointing straight ahead when the hip matures. Children with atypical stresses on their hip joints may never decrease the angle of anteversion as they grow, causing an apparent internal rotation of their hips when they are older, with the patellae facing inward rather than straight ahead.

Typically developing children, especially girls, can also have excessive anteversion. This peaks at 3 years of age, when some girls may appear "knock-kneed," and generally resolves as they grow older. Girls who run with their lower legs flailing outward may have excessive anteversion of their hips. This may resolve as they grow older and is not generally a cause for concern if their musculoskeletal system is otherwise normal. The angle of anteversion is important for the stability of the hip joint, especially in children with atypical musculoskeletal systems.

The Child With Developmental Dysplasia of the Hip

Developmental dysplasia of the hip (DDH), formerly called congenital hip dysplasia, refers to conditions in the developing hip that are apparent at birth or during early development, where the acetabulum and the femoral head are not aligned normally. Dysplasia refers to abnormal development or growth, in this case, of the acetabulum or proximal femur. Examples of dysplasia affecting the hip include a small or shallow acetabulum or a slanted acetabular roof (Chung, 1981). Common conditions diagnosed as DDH include a subluxed or dislocated femoral head. Teratologic hip dysplasia is a less common type of dysplasia caused by severe prenatal abnormalities, such as arthrogryposis or myelomeningocele, which affect prenatal development and positioning. Associated problems with DDH include cervical torticollis (Hummer & MacEwan, 1972), facial deformities, postural scoliosis, and foot deformities, such as metatarsus adductus or calcaneovalgus (Dunn, 1976).

Incidence and Cause

Hip dysplasia or subluxation occurs in 1 out of every 100 births in the United States. Hip dislocation occurs in 1 out of 1000 births in the United States (Mubarak, Beck, & Sutherland, 1986; Ramsey, 1973). The ratio of girls to boys is 6:1, and the left hip is affected twice as often as the right. It is thought that the left leg is more affected because in most fetal positions it is the left leg that is wedged in an adducted position against the mother's spine (Chung, 1981).

Cultural practices of swaddling and carrying infants is thought to affect the extreme diversity of DDH in various countries. For instance, DDH is relatively common in Japan and among the Native American populations. Both groups swaddle the infant's legs in extension and adduction, either by wrapping the legs together (Japan), or by strapping the infant onto a cradleboard (Native American). The incidence of DDH is low in countries such as China, where parents carry infants with hips abducted and flexed around the parent's waist or back.

Typical DDH usually develops in the last trimester of pregnancy. Tight in-utero positioning, such as a breech position, or being constricted by firm abdominal muscles in a primagravida mother may cause the hip to dislocate. Girls are thought to be more commonly affected because more girls than boys present as breech deliveries. A female infant is also more susceptible to the maternal hormone relaxin, which causes ligamentous laxity in the mother during the last trimester of pregnancy to aid in delivery. All these factors, as well as a family history of DDH, may be related to the development of the disorder.

Clinical Features

Affected newborn infants will have asymmetrical hip abduction in flexion, with the affected side being tighter. They may have asymmetrical groin or buttock skinfolds; pistoning, or movement of the femur in and out of the hip socket with manual traction; or apparent femoral shortening on the affected side. Diagnosis by x-ray examination is difficult or impossible in an infant younger than 6 to 8 months because of the lack of ossification of the joint. Ultrasound is increasingly being used to supplement clinical diagnosis for very young infants.

Most newborns are screened for DDH using a Barlow or Ortolani test. The Barlow test involves the examiner moving the infant's hip into flexion and abduction, then slowly moving it back into adduction with pressure directed posteriorly. If a click is felt, the femur may be slipping out of the acetabulum or sliding over the posterior border of the acetabulum indicating instability. The Ortolani test involves first placing the hip in adduction and flexion with posterior force applied. When the hip is subsequently moved into abduction with slight traction, a click will usually be felt as the dislocated hip slides back into the socket.

A child with a positive Barlow or Ortolani sign may have one of several grades of DDH, which are summarized in Table 4-1. Initial treatments are similar for grades 1 through 3, but infants with teratologic DDH always need surgery to reconstruct the joint.

Treatment

Conservative treatments for DDH will be most effective for infants whose subluxation or dislocation have been discovered and treated early, within the first 6 months of life (Chung, 1981).

During this period the femoral head and the acetabulum continue to grow at a relatively fast pace, allowing optimal remodeling. After the first 18 months of life, conservative treatment is not likely to be effective (Salter, 1961).

Conservative treatment involves maintaining the hip in flexion and abduction through bracing, splinting, or diapering until the hip has adequately remodeled. The most conservative treatment is multiple diapering. The child is placed in two to three diapers holding the legs in abduction, and parents are instructed to position the infant in hip flexion as well. If symptoms persist after several weeks, a brace such as the Pavlik harness is used (Figure 4-11). This harness holds the infant in a position of moderate hip abduction and flexion, yet allows spontaneous

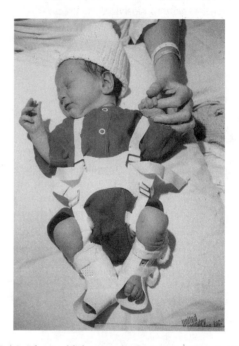

Figure 4-11 The Pavlik harness looks intimidating, but it is relatively gentle as it holds an infant's hips in abduction and flexion.

TABLE 4-1	Types of Developmental Dysplasia of the Hip in Infancy	
Type	**Definition**	**Treatment considerations**
Dysplasia	Acetabulum may be shallow or small with poor lateral borders. Acetabular dysplasia may occur alone or with any level of femoral deformity or displacement.	The hip must be kept abducted and flexed with the femoral head centered in the acetabulum. In this position the acetabulum will continue to deepen, maintaining a correct shape, and the ligaments and joint capsule will tighten to provide extra joint stability.
Subluxatable	The femoral head can be partially displaced to the rim of the acetabulum. It slides laterally, but not all the way out of the socket.	
Dislocatable	The femoral head is in the socket, but it can be displaced completely outside the acetabulum with manual pressure.	
Dislocated	The femoral head lies completely outside the hip socket but can be reduced with manual pressure.	
Teratologic	The femoral head lies completely outside the hip socket and cannot be reduced with manual pressure. Deformity of the joint surfaces is significant; it is usually related to another severe developmental anomaly, such as arthrogryposis or myelomeningocele.	Surgery will be needed to reconstruct the joint. The child may have pain with some hip movements and will probably have significant limitation in some ranges of motion (most likely abduction and extension).

kicking and movement of the legs. It is important not to hyper-abduct or hyperflex the hip because this can cause complications such as avascular necrosis resulting from excessive pressure on the femoral head. Allowing spontaneous movement also reduces the possibility of avascular necrosis. The infant usually wears the Pavlik harness for 24 hours per day for 6 to 12 weeks, then reduces wear to 12 hours per day for 3 to 6 additional months, until both clinical and radiographical signs are normal. Particular protocols will vary from center to center.

More aggressive treatment of the dislocated hip, usually for a child older than 18 months, may involve traction for several weeks either at home or as an inpatient in the hospital to reduce pressure through the femoral head and relax contracted muscles in an attempt to align the joint surfaces. In a child over 2 years closed or open reduction is always indicated. If the hip is able to be reduced manually after traction (closed reduction), casting is used to maintain joint alignment while the joint capsule and ligaments tighten to support the joint. If the hip is not able to be aligned manually or redislocates easily, surgery (open reduction) is necessary to obtain and maintain the desired correction in joint alignment. Surgery may involve soft tissue releases of contracted adductor muscles, as well as modification of joint angles through cutting and realigning the pelvis or femoral head. Common surgical procedures to the femur and pelvis are outlined in Table 4-2. Protocols vary across the country, but after surgery the child is generally placed in a spica cast for 6 to12 weeks, usually with a progressive cutting back of the cast to allow greater movement as time passes (Figure 4-12).

The child may be casted with both hips in extension, moderate abduction, and knee extension. Usually the cast on the uninvolved leg is cut back to above the knee after 4 to 6 weeks to allow free knee movement. Then the cast is cut back on the uninvolved side to the hip, allowing full hip movement, but continuing to secure the pelvis. After several more weeks, the cast on the involved leg may be cut back to above the knee, and finally, removed altogether.

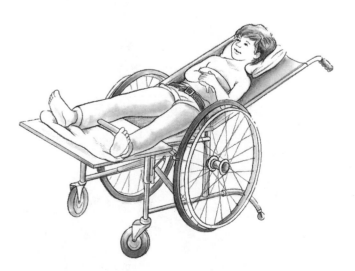

Figure 4-12 The child in a spica cast is fairly limited in voluntary movement and mobility.

Physical Therapy Intervention

The PT may be involved with families of infants with DDH for teaching as well as direct intervention.

Pavlik harness. When parents are taught how to apply the Pavlik harness, it is important to ensure that the hips are placed in the correct position; too much flexion or abduction can cause excessive pressure through the femoral heads, leading to possible avascular necrosis. The child should be able to move the legs freely within the constraints of the harness.

Teaching family members how to apply the Pavlik harness can be an opportunity to familiarize parents with appropriate developmental interventions for their infant. Decreased sensory input or motor output as a result of wearing the harness has potential for causing developmental delays. Parents or others may be reluctant to pick up or move the child who is wearing a complicated positioning device because they fear hurting or dislocating the involved hip. It is important to assure parents that interacting socially and physically with their child is essential to the child's development. Teaching parents appropriate handling skills for picking up and carrying their infant can relieve some of the stress they may feel at first with the Pavlik harness.

The young child in a spica cast. A young child in a spica cast is also a challenge for parents and caregivers. The plaster cast may weigh as much as the child. A child who is heavy, stiff, and extended from the chest down is difficult to lift and carry short distances. Longer, away-from-home activities are even more difficult. Diapers are a challenge, and the cast itself needs protection and care to prevent it from deteriorating quickly. Even with good care, the cast becomes somewhat soiled, stained, and rank over time.

Giving the child the ability to do things independently is the best way to ensure appropriate developmental stimulation and minimize dependence and passivity. A young child with a spica cast fits well on a reclining adult wheelchair with the leg rests removed and pillows added. The use of anti-tippers ensures safety because the center of gravity is more posterior than if an adult were sitting in the chair. Alternate forms of mobility include a wagon with pillows and a wooden platform to support the child's abducted legs; a lawn cart, with an extension to support the cast if needed; and a large scooter board such as the ones used for automotive work, with the child either in the prone or supine position and supported with pillows. Other ways of promoting independence include giving the child the television remote control, arranging a plastic basin that can sit on the chest for washing and tooth care, settling the child in the family room rather than the seclusion of the bedroom, and giving the child a bell to signal for help if needed. An older child may be given access to the computer for homework or recreation.

Make small ankle puppet weights for young children. These can look like saddle sandbags with an additional torso and head attached to the connecting strap. The hanging-down portion of the sandbags form the legs of the puppet, and the sand can be carefully weighed to provide the appropriate amount of resistance. The puppet straddles the child's leg and provides a source of fun and games during weight training.

TABLE 4-2   Common Surgical Procedures for the Hip in Children

Type of surgery	Example	Disorder	Explanation
Myotomy	Figure A	CP	Soft tissue releases, usually of the adductor muscles, can reduce abnormal pressures that cause subluxation and potential dislocation of the femoral head.
Fixation in situ	Figure B	SCFE	A pin is driven through the femoral neck into the femoral head to stabilize the head on the neck.
Proximal femoral derotation osteotomy	Figure C	CP	The femoral head is rotated to decrease the angle of anteversion. This procedure is usually done with a varus osteotomy.
Proximal femoral varus osteotomy	Figure D	DDH LCPD CP	A wedge is cut out of the femoral neck so that the neck-to-shaft angle is reduced (the neck sticks out more from the shaft). The femur has increased stability because it can be seated more directly in the acetabulum with less tendency to slide out.
Innominate pelvic osteotomy	Figure E	DDH LCPD CP	If the acetabulum faces more anteriorly and laterally than normal, the hip is not stable in a normal weight-bearing position. This procedure rotates the acetabulum so that it faces more downward and provides more stability for the femoral head during weight bearing.
Pemberton pelvic osteotomy	Figure F	DDH LCPD CP	The acetabulum is deepened and rotated downward to provide more stability to the femoral head. This procedure is used for the younger child with a shallow, dish-shaped acetabulum.

CP, Cerebral palsy; *DDH,* developmental dysplasia of the hip; *LCPD,* Legg-Calvé-Perthes disease; *SCFE,* slipped capital femoral epiphysis.

Standing and gait training for the young child in a spica cast. The child who is old enough to stand may begin passive standing on the uninvolved leg or on both legs even while in the spica cast, depending on the stability of the joint and the type of surgery performed. If medically appropriate, passive standing can be done on a tilt table or supine stander where the child's weight can be supported unilaterally or bilaterally (Figure 4-13). Because of the equipment needed, the child will likely be either an inpatient in a pediatric hospital or at a school when the standing program is initiated. Monitoring the child's pain, blood pressure (if placed on bedrest for more than a week), as well as apprehension, when coming to an upright position is important. The child should always be performing an activity while standing. Appropriate activities include playing catch, coloring at a table, or watching television. Box 4-3 outlines handling strategies for a young child in a spica cast.

When the child is in the cast, maintaining functional range of motion and strength in joints that are not restricted is important. This can be achieved through developing and playing age-appropriate games to encourage active movement. Children may enjoy puppet shows (with foot and hand puppets), prone scooterboard races, upper extremity dancing, finger (or toe) painting, and playing catch. If the child is in school, classmates and teachers can participate in games; or the child can participate in a classroom activity such as painting at an easel, singing, or academic work. If the child is at home, siblings, neighbors, and parents can be recruited as playmates.

If the child can stand, crutches or a walker can help maintain balance or movement as well as strength and range of motion. Crutches should not be used for a child under 6 years old. A young child's balance is not adequate for the task of balancing on, or coordinating, separate crutches. A walker is much safer for a young child in any kind of a cast.

When teaching a young child or a child with mental retardation to use crutches, use the parallel bars before progressing to crutches. You may also find the use of a walker a helpful intermediate step between the bars and the crutches.

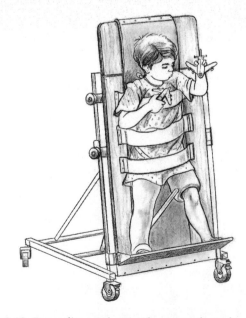

Figure 4-13 Depending on the specific surgery done, the child in a spica cast may be able to bear weight with help.

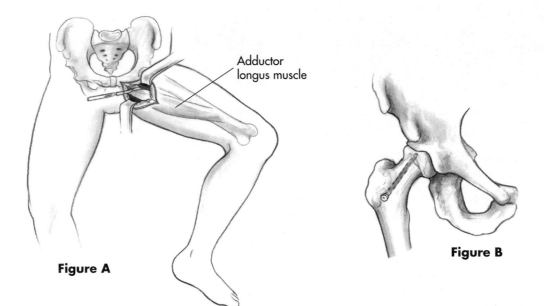

Figure A

Figure B

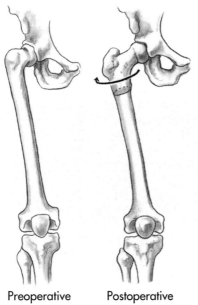

Preoperative   Postoperative

Figure C

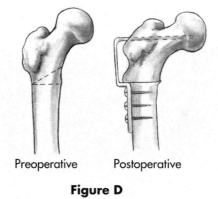

Preoperative   Postoperative

Figure D

Preoperative   Postoperative

Figure E

Preoperative   Postoperative

Figure F

BOX 4-3   Handling Strategies for a Child in a Spica Cast

Turning

1. Use proper body mechanics, getting up on the bed if needed to turn the child.
2. Seek help. It usually takes two people to safely turn a child who weighs more than 50 pounds (with the cast) in a spica cast.
3. Make sure that the child knows what will happen and is ready. Initially the child may be in significant pain. Think about pre-medicating the child 30 minutes before turning.
4. The child should be turned as one unit, in a "log roll." Do not twist the child's trunk during the turn.
5. Do not use the cast as a lever when turning the child. The cast should be grasped firmly with attention paid to preventing excessive pressure through the legs when turning the child.
6. The child should be positioned (if supine) with pillows under the head and shoulders and possibly under the legs until he or she is comfortable after being turned.

   If the child is in the prone position, pillows should be placed under the abdomen and chest.

   Make sure the edges of the cast are not digging into the child. Make sure any diapers are positioned appropriately to avoid accidents.

Lifting

1. Use proper body mechanics to lift a child (see Chapter 9, discussion of handling and positioning).
2. Obtain the help of another person or a mechanical lift if the child weighs more than 50 pounds (with the cast).
3. Always plan the lift thoroughly before actually lifting the child. You should know how you will lift, where your hand holds will be, where the child is going, and the reason for the lift.
4. Always get the child to help, even if the child is only counting 1, 2, 3 in preparation for the lift.
5. For a two-person lift, the person at the head is always in charge. This person will ensure the environment is safe, make sure the other(s) are ready, and will initiate the count.

Positioning

Supine

The head and shoulders should be supported with pillows. If the child is in a bed, a trapeze should be set up to allow the child in-

dependent weight shifts and to assist with transfers. The legs may need to be elevated slightly with pillows.

Prone

Pillows should be placed under the chest and abdomen of the child, with a small pillow under the head. The head of the bed could be elevated or the child could be placed on a wedge to allow the child to see the environment more easily.

Side-lying

Full side-lying position is not possible in a spica cast; however, in either the prone or the supine position, the child could and should be placed in a partial side-lying position. Pillows should be placed under one side of the child and cast to prop the child in a partial side-lying position. Make sure that the child and the cast are aligned and not twisted.

Mobility

Small child

An adult reclining wheelchair, with the legrests removed and possibly the armrests too, works very well. Make sure anti-tippers are on to prevent the chair from falling over backward because of the posterior shift in the center of gravity.

A wagon, lawn cart, or automobile scooterboard can be adapted to position and transport a child in a spica cast. A dolly (for carrying heavy boxes) or a tilt table are also acceptable mobility devices. Beware of the width of the cast and the narrowness of doorways.

A gurney or special cart can be used to transport a child in a spica cast. This type of device takes up a lot of room and is almost impossible to transport in a car.

Larger child

A hospital bed provides the most stable positioning and greatest potential mobility in the house for a larger child in a spica cast. An older child should always have a trapeze attachment on the bed frame to assist with transfers, bed mobility, and turning. The trapeze also helps maintain upper extremity strength and range of motion.

Another option is an adult wheelchair with elevating legrests and a wide board across the leg rests to support the width of the cast. The cast may need to be tied loosely to the frame of the wheelchair to prevent it from falling off.

Because transferring is so difficult with a large child, floor level mobility devices such as scooterboards are not recommended.

When the cast is removed, the child will need to learn or relearn balance and mobility in standing, especially if bedrest was required for the entire casting period. The child will need progressive gait training as gains are made in mobility skills.

Role of the PTA

The physical therapist assistant (PTA) may be working with a child either in the hospital for teaching shortly after birth or after surgery, at home for home care after surgery, or at school. The physical therapist is responsible for evaluating the child and, along with the physician and the team of people working with the child, deciding what types of intervention are appropriate. The PTA may provide strengthening and range of motion activ-

ities, progressive gait training, caregiver training for transfers, mobility and exercise, or consult for adaptive equipment and functional access for the child. Communication with the PT and the team on the progress of a child who is recovering from acute surgery is essential because needs change and problems may arise quickly.

The Child With Legg-Calvé-Perthes Disease

In children Legg-Calvé-Perthes disease (LCPD) causes degeneration of the femoral head from a disturbance in the blood supply, with subsequent regeneration of the femoral head. The disease

TABLE 4-3 Radiographical Stages in Legg-Calvé-Perthes Disease

Stage	Radiographical changes	Risk for deformity
Initial stage	Failure of the femoral head to grow because of lack of blood supply. Femoral head appears smaller that the opposite side. Medial joint space in the hip appears wider than the other side.	High risk for deformity in the femoral head and neck if not treated.
Fragmentation stage	The epyphisis appears fragmented. New bone is beginning to form on the old bone. Revascularization of the femoral head is occurring.	High risk for deformity in the femoral head and neck if not treated.
Reossification stage	Bone density returns to normal. The femoral head and neck may show changes in shape and structure.	At this stage no more deformity will develop. The femoral head and neck remodel somewhat.
Healed stage	The femoral neck and head retain any residual deformity from the repair process.	Residual deformity is left.

has a 2- to 4-year progression and is self-limiting, meaning that it always heals itself eventually. Milder cases do not always require treatment, but a physician should closely monitor the disease's progress through x-ray examinations and clinical evaluations.

Incidence and Cause

Legg-Calvé-Perthes disease occurs in boys four to five times more frequently than in girls (Chung, 1981; Barker, 1986). About 1 in 18,000 children will develop the disease (Molloy & MacMahon, 1966). Although girls develop the disease less frequently, they usually manifest symptoms at a later age and have a poorer prognosis than most boys. Children are usually between 2 and 18 years of age when the disease develops, with a majority of cases being boys between 4 and 8 years of age (Weinstein, 1990). LCPD is found more frequently in children of Northern European or Asian ancestry than in those of Native American, Polynesian, or African-American ethnicity. It occurs more often in children who are in urban rather than rural settings. Children who get LCPD are generally smaller than their peers, had a relatively low birth weight, and delayed bone age at the time of diagnosis. The disease expresses itself in both hips in 10% to 20% of cases.

Although the cause of LCPD is not known, it is now thought that certain children may be susceptible to developing the disease as a result of genetic predisposition or other factors. Current theories elaborate on various problems or variations in the anatomy that cause the blood supply to the femoral head to be interrupted. Some theories discuss recurrent synovitis of the hip as a precursor to LCPD; others describe multiple infarctions of arteries supplying the femoral head; and yet others discuss the particular anatomy of the blood supply to the femoral head, which is more fragile in boys and Caucasians than in other groups (Chung, 1981). Weinstein (1990) summarizes a more comprehensive theory that LCPD may be reflective of a generalized disorder of epiphyseal cartilage in children who are susceptible to the disease.

Clinical Features

A young child usually begins to limp with mild pain in the groin, medial thigh, or medial knee. Pain more distally is referred from the hip, but difficulties in diagnosis arise when this is not realized by a diagnosing physician. Some children can relate a specific traumatic incident that precipitated the pain. Because the pain is generally mild, children may not be seen by a physician until months after the onset. This delay is a problem because earlier treatment provides a significantly better prognosis. Other clini-

cal signs include decreased range of motion, especially in hip abduction and internal rotation; positive Trendelenburg (the pelvis drops lower on one side during gait because of muscle weakness); thigh, calf, or buttock atrophy from disuse; or limb length inequality from collapse of the femoral head on the affected side.

There are four stages to the disease process, as demonstrated radiographically, which demonstrates the cycle from the initial injury to complete healing (Table 4-3). During the course of the disease the femoral head stops growing because of inadequate blood supply; then the epiphysis fragments with some degree of collapse of the femoral head in most cases. Revascularization is apparent during this stage. When reossification occurs, new bone grows and, finally, the femoral head is reformed with some degree of deformity. The disease process takes from 2 to 4 years to complete (Chung, 1981).

Catterall (1971) has postulated four categories of severity of the disease, depending on the degree of epiphyseal involvement and extent of necrosis of the femoral head. Most children fall into category 1 or 2. Children with grades 3 or 4 are likely to have greater deformity of the femur with less congruence between the acetabulum and femoral head upon healing, and therefore more limitation in range of motion, residual pain, and decreased function. Prognosis depends on the age and gender of the child, the severity of the disease, and whether or not the femoral head has subluxated on the femoral neck. Prognosis is also dependent on obtaining adequate treatment in a timely manner to prevent or minimize deformity of the femoral head.

Follow-up studies have indicated that most children with mild or moderate disease have very good outcomes, at least for the first 40 years after the onset of symptoms. Longer term studies have demonstrated degenerative arthritis of the hip in most adults who had LCPD in childhood by the time they were 60 or 70 years old (Weinstein, 1990).

Associated problems of the child with LCPD include osteochondritis dissecans, a lesion affecting subchondral bone and the articulating surface of a joint. It is most common in the distal femur, but it has been seen in the proximal femur in a child with healed LCPD. Osteochondritis dissecans may or may not be symptomatic, but trauma or ischemia to the joint is thought to be a cause. It is frequently self-limiting and may not require treatment.

Treatment

Treatment varies for LCPD according to the severity of the disease, the stage of initiation of treatment, and the experience and predisposition of the orthopedic surgeon managing the case.

Some physicians advocate no treatment at all, feeling that because LCPD is a self-limiting disease, no treatment will affect its course. Most research, however, documents the effectiveness of early and/or vigorous treatment. The prevention of deformity, protection of growth plates, and prevention of degenerative joint disease through preserving the joint surfaces are the primary goals of treatment for children with LCPD. Containment of the femoral head in the acetabulum throughout the course of the disease process is key to achieving these goals, because it allows the femoral head to remodel in the acetabulum, preserving the joint congruence as much as possible. Containment of the femoral head can be accomplished in many ways.

Conservative treatment consisting of observation and monitoring, limitation of contact sports, and encouragement of swimming for range of motion exercise and strengthening may be all that is necessary for children with mild forms of the disease. For children with more vigorous disease processes, splinting with bedrest used to be the treatment of choice, but it has given way to more active splinting, allowing children to participate more fully in their lives and avoid 2 to 4 years of bedrest. Partial or non–weight-bearing on the affected leg using standard crutches for a period of time can be an effective treatment for children older than 5 years with mild disease, along with daily stretching to loosen contracted muscles.

It is important that family members be willing to provide daily exercise (Figure 4-14). Night- or daytime weight-bearing abduction splints, such as the broomstick, Petrie, or Toronto orthoses (Figure 4-15), allow a child to walk with crutches while maintaining the leg in abduction, which effectively contains the femoral head in the acetabulum to allow congruent reossification of the femoral head with the acetabulum. The problem with use of an orthosis is that treatment is usually long-term, up to several years; and the orthosis can significantly interfere with the child's daily functioning, not to mention self-esteem. One study comparing children with LCPD who had surgery with those who received bracing demonstrated that children who received bracing were more likely to be delayed in areas of academics and social and sexual behavior (Price, Day, & Flynn, 1988).

Surgery is a more aggressive method to treat LCPD. The goal of surgery is the same as that of more conservative treatments: containing the femoral head in the acetabulum during the healing process. Surgery is usually necessary for those children with Catterall grades 3 and 4 LCPD to affect adequate containment of the femoral head. The surgical procedure used will be either a varus osteotomy of the proximal femur, a pelvic osteotomy, or in severe cases, both. See Table 4-2 for a review of common hip surgeries, including those that may be used for LCPD. Children may require bracing even after surgery if the reossification is slow or if the femoral head begins to subluxate.

Physical Therapy Intervention

Physical therapy could be involved with the child with LCPD at various stages in the disease process in the clinic, hospital, home, or school. At initial diagnosis the child needs to be evaluated for range of motion, strength and functional skills. The family may need assistance learning range of motion or strengthening exercises, depending on the treatment decided on. The child's teacher may need to learn how to include the child who is wearing an abduction orthosis or using crutches into classroom activities and how to encourage mobility and activity in school. If the child

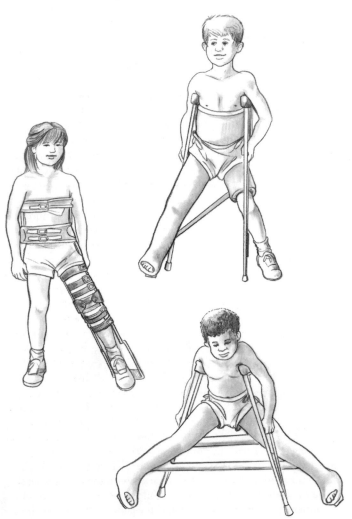

Figure 4-15 Abduction braces may be used in conservative treatment of Legg-Calvé-Perthes disease.

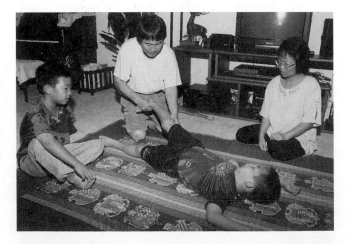

Figure 4-14 Aaron receives daily stretching from his father for hip extension, abduction, and hip internal rotation.

receives surgery and is immobilized in a spica cast, the family will need to learn how to turn the child over, lift the child, assist the child in strengthening and range of motion activities, and help the child gain independence in daily tasks such as self-help, recreation, and academic activities. The family may also need help learning how to transport the child, use a mechanical lift at home, and work with the school to accommodate the child's new needs. Once the child is out of a spica cast, regaining lost range of motion and strength and relearning ambulation skills become important. Monitoring and communication to other team members about pain, range of motion, and strength throughout the treatment process help the team make appropriate decisions regarding future treatment for the child.

Role of the PTA

The PTA may be responsible for any of the above activities except for evaluation. Monitoring of strength and range of motion in order to communicate regularly with the PT and the physician about the child's status is important. Therapy may be provided at home, school, or in the clinic. If the PTA is in a school situation and can work with the teacher to integrate strengthening and range of motion activities into classroom activities, an exciting challenge can be met. Designing classroom activities to encourage academic growth, as well as physical challenges, takes imagination and teamwork, as well as a teacher who is willing and able to participate fully in the design process.

The Child With Slipped Capital Femoral Epiphysis

Also called coxa vara, or epiphyseal hip fracture, slipped capital femoral epiphysis (SCFE) is a hip problem common to preadolescent and early adolescent children, especially children with delayed skeletal maturation and obesity. The femoral epiphysis slips, causing the femoral head distal to the epiphysis to slide off the femoral neck.

Incidence and Cause

SCFE occurs in 0.71 to 3.41 per 100,000 children (Leach, 1994). It occurs in boys two to three times more frequently than in girls. Children who are obese or very tall and generally heavy, those who have delayed skeletal maturation, and those who are between 9 and 16 years of age are most likely to have SCFE. African-American and Polynesian children are more susceptible than Caucasian children (Loder, 1996). Although bilateral slips are documented in only about 25% to 30% of cases, it is thought that they may occur asymptomatically in up to 60% of cases (Jerre, Billing, Hansson, Karlsson, & Wallin, 1996). SCFE occurs in boys about 2 years earlier than in girls, and its onset is related to the onset of puberty. Although its cause is unclear, hormonal influences are thought to play a part. The interplay between growth and sex hormones, which are influenced by puberty, is thought to influence the development of SCFE by weakening growth plates. A more comprehensive theory is that children have a predisposition for SCFE with growth plates that are weaker than normal, allowing usual stresses from gravity, weight bearing, and muscle activity to cause the slippage (Morrissy, 1990).

Clinical Features

Children usually present with an intermittent limp and pain in the groin, buttock, or thigh after some sort of trauma. They may lean toward the side of the injury during the stance phase of gait. Weakness in the abductor muscles on the affected side from guarding and disuse may cause a Trendelenburg gait. The leg is usually held in external rotation, and attempts to flex the hip result in external rotation as well. Limitations in range of motion may be seen in internal rotation, abduction, and sometimes flexion.

Three types of SCFE have been described. The *chronic* slip has a gradual onset with a progression of symptoms for 3 weeks or more. A particular episode of trauma may not be identified. This is the most common type of onset. An *acute* slip has a sudden onset of severe pain, which is usually precipitated by an episode of trauma. The trauma may be as mild as jumping off a table. The pain usually lasts less than 3 weeks before seeking medical assistance, and the child will have difficulty walking on the leg at all. In the third type of slip, the *acute-on-chronic,* the child may have had symptoms gradually building for more than 3 weeks, but then an episode of trauma causes an acute exacerbation of the symptoms. The child with this type of slip may not be able to walk on the affected leg.

The severity of SCFE is measured in grades of slippage. Chung (1981) describes four grades of slippage, three of which correspond to classic radiographic grades of slippage (Figure 4-16). Treatment varies somewhat for the different grades.

Treatment

The goals for treatment of SCFE are to keep the slippage or displacement to a minimum, to maintain hip range of motion and function, and to prevent degenerative changes in later years. A hip that has been determined to be in a preslip phase may be pinned in situ (see Table 4-2), or conservative treatment may be attempted, including non–weight-bearing status on crutches with attempts at weight loss and prohibition from athletics until the growth plates are fused. Radiographs every few months monitor the status of the hip; and if any slippage is observed, surgical pinning is done immediately.

For any degree of slippage surgery is almost always required, although casting in a spica cast may be attempted for mild slips as a conservative measure to prevent further slippage. Mild or moderate slips (grades 1 and 2) are usually treated by surgical pinning in situ. Bedrest and traction may be instituted to reduce hip pain and spasm before surgery. The surgical procedure for mild-to-moderate slips involves driving pins through the neck of the femur into the femoral head, but not protruding into the joint space. This method prevents further migration of the femoral head off the femoral neck, but it does not reduce the slippage that has already occurred. The pins can be removed after the growth plates have fused, at least 12 months after surgery. Remodeling of the femoral head and neck will help to reduce any deformity.

For moderate or severe slips an osteotomy to change the angle of the femoral neck to the shaft or manipulation to try to achieve a reduction of the slip may be done. Research has shown that most hips do better with pinning in situ rather than more vigorous surgical manipulations (O'Brien & Fahey, 1977). Other surgical procedures ranging from epiphysiodesis (inserting a bone graft into the epiphysis) to hip replacement in later life may

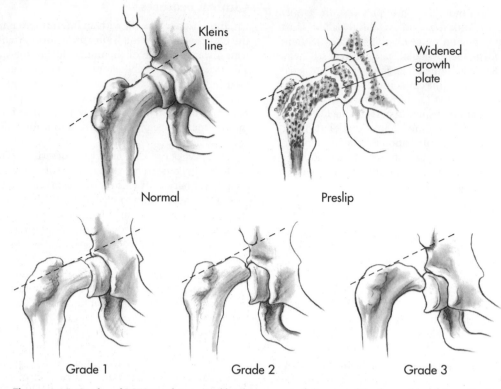

Figure 4-16 Grades of SCFE are determined by the amount of slippage of the femoral head from the femoral neck. *Preslip:* mild changes in the x-ray such as a widened growth plate. *Grade 1/mild slip:* the femoral head has slipped posteriorly and inferiorly up to one third the width of the femoral neck. *Grade 2/moderate slip:* the femoral head has slipped between one third and one half the width of the femoral neck. *Grade 3/severe slip:* the femoral head has been displaced more than one half the width of the femoral neck.

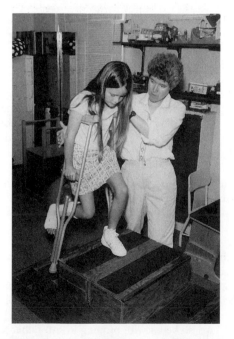

Figure 4-17 Teaching crutch-walking to a child can be different from teaching an adult.

be needed for more severe problems, especially those that develop complications. Hip replacement is not usually advocated for children because it does not usually last well with vigorous use over time.

Complications from surgery include chondrolysis, or breakdown and absorption of the cartilage surfaces of the joint, which causes joint space narrowing, stiffness, and pain; and necrosis of the femoral head from an interruption of the blood supply. Both complications increase the likelihood of significant joint degeneration in later years. Both complications are also more likely with severe slips. Complications can be minimized by ensuring that pins do not protrude into the joint space and irritate the joint surfaces. Attention to the placement of pins and care in reducing the femoral head displacement can preserve the blood supply to the femoral head. Because of the differences between the anatomy of the blood supply to the hip in girls and boys, girls are at less risk of necrosis of the femoral head than boys.

For hips pinned in situ, a child is usually up and ambulating on crutches with weight-bearing, as tolerated within 2 to 10 days after surgery. Crutches may be used for up to 3 months, with contact sports avoided until the epiphysis closes to preserve both the repaired hip and the opposite hip, which is at significant risk of slipping. More invasive surgeries may require hip spica casting and longer periods of immobility.

BOX 4-4   Teaching Crutch-Walking to Young Children

1. Gaining the confidence of young children before getting them up to learn to walk on crutches is important. This can be achieved by:
   a. Premedicating the child if pain is likely. Pain always occurs after surgery.
   b. Gaining the confidence of parents or caregivers whom the child trusts.
   c. Sitting and talking or playing with a child for a few minutes before getting the child up.
   d. Telling the child in a straightforward, but not scary way, what you are planning to do, and why.
   e. Being firm with your expectations, yet considerate of the child's feelings.
   f. Using toys, games, or music to engage the young child during the activity.
   g. Using appropriate safety equipment including a gait belt so you will not let a child fall or feel out of control.
2. Use appropriate appliances to help the child learn the skills.
   a. A child younger than 5 years will probably not be able to learn to use crutches, so a pediatric-sized, front-rolling or pickup walker may be most appropriate.
   b. Crutches and walker should be fitted before getting the child up.
   c. For a child with significant pain and/or fears, progressing from parallel bars to a walker to crutches may be most effective.
3. Involve the parent or guardian as much as possible.
   a. Teach the parent or guardian how to help the child get to a sitting position on the side of the bed and how to help the child stand using crutches or walker. The parent should be able to guard the child while walking on flat surfaces, uneven surfaces, and up and down stairs using crutches. Demonstrate the skills with the child, and then observe the parent doing it. It is very important that the parent be successful in learning these skills because the child may need help for several days after discharge until the skills are mastered.
   b. If the child is frightened and uncooperative with you, teaching the parent, grandparent, or sibling to help the child learn the skill is an alternative strategy.
4. Measuring for crutches or walker.
   a. The height of the crutches should be two finger widths shorter than the child's axillae. The height can be estimated, then fine tuned when the child first stands.
   b. The handpads of the crutches should be placed so that the child's elbows are slightly bent when standing with the crutches. This way, when the elbows are extended fully, the child will lift him or herself up off the ground slightly.
   c. A walker height should be between the child's waist and hip level. The height will depend on the child's skills and confidence.
5. Teaching ambulation skills.
   a. Standing up and sitting down in a chair should be the first skill that is learned.
      • From sitting, a child should hold the walker or crutches in one hand and place the other on the armrest or seat of the chair. The child should scoot his or her bottom to the front of the chair. Weight should be placed through the good leg while the arm pushes off the chair. The arm holding the crutches or walker should be used for balance only.
      • Sitting down should be accomplished using the same steps in reverse. Put the crutches or walker in one hand, reach back for the chair with the other hand, and gently lower to sitting.
   b. Walking on flat surfaces.
      • The weight-bearing status of the child should be ascertained and followed (none, partial, as tolerated). The child should firmly grasp crutches with hands. Elbows should be held close to sides to stabilize the crutch tops against the ribs. Weight should not be borne through the axillae but through the arms from the hands. Move the crutches forward, push down through the crutches and swing body either to the crutches or through them for a longer stride.
      • Guarding should be done from diagonally behind or next to the child. One hand is on the child's shoulder closest to you, and the other is on the gait belt. The priority is to help the child regain balance before a fall, not to catch the child once a fall is imminent.
   c. Going up and down stairs.
      • In going up or down stairs, the therapy provider or parent should guard the child diagonally from behind, or next to the child, in the same manner as on flat surfaces. Do not stand on a lower step than the child, facing up the stairs as a child descends, thinking that you can give the child more confidence and catch him or her if a fall occurs. This is a vulnerable position which puts you both in danger.
      • The "bad leg" and the crutches always move together. The child should go "up with the good and down with the bad." In other words, during ascent of stairs, the good leg moves up before the crutches and the bad leg; during descent of stairs, the bad leg and the crutches move down first together. Move only one step at a time. Do not attempt to take longer strides on stairs.

Physical Therapy Intervention

Physical therapy is generally helpful for children in the acute recovery phase after surgery. Appropriate equipment must be ordered and training provided for its use before the child can be discharged from the hospital. A wheelchair must be rented for a child, or appropriate-sized crutches purchased. If a child is going home in a spica cast, transfer training for parents, and teaching upper extremity exercises to the child to maintain strength and mobility are usually indicated. A home evaluation would be advantageous to assess the home accessibility and help the family determine care for the child at home. A hospital bed and mechanical lift may be needed for a few months to facilitate home care. A child must learn either crutch-walking or wheelchair mobility skills before going home from the hospital (Figure 4-17). See Box 4-4 for methods to teach crutch-walking to children.

Physical therapy consultation may be requested in school to accommodate the needs of the child either on crutches or in a wheelchair because of a large cast. Section 504 of the Rehabilitation Act of 1973 requires that schools accommodate needs of children whose medical conditions may interfere with their educational needs.

After a child comes out of the spica cast, progressive gait training is usually needed to facilitate independent mobility. Strength training and active and passive range of motion, may be needed to regain lost range of motion and strength. Because of funding issues, these services would likely be provided in an outpatient clinic rather than the home or school. It would be advantageous for the child if the therapy provider communicated with the child, family, and teacher to learn about stairs at home and school, uneven surfaces the child is likely to negotiate, and other obstacles that may be encountered throughout the day.

Role of the PTA

The PTA may be involved with the child with SCFE in the hospital as an inpatient or outpatient, home care, or at school. Ordering equipment, providing mobility training, teaching and monitoring range of motion and strengthening exercises, or consulting about environmental adaptations may all be needed interventions from the PTA. Communication with the entire team of people affected by the child's injury is very important to make appropriate decisions about equipment and activities. A dietitian, teacher, physician, and nurse may all be involved with the child and family. Behavioral issues of poor cooperation, poor motivation, and difficulty dealing with pain or adversity are not uncommon with children who have SCFE; and the teacher or family members may be able to offer good strategies to address these potential behavioral problems.

The Child With
Infectious Disease of the Hip

Several forms of infectious disease of joints can affect children as young as a newborn. The hip is a common site of infection, but these diseases may also attack other joints, particularly the knee. Hips are affected more in children than adults, probably because children have a better blood supply to the joint. In this section problems that osteomyelitis and sepsis may cause in children's hips are addressed.

Osteomyelitis

Osteomyelitis is an infection of bone and is most common in children from birth to 5 years of age. The most common sites of osteomyelitis in children are the distal femur and proximal tibia (knee), but it can also affect the proximal femur including the greater trochanter and femoral neck, as well as the innominate bone of the pelvis. It is caused by a bacterial microorganism such as *Staphylococcus, Salmonella, E. Coli,* and *Streptococcus,* and is usually spread through the blood rather than contracted directly through an open wound. Another site of infection, such as in a cut or scratch on the skin, can be the point of entry of the infectious agent into the blood.

Children generally develop a high fever, chills, pain over the affected bone, and swelling and tenderness over the site of infection. It is important to treat the bacterial infection immediately because bone destruction can occur rapidly and lead to lifelong problems of deformity and dysfunction.

Treatment includes immediate antibiotics, immobilization of the affected joint, and needle aspiration or surgical drainage of the infection. Children are usually admitted to the hospital for intravenous antibiotics and close observation to ensure that the infection does not spread to other bone sites.

Septic Joint

A septic joint often accompanies osteomyelitis, but it is differentiated from it because immediate aggressive treatment is even more imperative. It may also occur without osteomyelitis. A septic joint is similar to osteomyelitis, except the bacterial infection is in the joint itself rather than the bone. The joint surfaces, therefore, are at extreme risk of being destroyed by the infection, causing deformity and resultant dysfunction that could have lifelong consequences. The hip is the most common joint affected in young children. Infection can be introduced by an adjacent osteomyelitis; another infection elsewhere in the body, such as an ear infection; or an external agent introducing the infection directly into the joint, such as a needle or a surgical instrument during surgery. Infectious agents are the same as those for osteomyelitis, but *Haemophilus influenzae* can also cause septic arthritis in young children.

The child usually has a high fever and irritability and may refuse to walk or move the affected joint. The joint is warm, swollen, and is usually held in flexion. Older children and adolescents may present with milder symptoms.

Treatment involves immediate intravenous antibiotics, as well as aspiration and drainage of the infection. Children are admitted to the hospital for intravenous antibiotics, surgical drainage of the affected joint, and close observation.

Physical Therapy Intervention in Bone and Joint Infections

Physical therapy may be involved initially when the child is an inpatient in the hospital for gait training, strengthening, or parent training in lifting and carrying the young child (Figure 4-18).

Although the illness is orthopedic in nature, young children run the risk of developmental delays when significant sensory inputs, such as walking and actively exploring, are limited in their lives for extended periods. Therefore caregivers should be encouraged to foster independence in the child, to provide stimulation through reading and conversation, play with the child, and to nurture the child while movement is restricted. Because most children will catch up to their peers fairly quickly after a brief illness, these interventions are especially important for those who need extensive recovery time.

> Weighting the base of a rolling walker with sandbags can provide the extra stability a child needs to be successful at balancing with a walker.

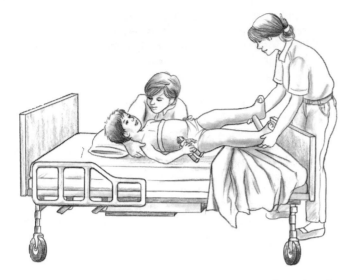

Figure 4-18 Lifting a young child in a spica cast can be tricky. The child's trunk and head should be supported fully, and the cast should be supported to prevent injury to the child or breakage of the cast.

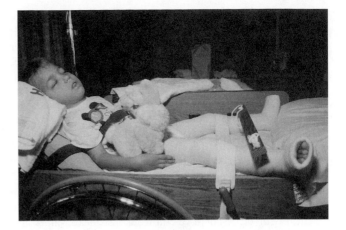

Figure 4-19 Andrew, a 5-year-old child with cerebral palsy, had bilateral adductor releases to prevent his hips from subluxing or dislocating. He is in bilateral full-length casts attached with a wooden bar to maintain abduction, sometimes called broomstick casts. He also had heel cord releases, which is why his ankles are casted at 90 degrees.

Physical therapy may work with children on a longer-term basis if joint or bone damage ensue from the initial infection. Gait training, strengthening, range of motion, and functional skills all need to be addressed in a child who loses function after an acute infection.

Developmental Disorders of Hip Development

Chronic disabilities of the neuromuscular system including cerebral palsy or myelomeningocele, as well as disorders of the musculoskeletal system including arthrogryposis and osteogenesis imperfecta, may affect a child's ability to bear weight, stand, or walk. Acquired neurological injuries, such as traumatic brain injury or early childhood spinal cord injury, can also affect a child's ability to bear weight through the lower extremities and use these limbs for mobility. Medical disorders affecting other systems in childhood can also affect the musculoskeletal system and include juvenile rheumatoid arthritis, sickle cell disease, or hemophilia. Children with these types of disabilities who have had significant limitations in standing and walking may also have atypical patterns of hip development. Atypical hip development may also be affected by abnormal muscle pull from spastic muscles. These children may be more susceptible to hip problems later in life, such as subluxation or dislocation, than children with typical motor experiences.

Children with cerebral palsy, in particular, have been documented to have more femoral anteversion, as well as a greater neck to shaft angle of the femur than children without cerebral palsy (Chung, 1981). Acetabulae of children with developmental disabilities are also generally more shallow than others. These differences have been postulated to be caused by the lack of typical stresses (weight bearing, muscle pull) on the joint, which in a growing child help to mold the femur and acetabulum as they develop. The excessive neck to shaft angle, shallow acetabulum, and excessive anteversion of the femoral head and neck cause the femur to be less stable in the acetabulum. Decreased structural stability plus asymmetrical muscle pull in a child with cerebral palsy can cause the femur to sublux or dislocate, especially during growth spurts when the bone to muscle length is changing (Figure 4-19).

Much has been written about the benefits of passive standing for children with cerebral palsy and other developmental disabilities. Stuberg (1992) described the benefits of standing on bone density in young children with cerebral palsy, finding that standing 45 minutes three times daily can prevent loss of bone density.

No studies have documented benefits of standing on hip alignment or hip geometry for children with cerebral palsy, myelomeningocele, or other developmental disabilities. Some PTs believe that passive standing in young children can improve joint angles to promote greater stability in the hip.

APPLICATIONS   Multicultural Aspects of Physical Therapy Intervention

Jordan, a 4-year-old Filipino-American boy recently diagnosed with Duchenne's muscular dystrophy, is always late for his physical therapy appointments at a medical center clinic. His large family usually arrives between 1 to 3 hours late and expects to be accommodated. Susan, his therapist, manages to fit them in, sometimes at the expense of her lunch hour; she harbors negative feelings about Jordan and his family for their lack of consideration. She struggles with providing appropriate treatment to Jordan who sometimes enjoys playing, but frequently acts out, refuses to cooperate, or hides in a corner of the room. The family members, who all come into the therapy room, are not effective at disciplining Jordan although they frequently discipline his younger brother who is also very active. The 2-year-old brother is made to sit quietly for the entire hour session. Jordan's mother and grandmother sit quietly during the session and listen to what they are told, but they ask no questions. Susan decides that they would not be able to do home exercises with him, so she gives them none. She feels ineffective with this family and frustrated.

What Is Culture?

Although many definitions of culture abound, most include the shared values, assumptions, and ideals of groups of people. Richard Brislin (1993) defined culture as the "ideals, values, and assumptions about life that are widely shared among people and that guide specific behaviors." Other features identified by Bris-

lin include that culture is created by people, transmitted from generation to generation, taught by respected elders through childhood experiences, not frequently discussed, and changes slowly. Although shared values exist for a long time in society and can be identified in oral and written traditions such as literature and the arts, many are invisible to the everyday eye.

Generally members of a culture can identify overt values about their own culture. These could include the value of family as a cohesive unit, education, physical strength, or beauty. Without some understanding of an individual's or a family's cultural perspectives, a health care provider from another culture can make mistakes in recognizing shared overt values. For instance, Jordan's family and Susan both appeared to value the American health care system. Susan works within the system, and the family is availing themselves of services she provides. Other more subtle values could be exerting their influence on Jordan's family, however, such as respect for authority rather than respect for

TABLE 4-4 Comparative Cultural Values and Assumptions*

Cultural consideration	European-American culture	Pacific cultures
Time orientation	Time is short. More concerned about the future. Being on time is important.	Time is plentiful. More concerned about today.
Family size and roles	Nuclear family is central.	Family includes extended family and the community. Children may live with other relatives.
Education	Academic education is highly valued.	Age and life experiences mean more than academic achievement.
Social orientation	Individual is important. Privacy and democracy are valued. Equality and informality are valued. Competition is the norm.	Relationships between people are important. Society is hierarchical with formal relationships. Social roles are ascribed by birth, inheritance, family name or role. Social relationships are cooperative.
Health	Disorders of the mind and body are separated. Technology and science are relied on for diagnosis and treatment.	Health is related to spiritual variables. A poor relationship with God may lead to birth defects, poor health. Native health practices are used to supplement Western medicine.
Child development	Individual children are nurtured, and children are expected to achieve. Child development monitored, and developmental milestones are noted.	Children are highly valued. Child development is viewed in terms of culturally relevant events. Delays in development may not be identified or seen as a problem.
Handling of conflict	Public agencies are intended to serve the people. Individuals must agitate to get what is rightfully theirs. Conflict is handled directly.	Conflict is dealt with through formal channels of elders, family relationships, or formal mediation.
Religious/ spiritual life	People have personal control over the environment and can direct their health and well-being. Many religions are practiced and tolerated.	Many people are Christian. The church is very important. Relationship with God is central.

*These values are presented in a simplified fashion to demonstrate that differences exist between cultural groups. Individual families' adherence to values presented can be affected by factors such as immigration status, social or class level, level of education, and rural or urban experience. Each family is unique, as are individuals within families. Values may differ significantly from those presented here.

the American health care system. Susan cannot assume that they share these values without more information.

Other values are more covert and may not be identified easily by members of a culture. Brislin called these values "assumptions." Jordan's family, for instance, felt that if they arrived within a few hours of their appointment, they were within a reasonable time limit. Susan, on the other hand, felt that they were significantly late. It is unlikely that either party would have recorded their version of timeliness in a list of values common to their culture. Other examples of covert values could include standards of cleanliness; public display of personal habits (belching, scratching) or intimate behavior (holding hands, kissing); and nonverbal communication including eye contact, posture, and physical distance in interpersonal encounters. Assumptions about cleanliness direct how frequently we bathe; those about personal habits affect our interpretation of observed behaviors; and assumptions about physical space direct how close we stand

to someone during a conversation. If these assumptions are not clear between people of different cultures, possibilities exist for misinterpretation.

The United States—A Cultural Melting Pot or a Pluralistic Society?

Because the emphasis in America is generally on the individual (Bhawuk, 1992; Hofstede, 1986), seeing the shared practices that form our culture is sometimes difficult. But as Hanson (1992) points out, "the cultural backgrounds and practices of immigrants from the British Isles and Western Europe, as well as the conditions and opportunities encountered in the new land, shaped the major cultural values and practices of the American people" (p. 71). Some European-American cultural values and assumptions are listed in Table 4-4, along with values and assumptions from several other cultural groups for comparison.

TABLE 4-4 Comparative Cultural Values and Assumptions—cont'd

Native American cultures	Latino/Hispanic cultures	Filipino culture
Time is plentiful. Time and place are settled, not changing.	Relaxed about time. Taking enough time with someone indicates respect. Hurrying indicates disrespect.	Although time commitments are honored, family and other commitments may take priority.
Family includes supportive friends and helpers. Elders and spiritual leaders are respected. Families may be nuclear outside the reservation and extended on the reservation.	Family is central. Spanish influence dictates traditional roles of the father as material provider and the mother as child care provider. Extended family may include godparents, neighbors, and friends.	Family is central, including several generations. The family is relied on for love, support, and refuge. It is the source of one's personal identity. Men and women have equal but different roles.
Education that incorporates native language, values, and traditions is valued.	Education is a route to acculturation and is valued as a path to success.	Academic education is highly valued.
Group life is primary. Individuals take responsibility for family and personal sphere.	Class is very important. People are very sensitive to interpersonal relationships. Collective style rather than individualistic style of family and community life is usually practiced.	Age, power, prestige, and wealth are important social considerations and dictate levels of authority.
Health has multiple causes, some of which may be spiritual. Tribal rituals and practices may be practiced to prevent or ameliorate ill health or disability.	Use of folkhealers is common. Disability may be seen as caused by evil thoughts or a hex from someone with jealous or covetous feelings.	Indigenous and modern health care are used simultaneously; however, people from rural areas tend to know more about and use folk practices more.
Children are respected and are taught autonomy at a young age. They participate in decision making and rituals with the family. These occasions may be marked with gifts.	Families are nurturing toward children and permissive and indulgent with young children. Children are not pushed into achieving. Girls are protected.	Children are loved and nurtured. Early years are characterized by indulgence and lack of adult anxiety about performance. School-aged children are expected to help at home and do well in school.
Group consensus is very important. Time is taken to hear and examine all aspects of an issue. Sometimes a third party can help with language or cultural interpretation.	Respecting others is important. Anger, aggression, and negative feelings are not tolerated in children. Authority is vested in older members of society and in males.	Harmony is essential. Achieving smooth interpersonal relationships can take precedence over tasks or conflict resolution. Individuals in authority are asked to help make decisions.
The interconnectedness of all things, with people being a small part of the larger fabric of the universe, is a central belief of many groups.	Many families with Latino cultures are Catholic. Folk beliefs regarding warding off evil are also widely practiced.	Because of Spanish influence, many families are Catholic. Others are Protestant, Islamic, and Buddhist. Ancient folk rituals may also be practiced.

American practices may differ from those of minority people who bring with them values and assumptions from their own culture. When cultures interact, both the dominant culture and the minority culture are affected.

The United States as a country was formed by people who had emigrated from other countries and has continued to accept immigrants from all over the world. Therefore the cultural mix is quite diverse. Our communities include members of immigrant or voluntary minority groups, involuntary minority groups who lived here before other immigrants arrived and were conquered, and those involuntary groups who were imported against their will (Ogbu, 1991). Involuntary minorities include Native American people, Native Alaskan people, Native Hawaiian people, some Mexican-American people, and many African-American people.

Many communities in the United States reflect significant diversity in their ethnic makeup. For example, in 1990 Los Angeles had a population of 52.8% white, 39.9% Hispanic, 14% black, 9.8% Asian or Pacific Islander, and 22.9% other ethnic groups. New York City's ethnic mix was 52.3% white, 28.7% black, 24.4% Hispanic, 7.0% Asian or Pacific Islander, 0.4% American Indian/Eskimo/Aleut, and 11.6% other groups. Smaller communities in states with a higher percentage of white members also have significant numbers of population with diverse ethnic characteristics. In most communities the percentage of the population of white members has dropped between 1980 and 1990, and the percentages of members of diverse ethnicities has increased (Universal Reference Publications, 1993).

The model of America as a melting pot where diverse cultures meld into one cohesive culture is changing to that of a pluralistic model, where many different cultures coexist, each maintaining its own unique qualities. Responses to the dominant culture by minority cultures can vary. Members of immigrant cultures may add features of the dominant American culture to their own, whereas members of involuntary cultures may resist the dominant culture to save their own (Ogbu, 1991). Native and immigrant cultural groups are experiencing a resurgence in ethnic pride; they desire to rediscover lost or faded cultural identity and recreate, strengthen, or maintain values and structures that perpetuate their ethnic origins.

Cultures tend to change and adapt over time, especially when exposed to different values that may challenge traditional beliefs. Henze and Vanett (1993) discuss this evolution as it affects Native Alaskan children trying to reconcile their native culture at home with the European-American culture at school. The authors maintain that a third culture emerges from this conflict and that the model of "walking between two worlds" is too simplistic. In Hawaii, a state with a native population, immigrant groups, and European-American groups, Hormann (1972) identified the development of a new local culture, which evolved as these groups lived together. Jordan's family, being immigrants from the Philippines, shared ethnic cultural values with other immigrant Filipinos. These values may have changed from traditional values in the Philippines.

Individuals are especially affected by challenges to traditional belief structures. Yang (1988) found that as Hispanic families moved to the city and were exposed to values that challenged their beliefs, traditionally strong family ties weakened.

Through these examples it is evident that the American diversity of ideals, values, and assumptions is not static; it is constantly changing with demographic, political, and economic evolution. The models of America as a melting pot or as a pluralistic society may not be adequate to describe the evolution of American culture, which is created by the coexistence and influence of different beliefs and practices on each other. Individuals and families from minority cultures may react differently from each other when exposed to the dominant American culture, depending on their own cultural history, individual personalities, and experiences. Health care providers must keep an open mind and be willing to get to know each individual and family to learn their unique perspectives.

Institutions and Changing Cultural Demographics

Institutions administered by the federal or state governments, as well as many private institutions, tend to reflect the majority culture. Examples of institutions in our society include hospitals, universities and colleges, large businesses, and schools. Values in these institutions usually reflect those in the dominant population. Think of your own acculturation through your schooling. Public and private schools for children expect certain behaviors, such as promptness, turning in work, striving to do one's best, and participating in class. By the time most of us graduate from high school we have learned these behaviors. These same behaviors are expected in college and in the work world, but we are not given as much support from employers, teachers, and administrators to develop these skills. It is assumed that we have learned these expected behaviors. If we are not successful in practicing them, we may not succeed in school, college, or in the business community.

Health institutions. Those who work in the health professions generally have certain values as well. These include that the American/Western system of health care is the best, physicians and other health professionals are to be respected, and patients must follow medical advice to get better. The "medical model" of identifying a health problem and solving it through drugs, exercise, or other therapy is widely accepted among Western health professionals. These assumptions may be significantly different from those of people who work in other settings or who are from diverse ethnic backgrounds. For example, the strategy of educators working with a child with a disability in the schools may be to identify what skills the child needs to succeed. Then services and supports are introduced to help the child develop the needed skills. This approach is different than identifying a child's problems and putting services into place to remediate the problems. Therapy providers who work in educational settings may have to examine their own values and assumptions to work effectively. Unless we all make an effort to recognize our own assumptions, we cannot begin to adequately serve people from backgrounds and in settings different from our own.

Cultural diversity. Institutions such as schools and hospitals reflect America's increasing social diversity, with European-Americans, African-Americans, Asian-Americans, Native Americans, Pacific-Americans, immigrants who are not yet Americans, and others, learning, working, healing, living and dying together. Because of changing demographics in the United States reflecting a significant increase in numbers of families with other than European-American roots (Hanson, 1992), multicultural education in the schools has become a catchword of the nineties. Many programs have been developed to assist students to become more culturally aware, teachers to be sensitive to cultural differences, and school curriculums to reflect the richness of community diversity. A need for these programs continues to exist, indicating that the cultural diversity existing in our communities is not yet reflected in the schools.

With the tightening of health care dollars, medical institutions have not been as responsive as schools to the increasing social diversity in our cities and towns. Community health clinics and those set up to serve specific minority groups, such as Native-American people, have been more responsive. However, the substandard health care that many of our ethnically diverse population receives indicates that there is widespread inequity and lack of sensitivity in the services provided.

Special education. Minority students are overrepresented in special education (MacMillan, Henrick, & Watson, 1988; Reschly, 1988; Turnbull & Turnbull, 1990). Reasons for this overrepresentation may include a higher poverty level among children of minority ethnicities affecting their performance in school (Gottlieb, Alter, Gottlieb, & Wishner, 1994), different learning styles among children of different cultural backgrounds (Bert & Bert, 1992; Tharp & Gallimore, 1988), and a conflict in values that may cause children to resist the values of the school (D'Amato, 1988; Ogbu, 1991; Yamauchi, Greene, Ratliffe, & Ceppi, 1996). Because of this overrepresentation, providers of services to children in special education are working with an increased number of children and families from ethnic backgrounds that are different from their own and with which they may be unfamiliar.

Legislation mandating close working relationships between service providers and families in special education, as well as families in early intervention for children of less than 3 years of age, was passed in the late 1980s (P.L. 99-457, 1986; P.L. 101-476, 1990). The legislation as it affects the practice of physical therapy in the schools and early intervention programs is explored in more detail in Chapter 5. Families are being included more now in the design and implementation of services for their children than in the past. Understanding the values and assumptions of the families we work with, as well as our own values and assumptions, is essential to provide services effectively to all children and their families. We must become more culturally sensitive.

Developing Cultural Sensitivity

When the concept of cultural sensitivity was first broached, it was felt that having information about cultural differences was enough to work effectively with people from different cultural groups. This approach is no longer seen as sufficient in becoming culturally sensitive. The application of cultural sensitivity extends beyond knowledge. Three components of cultural sensitivity are important: (1) knowledge of culture and cultural differences, (2) willingness to bring one's knowledge to interactions with people of different cultural backgrounds, and (3) the ability to take culture into account when interacting with people (Brislin, 1993).

Knowledge

Formal training programs using reading materials, guest speakers, and audiovisual supports can provide knowledge about specific cultures. Formal training programs can be helpful if a large ethnic minority group lives in one's service area or if there have been problems interacting with people from a specific ethnic group. Community leaders from the ethnic group in question may be very willing to assist in presenting information to the staff. Caution must be taken, however, when participating in informational workshops. Workshop presenters may present a "checklist" type of information that promotes token understanding, perpetuation of stereotypes, or generalizations about people from particular ethnic minorities. Informal sources of knowledge including talking to friends and neighbors; reading newspapers, magazines, and books; and talking to families during therapy can also be helpful in gathering information.

Knowledge must go beyond specific facts to an understanding of how people interpret specific behaviors. Jordan's mother, for instance, may interpret the therapist's coolness during the therapy sessions to appropriate professional aloofness and not be aware that there are interpersonal problems. She also may be aware that there is a problem but is not comfortable addressing interpersonal problems directly. Susan's understanding of Jordan's mother's interpretation of the events can help her plan the method to address the perceived problems. She can decide whether to discuss the family's lateness and Jordan's behavior problems with his mother directly, have the receptionist or program director discuss the issues with them, or approach the issue more indirectly in conversation. Susan's understanding of the family's cultural background can help her alleviate her own discomfort with the family in the most appropriate manner.

Willingness

Willingness to use this knowledge in interactions with people from cultures different from one's own implies a comfort level with your own ethnicity and ethnic practices, an acceptance and openness to attitudes and practices different from one's own, and a willingness to learn and make social mistakes. Introspection and group discussion, as well as more formal processes of learning specific practices of other cultures, may be helpful in assessing and developing the willingness to interact appropriately with others of different ethnicities.

Awareness of one's own culture. Because culturally specific principles are taught in early childhood and because of their "invisibility" in everyday life (everyone knows them; there is no need to talk about them), many people are unaware of their own cultural biases. It is therefore important to delve into one's own culture to find the values and assumptions that direct the choices one makes and responses to different situations. Accomplishing this is not as easy as it sounds. Each of us has several cultures in which we live. For instance, ethnicity, gender, work setting, living situation, and community all affect values and assumptions. Each of these factors affects our behavior in a given situation.

Gender is often unrecognized as a cultural group, but this example serves as an appropriate illustration. Years ago I used to come home from work in the evening at about the same time as my husband. Once in a while, we would have the following conversation:

HUSBAND: "Hi, how was your day?"
ME: (Sitting down in a chair) "I had a hard day. I'm really tired."

HUSBAND: "Oh, that's too bad. What's for supper?"

Many of the women reading this will probably experience the same emotions of frustration and anger that I had because I was expected to cook dinner no matter how I was feeling. My husband did not hear my cues and offer to cook dinner himself. Men reading this, however, may feel more sympathetic to my husband, who was surprised when I told him of my feelings. He asked why I did not just ask him to fix dinner. It was not until I read John Gray's *Men Are From Mars, Women Are From Venus* (1992) that I realized we were miscommunicating because of cultural differences. Rather than expecting him to recognize my verbal and nonverbal cues, I now am very explicit with my needs and ask him to fix dinner when I am tired. To his credit, he is always happy to do so!

Ability

It cannot be assumed that we all have the necessary skills to interact effectively with others of different cultural backgrounds. Developing these skills is important to provide effective intervention for children and their families. Formal training programs, which include role playing, using audio or videotapes of culturally sensitive interventions, and using scenarios that challenge commonly held beliefs and assumptions about people from other cultures can be very useful. Informal methods of developing cultural competence can include talking with coworkers and families and practicing specific skills during the work day.

Working With Children and Families

Hanson, Lynch, and Wayman (1990) point out specific information that is helpful when working with children and their families; it includes: (1) knowledge of cultural views of children and child-rearing practices, (2) family roles and structure, (3) views of disability and its causes, (4) health and healing practices, and (5) views of change and intervention. Learning cultural norms of the many different cultural groups with which you work may not be possible, but an open mind, awareness that others may think differently, and a willingness to learn through experience will allow you to learn as you go. Keep in mind that the development of cultural competence is not something that happens all at once, it evolves out of life experiences and is continually changing as your knowledge, level of experience, and comfort develop. It is a lifelong process.

Application to the Case Study

When Susan realized that cultural factors were affecting Jordan's therapy, she tried to find out more about his family by talking with them. She also talked with her friend who had been a social worker in the United States for 10 years but had grown up in the Philippines. The library offered some books that helped her learn more about life in the Philippines. It was important for her to become aware of the family's cultural values and assumptions in general and how their specific life situation may have influenced their application of these practices. She realized that their lifestyle in the Philippines, as well as their new lifestyle in the United States, influenced their values, assumptions, and cultural practices. She found out that Jordan's family moved to the United States from an urban area of the Philippines a year before he was born, and the maternal grandparents followed to join them after Jordan's brother was born 2 years ago. Because of time constraints, Susan was not able to research every aspect of their culture in depth, but an openmindedness and awareness of differences during conversations with the family on these topics helped her to be more sensitive to their perspectives.

When Susan gathered more information about Filipino culture, she was able to open up to the family. As the relationship progressed and Susan listened to Jordan's family, she learned information that helped her to evaluate her own feelings, the family's behaviors, and the appropriateness of the services that Jordan was receiving.

Cultural Views of Children and Childrearing Practices

In the Philippines large families are the rule, and children are the center of the family concerns and efforts. As Susan became more comfortable with the family, she learned how much Jordan's diagnosis affected the family. Because Jordan is the oldest son, many hopes and expectations were placed on him that he will not be able to fulfill because of his illness. With tears, his grandmother expressed her despair that the promise in her oldest grandson will not be fulfilled. His mother expressed a concern for her other children because the disease is hereditary and she is pregnant with her third child. Jordan's brother tested negative, but she is concerned about the baby she is now carrying. She is in the early stages of the pregnancy and has agonized over whether or not to terminate it if she finds that her child is a boy, as she has been advised by the medical profession. Her family is Catholic, and the church plays a large role is her decisions.

In the Philippines children are indulged as infants and toddlers, with a more authoritarian stance emerging as children approach school age. All family members take a role in raising children, but the mother may be the disciplinarian. Jordan, seen by his family as sick and disabled, is indulged even though he is approaching school age. The family is expecting the younger brother to act more grown up because his brother is disabled.

Based on this information, Susan changed her approach to the therapy sessions. Initial therapy time was now spent talking with the family while Jordan and his brother worked out their activity needs from their recent 2-hour bus ride to reach the Medical Center. Susan was able to listen to the feelings, concerns, and fears expressed by the family. She could share information with Jordan's mother and grandmother about muscular dystrophy and Jordan's future, to reinforce and elaborate what they had already been told. Although the family was still struggling with the emotional impact of Jordan's diagnosis, the relationship of trust that developed allowed them to listen to what Susan told them and communicate some of their fears. This time was also a good opportunity for Susan to reinforce ideas about home activities to preserve Jordan's functional skills as long as possible. Susan could then enter into play with Jordan and his brother and shape it into activities that addressed Jordan's therapy goals. Toward the end of the hour, Jordan allowed some direct handling by Susan and his mother for stretching and to demonstrate home activities.

Family Roles and Structure

Men and women have more equal status in the Philippines than in the United States, and families tend to live in extended groups. Relationships between people and hierarchy in the community is very important for Filipino families both in the Philippines and the United States. Community members have specific roles to fulfill in the Filipino community, which are important and help to maintain their status. Jordan's parents share responsibility for his care, although his mother does the day-to-day care because she is home with him. Grandparents also help in the home. As Jordan gets older and needs more personal care, such as help with bathing or toileting, his father may take a more active role. The family comes to therapy appointments as a group so they can all be informed of Jordan's progress and can support one another.

Views of Disability and Its Causes

In the Philippines disability is generally seen as a stigma. This view may be modified depending on whether the family lived in an urban or rural area and, after they moved to the United States, their level of acculturation into the American community as a whole. Disability is believed to be caused by natural or supernatural events, for example, eating the wrong things during pregnancy or divine retribution for sins against God. Having a disabled child can cause embarrassment in the Filipino community and may cause some loss of status. Jordan's father did not accompany the family to his therapy sessions, perhaps because of conflicts with his work, but also possibly because he was embarrassed to be seen with his disabled son and wanted to protect his status in the community.

Susan was able to communicate some of this information to other team members involved in Jordan's care. She recommended, with the family's support, that Jordan be discharged from the medical center outpatient therapy services as soon as he could be evaluated by the department of education and enrolled in a preschool classroom at his neighborhood school. There, therapists and teachers could work together to support his educational, emotional, behavioral, and gross motor needs as his disease progresses. The stress on the family of taking full day trips to receive physical therapy services would also be alleviated. Perhaps the community contact at the neighborhood school would allow his family to understand more of the American attitude toward disability and shift their own views to accommodate the new perspective. Education was highly valued by his family, and the prospect of Jordan starting school held out hope for the future.

Health and Healing Practices

In the Philippines Western medicine is used simultaneously with Filipino folk medicine. People from urban areas tend to rely more on the Western practices of doctors and drugs, whereas people from more rural areas have a stronger reliance on traditional healing practices. Folk healers may refer a family to a doctor if they have not yet been seen by the medical profession. Folk practices may include traditional healing such as Chinese oils, massage, and supernatural (faith) healing. Jordan's family did not discuss their use of Filipino healing techniques or healers with Susan or any other medical providers. They saw their use of healers as completely compatible with using the Western system of health care.

Views of Change and Intervention

The relationship between the family and the therapy provider is very important to the Filipino family. It is important for the health provider to maintain an authoritative role, yet be personable so that give and take can occur. Susan had to "be sensitive to the family's desire for acceptance and an appropriate level of emotional closeness, allowing for reciprocity which preserves the family's 'face' and dignity" (Chan, 1992). When Susan overcame her negative feelings and was more sensitive to Jordan's family's needs, the relationship was able to develop. The family became more of a partner in Jordan's therapy.

In the Philippines interventionists are expected to act in an authoritarian role and offer practical advice. Thus Jordan's family responded better to Susan when she took control of Jordan's behavior during the therapy session. They also responded when Susan finally gave them activities to do at home with him. They followed through on all his exercises even though it was difficult at times.

Language

Language differences can affect the provision of services to a family of differing ethnic background. Language differences imply not only speaking a different language, but also differing communication styles and habits. Although Jordan's family appeared to speak fairly good English, their actual language skills varied between Jordan's mother and grandparents. His mother spoke the best English, but her skills were limited by poor vocabulary. All of the family members relied heavily on nonverbal communication including body language, expression of eyes, and intuitive understanding. These realms of communication were outside Susan's experience, and she initially interpreted their silence as uncaring or unable to participate. Once she had made an effort to understand their communication styles and when she facilitated acquiring an interpreter for one or two sessions, she was able to understand more fully the family's concerns and better communicate her own goals to provide more effective therapy for Jordan.

Conclusion

To work more effectively with culturally diverse families, a therapy provider needs to (1) learn more about the family's culture, (2) be willing to change the approach to the family to accommodate their different beliefs and attitudes, and (3) learn how to interact differently in a way that respects a family's unique perspectives. Through these efforts a therapy provider can appropriately address a child's physical therapy needs, avoid frustration and negativity in a relationship, and learn in the process. The lifelong learning that working with culturally diverse families engenders can be stimulating and fulfilling.

Although a therapy provider's knowledge and skills regarding cultural diversity are important, it is the willingness to learn and the openness to other ways of thinking and acting that can make the difference in developing a relationship with a family from a different cultural background. Both formal and informal routes of information and training can be helpful, and the family members themselves can be a powerful source of information. With the increasing cultural diversity in our cities, towns, schools, and hospitals, it is important that we are all willing and open to develop the skills needed to work effectively with our diverse neighbors.

EXERCISES

1. Learn to walk on crutches, including areas of flat surfaces, stairs, and uneven surfaces.
2. Learn advanced crutch-walking skills, such as jumping or walking with no weight bearing through either leg.
3. Teach a school-aged child to use crutches. Share with your classmates some strategies that work to teach a young child to use crutches.
4. Work in a group with your classmates to position each of you upright on the tilt table and raise it to an upright position. How do you feel as you are coming to the full upright position? Can you think of some strategies to help a child cope with this situation?
5. Write an exercise program for a young child in a spica cast. What muscle groups will you include to strengthen? Why? How will you address the child's endurance? How will you structure the exercise program so the child will be more likely to comply?
6. Talk with someone who grew up in a different cultural context than you. Discover similarities and differences in your backgrounds, traditions, views of disability and health, and childrearing practices.

QUESTIONS TO PONDER

1. A teenager with cerebral palsy is a household ambulator with a rolling walker. He has pain in his right hip with ambulation. His physician has recommended a femoral osteotomy to prevent recurrent subluxation of the hip. The child will be in a spica cast for 8 weeks after surgery, will have a leg length discrepancy, and may lose his ambulation skills as a result of surgery. Should the family go ahead with the surgery or not? What do you need to consider to help the family make this decision? Is there a right or wrong answer?
2. A teenager with Legg-Calvé-Perthes disease is not compliant with her exercise program. She is not gaining back the strength and function that has been hoped. Should you make the effort to increase her compliance, or does she have the right to decide her own level of participation? What options do you have to increase her compliance?
3. Should families with diverse cultural orientations have to learn the language and culture of the dominant society, or should members of the dominant society accommodate to other's differences? Why or why not?

Annotated Bibliography

Rothstein, J. M. (Ed.). (1992). *Pediatric orthopedics: An American Physical Therapy Association monograph.* Alexandria, VA: American Physical Therapy Association.

This monograph from the APTA is a compilation of articles addressing pediatric orthopedics that were originally published in the December 1991 and January 1992 issues of *Physical Therapy.* Although not specifically addressing management of disorders of the hip, the articles discuss current treatments and assistive devices for children with disabilities ranging from scoliosis, juvenile rheumatoid arthritis, limb deficiencies, cerebral palsy, and myelomeningocele. Articles discuss newer procedures, such as the Ilizarov procedure for limb lengthening, as well as orthotics and prosthetics for children. This compilation of articles provides an excellent overview of physical therapy management techniques for children with a range of orthopedic disorders.

Lynch, E. W., & Hanson, M. J. (1992). *Developing cross-cultural competence: A guide for working with young children and their families.* Baltimore: Brookes.

This book describes cultural practices and beliefs of individuals from eight different ethnic backgrounds. These descriptions are useful in learning about the different cultures. They emphasize early intervention and working with families of young children with disabilities. The authors also discuss issues related to working with families of young children from different cultures, including culture identity, culture shock, and the development of cross-cultural competence. Although working with families of young children is emphasized, much of the information presented here is also applicable to families of older children or adults with disabilities.

References

Barker, D. J. P., & Hall, A. J. (1986). The epidemiology of Perthes' disease. *Clinical Orthopedics, 209,* 89.

Bert, C. R. G., & Bert, M. (1992). The Native Americans: An exeptionality in education and counseling. Miami: Independent Native American Development Corp. (ERIC Document Reproduction Service No. ED 351-168).

Bhawuk, D. P. S. (1992). The measurement of intercultural sensitivity using the concepts of individualism and collectivism. *The International Journal of Intercultural Relations, 16,* 413-436.

Brislin, R. (1993). *Understanding culture's influence on behavior.* Orlando, FL: Harcourt Brace.

Catterall, A. (1971). The natural history of Perthes' disease. *British Journal of Bone and Joint Surgery, 57,* 37-53.

Chan, S. (1992). Families with Filipino roots. In E. Lynch & M. Hanson (Eds.), *Developing cross-cultural competence: A guide for working with young children and their families* (pp. 259-300). Baltimore: Brookes.

Chung, S. M. K. (1981). *Hip disorders in infants and children.* Philadelphia: Lea & Febiger.

D'Amato, J. (1988). "Acting": Hawaiian children's resistance to teachers. *The Elementary School Journal, 88,* 529-542.

Dunn, P. M. (1976). Perinatal observations on the etiology of congenital dislocation of the hip. *Clinical Orthopedics, 119,* 11.

Gray, J. (1992). *Men are from Mars, Women are from Venus.* New York: Harper Collins.

Gottlieb, J., Alter, M., Gottlieb, B. W., & Wishner, J. (1994). Special education in urban America: It's not justifiable for many. *The Journal of Special Education, 27*(4), 453-465.

Jarre, R., Billing, L., Hansson, G., Karlsson, J., & Wallin, J. (1996). Bilaterality in slipped capital femoral epiphysis: importance of a reliable radiographic method. *Journal of Pediatric Orthopedics, British, 5*(2), 80-84.

Hanson, M. J. (1992). Families with Anglo-European roots. In E. Lynch & M. Hanson (Eds.), *Developing cross-cultural competence: A guide for working with young children and their families* (pp. 65-83). Baltimore: Brookes.

Hanson, M. J., Lynch, E. W., & Wayman, K. I. (1990). Honoring the cultural diversity of families when gathering data. *Topics in Early Childhood Special Education, 10*(1), 112-131.

Henze, R. C., & Vanett, L. (1993). To walk two worlds—or more? Challenging a common metaphor of native education. *Anthropology and Education Quarterly, 24,* 116-134.

Hofstede G. (1986). Cultural differences in teaching and learning. *The International Journal of Intercultural Relations, 10,* 301-320.

Hormann, B. L. (1972). Hawaii's mixing people. In N. P. Gist & A. G. Sworking (Eds.), *The blending of races* (pp. 213-236). New York: Wiley & Sons.

Hummer, C. D., & MacEwan, G. D. (1972). The coexistence of torticollis and congenital dysplasia of the hip. *American Journal of Bone and Joint Surgery, 54,* 6, 1255.

Leach, J. (1994). Orthopedic conditions. In S. Campbell (Ed.). *Physical Therapy for Children.* Philadelphia: W. B. Saunders.

Loder, R. T. (1996). The demographics of slipped capital femoral epiphysis: An international multicenter study. *Clinical Orthopedics* 322: 8-27.

MacMillan, D., Henrick, I., & Watson, A. (1988). Impact of Diana, Larry P., & P. L. 94-142 on minority students. *Exceptional Children, 54*(5), 426-432.

Molloy, M. K., & MacMahon, B. (1966). Incidence of Legg-Perthes disease. *New England Journal of Medicine, 275,* 988.

Morrissy, R. T. (1990). Slipped capital femoral epiphysis. In R. T. Morrissy (Ed.), *Lovell and Winter's Pediatric Orthopedics* (3rd ed.) (pp. 885-904). Philadelphia: J. B. Lippincott.

Mubarak, S. J., Beck, L., & Sutherland, D. (1986). Home traction in the management of congenital dislocation of the hips. *Journal of Pediatric Orthopedics, 6* (6), 721-723.

O'Brien, E.T., & Fahey, J.J. (1977). Remodeling of the femoral neck after in situ pinning for slipped capital femoral epiphysis. Journal of Bone and Joint Surgery (American), 59 (1), 62-68.

Ogbu, J. (1991). Immigrant and involuntary minorities in comparative perspective. In M. Gibson & J. Ogbu (Eds.), *Minority status and schooling: A comparative study of immigrant and involuntary minorities* (pp. 3-33). New York: Garland.

Price, C. T., Day, D. D., & Flynn, J. C. (1988). Behavioral sequelae of bracing versus surgery for Legg-Calvé-Perthes disease. *Journal of Pediatric Orthopedics, 8,* 285-287.

Ralis, Z., & McKibbin B. (1973). Changes in the shape of the human hip joint during its development and their relation to its stability. *British Journal of Bone and Joint Surgery, 55*(4), 780.

Ramsey, P. L. (1973). Early diagnosis and treatment of congenital hip dislocation. *Jefferson Orthopedic Journal, 2*(1), 37.

Reschly (1988). Minority MMR over representation and special education reform. *Exceptional Children 54:* 316-323.

Salter, R. B. (1961). Innominate osteotomy in the treatment of congenital dislocation and subluxation of the hip. *British Journal of Bone and Joint Surgery, 43,* 518.

Stuberg, W. A. (1992). Considerations related to weight bearing programs in children with developmental disabilities. *Physical Therapy, 72*(1), 35-40.

Tharp, R. G., & Gallimore, R. (1988). *Rousing minds to life: Teaching learning, and schooling in social context.* New York: Cambridge University Press.

Turnbull, A. P. & Turnbull, H. R. (1990). *Families, professionals, and exceptionality: A special partnership.* New York: Macmillan.

Universal Reference Publications. (1993). *America's top-rated cities: A statistical handbook, Vol. 2.* Boca Raton, FL: Author.

Walmsley, T. (1915). The neck of the femur as a static problem. *Journal of Anatomy and Physiology* 10,314.

Weinstein, S. L. (1990). Legg-Calvé-Perthes disease. In R. T. Morrissy (Ed.), *Lovell and Winter's pediatric orthopedics (3rd ed.)* (pp. 851-884). Philadelphia: J. B. Lippincott.

Yamauchi, L. A., Greene, W., Ratliffe, K. T., & Ceppi, A. (1996, April). *Native Hawaiians on Moloka'i: Culture, community and schooling.* Paper presented at the meeting of the American Educational Research Association, New York, NY.

Yang, K. S. (1988). Will societal modernization eventually eliminate cross-cultural psychological differences: In M. Bond (Ed.), *The cross-cultural challenge to social psychology* (pp. 67-85). Newbury Park, CA: Sage.

5

Developmental Orthopedic Disorders

CASE STUDY — Camila, A Young Girl With Juvenile Rheumatoid Arthritis

"Mommy, you stand over there, and, Meghan, you stand over there." Camila pointed to two areas of the patio and directed her mother and a neighbor to hold onto two ends of a long jump rope. She stood carefully in the middle. "I'm ready now, swing!" As the rope came up over her head, she jumped, her feet barely leaving the ground and the jump rope catching on her ankles. "No! Do it again!" she shouted, standing stubbornly in the middle of the jump rope and waiting for it to swing. The next time the rope swished under her feet in perfect timing for one jump, but it caught one ankle as it lagged too late for the second jump. "Again, again, please." She looked pleadingly at her mother. The rope swingers exchanged glances, smiled, and swung again and again as Camila tried to master the skill of jumping rope (Figure 5-1).

Early Childhood

Camila was the first child of her Brazilian mother, Marizete, and American military father, Kenneth. Even when she was pregnant, Marizete worried about her unborn child. Around 10 weeks into the pregnancy, the baby turned and Marizete had some spotting. The doctor told her not to worry. During an early diagnostic ultrasound the power shut off in the middle of the procedure, and Marizete worried that maybe the baby had received an electric shock. The fetus did not move much, but Marizete's English was not good enough to express her concerns to her doctor. So she waited and worried. Camila was born 2 weeks early via Cesarean section. She was a big baby, weighing 7 pounds and 8 ounces at birth. Kenneth was away at this time on a 6-month sea duty and did not meet his daughter until she was 5 months old.

Marizete was very happy and proud of her beautiful daughter. She wrote Kenneth and sent him pictures of Camila. Her fears subsided as Camila learned to suck on her fist at 2 weeks old and sucked her thumb at 1 month. Then at 1 month old, Camila's foot got caught in the car door by accident. Marizete was horrified, but the doctors assured her that the baby's foot was fine. Marizete watched carefully, and the bruises healed. She relaxed again as Camila gained more skills, learned to roll over, and played with toys.

When Camila was 6 months old and her father was stationed in the Persian Gulf, Marizete's worries returned. Camila started having fevers and a rash that looked like little pimples on her chest and stomach. The doctors could find no reason for the fevers, and Camila's growth was slowing down according to her 6-month well-baby checkup.

She gradually recovered from the fevers, and she learned to stand at the coffee table when she was only 7 months old. Her mother was very proud and wrote to Kenneth describing Camila's exceptional skills. By 9 months of age Camila was putting her feet up in the air to be kissed by mom. Kenneth was home then and could witness this wonderful skill for himself. Marizete still had nagging worries about her daughter though. Camila cried frequently and Marizete could not always console her.

When she was 10 months old, Camila stopped standing. Marizete felt that Camila was trying to stand, but that she was hav-

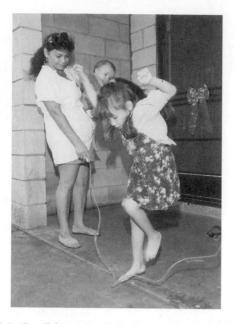

Figure 5-1 Camila's mother helps her to develop balance and strength through play.

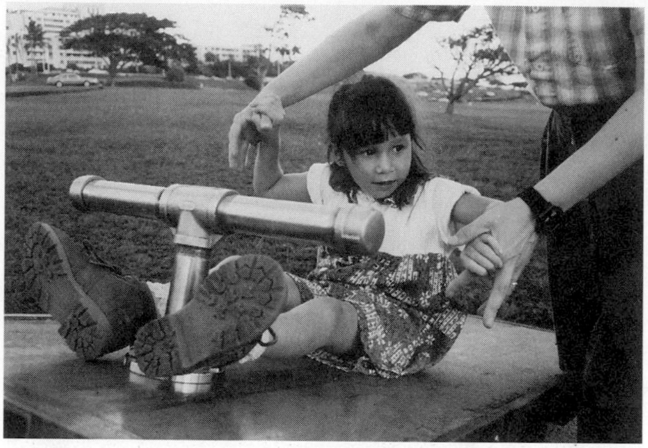

Figure 5-2 Camila's abdominal muscles are not strong enough for her to sit up without help. Working on outdoor athletic equipment can be fun and a change from the same old routine.

ing pain; her feet also seemed swollen. Although Kenneth thought that Marizete was overreacting, Marizete took Camila to the doctor anyway; she was told that Camila had normal feet and the swelling was from mosquito bites. When she was 11 months old, Camila developed a more prolonged fever. Her fever was very high at night; although still elevated, it was lower during the day. Her legs felt cold all the time. At first the doctor told Marizete that Camila had bronchitis and gave her antibiotics, but the fevers continued. When Marizete insisted that the doctor check her further, x-ray examinations were done of her feet, and she was referred to a hematologist. Finally a diagnosis was made of pauciarticular juvenile rheumatoid arthritis (JRA).

Although Marizete felt that her concerns were finally being taken seriously, she was devastated about her daughter's diagnosis. She was told that Camila had a 50% chance of growing out of her illness by the time she was 5 years old. She was referred to a rheumatologist who specialized in treating children and to a physical therapist (PT) and an occupational therapist (OT) with experience in treating children with JRA.

Marizete kept Camila at home rather than sending her to daycare or preschool so she could care for Camila and give her the attention she needed. Because Marizete was not comfortable driving, an OT and a PT alternated weeks coming to their home to provide therapy when Camila was less than 3 years old. Marizete gave her daughter naprocyn twice a day and did the strengthening and stretching exercises with her at home that the therapists suggested. At 2 years old Camila walked fairly well with a normal two-year-old gait pattern. As she grew older, however, her joints stiffened and her gait pattern changed. She started to walk without bending her left knee, especially in the morning when she felt the most stiff. She fell frequently, and her mother worried about her playing with other children. The family had a large dog at home that made Marizete nervous, but the dog was very careful with the fragile child. Camila's diagnosis was changed to polyarticular JRA when more joints became in-

flamed. Camila's medication was changed to methotrexate once a week, but she did not have much improvement. Camila was outgoing and active and became frustrated when she faced physical limitations from the JRA.

When Camila was 3 years old, her mother started taking her to the hospital weekly for therapy services. Transporting her there every week was difficult because it was a 40-mile drive each way, and Marizete was not comfortable driving in the city; but she did the best she could.

Camila enjoyed swimming in the pool that was available to residents of their apartment complex. The therapist told her mother that swimming was very good exercise for Camila, so they tried to swim on the days that were warm enough. Camila wore inflatable cuffs on her upper arms and was fairly independent in the water with supervision. Marizete also made sure that Camila got outside everyday to walk and play in the park or to play with neighborhood children (Figure 5-2). Camila became good friends with one child, and they played frequently at each other's homes. Marizete also took the children for picnics to the beach.

By the time Camila turned 4 years old, both wrists were subluxed, several fingers had deformities, and she had a very stiff gait. She wanted to be able to do everything, however, and ran using a hopping motion. Both parents encouraged Camila to do whatever she wanted, although her mother was more protective. Her parents gave her an electric jeep to drive around the neighborhood when they went for walks. She was a daredevil in it, but she never had a serious accident (Figure 5-3).

Camila's younger brother Cody was born in the middle of her fourth year. His arrival started a series of changes for Camila, which included starting kindergarten and, a few months after that, moving to a larger apartment in a new neighborhood and a new school. Her father also retired from the military during this year, and the family had to decide whether they would stay in the same state or move closer to family members in another state. He was able to obtain a well-paying civilian job with the military as a jet mechanic, however, and they decided to stay for awhile.

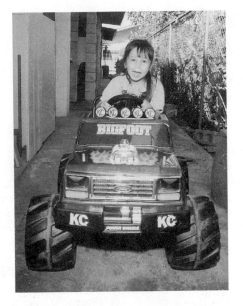

Figure 5-3 Camila's electric vehicle allows her freedom to roam the neighborhood.

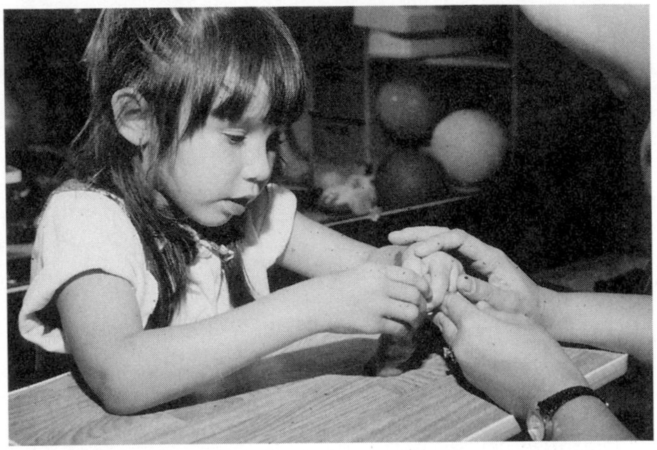

Figure 5-4 Although Camila's joints are unstable, she needs to improve strength in her intrinsic hand muscles to help her with daily tasks such as brushing her teeth or cutting with scissors. Therapeutic putty is a fun medium to work with!

BOX 5-1 School Activities and Accommodations for Camila

1. Adapted learning tools will be provided for Camila, including large pencil grips, large eraser that she can hold with her fist, adapted scissors, and large-diameter crayons.
2. Her workstation will be adapted so that Camila is closer to her work without having to use excessive neck flexion. An angled desktop with a clip that holds her work and a trough for her writing/coloring utensils will be provided.
3. A thick carpeted area for floor sitting will be provided for the entire class. In this way Camila will not be singled out to sit on a soft cushion when the class sits on the floor.
4. Camila will wear thick-soled shoes to school to protect her feet during outdoor activities.
5. The teacher will be aware of Camila's limitations in gross motor activities and will modify activities that Camila is unable to do, such as creeping on hands and knees, bear walking, tip-toeing, and somersaults, to activities that will challenge balance, strength, and coordination, such as giant steps, side stepping, side skipping, obstacle courses, gliding, and rolling.
6. The school nurse will give Camila her medication when needed.

Camila at School

Camila was young for her kindergarten class; her birthday fell just before the end of December. She was also small for her age and more physically fragile than her classmates. However, she was friendly and eager to participate fully in whatever kindergarten had to offer.

Because of her medical needs, Camila was tested by special education for related services needed to support her educational program, as well as her needs for educational support (Figure 5-4). Cognitively she was age appropriate; and although she had some gross motor and fine motor delays related to her arthritis, she was close enough to age level in many of her skills to preclude her qualifying for physical therapy services. Her speech articulation was found to be immature, resulting in initial approval for speech-language therapy, but these services were never provided. By the time her, individualized education program (IEP) meeting was held 3 months after school started, the team believed that her speech had improved enough that she no longer qualified for services. The school district decided that Camila did not qualify for direct occupational therapy services, but they agreed to monitor her needs intermittently to ensure that she was maintaining the skills necessary to participate in school.

Camila enjoyed school very much. She liked the academic portion of school and the social exposure as well. She became enamored with drawing and felt a keen sense of accomplishment when she could write letters and her name! She made cards and drawings for relatives and friends. She was very outgoing in school and enjoyed participating in the Thanksgiving presentation for family and friends. She had a role singing with her class. After Thanksgiving Camila's family moved to a new neighborhood so they could live in a larger apartment. Camila had to change schools and leave behind many of her new kindergarten friends. Her mother was pleased with Camila's new teacher and her new school, however. Camila quickly made new friends, although she missed her best friend from her old neighborhood and her previous teacher, whom she had liked.

Camila's new teacher wanted to learn what Camila could and could not do. She asked Marizete for information about JRA and about Camila's disease process specifically. Marizete asked Camila's PT to come in and speak with the teacher about what would help her in the classroom. Box 5-1 summarizes some of the activities and accommodations that were developed by the PT, the teacher, and Marizete working together. Unfortunately

BOX 5-2   Physical Therapy Evaluation Summary: Camila

Social and Medical History
Addressed in the Case Study.

Range of Motion
All within normal limits (WNL) except for limitations in the following:

Upper extremities
Wrist flexion: 70 degrees on right; left is WNL
Wrist extension: 45 degrees on left; right is WNL
Wrist ulnar and radial deviation: both limited on left 5 to 10 degrees; WNL on right
Forearm pronation and supination limited 5 to 10 degrees, left more than right
Left hand fingers: -20 degrees index DIP extension; -10 degrees ring PIP extension
Right hand fingers: -20 degrees ring MP extension; -15 degrees little PIP extension

Lower extremities
Bilateral decreased passive midfoot mobility; slight forefoot adduction, left >right
Slight flexion deformities toe PIP and DIP joints

Posture
Anterior pelvic tilt with resultant slightly excessive lumbar lordosis in standing position.
Both hips in internal rotation in standing position.

Muscle Strength, Tone, and Bulk
Muscle tone is WNL. Strength is difficult to assess because of Camila's age. It is generally fair- to fair+ throughout with specific difficulties noted in hip extension against gravity (F+), knee extension against gravity (G-), ankle plantarflexion against gravity (F-), and toe extension against resistance (F+).
Muscle bulk is lean throughout with girth measurements lower on all aspects of the left lower extremity than on the right by approximately 0.5 to 1 cm.

Reflexes and Developmental Reactions
Camila has functional static balance skills in sitting and standing. In standing her dynamic balance is only fair, with reactions tending to be slightly delayed, and overcompensation for slight challenges to her balance. Because of decreased strength and joint stiffness, she is unable to complete some age-appropriate balance activities such as walking on a balance beam without support.

Gait
Camila walks with a stiff-legged gait. She has excessive arm swing and tends to circumduct her left hip rather than swinging it straight through. Upper extremities tend to move into a mid-guard position, especially when she is feeling insecure. In the morning Camila walks with her left leg stiff at the knee. She is able to do a modified run, which is asymmetrical, with her jumping off a stiff left leg and pushing off on a bent right leg. Occasionally she is able to run more symmetrically.

Functional Skills
Camila can ascend stairs using the railing with a step-to (mark time) pattern leading with her left foot. When descending the stairs, she leads with her right leg and uses the railing for upper extremity support. With effort she is able to manage a symmetrical gait ascending 3 to 4 steps in an alternating pattern without using the railing. She can ride a bicycle with training wheels at least 20 feet on a level surface and is able to get on and off the bicycle independently. She can jump with both feet only briefly leaving the ground at the same time, but the left foot trails significantly and sometimes does not leave the ground. She can throw and catch an 8- to 9-inch ball and can throw (but not catch) a 3-inch ball. She can run as described above. She can stand on one foot briefly but is not yet able to skip.

Adaptive Equipment
- Bilateral custom foot orthotics worn inside her shoes to provide arch support, forefoot alignment, and toe alignment
- Bilateral resting hand splints that position the wrists in dorsiflexion and support appropriate alignment of the fingers for nightwear
- Day splint for the left wrist to maintain dorsiflexion and neutral lateral deviation to counteract tendency for ulnar deviation and flexion

Activities of Daily Living
Camila's self-care skills are generally age-appropriate, except for not being able to fasten small buttons or snaps. She needs extra time to fasten large and medium buttons as well. She needs help with teeth brushing for thoroughness because of weakness, poor wrist stability, and her age. She sometimes needs help to turn faucets on or off.

Summary
Camila is a bright, active child with significant joint deformities, especially in her wrists and fingers, for a child of this age. She has delays in gross motor skills resulting from difficulties in standing balance and jumping skills; she has limitations in fine motor skills requiring strength and mobility of her wrists and fingers such as cutting, pulling, and pinching. Camila has a vivid imagination and a strong will.

DIP, distal interphalangeal joint; *MP,* metacarpal phalangeal joint; *PIP,* proximal interphalangeal joint.

Camila was not able to obtain any services from occupational therapy through the school or the medical center, so her PT addressed her fine motor needs as well as her gross motor needs.

Camila's Physical Therapy

Camila continued to see her PT weekly. The military paid for Camila's therapy and medical services, even after her father's discharge. During her therapy sessions Camila played games and did exercises to help her maintain her range of motion and strength. The therapist informed the physician and the parents of any changes and adapted her therapy as needed. This was important because Camila rarely complained of pain. She obviously had pain because of the changes in her gait, her joints, and how she performed tasks such as climbing or running. Her mother thought that Camila did not complain because she did not like to go to the doctor. Camila did not like to talk about her arthritis or how she felt. She preferred to ignore her illness and to focus on activities and events that were fun. Her mother had to guess by Camila's actions how she was feeling. Marizete was taught exercises to do at home with Camila, as well as precautions to help keep Camila's joints healthy for as long as possible. The therapist also monitored Camila's resting wrist splints that she wore at night. Camila did not like to wear these splints, so her mother would come in after Camila was asleep to put them on. Box 5-2 summarizes the PT's most recent evaluation. Box 5-3 elaborates

some of the home exercises that Marizete was taught to do with Camila since she was diagnosed at the age of 1 year.

Some examples of games she played with the PT included "catch" with a fabric "loop"-covered ball on paddles that were covered with "hook" fabric (Figure 5-5). Camila wore 1-pound weights on her forearms when she played this game. Through

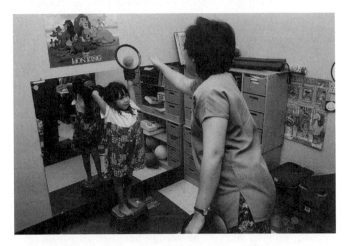

Figure 5-5 Games during therapy help Camila improve her dynamic standing balance and her range of motion. Cuff weights add extra resistance.

BOX 5-3 Home Exercises for Camila

1-2 Years Old

1. Sit Camila on your lap facing you. Gently bounce her up and down on your knees while tipping her side to side slowly as you sing to her. This exercise will encourage her to use her own trunk muscles to straighten up to make them stronger.
2. Encourage Camila to reach up for toys, food, and other items so that she reaches her arms up above her head and goes up on her toes. This movement will help her to keep her shoulders flexible and will strengthen her calf muscles.

2-3 Years Old

3. Encourage Camila to walk and push her own stroller as far as she can. Do not always carry her when she asks; push her a little to develop her strength and endurance.
4. Play ball with her. Use a soft, flexible ball that she can easily grasp. Encourage her to squeeze the ball between her forearms and squeeze it with her fingers. Help her roll the ball all over her body and all over your body. These activities will help her develop strength in the small muscles of her hands (by gripping the ball), strengthen her shoulder muscles (by squeezing the ball between her forearms), and move her arms through their complete range of motion (by rolling the ball over her body).

3-4 Years Old

5. Play games such as "follow the leader" with Camila. Include activities such as marching with high steps, side stepping, turning around with each step, squatting to touch the ground or pick something up off the ground, and standing on one leg.

6. Play ball with Camila. This can include kicking a soft ball back and forth to each other, playing catch with a soft 6- to 8-inch ball, or even rolling a ball to each other while sitting on the floor. All these activities will help Camila to develop her strength, balance, and motor coordination.

4-5 Years Old

7. Take Camila someplace where she can ride her bicycle for a long distance on a flat surface safely (e.g., park, track, sidewalk). Make sure that she is wearing her helmet and that the training wheels are secure so she will not fall. Knee pads or long pants are suggested to avoid injury if she should fall. Encourage her to ride around obstacles, ride fast enough so that she gets out of breath, and ride for a long time. You can be on your bicycle with her, encouraging her; you can be an obstacle, allowing her to chase you; or you can chase her. This activity will help Camila develop some strength in her legs, endurance for sustained physical exertion, and motor coordination through riding and steering her bike.
8. Help Camila learn to pump a swing. If needed, you can put a soft foam "handle" around the chains or rope of the swing so she can grip it better. You can use foam insulation or pipe insulation, which is usually available at the hardware store. If you use it, make sure that you wrap duct tape around it securely so it does not come off in her hands! Then she can learn to pump with her trunk and legs to get the swing to go higher. This activity will help her improve her balance, and strength in her arms, trunk, and legs.

playing she could improve her arm strength as well as her active range of motion by reaching for the ball. When Camila stood on a low bench to play, the game also helped her to improve her balance. Another of her favorite games was working on a felt board. Small shapes and figures of colored felt could be placed on a fabric board. The board was put at the top of a flight of steps, and Camila wore 1-pound weights on her ankles as she traveled up and down the steps to place all the figures on the board and create her own scene. The therapist helped keep Camila's interest in the activity by talking with her about the scene she was creating. She also closely monitored Camila's frustration and fatigue levels and modified the activity if needed.

Camila at Home

At the new apartment Camila shared a room with her baby brother, Cody. The apartment was one of several in a large house in a residential neighborhood. Other children lived in the house as well, and Camila soon became friends with a 3-year old boy who thought she was wonderful. On a narrow paved area at the side of the house and a wide area at the front of the house, Camila would ride her bicycle with training wheels or drive her electric jeep after school. She liked to hold her baby brother in her lap while she drove her jeep, although her mother hovered closely when allowing this at all! Camila preferred to go on walks through the neighborhood with her parents rather than stay in the yard.

Camila's dream was to go ice and roller skating, but her mother resisted taking her because she was afraid she would fall and injure herself (Figure 5-6). For Christmas her father brought home a pair of inline skates. Camila was thrilled! They came with a helmet, elbow and knee pads, and wrist guards, which her mother insisted that she wear. Camila did not have the strength, balance, or skill level at first to skate without her mother or father holding tightly to her; but she aspired to skate without any help at all. Her mother was nervous about supporting Camila by holding her hands because of the risk of increased joint damage at her wrists and fingers, so she supported her at her trunk holding under her arms from behind. Although this was difficult and awkward for both of them, it was safer for Camila's joints. Marizete was not comfortable with this activity of Camila's at all, but she yielded to her daughter's pleading demands and hoped that no injuries would occur.

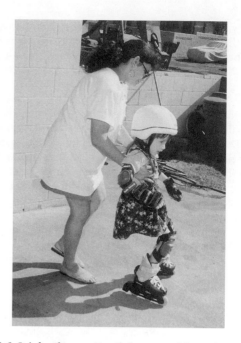

Figure 5-6 It is hard to see Camila because of the pads, but at least her joints are somewhat protected against a fall on concrete when learning to roller skate.

At her fifth year checkup, Marizete asked the doctor about Camila's prognosis with the JRA. Her pain and joint deformities seemed to be getting worse, not better. When Camila had first been diagnosed, she had a 50% chance of growing out of the disease; and Marizete wanted to know what Camila's present chances were. The doctor replied that he didn't know. Marizete took a deep breath and glanced over at her little daughter. Camila was limping across the waiting room, holding her left leg stiffly. She held her arms up at her sides and carried a toy between her forearms. Her wrists were obviously subluxed. Camila was singing to her 8-month-old brother, grinning as she brought him a toy. She leaned down beside Cody, who was sitting on the floor, and tried to teach him to suck his thumb. Cody preferred to suck his fingers, but Camila had been trying to get him to change. Marizete smiled. What a determined little girl!

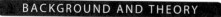

BACKGROUND AND THEORY

Some children are born with, or develop during childhood, orthopedic disorders that extend beyond one joint. The disorders may be primarily orthopedic in nature or may also be related to a neurological process. These disorders can affect development in many domains. Multiple joints and limbs may be involved with diverse effects, depending on the cause and process of the disability or disease process itself and whether the disorder developed in utero or in early childhood. Functional skills such as mobility, self-help, grasping, or sitting may be impaired. Neurological or medical conditions related to the orthopedic impairment may cause problems with attention, schoolwork, or social behaviors. The therapy provider may work with children with any

of these disabilities in a school, a clinic, a hospital, or at home to help address functional limitations caused by their disorder.

This chapter addresses the developmental disorders of congenital limb deficiencies, spina bifida, arthrogryposis, and JRA. Although spina bifida is classified as a developmental orthopedic disorder in this book, it is usually classified primarily as a neurological disorder. The orthopedic nature of the consequences of the neurological deficits, however, make it fit equally well in this chapter. The incidence, etiology, and clinical presentation of these disorders are discussed, as well as the role of physical therapy, in general, and the physical therapist assistant (PTA), specifically, in their management.

A case study of Camila, a young child with JRA, demonstrates some of the practical problems a child with JRA faces when starting school. A special section on the changing role of physical therapy in school addresses laws related to the provision of related services in school, differences between a medical and an educational model of intervention, and the effects of ideas such as inclusive education on the provision of physical therapy in schools. The importance of working in teams and models of intervention such as consultation and collaboration are also discussed.

Congenital Limb Deficiencies

Children with congenital limb deficiencies (CLD) or amputations may be affected minimally, such as having two fingers fused together, or greatly, such as missing all or most of their limbs. Children missing portions of even one limb need to make substantial adaptations to achieve functional skills as growth and maturation occur. This section defines a classification system for limb deficiencies and outlines the role that physical therapy plays in helping children achieve functional skills.

Causes

When genetics plays a key role in congenital limb deficiencies, other abnormalities, such as cleft lip and palate, small mandible, and thoracic and spinal deformities, may also occur. Many different genetic syndromes have been implicated in patterns of skeletal abnormalities in children (Jones, 1988), but in 60% to 70% of cases, the cause is unknown (Brent, 1985).

Environmental influences are thought to cause 10% of limb anomalies. The limb buds develop during the third to seventh weeks of embryonic development. Development occurs in distal structures first, then in proximal structures a few days later. Any teratogenic influence during this period may have catastrophic effects on the developing limb. The manifestation of the deficiency depends on the exact time of the introduction of the teratogen during development. Known teratogens include certain drugs, irradiation, viral infections, and some contraceptives.

A well-known teratogen causing limb deficiencies is the drug thalidomide, which was prescribed in the late 1950s and early 1960s for nausea in early pregnancy. Mothers used the drug during a vulnerable period of development for their fetuses. This drug was sold and prescribed in third-world countries even after its effects were recognized, and it was banned in Europe and the United States. Therefore young adults with thalidomide-induced limb deficiencies in the Philippines and other developing countries are generally younger than their counterparts in Europe and the United States (Figure 5-7).

Clinical Features

Classification. Although other methods have been used to describe congenital amputations, the international standard, which was published by the International Society for Prosthetics and Orthotics (ISPO) in 1973 and modified in 1989, is generally accepted throughout the world. Older methods including Greek terminology or classification based on embryological failure have been abandoned in favor of the ISPO standard, which reflects

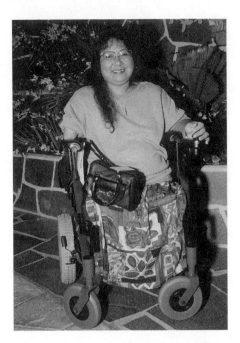

Figure 5-7 This young woman from the Philippines developed congenital limb deficiencies in three limbs after her mother took thalidomide for nausea during pregnancy. She has recently learned to drive with custom-adapted equipment.

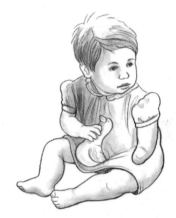

Figure 5-8 A child with a transverse limb deficiency of the upper extremity.

anatomical classification and is easily applied to radiological studies.

Two major groups are identified: those with transverse deficiencies and those with longitudinal deficiencies. A transverse deficiency describes a limb that has developed normally to a certain point, with structures beyond that point missing. For example, a child's upper extremity has a fully developed humerus but no ulna, radius, carpal, metacarpals, or phalanges, except for perhaps some residual nubbins (Figure 5-8). This below-elbow type is the most common transverse deficiency. Most transverse deficiencies are unilateral.

A longitudinal deficiency describes a limb that is missing elements in the long axis of the limb. An example of a longitudinal deficiency is a child who is missing the radius and thumb in one

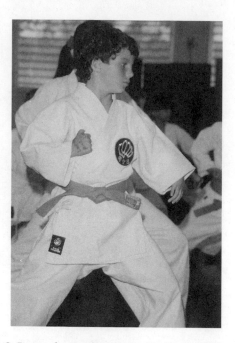

Figure 5-9 Ryan, a boy with a longitudinal limb deficiency of his upper extremity, can participate in karate with some modifications. He also pitches on his baseball team.

upper extremity, with the ulna, carpals, and other digits present (Figure 5-9).

Children may have one or more limbs with any level of deficiencies. From 20% to 30% of children with CLD are affected in more than one limb (Tooms, 1985), but the level may vary between affected limbs. For example, a child may be missing a radius and thumb in the right arm and missing only a few phalanges in the left arm.

Clinical presentation. Clinical presentation of CLD varies according to whether it is transverse or longitudinal, the level of the deficiency, and the number of deficiencies or limbs affected. Certain problems, such as ligamentous absence or laxity, absence of supporting structures such as bones and muscles, soft tissue contractures, or muscle weakness caused by a decreased lever arm or decreased length-to-strength ratio of the muscle, may impact the functional skills of children with CLD.

Several patterns of limb deficiencies have been identified and classified. One type of lower extremity limb deficiency is proximal femoral focal deficiency (PFFD). Proximal femoral absence or hypoplasia (underdevelopment) is accompanied by varying involvement of the acetabulum, femoral head, patella, tibia, and fibula. Aitken (1969) described four classes (A through D) of PFFD, depending on the extent of involvement of the structures (Table 5-1). The incidence of this type of CLD is one in 50,000 live births (Herzenberg, 1991). Clinical presentation of a child with PFFD is with the thigh abducted, externally rotated, and flexed. The child may have hip and knee flexion contractures. The foot is held in equinus; because of the shortened femur, the foot may be at the level of the opposite knee or may be amputated to allow for a better prosthetic fit (Figure 5-10). Associated problems may include scoliosis, patellar absence, femoral bowing, and congenital arm amputation (Chung, 1981). This disability occurs bilaterally about 15% of the time.

Aitken Classification of PFFD

TABLE 5-1	
Class	**Description**
A	• Femoral head present • Acetabulum normal • Short femoral segment • Femoral head is in acetabulum • Contiguous femur • Subtrochanteric varus angulation • May be subtrochanteric pseudoarthosis
B	• Femoral head present • Acetabulum may be dysplastic • Femur shortened • Femoral head is in acetabulum • No bony connection between head and shaft of femur
C	• Femoral head absent or represented by bony remnant (ossicle) • Acetabulum severely dysplastic • Femur shortened, usually tapered proximally • Femoral head not in acetabulum • Femoral shaft and bony ossicle may be connected by bone
D	• Femoral head absent • Acetabulum absent • Femur shortened and deformed • No connection between femur and pelvis

PFFD, Proximal femoral focal deficiency.

Another pattern of disability involves presentation of a fully formed distal portion of the limb and missing proximal portions. The child may have a normally formed shoulder with a hand attached. The humerus, radius and ulna are missing. A comparable deficiency in the lower extremity is exemplified by the child with a fully formed pelvis, absence of the femur, tibia and fibula, and a fully formed foot. This type of deficiency was formerly called phocomelia, based on time of embryological insult; but it is now classified as a transverse deficiency. The pattern of deficiency can be explained by the fact that distal structures are formed before proximal structures embryologically.

Treatment

Surgical treatment of the child is directed at enhancement and preservation of functional skills for the child with CLD.

Amputation. For a child with CLD in an upper extremity, amputation is not generally indicated. A surgical amputation may provide more stability and function for a child with a lower extremity CLD, however. If one lower extremity is significantly shorter than the other and a foot deformity exists that precludes stable weight bearing, amputation of the foot may allow use of a lower extremity prosthesis for standing and walking.

Arthrodesis. Other types of surgery useful for a lower extremity CLD include knee arthrodesis or fusion to allow increased stability of the limb, especially if the femur is significantly short, such as in a child with PFFD.

Rotationplasty. For children with good ankle and hip mo-

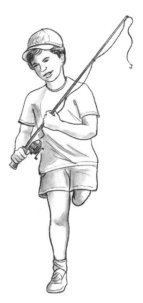

Figure 5-10 A child with proximal femoral focal deficiency.

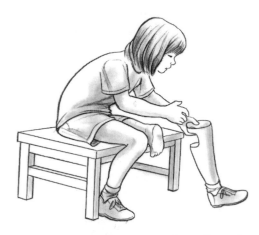

Figure 5-11 The child with a rotationplasty allows the ankle to function as a knee joint.

tion, a rotationplasty may be a functional alternative to increase function. The knee joint is removed by excising the distal femur and proximal tibia; then the entire lower leg is rotated 180 degrees. This allows the ankle joint to act as a functional knee, and a below-knee prosthesis can be used (Figure 5-11). Functional skills are greatly enhanced with a below-knee prostheses, with improved weight bearing through the existing foot; the child can usually participate in sports and recreational activities. A negative effect of a rotationplasty is reduced cosmesis. The child and family need to become accustomed to the foot facing backward. Also, if the surgery is performed on a child younger than 10 years, it may need to be repeated because of spontaneous derotation or the development of a varus deformity of the knee in children without a fibula (Chung, 1981).

Tendon transfers. For children with longitudinal deficiencies of the upper extremities, tendon transfers may allow more functional hand use. An opposable thumb is necessary for a pincer grasp to pick up and manipulate objects and for a strong grip. Appropriate tendon transfer surgery allows surgeons to either create an opposable digit or to improve function in existing structures.

Physical Therapy Intervention

Physical therapy for children with CLD is directed toward helping the child develop appropriate functional and developmental skills while reducing any secondary impairments, such as soft tissue contractures. Depending on the age of the child, the extent of the limb deficiency, and the intervention needed, therapy may be provided in the home, at school, or in an outpatient rehabilitation clinic. The therapist should be working with a team of individuals—including the family, child, orthopedic physician, prosthetist, OT, and teacher—to assess in what environments the child needs to function and what skills the child needs to develop. The team can help to develop or identify natural activities for the child to practice functional skills in a supportive environment.

Physical therapy for the infant and toddler. Therapy goals for young children should be appropriate for their developmental age. Very young infants should be seen primarily to teach caregivers how to handle the child to encourage normal exploration and learning through movement. Encouraging symmetrical movements, weight bearing, and posture during the infant years are important for an infant with an intrinsically asymmetrical limb deficiency. Symmetrical strength, orientation, and range of motion can be facilitated by encouraging reaching with bilateral upper extremities, rolling to both sides, pushing up to sit from both directions, turning and reaching to both sides in sitting, and weight bearing through all extremities in a variety of positions.

Many children with congenital limb deficiencies can benefit from a prothesis to improve their functional skills. Research has shown that children who learn to use prosthetics early develop greater motor development than children who are introduced to prosthetics at a later age (DiCowden, Ballard, Robinette, & Ortiz, 1987). As the child begins to sit independently and to bear weight through the lower extremities, the prosthesis can be introduced. Therapy may need to be more frequent when the prosthetic device is introduced to teach caregivers how to use and care for it, as well as how to encourage normal developmental activities while using the device.

A child with an upper extremity limb deficiency should be fitted with a preliminary prosthesis by the time the child is 6 to 8 months old. This is the developmental stage when the child is sitting without support and using hands to reach and play with toys. Because an upper extremity prosthesis changes the child's balance in sitting, it may require a period of adjustment. Becoming accustomed to the changes in balance and tolerating the device are initial goals. A child may ignore the prosthesis initially but gradually will begin to use the device for weight bearing when pushing up to a sitting position or propping to reach for toys with the other hand. The child may begin to use the device to move or hold larger toys that do not need grasping.

A young child with PFFD or another type of lower extremity limb deficiency should be fitted with a preliminary lower extremity prosthesis by the time the child is at a developmental age to stand. By 8 to 10 months of age a typically developing child is usually pulling to stand at furniture and may be beginning to "cruise." If surgery is necessary to amputate a nonfunctional foot

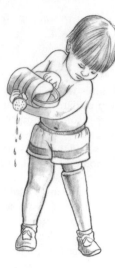

Figure 5-12 A young child is usually fitted with a preliminary lower extremity prosthesis that does not have a knee joint. Using the device, a child can experience initial weight bearing and can explore the environment.

that would otherwise impede function, or if surgery is necessary to fuse the knee, it is performed at this age. When the surgical sites heal, a preliminary prosthesis with no knee is fitted to the child; the child is encouraged to bear weight through both legs while playing (Figure 5-12).

> ☀ If you are working with a child who is included in a regular education class, offer to lead a group activity for the entire class, and teach the educational assistant (EA) in the classroom to help the student or students who need assistance. In this way you can integrate therapy activities into a class with even a very resistant teacher and teach the EA essential skills that will be useful even when you are not there.

Physical therapy for the preschool and early school-aged child. When the child enters school, the therapist can meet with the teacher to help adapt the environment or the activities in the school for the child. Some examples of adaptations that may be necessary or helpful include raising or lowering the chair height so that the child can have the optimal angle for writing or drawing with an upper extremity prosthesis, forming the tables or desks into islands so the child using crutches does not need to negotiate individual tables or desks, or adapting circle games so the child using crutches can play. The teacher also needs to learn how to assist the child in donning and doffing the prosthesis.

When the child begins to play with toys with both hands, a simple terminal device ("hand") that will grasp and release objects can be introduced. A child may begin to learn to use a terminal device by 15 to 18 months of age (Figure 5-13). By 3 or 4 years a child should learn how to operate the elbow in an above-elbow prostheses. A dual cable system allows the child to flex and extend the elbow, and to pronate and supinate the forearm.

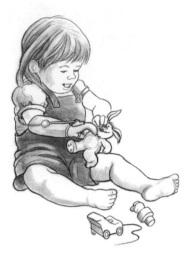

Figure 5-13 A child will learn to use the terminal device on an upper extremity prosthesis first to release and then to grasp objects.

By the time a child with a lower extremity limb deficiency approaches 3 years of age, he or she may be ready to learn to operate a simple prosthetic knee. A child may need to use a walker when first walking with a prosthesis but will progress to walking independently as balance and skill improve. A walker may help the child who is learning to use a lower extremity prosthesis to maintain the trunk in an erect posture and to use a full reciprocal gait pattern. Children younger than 5 years are not generally able to use crutches.

A myoelectric upper extremity prosthesis is operated by electrical signals from residual muscles, which activate electrodes in the socket. The electrodes activate a motorized hand. If a child is to operate this type of device successfully, it should be introduced by the time the child is 5 to 6 years old (Sauter, 1989). This type of device is more cosmetically acceptable, but it is heavy and expensive. The benefits and potential problems of this device should be weighed carefully by the entire team, especially the family, before a decision is made on its use.

The therapist should be monitoring the fit of the prosthetic device, range of motion of related joints, and strength of related muscles to ensure optimal functional skills. Skin problems related to poor fit may take a long time to heal and may have an adverse affect on the child's perception of the prosthesis. The therapist should be working closely with a prosthetist during the child's growing years.

Role of the PTA with the infant, toddler, preschool, or early school-aged child. The PTA may work with the PT to teach the young child with CLD developmentally appropriate movement transitions and mobility skills, such as rolling, pulling to stand, and walking. In a transdisciplinary situation the PTA will also be working on reach and grasp, self-care skills, and language and communication with the young child. The child may or may not be using a prosthesis. Services may be provided in the home, clinic, or school.

Physical therapy for the school-aged child and adolescent. Therapy for a school-aged child or adolescent should be focused on problem-solving to help the child participate in activities with peers. Most children will be fairly good at problem solving for themselves. Family members, by this time, will also be veteran

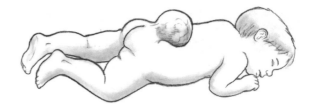

Figure 5-15 An infant with a myelomeningocele looks as if he has a sac on his back.

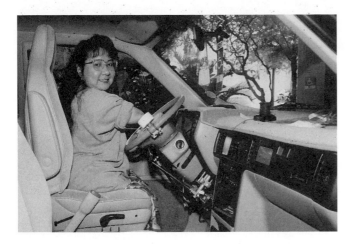

Figure 5-14 Lourdes, a young woman with three limbs congenitally amputated, worked hard with a team to learn to drive with adapted controls.

problems solvers. History provides some excellent role models for children with limb deficiencies; for example, Jim Abbott, a professional baseball pitcher for the California Angels who has a transverse amputation of one arm. Children can accomplish almost anything.

A young child will usually use a prosthesis if it is purchased for him or her, if adults help the child learn to use it, and if adults supervise and support its use. When the child grows older, the prosthesis may be too cumbersome, energy intensive, or cosmetically unappealing to use on a regular basis. The child, especially one with a bilateral upper extremity deficiency, may develop other means of achieving functional goals. The child may learn to use feet, mouth, or chin for dressing, feeding, grooming, or completing schoolwork. Other forms of assistance such as computers, service animals, or attendants may prove to be more energy efficient than a prosthesis.

As a child grows older, advanced gait activities such as running, jumping, and skipping can be mastered. Children with below-knee prostheses will master these skills more easily than those with above-knee prostheses, who need to learn to control the extra knee joint. An older child may decide that a lower extremity prosthesis is too much work and may prefer to use forearm crutches for mobility. This is especially true for children with an above-knee prosthesis (see Chapter 12, Case Study: Caroline, A Girl Recovering From Cancer). Their wishes should be respected.

As a child grows into an adolescent, other challenges, including learning to drive, dating, and playing competitive sports, may arise. The adolescent with a prosthesis may be able to compete, depending on the sport, with athletes without amputations. Another avenue for athletic participation is the Paralympics, the international sporting event for athletes with disabilities that has been held in parallel with the Olympics for the last two Summer Olympics (Barcelona in 1992 and Atlanta in 1996). The Paralympics are gaining increased recognition as an elite athletic venue (Scheck, 1996).

Learning to drive may be accomplished by using adapted controls, which would vary depending on the limb(s) affected and the capabilities of the learner. The Americans with Disabilities Act (ADA) guarantees that people with disabilities can rent vehicles,

and many car rental agencies are making adapted hand controls available to those who need them (Tatum, 1996). Some creativity and patience may be needed, however, both to adapt a private vehicle and to rent a car or van with adapted controls. The resources of a rehabilitation center with adapted driving instruction may be helpful to decide which adaptations would be appropriate and to learn specific skills to drive safely (Figure 5-14).

Role of the PTA with the school-aged child and adolescent. Problem solving, checking prosthetic fit, and communicating with team members are important activities during this time. A child may need training when learning to use a new or more advanced prosthesis, strengthening exercises to learn new skills, or range of motion to try to correct contractures that have developed. The PTA can be an important member of the team working with a child and family as a child moves through elementary school and high school and approaches many of the challenges leading to adult life.

The Child With Spina Bifida

Myelodysplasia, myelomeningocele, congenital spinal cord defect, and *neural tube defect* are all terms used to describe spina bifida, a group of congenital malformations of the vertebrae and spinal cord. Spina bifida refers to malformed vertebrae (spina) that do not close completely and look as if they have divided in two (bifida). The malformed vertebrae may not be visible, and the infant appears normal at birth. This type of lesion is called occulta, or not visible. The malformed vertebrae may allow tissue to protrude from the spinal canal and form a sac, either skin covered or not, which may contain nerve tissue. This type of lesion is called aperta, or visible (Figure 5-15). The sac is called a meningocele if it does not contain functional nerve tissue and myelomeningocele if it contains damaged nervous tissue. Children with a myelomeningocele generally have some degree of paralysis of their legs because of nerve damage. (Table 5-2 presents a description of the different types of spina bifida and associated problems.) Most of the information in this section addresses the problems of children who have myelomeningocele, because they have the most serious neurological damage, more severe orthopedic problems, and need the most help throughout life.

A range of disabilities can occur from this congenital defect, depending on the level of the defect, its severity, and associated problems such as club foot, hydrocephalus, and paralysis. Children with spina bifida grow, change, and develop, and they need changing supports as they mature. The PTA can provide many of these supports to the child and family.

TABLE 5-2   Classification of Spina Bifida

Spinal defect	Neurological classification	Level of disability	Functional prognosis
Occulta (not visible)	No tissue protruding from non-fused spinous processes	None	Excellent. Usually no neurological or orthopedic problems.
Acculta (visible)	Meningocele—although tissue protrudes in a sac, neurological tissue is rarely involved	None	Excellent. Usually no neurological or orthopedic problems.
	Myelomeningocele—abnormal neural elements are part of protruding sac	Depends on levels of involvement	Innervation of neck, upper limb, shoulder girdle, and trunk musculature.
		Thoracic levels	No volitional lower limb movements are present. For lesions below T10, lower trunk muscles may be weak. Will need to use a wheelchair for mobility. Likely to develop hydrocephalus.
		L 1-2	Weak hip movements. May develop dislocated hips. With assistive devices Knee-ankle-foot orthosis [KAFO], crutches, walker) may ambulate short distances, especially when young, but will need wheelchair for longer distances. No bowel and bladder control. Likely to develop hydrocephalus.
		L 3	Strong hip flexion and adduction; some knee extension. Will need KAFO and crutches for household and short-distance community ambulation and a wheelchair for longer distances. No bowel and bladder control. Likely to develop hydrocephalus.
		L 4	May have some active knee flexion and ankle dorsiflexion with stronger knee extension. Community ambulation with ankle-foot orthosis (AFOs) and crutches. May develop foot deformities. May need a wheelchair for long community distances. No bowel and bladder control. Less likely to develop hydrocephalus.
		L 5	Weak hip extension and abduction. Good knee flexion against gravity. Weak plantarflexion with eversion and strong dorsiflexion with inversion may lead to foot deformities. Can walk with no orthoses but needs crutches for long distances because of fatigue. Can use a bicycle. No bowel and bladder control. Less likely to develop hydrocephalus.
		S 1	Improved hip stability leads to independent walking without support. Weakness in hip abductors and plantarflexors lead to gait deviations. No bowel and bladder control. Good ambulation with weak push-off and decreased stride length with rapid movement. May have impaired bladder and bowel control. May need foot orthoses for support.

Incidence and Cause

Spina bifida occurs in approximately 1 of every 1000 births in the United States. It has a higher incidence in certain ethnic groups, including the Irish and individuals of Irish descent in the United States, whereas black Africans and Japanese have a significantly lower incidence than average, only 0.3 per 1000 births. In 1966 the incidence was 2 to 3 per 1000 births in Great Britain, but this rate has decreased substantially in succeeding decades (Eckersley, 1993). The incidence of spina bifida has been decreasing worldwide over the last 40 years. Although the reasons for this decline are not clear, it is thought to be at least partially the result of attention to nutritional deficiencies, which may predispose individuals to this spinal cord defect. Other rea-

sons for the decline include better prenatal testing, leading to termination of some pregnancies in which the fetus has spina bifida.

Spina bifida is associated with several genetic syndromes, but no gene for the defect alone has been identified. Genetic predisposition is thought to play a role, however. Nutrition is also thought to be a factor in the development of this defect. Several studies have demonstrated that maternal deficiency of folic acid is associated with spina bifida, and research has demonstrated that women who are treated with folic acid have less chance of having a second infant with the defect than those who were not treated (MRC Vitamin Study Research Group, 1991).

Environmental influences also can cause spina bifida. The

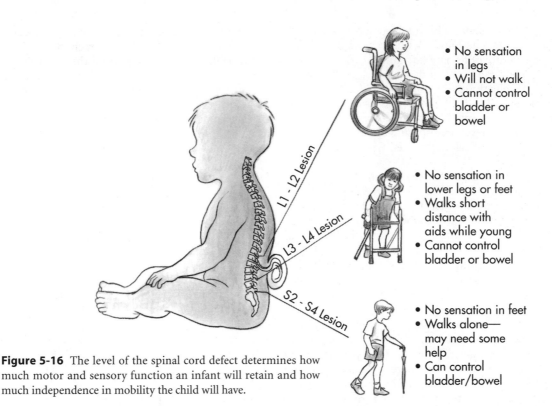

- No sensation in legs
- Will not walk
- Cannot control bladder or bowel

L1 - L2 Lesion

- No sensation in lower legs or feet
- Walks short distance with aids while young
- Cannot control bladder or bowel

L3 - L4 Lesion

- No sensation in feet
- Walks alone— may need some help
- Can control bladder/bowel

S2 - S4 Lesion

Figure 5-16 The level of the spinal cord defect determines how much motor and sensory function an infant will retain and how much independence in mobility the child will have.

embryonic neural tube closes about 4 weeks of gestation. Teratogen exposure earlier than this point in the pregnancy is thought to interrupt the normal closure and cause the defect. Defects can occur at any point along the embryonic neural tube, including the skull and C1 through the entire spinal cord. Excessive maternal alcohol intake during the first trimester can cause spina bifida and fetal alcohol syndrome. Women who take valproic acid or some other anticonvulsant medications for seizures during the first trimester have been shown to produce children with an increased risk of spina bifida.

Prenatal diagnostic techniques, which can identify a fetus with myelomeningocele, can also help preserve the optimal function of these children during the birth process. If an infant is detected with a myelomeningocele and has innervation to allow knee and ankle function, a cesarean section can spare the myelomeningocele the trauma of a vaginal delivery, thus preserving some of the infant's nerve function. Immediate surgery to close the defect can prevent infection and other complications, which may lead to decreased function. Because of ultrasonography and quick surgical responses, some spinal nerves of infants who are born with spina bifida can be spared and infections can be prevented, allowing children better function throughout their lives.

Clinical Features

Severity of defect. Physical presentation of a child with spina bifida at birth varies according to the level of the lesion, the severity, and the associated problems. Children with an occulta, or nonvisible defect, may have a hairy area or fat pad at the base of their spine. These children generally have no paralysis and move their legs normally. Children with an aperta, or visible defect, have a fluid-filled sac protruding from their spine. In the case of a meningocele there is no nervous tissue in the sac, and the child is not likely to have neurological damage. For those children with a myelomeningocele, this fluid-filled sac contains the deformed spinal cord and ineffective spinal nerves distal to the defect. The sac is made of a thin, fragile membrane. Infection can easily be introduced to the spinal cord and brain. Surgery to repair the defect closes the sac and protect the spinal cord by covering it with muscle and skin. Infants with a myelomeningocele have paralysis of muscles innervated both at the site of the defect and below it.

Level of defect. The level of injury determines the mobility the infant will have in the legs and at the hips, knees and hips, or ankles, knees, and hips. Most defects occur in the thoracic or lumbar region of the spine; the higher the site of the defect, the greater the extent of paralysis. The level of the defect can predict the later motor function of the child (Figure 5-16). Sensory impairments also result from the malformation of the spinal cord. The child may lack all sensation in areas below the level of defect, or some areas may be spared. Light touch, deep pressure, temperature, pain, and proprioception may all be impaired.

Associated problems. Problems associated with spina bifida include orthopedic impairments, intellectual impairments, and physiological difficulties from anatomical impairments.

Orthopedic deformities from lack of movement in utero and muscle imbalances, such as club feet, bowed long bones, hip flexion contractures, and dislocated hips, are common in children with spina bifida. Cleft palate is sometimes associated with spina bifida. Other possible orthopedic problems include a scoliosis or kyphosis caused by the structural deformities in the spinal vertebrae or an imbalance of muscle pull at different spinal levels. Spinal deformities may be present at birth or may develop as the child grows.

Incontinence of bladder or bowel is common, depending on

the level of the defect. Abnormalities of the urinary tract include fused or absent kidneys and missing ureters, complicating the already difficult control of urinary tract functions.

Obesity is a common problem developing in children with spina bifida, especially those with thoracic and high lumbar lesions. The reasons for the development of obesity include a decreased activity level for children with lower extremity paralysis and a lower metabolic level predisposing them to gain weight with the same number of calories as their typically developing peers.

Osteoporosis is another problem in children who do not bear weight through their legs or walk or run for mobility. Three predisposing factors can promote bone loss: (1) lack of weight bearing and normal muscle pull through the long bones; (2) seizure medications, which tend to leach calcium from the bones; and (3) inadequate vitamin D production for children who are not adequately exposed to sunlight. Any one or a combination of these factors may cause many children with spina bifida to be prone to fractures. Care must be taken with handling to minimize fractures.

Skin breakdown is common among children with lack of sensation through their hips, buttocks, or feet. Causes of the skin breakdown can be excessive pressure over bony prominences such as the greater trochanter, ishii, sacrum, or heels; pressure related to orthotics or casts; abrasions or burns that are not treated because the child is not aware of them; or skin maceration from urine or stool. Ninety-five percent of children with spina bifida experience some form of skin breakdown before they reach adulthood (Shurtleff, 1986).

Both specific and general learning problems are prevalent. Visual-perceptual problems, clumsiness, and low or low-average intelligence are common. Two thirds of children with spina bifida have intelligence in the normal range, and one third may have retardation, usually mild (Charney, 1992). Intellectual problems may be caused by hydrocephalus.

Language differences, including "cocktail-party speech," also known as hyperverbal behavior, are common with children who have spina bifida. Children with cocktail-party speech use sophisticated language, especially greetings and social language, demonstrating good vocabulary and sentence construction skills. Their repetitive use of the same phrases, meaningless use of language, and inappropriate utterances soon demonstrate rote rather than meaningful speech, reflecting poor intellectual understanding of the contexts and use of language.

Hydrocephalus. Hydrocephalus can be caused by an associated deformity of the hindbrain called Arnold-Chiari malformation type II, in which the cerebellum and part of the brain stem are displaced downward toward the neck. Almost all children with myelomeningocele have an Arnold-Chiari malformation. This malformation interferes with the normal flow of cerebrospinal fluid around the brain and spinal cord and causes a build-up of the fluid in the ventricles of the brain called *hydrocephalus* (water-brain). From 60% to 95% of children with spina bifida will develop hydrocephalus. If not treated, hydrocephalus can cause severe mental retardation because the growing volume of fluid in the ventricles of the brain compresses the brain tissue against the hard cavity of the skull, causing irreparable damage. The usual treatment is to place a shunt between the ventricles in the brain to the peritoneal cavity. This is called a ventriculoperi-

toneal shunt (Figure 5-17). The higher pressure of the fluid in the brain causes it to flow through the flexible plastic tubing, through a one-way valve, into the lower pressure of the abdomen. The excess fluid is harmlessly absorbed in the abdomen. The shunt may drain into the atrium of the heart, where it is absorbed directly into the bloodstream, and in this case would be called a ventriculoatrial shunt.

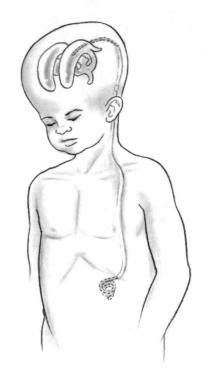

Figure 5-17 A ventriculoperitoneal shunt drains fluid from the enlarged ventricles of the brain to the peritoneal cavity. A coiled tube in the peritoneum will lengthen as the child grows.

Signs of Shunt Malfunction*

BOX 5-4

Irritability
Headache
Vomiting
Lethargy
Fever
Bulging eyes
Sleeping more than normal; difficulty in arousal
Change in behavior
Change in seizure activity
Change in visual acuity
Change in coordination
Change in muscle tone
Change in continence
Change in appetite

*Any of these changes should trigger an urgent call to the parent or the physician to assess for shunt malfunction.

Complications of shunt placement include either blockage of the shunt, causing the fluid not to drain properly, or infection of the shunt, causing a blockage as well as introducing infection into the brain. All therapy providers and teachers should be aware if a child has a shunt and be watchful for signs indicating problems with its functioning (Box 5-4). Signs of blockage may include a change in personality, sleepiness, lethargy, vomiting, headache, and irritability. Infection could also be signaled by these indications, as well as fever. If any of these signs is detected, getting the child to a physician as soon as possible is important. Delay could cause severe illness, brain damage, or death.

Seizures may develop in children with hydrocephalus. Their development is frequently related to a shunt infection and may be short-lived, or it may require lifelong treatment with anti-seizure medications.

Cranial nerve involvement causing strabismus, swallowing difficulties, or weak vocal cords may result from pressure on the cranial nerves from hydrocephalus or the Arnold-Chiari malformation.

Medical Treatment

Surgery. Surgical treatment to repair a myelomeningocele is needed either immediately or within the first few weeks of life. The primary purpose of the surgical repair is to reduce the threat of infection through the thin sac surrounding the site of the defect. A secondary purpose is to preserve any spinal nerves that could be damaged through trauma or pressure. Although it is unlikely that any of the nerves in the sac remain functional, early surgery holds the best hope to preserve what function there is.

Surgery may also be necessary to address some of the other defects associated with spina bifida such as cleft palate, kidney malformations, severe scoliosis, or dislocated hips. Clubfeet are generally treated with serial casting in the newborn period to avoid later surgery. Orthopedic surgery is generally delayed until the child is older and able to tolerate the surgery and recovery period better; also, the bones will have matured from the cartilaginous newborn bones to those that have more bone tissue. For those children with hydrocephalus, a shunt needs to be surgically placed as soon as any increased pressure is detected in the cerebrospinal fluid. The timing of such surgery depends on the severity of the abnormality, the health of the child, and the medical urgency.

Drugs. Medicines to control seizures, such as phenobarbital, carbamazepine (Tegretol), or phenytoin (Dilantin), are given if the child develops a seizure disorder. Sometimes combinations of seizure medications are more effective than one given alone. Manipulation of the drugs and dosages may be tried before the optimal combination and dose are decided on for seizure control. These drugs all have serious side effects, which are discussed in Chapter 12.

If the child has a blocked shunt or poorly controlled hydrocephalus for other reasons, drugs to decrease the volume of cerebrospinal fluid such as furosemide (Lasix), acetazolamide (Diamox), or dexamethasone (Decaden) may be given. These drugs are generally a short-term, stop-gap measure rather than a long-term solution to the problem. Other drugs that may be necessary include antibiotics for infection control, rectal suppositories for bowel evacuation, and supplementary calcium to reduce the effects of osteoporosis.

Physical Therapy Intervention

Physical therapy goals for the child with spina bifida include promoting age-appropriate functional skills and reducing secondary impairments such as contractures, fractures, and obesity, which could interfere with developmental skills. The physical therapy provider may work with a child with spina bifida in a clinic, hospital, home, or school, depending on the age, medical condition, and needs of the child.

Physical therapy for the infant and toddler. Early intervention generally focuses on the prevention of contractures and skin breakdown, as well as maximizing the child's developmental skills. Another primary goal is to teach parents to meet their child's medical needs while feeling comfortable handling and interacting with their child.

Positioning is important to reduce the threat of contracture, which could limit function in later life. The child with spina bifida tends to keep the lower limbs in hip abduction and external rotation, as well as flexion at the hips and knees and ankle plantar flexion. Overuse of this position, sometimes called "frogged legs," can cause contractures, which will limit the child's ability to sit or stand later. Placing towel rolls or stuffed animals lateral to the child's legs in infant seats, car seats, and strollers can keep the hips more aligned in a neutral position. If the child's hips need to be positioned in abduction and flexion because they are subluxing or dislocatable, this positioning takes precedence over a neutral alignment.

Health care activities such as watching for problems with a shunt, giving appropriate medications in a timely manner, observing skin, addressing feeding difficulties, and providing for bowel and bladder care may overwhelm parents, at least initially. Parents should be encouraged, however, to actively interact with their child through age-appropriate vigorous play, moving the child through space, challenging the child's balance and equilibrium, and allowing the child to become comfortable with movement. Active play also encourages development of strength and range of motion through the trunk and arms, which is especially important for a child with spina bifida.

Caregivers and therapy providers must always be aware of the child's lack of sensation, lack of ability to support flaccid joints,

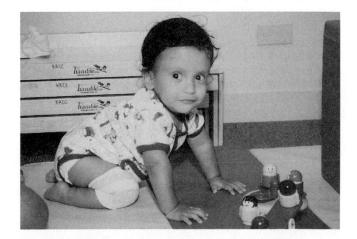

Figure 5-18 Ronnie's mother used tube socks to make protective knee pads for him.

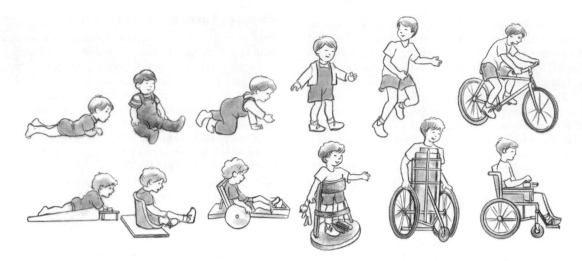

Figure 5-19 Adaptive devices can help the young child with spina bifida reach major motor milestones at the same time as peers.

and the fragility of the bones caused by osteoporosis. Supporting flaccid joints, while encouraging use of existing strength and skills, help a child safely develop balance and mobility skills. Orthoses, adaptive equipment, or manual support are all means to protect bones and joints. Protective devices such as knee pads, long pants, or protective shoes help to prevent skin abrasions from early mobility attempts (Figure 5-18).

Helping a child learn to sit, change positions, and move around the environment independently can include creating or finding appropriate assistive technology, strengthening innervated muscles, facilitating adequate range of motion, and developing confidence and skills in the child and family. A young child with spina bifida should be provided the means to accomplish age-appropriate tasks such as sitting, exploring the environment, and standing independently. Adaptive devices exist or can be created to meet these needs (Figure 5-19).

Role of the PTA with the infant or toddler. The PTA may work in conjunction with a PT in an early intervention program. Services may be provided at the center or in the home. The PTA may also see a child with spina bifida who has an acute medical problem and is in the hospital. Encouraging early movement and developmental skills through games and play assists the infant or toddler to develop strength through the trunk and upper extremities, as well as learn to be comfortable with movement. Monitoring the use and fit of assistive devices such as floor carts, ankle-foot orthoses, or even body jackets for children with a high-level lesion is important. Group activities encourage socialization, especially among toddlers with and without disabilities. Communicating with parents, therapists, and teachers about the child's developing skills and needs is an important function of a therapy provider who sees the child regularly.

Physical therapy for the preschooler and early school-aged child. As a child begins to interact with peers in more structured environments such as school or recreational settings, more creativity in adaptations to allow the child to participate may be necessary.

The child may ambulate with crutches or a walker, may use orthoses for lower extremity support, or may use a manual or powered wheelchair for mobility. Which devices are most ap-

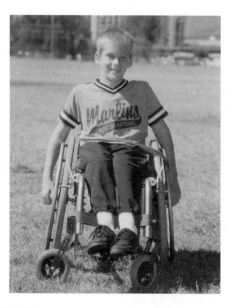

Figure 5-20 This young man recently underwent surgery for scoliosis and is observing his team's baseball games for a few more weeks until he is allowed to play again.

propriate depends on the strength and functional skills of the child, the judgment and sensory capabilities of the child, the needs and desires of the child, and the resources available. Means of mobility may change from circumstance to circumstance. For instance, a child may find more independence using a wheelchair during a baseball game and using crutches in the classroom. As the child ages, he or she may abandon orthoses and crutches for the ease and decreased energy expenditure of a wheelchair.

During the elementary school years surgical procedures to stabilize a scoliosis or a dislocating hip may be necessary (Figure 5-20). Rehabilitation from surgery may take weeks or months and may include strengthening, range of motion, relearning mobility skills in a wheelchair, or ambulation with assistive devices. Adapting and expanding assistive devices is necessary, including lower extremity orthoses, walkers, and wheelchairs, as well as self-care devices such as shower chairs, adaptive grooming aids, and transfer bars as the child grows and the needs change.

During early childhood, measures are taken to prevent contractures through proper positioning. Children with spina bifida often need special education services because of poor visual perception or other learning difficulties. Working with the special education and classroom teacher to ensure good classroom and wheelchair positioning can help prevent contractures.

School settings are also essential for developing social skills in a school-aged child. Receiving services in a special education room can isolate a child from peers and prevent friendships from forming. Awareness of these issues can spur a physical therapy provider to work with school personnel to set up mechanisms to support friendships, including developing networks of peer tutors or "helpers"; creating recess games where all students are included; using the "buddy system" for field trips, assemblies, or classroom activities; and providing opportunities for children to interact in circumstances other than school such as church, sports, and youth groups. Therapy services can be provided in inclusive settings through games and activities that are fun for all children. Physical therapy should not interfere with the development of peer relationships but should complement these efforts.

Role of the PTA with the toddler or early school-aged child. The PTA usually works with the child with spina bifida in school, in the hospital, or in the outpatient clinic after surgery. Responsibilities in school include assisting the teacher to integrate motor activities for the child into the daily curriculum, developing group activities at recess or in the classroom, and helping the child develop increased independence in transfers, toileting, and mobility around the school. Monitoring strength and range of motion can indicate if problems are developing; including activities for strengthening and maintaining or increasing range of motion for functional tasks into daily routines ensures optimal outcomes for the child. Setting up an IEP for individual physical therapy services once or twice per week will probably interfere with social or academic activities, but training classroom aides, teachers, or peers to assist the child during natural events of the day is functional and meaningful.

The PTA may also work with the child in an acute or rehabilitation setting. Efforts in these settings are directed toward developing functional skills, such as transfers or mobility skills after surgery. The PTA may implement protocols after surgery for increasing or maintaining range of motion, strengthening, or developing functional skills. The PTA may help the child learn to use new equipment, such as a reciprocating gait orthosis or a parapodium. Treatment in medical settings should be short term, with the activities turned over to individuals at the school and home once the child develops a certain level of skill. In this way skills can be generalized to the natural environment (Figure 5-21).

Physical therapy for the older school-aged child and adolescent. Most older children and adolescents no longer need direct physical therapy services to work on self-help or mobility skills; however, they still need help adapting equipment for growth and problem solving to help them participate in activities and events that are important to them. Many older children and adolescents who have higher spinal lesions and associated problems still need help with self-help tasks such as transfers, toileting, and dressing (Figure 5-22). Classroom aides need to be trained to use mechanical lifts for transfers, to position children in standers, and to

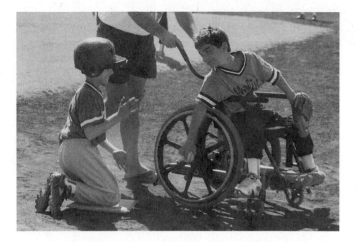

Figure 5-21 Picking up a ball from the ground and throwing it to a teammate develops balance, strength, and range of motion—even if the runner is safe!

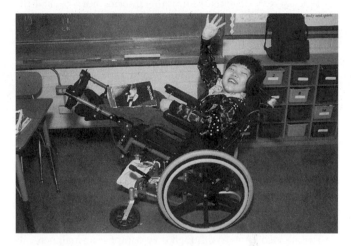

Figure 5-22 Joshua rests in a tilted position to decrease his lower extremity edema. He needs help for mobility at school because of impaired vision. He uses a condom catheter for urine, and his mother made a special cover for his urine bag, which hangs from his wheelchair.

provide training and guarding during gait activities. Many older children with spina bifida have abandoned long leg braces and ambulation as they get heavier and walking requires more energy.

Adolescents with learning disabilities can be included in regular education classrooms, even in junior high and high school. Encouraging children to plan and make decisions about their day, both in and out of school, is important to give them life skills that will be useful for the present and future. Many children with disabilities are overtly or subtly encouraged to be dependent on others and need to develop independence in social and vocational situations to be successful in later life. Physical therapy providers can help in this process by giving adolescents choices about how much and what form of therapy they need. The child should be an active member of his or her own team and should be involved in making choices.

The Child With Arthrogryposis Multiplex Congenita

Arthrogryposis multiplex congenita (AMC) is a syndrome present at birth that consists of severe nonprogressive joint contractures and muscle weakness. Arthrogryposis may take a number of forms, depending on the limbs involved and the extent of disability. It can range from mild cases, in which only two or three joints are affected, to severe cases, in which major joints in all of the extremities, as well the spine, are involved.

Incidence and Cause

The incidence of AMC is 1 in 3000 births (Hall, 1992). The incidence may be higher in Central and South America than in Europe and North America (Werner, 1987).

AMC has multiple causes, including genetic, environmental, and unknown influences. Cases can be classified according to an initial problem in the nervous system (neurogenic) or of muscle origin (myogenic). Many cases of neurogenic AMC are thought to be caused by degeneration in the anterior horn cells of the spinal cord leading to muscle weakness in utero, with subsequent joint immobilization because of decreased fetal movement. Myogenic cases have the same mechanism; muscle weakness causes decreased movement in utero, with resultant joint deformities.

Maternal fevers of greater than 100° F in the first trimester of pregnancy have been linked to some cases of AMC. Other causes are thought to include maternal viral infections in the first trimester, vascular compromise between mother and fetus, and a septum in the uterus or decreased amniotic fluid causing decreased space for the developing fetus. An autosomal dominant genetic defect has been demonstrated to cause at least one form of the over 150 forms of congenital joint contractures documented (Bamshad et al., 1994). This distal form of AMC, which affects primarily the hands and feet, is thought to make up 7% of all the AMC cases (Hall, Reed, & Greene, 1982). Other genetic causes are also known, although they compose a small percentage of cases of AMC.

Clinical Features

The most obvious clinical feature of a newborn with AMC is the joint deformity of the child's extremities. Although patterns and severity of joint deformities vary, at least two joints are usually affected, even in mildly affected children. Many children with classic arthrogryposis, however, have all joints in their extremities affected. Two classic patterns of joint deformity occur in those infants most severely affected. In the first pattern the child's upper extremities are held in internal rotation at the shoulders, extended elbows, and flexed and ulnarly deviated wrists. The lower extremities are held in abduction and external rotation with knee flexion and a clubfoot deformity of the feet. In the second pattern the arms are also held in internal rotation at the shoulders, with the wrists flexed and ulnarly deviated, but the elbows are flexed rather than extended. The lower extremities also have clubfoot deformities, but the hips are held in flexion and the knees in extension (Figure 5-23).

The affected extremities are characterized by tubelike joints, with no creases across the joint surface. Dimpling of the skin may be present over joints. The skin is thin with little subcuta-

neous tissue, and the limbs are cylindrical. Muscles are atrophied with some muscle groups absent. Joints are rigid with some joints subluxed or dislocated, especially the hips or knees.

Children with AMC may have associated problems of scoliosis, hemangiomas, congenital heart disease, facial abnormalities, respiratory problems, abdominal hernias, or feeding disorders because of abnormalities of the jaw and tongue. Failure to thrive and constipation may be a result of feeding problems. Sensation is intact, and children with AMC have normal intelligence and speech.

Treatment for the Infant

Medical intervention. Medical treatment focuses on orthopedic surgery to allow optimal function of the extremities for self-care and mobility. An assessment determines whether the child's contractures cause functional problems in sitting, standing, moving or using hands to eat, learn, or work. If surgery is indicated to improve the child's functional skills, it is timed to be of maximum developmental benefit to the child. Surgery for the lower extremities is usually performed before the age of 2 years and is timed when a child is developmentally ready to stand. In this way the child's desire to stand will assist the stretching and weight bearing needed to maintain surgical correction.

Surgery for the legs is usually directed at making the hips mobile for walking, reducing excessive knee flexion contractures, and allowing a foot flat position for standing and walking. Surgery is usually performed to reset a dislocated hip if only one hip is out, and the other is properly seated in the acetabulum. Relocating the dislocated hip provides a level pelvis for standing, walking, and sitting. This reduces chances for development of scoliosis and allows for improved function. If both hips are dislocated, surgery to reduce the dislocations may not provide enough benefit to the child and is not usually done. Relocating

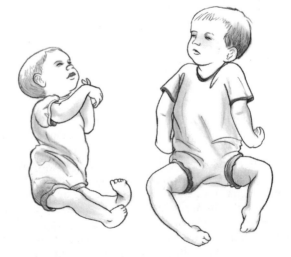

Figure 5-23 Common limb contractures of children with severe arthrogryposis multiplex congenita include patterns of flexed upper extremities with extended lower extremities and extended upper extremities with flexed lower extremities. Common contractures to the two patterns include internal rotation at the shoulders, flexed and ulnarly deviated wrists, and clubfeet.

hips may cause stiffness and pain and may reduce the mobility of the hips, rather than improving function. Surgery to improve knee function may involve a capsulotomy (resecting the joint capsule to improve range of motion), tenotomy (cutting tendon[s] to improve range of motion), osteotomy (cutting the bone to realign the joint angle and change the arc of motion), or tendon transfer to allow muscles optimal length and angle to move a joint through its available range. Knee surgery is not usually done until a child is already walking and an accurate assessment of the benefits and risks is performed. Serial casting is usually initiated at birth to reduce clubfeet; but if surgery is needed, it is timed for when the child is first standing.

Surgery for the upper extremities is performed later than that for the lower extremities. The goals of surgery for the upper extremities include optimizing functional skills, such as hand-to-mouth for feeding, and upper extremity range of motion for dressing and toileting. Since the early school-age years provide motivation to use hands and arms for functional tasks, surgery is generally performed at this time. Shoulder contractures are not usually addressed surgically; however, fusing one elbow in flexion for feeding, toothbrushing, and other tasks and the other in extension, for dressing, toileting, and other tasks has proven to be functional for some children. Tendon transfers can help to create strength for elbow movements to improve skills. Wrist deformities may also be addressed surgically fusing in either flexion or extension for improved function.

Scoliosis is usually managed conservatively with bracing unless the curve progresses to 50 degrees or beyond. Surgery is then necessary to stabilize the progression.

Physical therapy intervention. Physical therapy goals for the child with AMC include functional active and passive range of motion, adequate strength to achieve functional skills, transition and mobility skills, and ability to participate in inclusive activities at home and school and in the community.

Physical Therapy Intervention for the Infant, Toddler, and Preschooler

The physical therapy provider works closely with the orthopedic surgeons, the family, and the rest of the team to make decisions regarding the necessity, timing, and type of surgical intervention. Vigorous stretching and splinting may be tried before any surgery is performed to increase range of motion. Stretching and splinting are used throughout childhood to minimize development of further contractures and to optimize range of motion and functional skills. Infants and young children whose bones and joints are developing at a rapid pace may benefit more from these techniques to improve range of motion than older children. Splinting and vigorous range of motion can counteract some of the deforming effects of in-utero positioning and allow more normal limb positioning as the child grows. One limitation of these techniques is that small children do not generally tolerate vigorous stretching well. Another limitation is that although gains in range of motion can be made using vigorous stretching and splinting, they may not be maintained over time; and surgery may eventually be required to correct the contractures more permanently.

Splinting is frequently used to maintain joint range obtained via surgery. Physical therapy will make and monitor the splints

for fit, pressure, and function. Splinting may also be used to enhance hand function. A universal cuff can be placed over a child's hand to hold a spoon, pencil, or toy (Figure 5-24). A child may be able to move the arm grossly from the shoulder to write, eat, or play—even if elbow and wrist strength and range of motion are limited.

Helping a child develop strength and skills to sit without support or to move without assistance can be done using developmentally appropriate games and activities. The Swiss ball is a wonderful tool to use to develop balance skills and trunk strength while working on range of motion and providing vestibular input. Many young children are afraid of being on the ball, which is understandable given the lack of stability sitting on a ball provides! A level of trust between the therapy provider and the child and a firm control of the ball are absolute necessities for using this tool with young children. Ball work can be integrated into classroom activities by creating group games using the ball, inventing "ball olympics" for all children to compete and develop skills, or working with the child on the ball in a more passive way such as while listening to a story.

Helping a child with AMC achieve mobility is one of the greatest challenges and satisfactions a physical therapy provider can address. Early mobility can be achieved by rolling or scooting along the floor. When a child is ready to walk, depending on the level of disability, crutches or a walker with custom supports for upper extremity deformities may be all that is needed. Lightweight braces and assistive aids, such as crutches or a walker made from aluminum or PVC piping, can help the child be more successful. Individual accommodations for strength, joint contracture, and age need to be made. These may include custom thermoplastic forearm supports for the walker or crutches, straps to provide stability, or a custom height for the device (Figure 5-25).

If a child has deformities significant enough that a wheelchair is needed for mobility, the child will probably not be able to propel the chair manually. Power mobility should be seriously considered for even a very young child with AMC. With appropriate supervision children as young as 2 years have been known to use power mobility effectively. Power mobility allows the child to explore the environment and develop cognitive and social skills more fully than a child dependent on others for mobility. As the child gets older, independent mobility allows for greater autonomy at school and home. The child's home needs to be evaluated carefully for powered mobility. Besides architectural considerations, a family's perspective and ability to care for the expensive equipment should be considered. If the home is not accessible, a power chair made available to the child at school may foster independent thinking and social skills in a child who is able to think and make decisions independently. Child-friendly mobility devices, such as commercially available electric cars for children, can sometimes be modified for the child with severe deformities and may be less expensive than a power wheelchair.

The therapist needs to work closely with other team members to address other environmental modifications, which will help the child participate fully in school. A floor sitting device for a child in daycare or preschool can help the child participate in circle time or other floor activities if independent sitting has not been achieved. A chair with arms to help with sitting balance or an angled desk top may help the child be more successful at writing and drawing tasks. Early use of a computer can help the child learn academic subjects, write papers, and turn pages of a

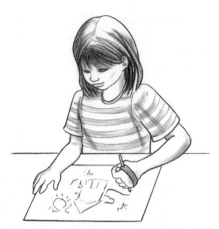

Figure 5-24 This child uses a universal cuff to hold a crayon.

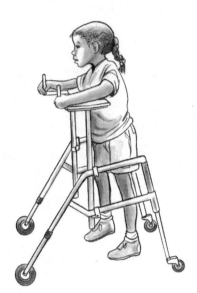

Figure 5-25 A child with arthrogryposis multiplex congenita may need custom adaptations to a mobility device to accommodate for contractures.

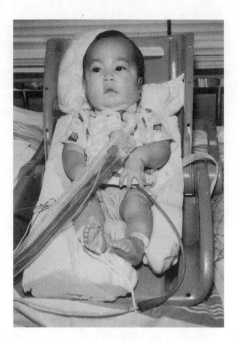

Figure 5-26 This child has arthrogryposis with other anomalies. She is ventilator dependent and must live in the hospital during her infancy. The light in her eyes tells us that she is very aware of her surroundings. She has been molded for a custom seating device to help her sit up.

book. Computer access technology, such as switches, on-screen keyboards, and trackballs, can help a child be successful with this learning tool. The therapist is an integral part of the team making decisions about technology use and positioning for the child with AMC (Figure 5-26).

Role of the PTA with the young child. The PTA is involved with the young child with AMC in an infant program, preschool, or early school setting. Home-, hospital-, or clinic-based therapy may be provided if the child has acute medical needs, such as recent surgery, or more chronic medical needs, such as feeding or respiratory problems.

The PTA designs activities to meet the goals set out by the PT and the team working with the child. Stretching, strengthening, and mobility skills need to be integrated into the child's daily routines. Brainstorming with other members of the team and troubleshooting to design methods to allow the child to be included in classroom and home activities and to participate in self-care activities such as feeding, toileting, and dressing are

challenges that can be faced together. Parent teaching in the areas of handling, stretching, and development of independent skills may be an important component of therapy services for the young child with AMC.

Physical Therapy Intervention for the Older Child and Adolescent

Because older children do not grow as fast as younger ones, stretching and splinting are not as helpful in changing limited range of motion. However, these techniques are still indicated for maintaining current range and preventing loss of range, which may affect functional skills. Older children can be taught to do their own stretching with straps and other aids and to monitor their own splints.

Older children and adults may develop secondary problems related to overuse of functional muscles or joints, such as arthritis, carpal tunnel syndrome, or tendonitis. Treatment for pain and stiffness may help these children preserve functional skills. Children who were ambulating during their younger years may find that a wheelchair provides the most efficient means of mobility as they grow older and bigger; secondary problems cause pain and weakness. Power mobility may then be explored as a mobility option if it was not adopted in earlier childhood.

During adolescence children are exploring social and vocational independence. Working with children and families to create workable accommodations for transportation, work situations, and social opportunities can help children move beyond dependency and into an independent lifestyle. Transition from school to the workplace can be a major life task and entails co-operation between various agencies, including the Division of Vocational Rehabilitation (DVR); rehabilitation facilities where adapted driver training is provided; durable medical equipment suppliers; and schools, workplaces, and recreation centers. These issues are not unique to a child with AMC, but the solutions need to be tailored to each child's unique needs. The PT can be an essential member of any transition team and aid in problem solving issues of positioning, mobility, and access.

Volunteer arrangements, as for any adolescent, can help an agency or company see the skills and capabilities of the child and look past the obvious disability. They can also create opportunities to try accommodations, which may help the adolescent be more effective at work tasks. Accommodations may be as simple as rearranging an office space to make it accessible or adapting a joystick or tray on the wheelchair. They may be as complicated as building ramps, making bathrooms accessible, or providing sophisticated electronic equipment to help a child access and use a computer. The Americans with Disabilities Act (ADA), passed in 1990, requires that reasonable accommodations be made to allow individuals with disabilities to work. Of course, a fine line needs to be walked between advocating for individual rights and alienating those who may hire the adolescent with a disability.

Role of the PTA with the older child and adolescent. The PTA may be an active member of the team working with the child. The PTA may provide equipment adaptation; train the child in specific skills for success in school, job, or social situation; or treat pain and stiffness related to arthritis or other overuse syndromes. Open communication with the child, the PT, and the team can ensure optimal outcomes.

The Child With Juvenile Rheumatoid Arthritis

Juvenile rheumatoid arthritis (JRA) is the most common chronic rheumatic disease of childhood. A rheumatic disease is characterized by inflammation of connective tissue. Inflammation commonly occurs in joints (arthritis), but it can also occur in other systems of the body, including the iris of the eye, lungs, or heart. Although classified as one disease, JRA actually includes several variations of disease, each of which has different clinical symptoms, somewhat different management strategies, and a different prognosis. A child with JRA may have symptoms that range from slight disability, with one or two affected joints, to severe disability, with not only pervasive joint inflammation but also organ inflammation.

Two main types of classification are used for JRA throughout the world. A rheumatic disease is classified as JRA by the American College of Rheumatology (ACR) if, (1) it occurs in children younger than 16 years, (2) arthritis is present in one or more joints for longer than 6 weeks, and (3) other diseases have been excluded (Prieur, 1994). Children with JRA may or may not have a positive rheumatic factor in their blood. A class of rheumatic disease in children called spondyloarthropathies is not included in the ACR diagnosis of JRA. These diseases are mentioned in Table 5-3 with common treatment approaches, but they are not addressed in depth in the text. The European League Against Rheumatism (EULAR) defines juvenile chronic arthritis (JCA) similarly to the ACR's definition, except that if a child has positive rheumatic factor, he or she cannot be diagnosed with the juvenile form of arthritis. The EULAR also include some rheumatic diseases that the ACR excludes, notably, the spondyloarthropathies. In the United States the ACR terminology and definition for JRA are used; in Europe the EULAR terminology of JCA and definition are used.

Incidence and Cause

Almost 14 cases of JRA are diagnosed each year per 100,000 people (Towner, Michet, O'Fallon, & Nelson, 1983). It is estimated that approximately 200,000 cases of JRA exist in the United States (Cassidy & Nelson, 1988).

Although multiple factors are thought to influence the development of JRA, no definitive cause is known. It is thought that

TABLE 5-3 Spondyloarthropathies in Children

Spondyloarthropathies	Age of onset	Description and common treatment approaches
Ankylosing spondylitis	Adolescence (boys > girls)	May begin with pauciarticular arthritis in childhood or back pain in adolescence. Can lead to general arthritis and in severe cases to ankylosis or fusion of the spine. Treatment includes drugs similar to those used in juvenile rheumatoid arthritis to decrease inflammation and swimming and gentle exercise to maintain range of motion and strength.
Psoriatic arthritis	9-10 years (girls > boys)	Arthritis that involves primarily the distal joints of the hands with psoriasis. Girls are affected more commonly than boys. Is usually a mild disease but may lead to general joint destruction. Management is similar to that of other forms of arthritis.
Reactive arthritis	Variable	Also known as Reiter's syndrome. Three "corners" of syndrome include urethritis, ocular disturbances, and arthritis. May be a brief illness with complete recovery or may have long-term sequelae.
Inflammatory bowel disease	Variable	Arthritis may be the presenting complaint in children with ulcerative colitis or Crohn's disease. Abdominal cramping, diarrhea, weight loss, unexplained fever, and pauciarticular arthritis are common symptoms. Septic joints, especially the hip, can occur. Treatment varies according to symptoms.

the etiology is multifactorial and that a viral or bacterial infection may trigger an autoimmune reaction. Children who develop JRA may have a genetic predisposition for this type of response. Because of the high fevers initiating systemic JRA, this type is especially thought to be triggered by an infection. The mechanism of JRA is an autoimmune reaction. The child's own immune system fights against connective tissue, causing inflammation and resulting pain and stiffness, especially in the joints.

Clinical Features

Presentation of JRA can vary according to the type of JRA a child is demonstrating, the child's individual responses, and whether the inflammation is in an acute or chronic manifestation. Symptoms may include fever, rash, joint inflammation, swelling, and malaise. An inflamed joint is characterized by fusiform swelling (fatter at the middle than the ends), warm temperature, limitation in range of motion, and pain with palpation or movement. Associated muscles may be atrophied, indicating a chronic disease process. Children who have been affected by joint inflammation for some time may demonstrate joint contractures, weakness, stiffness, reluctance to move, and a particular dependence on caregivers bred from years of pain and difficulty helping themselves. Children may have increased stiffness in the mornings from the immobility of sleeping at night. Cold may aggravate pain and stiffness, and heat may relieve symptoms.

JRA can be classified into three primary subtypes: oligoarticular (known as pauciarticular), polyarticular, and systemic.

Oligoarticular JRA.   There are two subtypes of oligoarticular JRA. The most common type occurs primarily in girls in early childhood, with the peak age of diagnosis being 2 years. From 40% to 60% of children with JRA have this subtype. Children with oligoarticular JRA develop arthritis in less than five joints, with the knee being most commonly affected. Ankles, fingers, elbows, and wrists are also commonly affected.

Because very young children cannot vocalize their complaints, a common presentation is that previously ambulatory children stop walking or begin to limp. Parents notice that one or more joints are swollen and warm and may have limited movement. Usually the joints involved are asymmetrical throughout the body. The involved joint usually differs from its uninvolved counterpart in girth, range of motion, and temperature.

Children with early-onset oligoarticular arthritis have an excellent prognosis, with less than 15% having joint destruction and disability 15 years after initial diagnosis. Sequelae can include leg length discrepancy resulting from premature closing of the growth plate in the knee and subluxation of joints; in some children the disease progresses to a polyarticular form that leads to widespread joint destruction and disability. The course of the disease can last from several months to several years. Twenty percent of these children, however, develop iritis, a chronic inflammation of the iris. This is a serious complication that can lead to visual impairment or blindness if not treated.

The other subtype of oligoarticular JRA occurs primarily in boys older than 8 years. These children usually have arthritis (inflammation) or arthralgia (pain) in one or more joints in the lower extremities in an asymmetrical pattern. Affected joints may include hips, knees, ankles, toes, and, rarely, upper extremity joints. Boys with the antigen HLA-B27 in their blood are likely to have a form of arthritis called spondyloarthropathy. A few years after the onset of joint pain and inflammation, low back pain begins. The disease process is similar to a condition in which adult men develop ankylosing spondylitis in the third decade of life with progressive arthritis and pain in the sacroiliac joints, hip girdle, and spine. Pain is worse in the mornings and at night. Back range of motion is limited, and the lumbar lordosis becomes flattened. Inflammation of the costovertebral joints can lead to decreased chest expansion. The disease course for these children is more severe than for those with simple oligoarticular JRA. Although affected children may lose some spinal range of motion, the pain can be managed with medications, and peripheral joint destruction or chronic iriditis is rare. The children may develop an acute form of iriditis that can be treated and does not usually lead to visual impairment.

Polyarticular JRA.   Polyarticular JRA occurs in 30% to 40% of children with JRA. There are two groups of children with polyarticular JRA, classified by the age of onset. The first group develops symptoms in early childhood, usually between 1 and 3 years of age. The second group develops initial symptoms in early adolescence and has a poorer prognosis, especially if children have a positive rheumatoid factor in their blood. Onset may be slow, with gradual joint pain developing, or it may be more acute with a low-grade fever and acute joint pain in multiple joints. Each child will have five or more joints affected, usually significantly more. The distribution of joint involvement will usually be symmetrical, with knees, ankles, elbows, wrists, and the small joints of the hands involved. The temporomandibular joint, cervical spine, hips, and shoulders may also be involved. More girls than boys develop this form of JRA. Of those children with a positive rheumatic factor, 50% will develop severe arthritis with erosive joint changes (Figure 5-27).

Systemic JRA.   The least common form of JRA, called *systemic onset*, occurs in 10% to 20% of children with JRA. Onset is acute, with high spiking fevers, sometimes even before joint pain becomes apparent. It commonly begins between 5 and 10 years of age, but it can begin any time in childhood. A rash over the

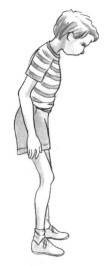

Figure 5-27 The posture of a child with polyarticular juvenile rheumatoid arthritis demonstrates the typical flexed spine and extremities, forward head, and shortened chin.

trunk and proximal extremities is sometimes seen. The rash may be more apparent during the regular fever spikes once or twice each day. Other acute symptoms may include enlargement of the liver and spleen; swollen lymph nodes; and inflammation of the lungs, heart muscle, or pericardium. Muscle pain (myalgia) frequently accompanies the fevers. The fever and muscle pain may last a few to many months, with joint pain frequently developing later in a few to many joints. The joint pain may lessen as the acute symptoms subside, but in 50% of the cases it continues, causing persistent and severe arthritis. From 25% to 50% of children with systemic JRA develop joint destruction, which can lead to significant disability.

Medical Treatment

Pharmaceutical management. Pharmaceutical management of JRA consists of trying to control the inflammation without overwhelming other body systems. Table 5-4 lists common drug treatments. The first level of treatment consists of aspirin and other nonsteroidal antiinflammatory drugs (NSAIDs). Although aspirin and some other NSAIDs are available over the counter, the side effects of high doses can be severe, including stomach irritation and tinnitus (ringing in the ears). Although high doses of aspirin can be effective, Reye's syndrome can be a sequela of using aspirin in children; therefore other NSAIDs such as naproxen or tolmetin are more commonly prescribed. Inflammation in 50% of children with JRA can be managed with these drugs along with other supportive measures such as physical therapy and psychosocial support (Arthreya & Cassidy, 1991).

The next level of medical management includes a class of drugs called slow-acting antirheumatic drugs (SAARDs). These may include gold salts, antimalarial drugs such as hydroxychloroquine, or penicillamine and sulfasalazine. These may be used in addition to the NSAIDs to provide improved relief of inflammation. The drugs in this class are called slow acting because it takes several months of administration before results are seen. Side effects may be very serious, and children taking these drugs are monitored closely.

Corticosteroids compose the next level of drug therapy for use with those children with very severe, poorly controlled symptoms. These may be administered systemically, opthalmically for inflammation in the eye, or injected into the joint space for specific joint inflammation. The side effects of steroid use can be severe and range from infection, osteoporosis, growth retardation, weight gain, and sterility. Therefore these drugs are used for only the most severe cases, and the dosage is controlled carefully to ensure that the child receives the smallest effective dose.

For children whose symptoms are still not able to be controlled and whose disease may be life threatening and include inflammation of vital organs such as the heart and lungs, newer drugs, including immunosuppressive agents and cytotoxic agents such as cyclosporine A, are being tested. These drugs generally have severe side effects, with the exception of methotrexate, a cytotoxic agent that has been extensively tested on children and found to be generally safe. Seventy percent of children who take methotrexate have a positive response, and this drug is gaining widespread use in early management of the disease process (Willkins, Watson, & Paxson, 1980).

Surgical management. Surgery is used to manage severe joint disease, prevent deformity, correct deformity, improve function, or decrease pain. Synovectomy, or removal of the inflamed synovium in affected joints, is a controversial procedure. The Arthritis Foundation and the American Rheumatology Association sponsored research on the long-term effects of synovectomy and found that in adults the surgery had little long-term value (Arthritis Foundation Committee on Evaluation of Synovectomy, 1988). In some cases this surgery may be effective, especially those in which one or several large joints are involved and where a short-term gain in pain relief is sought; but in general, the study found that short-term positive results eroded over time.

Soft tissue releases can be effective in increasing range of motion, decreasing contracture, relieving pain, and producing improved joint alignment. They are most effective at the hip and knee to improve function. By realigning joint surfaces, soft tissue surgery may avoid later surgery necessary to reconstruct joints. Physical therapy is required postoperatively to maximize the surgical outcome through stretching, splinting, and positioning. A child with JRA should not be immobilized for an extended period during the recovery phase to prevent joint erosion and possible fusion. A continuous passive motion machine (CPM) may be used to restrict motion of the joint but prevent deterioration of the joint surfaces with resultant loss of range of motion caused by immobility.

More invasive surgeries such as osteotomy (realigning the bone), epiphyseodesis (fusing the growth plate), and total joint arthroplasty (joint replacement) may be necessary to address

TABLE 5-4 Drug Treatments for Juvenile Rheumatoid Arthritis

Class of drugs	Examples of drugs	Side effects
Aspirin and nonsteroidal antiinflammatory drugs (NSAIDs)	Naproxen, tolmetin, ibuprofen, indomethacin, fenoprofen, aspirin	Stomach irritation, tinnitus, Reye's syndrome (aspirin only), rash, headache, dizziness, renal toxicity, edema
Slow-acting antirheumatic drugs (SAARD)		
Gold salts		Sepsis, rash, thrombocytopenia, kidney problems
Antimalarial drugs	Hydroxychloroquine, penicillamine, sulfasalazine	Eye problems, thrombocytopenia, anemia, kidney problems, rash
Corticosteroids	Prednisone	Infection, osteoporosis, growth retardation, weight gain, sterility
Immunosuppressive and cytotoxic agents	Cyclosporin A Methotrexate	Liver disease, bone marrow suppression, pneumonitis

specific orthopedic problems. An osteotomy at the hip or knee may be necessary to create a more functional joint position without interfering with the joint surfaces directly. Surgeries, including some osteotomies, that require immobilization are generally contraindicated for a child with JRA.

Joint fusion in distal joints, such as the wrist or finger joints, may be allowed to occur naturally in a functional position. Surgical fusion in a child with JRA is not usually indicated. Epiphyseodesis may be necessary to correct discrepancies in leg length. Total joint replacements may be required to improve function in a child with severe hip or knee destruction. Because of the limitations of the joint prostheses themselves and potential complications such as prosthetic loosening and infection, total joint replacement surgeries are delayed as long as possible, preferably at least until skeletal maturity. Any surgical intervention requires intensive physical therapy for rehabilitation.

Physical Therapy Intervention

Children with JRA may undergo physical therapy in the hospital clinic, at home, or at school. Therapy may be indicated during a flare-up of symptoms, before or after a surgical procedure, or for chronic problems such as limitations in joint movement, weakness, or difficulty with daily tasks. Ideally physical therapy participates as part of a team of individuals who share the management of the child's disease process. Other team members include the child, family members, teacher, physician, OT, nutritionist, nurse, and others who may be called in to help with specific issues.

Develop a "pain scale" for use with children with chronic pain, including children with JRA. This will give you an idea of the child's subjective levels of pain and help you guide therapy for that day. Depending on the age of the child, a pain scale can be numbered, with 0 being no pain and 10 being unbearable pain. A younger child may respond more effectively to fewer choices, so animals or colors may be more useful. For instance, the pain is "as big as a guinea pig," "as big as a lion," or "as big as a mammoth."

Use of pain modalities. Pain and stiffness are integral to JRA. Pain is usually the first presenting symptom and, together with stiffness, is the leading cause of future contractures and loss of function. Therefore pain and stiffness need to be treated, even in very young children. Medical treatment with NSAIDs and other drugs can be highly effective at reducing the inflammatory process of JRA, thereby reducing pain and stiffness. Therapists have also used other modalities for decades to treat these ills. Heat in the form of paraffin, ultrasound, warm water, and heat lamps have been shown to reduce pain and stiffness in adults. Cold has been demonstrated to be effective in reducing swelling. Care must be taken in using these modalities with young children, however. Children's bones and joints are different from those of adults. They have growth plates that are susceptible to damage from ultrasound. Children's skin is very sensitive; a child

may not be able to state when something is too hot or too cold, which causes the child to be at risk of skin damage from paraffin, heat lamps, hot water, or ice packs. The benefits of these modalities need to be weighed against their risks in children, and input from the medical team should be obtained before decisions are made. It may be that paraffin or ultrasound provide the most relief for a child, and the benefits of each outweigh the risks in certain cases. Such choices should be based on a team decision, however, with the parents fully informed of the risks.

Splinting. Splints may be helpful to prevent or decrease contracture related to joint subluxation or caused by pain and decreased active movement. Even very young children who are at risk for developing contracture may benefit from night splinting of knees, ankles, wrists, and hands. These splints are generally resting splints, rather than dynamic splints. Use of night splints is designed to prevent contracture from passive positioning. Older children may benefit from splinting to prevent contracture or to protect joints that are at risk for trauma. Orthotics may help to position feet for more functional and pain-free weight bearing. An orthotist or a therapist with specialized training may make splints and orthotics. See Chapter 6 for a more detailed description of splints and orthotics.

Stretching. Stretching is a common treatment modality to reduce shortened muscles and contracted joints. It may be effective at lengthening shortened tissues, but care must be taken to protect joints. Subluxation at the wrist, knee, and other joints is common in a child with severe arthritis; and stretching can traumatize inflamed joints, causing subluxation or dislocation, if care is not taken. Before stretching, the joint tissues should be warmed up through light exercise, modalities, or passive range of motion. The joint should be supported on both sides, and the tissues should be stretched gently. The lever arm should be short; in other words, the limb should be supported close to the joint itself. Attention should be paid to the cues of the child for pain and discomfort. Whenever possible, the joint should be stretched through active rather than passive motion. For example, a child can kick a soft foam ball to get active knee extension instead of passively stretching the knee into extension. Appropriate positioning can also prevent contracture. For instance, the use of night splints, appropriate seating to maintain good posture, and pillows to support limbs in extension at night all may be effective for maintaining range of motion. These methods may be used alone or in conjunction with a stretching program to prevent contractures in a child with JRA.

Physical therapy for the toddler and preschool child. Although splinting, modalities and exercises for pain relief, improving range of motion, and strengthening are often called for in treating a young child with JRA, boredom or intolerance is often the result if these services are provided in the same way as for adults. By embedding stretching, strengthening, and pain relief into activities that are appropriate for the specific age of the child, productive therapy is more likely to take place. If the therapy provider can shift the perspective even further from the "medical model" of treating symptoms and focus on what the child needs to be able to do developmentally, therapy activities will emerge from the activities themselves.

For example, a 2-year-old child with oligoarticular JRA is developing a flexion contracture of her right knee, has stopped ambulating, and is not tolerating hands-on therapy because of pain. She also has stiffness and pain in her left elbow, but she does not allow anyone to touch her arm. Her therapy goals include increasing the active and passive range of motion of her right knee and left elbow so that she can stand independently with both legs fully extended and can reach for toys with a fully extended elbow on the left. Other goals include walking independently and squatting to pick up toys from the floor. The parents are reluctant to do stretching at home because the child is becoming so afraid of pain that she starts to cry when they approach her to do her exercises. Her medical insurance company, however, allows direct therapy only once per week.

Developmentally this child is starting to match shapes and colors, is enjoying manipulating objects such as crayons and puzzle pieces, and is beginning to be more assertive to gain some mastery over her environment. She also loves rough-and-tumble play.

The therapist provides an easel with felt shapes on a formboard. She provides steps with a railing to climb up to reach the easel and begins to make a scene on the formboard while describing what she is doing. The child becomes interested, creeps over to the easel, and pulls herself to a standing position next to the steps. She carefully climbs up the steps while holding the railing and reaches up for the felt pieces. The child then shifts her weight from one foot to the other, reaches up onto her tiptoes while putting the "sun" in the "sky," and gradually allows the therapist to "help" her reach and place the felt forms. After awhile the child can stand without holding on as she places the felt pieces on the board. She squats to pick up felt pieces from the steps. She imitates the therapist, demonstrating what the sun, the rain, and the wind might look like, getting vigorous active range of motion of her legs and arms in the process. When she tires of the formboard, she allows a singing activity to turn into dancing. The therapist shows her father how to hold his daughter while dancing with her to provide stretching to her knee and elbow. The tango and the rumba turn into gentle rough-and-tumble play on the floor, where the child undergoes further stretching in the guise of a tickling game. The therapist is very careful to watch the cues of the child and never to allow the fun to cross the line into discomfort or pain. Although the therapist had ideas planned before the therapy session, the therapist followed the lead of the child, using creativity and inventiveness with developmental activities to further therapy goals.

Night splints at home, warm baths in the morning with special "games" of riding puppet animals on her feet for stretching and strengthening, and nightly dancing with Dad help her parents have fun with their child, yet allow them to support her rehabilitation needs at home.

Role of the PTA with the young child. The PTA needs to be creative with a young child, keeping both developmental and rehabilitation priorities in mind to develop activities that promote therapy goals, model for parents and siblings, and encourage a positive relationship between the PTA and the child. Developing a routine with several enjoyable activities during the therapy session, as well as allowing creative alternatives, can help the child become more comfortable in the therapy situation over time. All activities should be directed toward the child's therapy and developmental goals. Interjecting new games, toys, and new ways to use old materials can be helpful with this process. Using a toy the child brings as a transitional object to lessen his or her anxiety in the therapy setting can also help. Parents and siblings can actively participate in the therapy session and provide games,

routines, or activities that the child enjoys at home; these may also help the child become more comfortable.

When making splints, the PTA should include the child by providing some soft splinting material to play with or by making a small splint for a toy or doll. These activities may encourage the child to assist with the splinting process rather than resist it.

Physical therapy for the young school-aged child. Therapy for the young school-aged child may be provided in school or in the clinic. Therapy goals may include relief from pain or swelling; prevention or decrease of contractures; strengthening; and improvement of functional skills such as walking, sitting, climbing, running, jumping, skipping, or moving from one position to another. Functional skills should include those necessary in a school environment such as writing, climbing stairs, or sitting comfortably in a chair for several hours. Most young school-aged children with JRA are ambulatory, although some may use assistive devices such as a cane or crutches.

Although facilitating the activity of children and their involvement with peers is important, protection of fragile and painful joints is essential. Activities that offer potential trauma to joints, such as skiing, ice skating, roller skating, surfing, jogging, trampoline jumping, diving, and tennis, need to be evaluated carefully to weigh the benefits versus the risks to the child from joint trauma. The child and parents need to be informed about the risks of trauma, and the choices of the child and family should be respected. Therapy should avoid potentially traumatic activities such as jumping on small trampolines or jogging. Bicycling, swimming, or group and individual exercises using the Swiss ball are preferable to activities that cause repetitive trauma to joints.

The therapist is likely to be on a team that supports the child with JRA in school. In this setting the therapy emphasis is on supporting the child's education rather than treating medical problems. Responsibilities may include helping the physical education teacher to adapt the curriculum for the child with JRA; helping the teacher adapt the desk, chair, and classroom environment for the child; and teaching and supervising exercises for mobility, strengthening, or stretching. It is unlikely that the school-based therapist will be providing activities for acute pain relief or to decrease swelling from acute exacerbations of the disease. These activities would more likely occur in an acute outpatient clinic.

Role of the PTA with the young school-aged child. The PTA may work in a clinic, where a child with JRA is followed up for treatment of acute or chronic problems, or in a school setting, where the approach and goals are somewhat different. In either case the responsibility is to work with other team members to accomplish therapeutic or educational goals that are functional for the child. Flexibility and creativity to adapt equipment and environments or to create activities to further therapeutic or educational goals are essential. Goals may include climbing in and out of the bathtub independently, climbing stairs while holding the railing with one hand, sitting upright with good posture in a school chair, or reaching to scrub the upper back during bathing. Songs, dances, group activities with the Swiss ball, and individual exercise routines may be effective if the child is seen for individual therapy sessions. If the PTA's role is that of a classroom consultant, teaching the teacher and the child strategies to accomplish difficult tasks, such as how to use adaptive equipment in the classroom or how to get down to the floor for story time, can be most functional. Keeping educational goals in mind helps the PTA to design activities that provide the most benefit to the child in an educational setting.

> ☀ It often helps to talk with team members individually *before* a meeting in which you want to bring up a new idea or strategy. If you brief the individual members beforehand, the information or idea is not a surprise, and you have more likelihood of getting cooperation from the team. You will also have already heard some of the problems individuals will bring up and you will have had a chance to address them.

Physical therapy for the older child. Older children may have been coping with the pain and disability of JRA for several years, and their goals will differ from those of younger children. Older school-aged children and adolescents may have goals that range from dancing at the school dance, hiking with their family, walking between classes at school, and looking less different from their peers. Other goals may include reducing pain and contractures to allow the child to function more fully. These children generally tolerate stretching and pain relief modalities, such as paraffin or ultrasound, better than younger children and may be willing to do a regular exercise routine to work toward a personal goal. Assessing what the child would like to accomplish with therapy is important, especially for older children. Giving the adolescent control over therapy goals and activities encourages greater compliance and assistance in developing the crucial relationship between therapist and child that is necessary for progress. Therefore the child should have an active role in scheduling the therapy sessions, as well as in deciding the content, with input from the therapist, teacher, physician, and parents.

Role of the PTA with the older child. The older child with JRA is generally aware of which therapeutic intervention is helpful and will already have specific goals. The older child may need therapy only during acute exacerbations or to achieve certain goals. The PTA should work to develop a relationship of trust and mutual respect so that therapy sessions are fun and productive.

APPLICATIONS   The Changing Role of the School-Based Physical Therapist

IRENE R. McEWEN

PTs have worked with children in schools for almost as long as physical therapy has been a profession (Effgen, 1994). During the early years, however, not all school districts had programs for children with disabilities, and districts that did have programs often considered only children with mild disabilities to be "eligible" to go to school. Then in 1975 Congress passed Public Law (PL) 94-142, the Education for All Handicapped Children Act. The law, resulting from two decades of civil rights legislation and changing social policy, required states to provide a "free and appropriate public education" (FAPE) for all children with disabilities, regardless the severity of their disabilities. In 1991 Congress passed PL 102-119, which changed the name of the law to the Individuals with Disabilities Education Act (IDEA). One section of IDEA, Part B, addresses the needs of students with disabilities aged 3 to 21 years (or older in some states). Another section of the law, Part H, addresses early intervention programs for infants and toddlers age birth through 2 years and their families.

Part B of IDEA has many provisions that pediatric clinicians need to understand, not only when they work in schools but also when they work with children with disabilities who might be referred for school services. Children can receive physical therapy under IDEA either as a related service or, in some states, as special education. Special education is defined by IDEA as "specially designed instruction, at no cost to the parents, to meet the unique needs of a child with a disability" (34 CFR § 300.17*). Related services are defined as transportation, physical therapy, and other services "that are required to assist a child with a disability to benefit from special education" (34 CFR § 300.16).

Box 5-5 lists these definitions along with some of the other major provisions of IDEA.

Deciding Who Should Get Therapy in School: A Process

For most students who receive physical therapy in school it is a related service. The required link between physical therapy as a related service and "benefit from special education" has created much confusion and controversy over the years, as parents, administrators, therapists, and teachers have tried to decide which children should receive physical therapy for what purposes in school. Should children receive therapy only to help them with reading, writing, and mathematics? Should children with the most severe disabilities get the most therapy? Should children over a certain age be "ineligible" for hands-on therapy? Who should decide if a child needs therapy at school? Therapists? Physicians? Parents?

As with many of the other provisions of the law, IDEA gives only general direction for making decisions about physical therapy services. More specific direction has evolved as a result of court cases and clarification of "best practices" in both physical therapy and special education.

In general, any student who is eligible for special education can receive physical therapy *if* the student's educational team decides that the student needs physical therapy either to achieve educational goals or to have access to or participate in the educational environment (Giangreco, 1995). The educational environment includes not only classrooms but also other school and out-of-school settings, such as playgrounds, community-based instruction sites (Falvey, 1989), and vocational placements (Figure 5-28). Some therapists and administrators have attempted to develop other criteria to determine who should receive therapy, such as requiring the student to have a certain amount of

---

*"CFR" stands for Code of Federal Regulations, title 34 pertains to education regulations, and part 300 covers "assistance to states for education of handicapped children." The last number refers to the section within part 300. The regulations are published by the Office of the Federal Register, National Archives and Records Administration, and are available through the U.S. Government Printing Office, Washington, DC.

Definitions of Selected Major Provisions of the Individuals With Disabilities Education Act

BOX 5-5

Categories of Disability

Autism, deaf-blindness, deafness, hearing impairment, mental retardation, multiple disabilities, orthopedic impairments, other health impairment, serious emotional disturbance, specific learning disability, speech or language impairment, traumatic brain injury, and visual impairment including blindness. For children ages 3 through 5 years, states may choose to use the category of developmental delay, rather than label a child with a particular disability. *34 CFR § 300.7*

Special Education

Specially designed instruction, at no cost to the parents, to meet the unique needs of a child with a disability, including:
(1) Instruction conducted in the classroom, in the home, in hospitals and institutions, and in other settings; and
(2) Instruction in physical education.
The term includes speech pathology, or any other related services, if the service consists of specially designed instruction, at no cost to the parents, to meet the unique needs of a child with a disability, and is considered special education rather than a related service under state standards. The term also includes vocational education if it consists of specially designed instruction, at no cost to the parents, to meet the unique needs of a child with a disability. *34 § CFR 300.17*

Related Services

Transportation and such developmental, corrective, and other supportive services as are required to assist a child with a disability to benefit from special education; includes speech pathology, audiology, psychological services, physical and occupational therapy, recreation (including therapeutic recreation), early identification and assessment of disabilities in children, counseling services (including rehabilitation counseling) and medical services for diagnostic or evaluation purposes. The term also includes school health services, social work services in schools, and parent counseling and training. *34 § CFR 300.16 (a)*

Physical Therapy

Services provided by a qualified physical therapist. *34 CFR § 300.16(b)(7)*

Individualized Education Program (IEP)

The IEP for each child must include: (1) a statement of the child's present levels of educational performance; (2) a statement of annual goals, including short-term instructional objectives; (3) a statement of the specific special education and related services to be provided to the child and the extent that the child will be able to participate in regular educational programs; (4) the projected date for initiation of services and the anticipated duration of the services; and (5) appropriate objective criteria and evaluation procedures and schedules for determining, on at least an annual basis, whether the short-term instructional objectives are being achieved. *34 CFR § 300.346*

Least Restrictive Environment

To the maximum extent appropriate, children with disabilities, including children in public or private institutions, or other care facilities, are educated with children who are nondisabled; and that special classes, separate schooling, or other removal of children with disabilities from regular classes occurs only when the nature or severity of the disability is such that education in the regular classroom with the use of supplementary aids and services cannot be achieved satisfactorily. *34 CFR § 300.550(b)*

Zero Reject

All children have a right to a free and appropriate education, regardless of the nature or the extent of their disabilities.

---

delay in motor skills or have cognitive skills at least equal to motor skills (Carr, 1989; Notari, Cole, & Mills, 1992). Such types of decision-making mechanisms have been determined to be unlawful, however, if they categorically deny services to students and prevent students' educational teams from making decisions based on the unique needs of students (Rainforth, 1991).

To be eligible for special education and related services, children must have one of the 13 categories of disability defined by IDEA (see Box 5-5) *and* the disability must adversely affect educational performance. If the disability does not affect educational performance, students may still qualify for physical therapy services and civil rights protections under Section 504 of the Rehabilitation Act of 1973. Under this act a student could receive physical therapy at school if it is needed to accommodate for the student's disability (Rapport, 1995). Camila, the child with JRA who is described in the case study in this chapter, might qualify for school-based physical therapy services under Section 504 if she needs services to accommodate mobility limitations, for ex-

ample, or restricted hand function. If her disability affects her academic performance but special education services are not needed for anything other than therapy, she could receive physical therapy as special education (rather than as a related service) if she lives in a state that permits it. Given a choice, states usually prefer to serve students under IDEA, rather than under Section 504, because they receive federal funds for students served under IDEA (although not enough to cover costs); they are not reimbursed for students served under Section 504.

Deciding on a Student's Educational Program

Most students who receive physical therapy services at school qualify for services under IDEA. IDEA requires that a team decide what a student's educational program will be and that the program be documented on an IEP. The team always includes a student's parents and teachers; it may include the student and others who are involved with the student or who might be needed

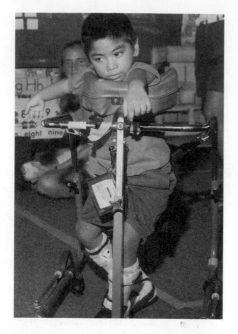

Figure 5-28 Joshua can walk around his classroom by himself.

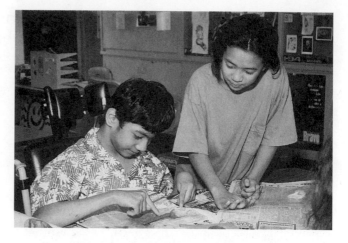

Figure 5-29 Cyril gets help from his friend in art class.

to be involved, such as a PT (Rainforth, Macdonald, York, & Dunn, 1992). As specified by the definition of "special education," a student's educational program must be individualized and designed to meet the student's unique needs. For this reason educational programs of students with disabilities vary widely. Some students, for example, might only need some extra help with reading and mathematics, whereas other students with more severe disabilities might need to learn basic self-help and communication skills.

While it is not specifically stated in the IDEA, a persuasive case can be made . . . that the unique educational needs of a child with a disability encompass much more than mastery of academic subjects. Rather, unique educational needs should be broadly construed to include academic, social, health, emotional, physical and vocational needs (Gorn, 1996, p. 3:15).

After reviewing a student's strengths and needs, the team decides what the student's educational goals and objectives will be. The objectives need to be measurable, and they usually cover a year's time. Current best practices in special education and related services require goals and objectives to be discipline free, functional, age appropriate, and meaningful to the student and family (Giangreco, 1995). Students do not have classroom goals, physical therapy goals, occupational therapy goals, and speech goals; rather, the team agrees on overall goals and objectives that it believes are important for the child to achieve (Figure 5-29). Andrew, a 5-year-old with cerebral palsy described in the Chapter 7 Case Study, for example, might have the following three functional, age-appropriate, and discipline-free goals:

- Andrew will sit on his carpet square during opening circle and use his communication device to answer correctly four questions without losing his balance and falling over on 10 consecutive school days by (date).
- Andrew will drive his power wheelchair from his classroom to the cafeteria without assistance in 5 minutes or less on 10 consecutive school days by (date).

- When given two nickels, dimes, pennies, and quarters, Andrew will indicate the correct coins to purchase his milk on 10 consecutive school days by (date).

Andrew would have more than three objectives on his IEP, but all would be similarly functional and chronologically age appropriate. Functional and chronologically age-appropriate goals are in contrast to developmentally based goals, such as improving trunk control, rolling with rotation, half-kneeling, or standing on one foot. Developmentally based goals were sometimes written for students in the past, but these goals rarely lead to achievement of meaningful skills, such as going to the cafeteria independently or feeding oneself (Brown et al., 1979; Harris, 1991). About the only time that developmentally based goals might be appropriate is for infants, for whom the typical developmental sequence is age appropriate, or for young children with mild developmental delays who may reach the stage of their typically developing peers.

Deciding on School Placement

After the goals and objectives are written, the team decides which school placement is likely to be the most effective in helping the child to achieve the goals and objectives. IDEA requires that children go to school in the least restrictive environment (LRE), which means that to the extent appropriate children with disabilities attend school with children who do not have disabilities (Figure 5-30).

Neither a child's category of disability nor the services needed can dictate the most appropriate placement. A child who qualifies for special education because of multiple disabilities, for example, cannot automatically be placed in a classroom for children with multiple disabilities; nor can a child who needs physical therapy be placed in a school because therapy is available only in that location. Students must be placed in the LRE in which they can achieve their goals. Services need to follow the student to whatever location is selected.

Increasingly, students with disabilities, including those with severe disabilities, are being placed in general education classrooms in their own neighborhoods (Giangreco, Cloninger, & Iverson, 1993; Taylor, 1988). This placement does not mean they are thrown in to "sink or swim." Rather, students must receive the supplementary aids and services that they need to achieve

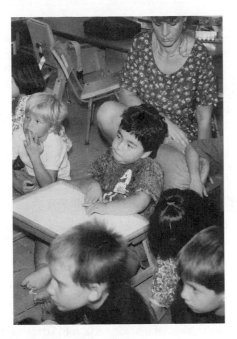

Figure 5-30 Rik can join the other children on the floor with help from equipment and his educational assistant.

their individualized goals and objectives. Often this means that a special education teacher will consult with the classroom teacher to modify curriculum and materials and that related services, such as physical therapy, will be provided in the general education setting. Even students with severe disabilities can make significant gains when they participate in good general education classrooms and have peer models without disabilities; the typical peers also often benefit from their interactions with students with disabilities. Andrew's team decided that he could best achieve his goals in the kindergarten class in his neighborhood school.

Deciding What Services a Student Needs

After a student's placement has been decided, the decision of who will do what to help the student achieve the goals and objectives and provide the necessary supports is the next step in the process. This decision needs to be based on not only the student's program and needs but also the experience and skills of the teachers (general and special education) and the rest of the educational team.

Considering Andrew's objectives, if he does not have the sitting balance necessary to sit on his carpet square and use his hands to select symbols on his communication device, he might need a PT or a PTA to help him improve this skill. On the other hand, if the educational assistant in his classroom has learned how to help Andrew sit on his carpet square and practice with the communication device while maintaining his balance, he might need therapy services only to monitor this objective and provide assistance if needed. If Andrew has not yet learned to use the communication device but his teacher has the skills needed to program the device and teach him to use it, he may not need the assistance of a speech-language pathologist. Another student, however, with a similar objective but a different

teacher might need speech-language services. As another example, if Andrew has a power wheelchair and his teacher or classroom assistant knows how to help him learn to drive, he may not require the services of a PT or PTA to achieve the mobility objective. If he does not have a chair, however, he may need physical therapy services to acquire an appropriate chair. If his family and classroom team do not know about power chairs or how to teach him to use one, consultation by a PT or PTA probably would be necessary.

In addition to helping students achieve their goals and objectives, PTs and PTAs often provide services that help a student have access to or participate in the school program. Andrew, for example, uses a stander during the day at school to prevent knee and hip flexion contractures and to promote gastrointestinal function. Standing in a stander is not something Andrew will learn, so it is not written as a goal or objective on his IEP; however, it is something he needs to do to be able to spend the day at school. Physical therapy services might be needed to find and fit an appropriate stander, develop a schedule for standing with his teacher, and teach the classroom assistant to transfer Andrew to and from the stander. If Andrew already had a stander in the classroom and the assistant knew how to transfer him, the PT or PTA might need to monitor his standing only occasionally to be sure that the stander still fits him and is being used appropriately.

Giangreco and his colleagues (1993) describe five categories of general supports that students might require to have access to education or to participate in an educational program: (1) personal needs (e.g., feeding, clean intermittent catheterization, or medication); (2) physical needs (e.g., positioning, managing equipment, or environmental modifications); (3) sensory needs (e.g., Braille or sign language); (4) teaching others about the student (e.g., teaching classmates or staff how to help the student); and (5) providing access and opportunities (e.g., arranging community-based experiences, or providing access to general classroom activities). Depending on the needs of the student and the skills of other school personnel, physical therapy services might be required to provide some of the necessary supports. Supportive services are documented on the IEP, along with services that directly help students to achieve their goals and objectives.

Deciding on the Type of School-Based Physical Therapy Services

In schools, just as in clinics, hospitals, and other settings, clinicians must select service delivery methods that are most likely to help a child achieve his or her functional goals. Traditionally therapists, parents, teachers, and many others have believed that hands-on therapy is better than other types of service delivery. As service providers have become more aware of motor learning principles, however, they have started to place greater emphasis on working with parents and others who are with the children for hours each day to help them implement intervention with children, regardless of the service setting (McEwen & Shelden, 1995). Working with parents and others who interact regularly with children supports several motor learning principles:

1. To learn motor skills, children need many opportunities to practice throughout the day. If parents and teachers help a child transfer to the toilet several times a day, for example, the skill will be learned more quickly than if the child practices transferring only during therapy sessions.

2. Children are more likely to use motor skills that are practiced in environments in which they actually use them. A child who practices transferring to the toilet is more likely to be able to do a toilet transfer when it is needed than a child who practices transferring to a mat table.

3. Practicing a motor skill throughout the day is more effective than practicing the skill the same number of times in one session. A child who practices transferring five times throughout the day is more likely to learn the skill than a child who practices transferring five times during one therapy session.

Sometimes hands-on therapy is necessary, particularly when students are learning new skills and the clinician needs to identify the best way to help the child to learn. Imagine that Andrew, the 5-year-old with cerebral palsy, is learning to move into a sitting position from lying on the floor so he can sit on his carpet square with the other children for opening circle. The physical therapy clinician may need to work with Andrew outside of opening circle time to find the best way for him to get into a sitting position, particularly if he finds it difficult and he is not clear on how to accomplish the task. Once a likely method is identified, Andrew needs to practice during circle time; the classroom teacher and/or assistant needs to be able to assist him appropriately every day. To identify how to help Andrew improve his sitting balance, the PT or PTA could work with Andrew during circle time, integrating his sitting practice into the flow of the circle activity. Again, once the methods have been determined, someone who is always present during opening circle needs to be taught to help Andrew so he has an opportunity to practice every day. An even better situation would be if he had several opportunities to practice every day; so in collaboration with the teacher, other times should be identified when Andrew can practice sitting while participating in classroom activities.

As some of the possibilities for Andrew's physical therapy program suggest, schools can be an excellent place for children to learn meaningful and functional skills. Since schools are natural environments, it is easy to evaluate students' functioning in real-world situations and to arrange practice so it promotes motor learning. These steps are more difficult in many clinical settings. Because educational goals can be any goals that a student's education team thinks are important, there are few skills that are not appropriately taught at school if the team agrees they are an educational priority for a child. Sometimes people try to differentiate "educational" therapy from "medical" therapy, but few goals are inherently medical or educational, and no methods of service delivery are inherently medical or educational. Whatever the service setting, teams need to identify meaningful, achievable goals and use methods that are most likely to achieve them (McEwen & Shelden, 1995).

EXERCISES

1. Work on a finite task with a small group of your classmates (write a poem, short story, or a SOAP note). After the task is complete, discuss the dynamics of your "team." Did each of you work on a portion of the task, then come back together? Did you write the entire thing together? Would a different size group of individuals have made a difference? Would a different type of task have made a difference? What did you learn about yourself and how you work in a team?

2. Write a treatment plan for a 5-year-old girl with oligoarticular JRA. Her right knee is swollen and painful. Her goal is to walk 50 feet without limping. List five different activities you might do to help her achieve her goal. Justify why each activity will help her achieve the goal.

3. A 4-year-old boy with AMC is being trained to drive a power wheelchair. His goals are to drive 10 feet in a straight line and to turn right and left within 5 seconds of your command. What activities would you do with this child to help him achieve his goals?

QUESTIONS TO PONDER

1. A grandmother of a 6-year-old with severe AMC tells you that her primary goal is to see her granddaughter walk. The therapist and the physician have both told you that this child will never walk. How would you respond to the grandmother's statement? Why?

2. Folic acid supplements were thought to be a preventive for spina bifida years before the public was educated about it. Until research showed that folic acid could decrease the incidence of spina bifida, some thought that it was irresponsible to recommend taking it. What are your feelings about this? What if folic acid had not ultimately been shown to prevent spina bifida? What if it had had serious side effects?

3. An adolescent with severe JRA wants to engage in a moderate hike of 3 to 4 hours up the side of a mountain and back down. You are concerned about potential trauma to his joints but want to respect his initiative. Should he go on the hike or not? Should he train for the hike and do it later? Why? Whom would you consult to get more information?

4. You think a 5-year-old boy with bilateral lower extremity limb deficiencies has the potential to use power mobility. His house is not accessible to a power wheelchair, and you are concerned about his family's ability to care for the chair. What should you do?

Annotated Bibliography

Werner, D. (1987). *Disabled village children: A guide for community health workers, rehabilitation workers, and families.* Palo Alto, CA: Hesperian Foundation.

This comprehensive, lay-oriented book covers topics related to working with children with disabilities who live in rural areas and have little support. Simple explanations of diagnosis and treatment of common disabilities, including cerebral palsy, juvenile rheumatoid arthritis, muscular dystrophy, scoliosis, clubfoot, and Down syndrome, are accompanied by simple drawings illustrating most concepts. Suggestions for common therapeutic activities, such as providing range-of-motion exercises, treating pressure sores, and helping children stand, walk, and learn self-help skills, are described simply and are illustrated with accessible line drawings. Descriptions of how to build simple adaptive equipment with locally available materials and how to work with a community of individuals to promote rehabilitation, social integration, and the rights of disabled children in a village setting are useful and practical. The Hesperian Foundation (P.O. Box 1692, Palo Alto, CA 94302) allows copying and adaptation of any or all parts for local needs, provided that distribution is free of charge. This book is a gold mine. It is easily accessible to parents, teachers, and health professionals. It is available in many languages for a nominal fee. Any professional who works with children in rural settings should have a copy of this book—if only to give away!

References

Aitken, G. T. (1969). Proximal femoral focal deficiency: Definition, classification, and management. In *Proximal femoral focal deficiency: A congenital anomaly.* Washington DC: National Academy of Sciences.

Arthreya, B. H., & Cassidy, J. T. (1991). Current status of the medical treatment of children with JRA. *Rheumatic Disease Clinics of North America, 17,* 871-889.

Arthritis Foundation Committee on Evaluation of Synovectomy. (1988). Multicenter evaluation of synovectomy in the treatment of rheumatoid arthritis: Report of results at the end of five years. *Journal of Rheumatology, 15,* 764.

Bamshad, M., Watkins, W. S., Zenger, R. K., Bohnsack, J. F., Carey, J. C., Otterud, B., Krakawiak, P. A., Robertson, M., & Jorde, L. B. (1994). A gene for distal arthrogryposis type I maps to the pericentromeric region of chromosome 9. *American Journal of Human Genetics, 55,* 1153-1158.

Brent, R. L. (1985). Prevention of physical and mental congenital defects: The scope of the problem. In M. Marios (Ed.), *Progress in clinical and biological research* (*Vol. 163A,* pp. 55-68.) New York: Alan R. Liss.

Brown, L., Branston, M. B., Hamre-Nietupski, S., Pumpian, I., Certo, N., & Gruenewald, L. (1979). A strategy for developing chronological age-appropriate and functional curricular content for severely handicapped adolescents and young adults. *Journal of Special Education, 12,* 81-90.

Carr, S. H. (1989). Louisiana's criteria of eligibility for occupational therapy services in the public school system. *American Journal of Occupational Therapy, 43,* 503-506.

Cassidy, T., & Nelson, A. M. (1988). The frequency of juvenile arthritis. *Journal of Rheumatology, 15,* 535.

Charney, E. B. (1992). Neural tube defects: Spina bifida and myelomeningocele. In M. L. Batshaw & Y. M. Perret, *Children with disabilities: A medical primer* (pp. 471-488). Baltimore, MD: Brookes.

Chung, S. M. K. (1981). *Hip disorders in infants and children.* Philadelphia: Lea & Febinger.

DiCowden, M., Ballard, A., Robinette, H., & Ortiz, O. (1987). Benefit of early fitting and behavior modification training with a voluntary closing terminal device. *Journal of the Association of Children's Prosthetic Orthotic Clinics, 22,* 47-50.

Eckersley, P. M. (Ed.). (1993). *Elements of paediatric physiotherapy.* New York: Churchill Livingstone.

Effgen, S. (1994). The educational environment. In S. K. Campbell (Ed.), *Physical therapy for children* (pp. 847-872). Philadelphia: W. B. Saunders.

Falvey, M. A. (1989). Introduction. In M. A. Falvey (Ed.), *Community-based curriculum: Instructional strategies for students with severe handicaps* (pp. 1-13). Baltimore: Paul H. Brookes.

Giangreco, M. (1995). Related services decision-making: A foundational component of effective education for students with disabilities. In I. R. McEwen (Ed.), *Occupational and physical therapy in educational environments* (pp. 47-67). Binghamton, NY: Haworth Press.

Giangreco, M. F., Cloninger, C. J., & Iverson, V. (1993). *Choosing options and accommodations for children: A guide to planning inclusive education.* Baltimore: Paul H. Brookes.

Gorn, S. (1996). *The answer book on special education law.* Horsham, PA: LRP Publications.

Hall, J. G. (1992). Arthrogryposis. In A. E. H. Emery & D. L. Rimoin (Eds.), *Principles and practice of medical genetics* (2nd ed.). Edinburgh: Churchill Livingstone.

Hall, J. G., Reed, S. D., & Greene, G. (1982). The distal arthrogryposes: Delineation of new entities—review and nosologic discussion. *American Journal of Medical Genetics, 11,* 185-239.

Harris, S. R. (1991). Functional abilities in context. In M. J. Lister (Ed.), *Contemporary management of motor control problems: Proceedings of the II STEP Conference* (pp. 253-259). Alexandria, VA: Foundation for Physical Therapy.

Herzenberg, J. E. (1991). Congenital limb deficiency and limb length discrepancy. In S. T. Canale & J. H. Beatty (Eds.), *Operative pediatric orthopedics.* St. Louis: Mosby.

Jones, K. L. (1988). *Smith's recognizable patterns of human malformation.* Philadelphia: W. B. Saunders.

McEwen, I. R., & Shelden, M. L. (1995). Pediatric therapy in the 1990s: The demise of the educational versus medical dichotomy. In I. R. McEwen (Ed.), *Occupational and physical therapy in educational environments* (pp. 33-45). Binghamton, NY: Haworth Press.

MRC Vitamin Study Research Group. (1991). Prevention of neural tube defects: Results of the Medical Research Council Vitamin Study. *Lancet, 338,* 131-137.

Notari, A. R., Cole, K. N., & Mills, P. E. (1992). Cognitive referencing: The (non)relationship between theory and application. *Topics in Early Childhood Special Education, 11*(4), 22-38.

Prieur, A.M. (1994). Chronic arthritis in children. *Current Opinion in Rheumatology, 6,* 513-517.

Rainforth, B. (1991, April). OSERS clarifies legality of related services eligiblity criteria. *TASH Newsletter,* p. 8.

Rainforth, B., Macdonald, C., York, J., & Dunn, W. (1992). Collaborative assessment. In B. Rainforth, J. York, & C. Macdonald (Eds.), *Collaborative teams for students with severe disabilities: Integrating therapy and educational services* (pp. 105-155). Baltimore: Paul H. Brookes.

Rapport, M. J. (1995). Laws that shape therapy services in educational environments. *Occupational and physical therapy in educational environments* (pp. 5-32). Binghamton, NY: Haworth Press.

Sauter, W. F. (1989). Electric pediatric and adult prosthetic components. In D. J. Atkins & R. H. Meier (Eds.), *Comprehensive management of the upper-limb amputee* (pp. 121-136). New York: Springer-Verlag.

Scheck, A. (1996). The games: All for one? *TeamRehab, 7*(8), 24-29.

Shurtleff, D. B. (1986). Decubitus formation and skin breakdown. In D. B. Shurtleff (Ed.), *Myodysplasias and exstrophies: Significance, prevention, and treatment* (pp. 299-312). Orlando, FL: Grune & Stratton.

Tatum, L. (1996). Behind the wheel: Hand controls for rental cars. *TeamRehab,7*(8), 33-37.

Taylor, S. J. (1988). Caught in the continuum: A critical analysis of the principle of the least restrictive environment. *Journal of The Association for Persons With Severe Handicaps, 13,* 1-53.

Tooms, R. E. (1985). Acquired amputations in children. In J. H. Bowker & J. W. Michael (Eds.), *Atlas of limb prosthetics: Surgical, prosthetic, and rehabilitation principles* (2nd ed.). St. Louis: Mosby.

Towner, S. R., Michet, C. J., O'Fallon, W. M., & Nelson, A. M. (1983). The epidemiology of juvenile arthritis in Rochester, Minn. *Arthritis and Rheumatism, 26,* 1208.

Werner, D. (1987). *Disabled village children.* Palo Alto, CA: Hesperian Foundation.

Willkins, R. F., Watson, M. A., & Paxson, C. S. (1980). Low-dose pulse methotrexate therapy in rheumatoid arthritis. *Journal of Rheumatology, 7,* 501.

Other Orthopedic Disorders

6

Tyler, An Infant With Congenital Torticollis and Erb's Palsy

Tyler grinned at his mother. His whole face lit up when she smiled back at him. Leinani sang to him as she put both of his hands on his knees and rolled his body gently side to side. When he was lying on his side, she picked up his hips and slid him toward her so that his neck stretched to the side. She repeated this several times, singing and smiling at Tyler. He smiled throughout his exercises.

Tyler's mother put him in the infant swing, and he tilted his head to one side to watch the toys that were hanging from the bar of the swing. Swinging back and forth, back and forth, he finally fell asleep.

Family History

Leinani and Ivan met 3 years before Tyler was born, when she was 16 years old and he was 20 (Figure 6-1). They have been living together for 1 year. Although Leinani did not finish high school in Hawaii, she took and passed the test for her Graduate Equivalency Diploma 1 year ago. Leinani was working as a hostess when she became pregnant with Tyler. Ivan has worked for a food service company for the past 5 years. He enjoys his job and

eventually would like to go to cooking school to get a degree to allow him to become a chef.

Leinani and Ivan have been living with family, and they have close relationships with their extended family members. Both of them come from large families and are part Hawaiian. Family is very important to them. Tyler is the first grandchild in Leinani's family.

The pregnancy was uneventful except for an episode of kidney stones. Leinani was in the hospital for 3 days and had a temperature of 105° F during this illness. Leinani took a class to teach her how to take care of her infant after he was born, but she and Ivan did not take childbirth classes. She did not think that childbirth classes would help make the birth easier. Six months before Tyler was born, Leinani applied to the Hawaii Department of Human Services for Medicaid health coverage for herself and her unborn baby. Ivan receives health coverage through his job.

Ivan and Leinani were moving from one family home to another the weekend that her labor started. Later Leinani's aunt told her of a dream she had the night before Tyler was born. She dreamed of a bird with a broken wing.

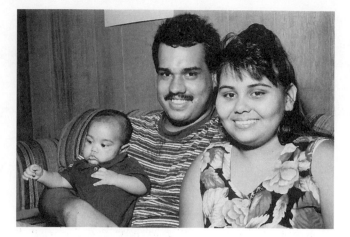

Figure 6-1 Family portrait.

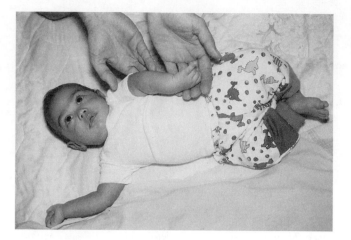

Figure 6-2 Tyler's left arm, which is affected by the Erb's palsy, is held in extension, adduction, and internal rotation.

Birth History

Leinani was at home when her contractions started. She waited 4 hours before Ivan took her to the hospital. She was put into a labor room that she hoped would also be the delivery room. Luckily, the labor room was large because both her family and Ivan's family came to support them. Leinani's sister acted as a labor coach, and her mother, father, brother-in-law, friend, the friend's daughter, Leinani's two aunts, and younger cousin were also there for support. Ivan's aunt was there, too. In total there were a dozen people besides medical personnel in the labor room.

Labor progressed slowly, and it seemed that she spent hours at only 5 cm of dilation. The infant was face up and would not turn over, no matter what position Leinani tried. Finally, the doctor decided to use oxytocin to augment the contractions so that the delivery could progress. After at least 24 hours in the labor room, Leinani finally reached full cervical dilation.

Leinani was moved to the delivery room and given an epidural anesthetic. Ivan and her sister were allowed to come with her. She remembers her sister staying at her side, holding her hand, and Ivan pacing the length of the room. The doctors used forceps to try to turn the baby. For 45 minutes they prodded, twisted, and turned, trying to get the infant to turn over. Leinani remembers kicking two different doctors without meaning to. She still had feeling and movement in her legs. Although her perineum was numb, the forceps were uncomfortable and she could feel pressure. The doctors were unsuccessful in turning the infant, and they finally decided to let the infant be born "sunny side up." They gave Leinani a long episiotomy to make room, and Tyler was delivered at 4:49 PM. He was 20 inches long and weighed 6 pounds, 4¾ ounces.

When Tyler was born, he was not moving his left side (Figure 6-2); nor was his left arm moving. He also seemed to have paralysis of the left side of his face. He was so stressed during the delivery that he had aspirated or breathed in his own meconium, the tarry first stool of a newborn. The doctors were concerned that he might have a fracture of his collar bone. For all these reasons he was immediately rushed to the neonatal intensive care unit (NICU) so that he could be closely monitored. He was breathing on his own, and his color was good. He was put in an Isolette for temperature control with an intravenous line for an-

tibiotics and a heart rate monitor. By the first evening Tyler's face looked more symmetrical, and he was moving his left leg, but he still was not moving his left arm. Radiographs showed that his collar bone was not fractured. His face was bruised and cut from the forceps, including one deep cut below his ear.

Leinani stayed in the hospital for 3 days. She was finally able to hold her son after 2 days had passed. After 5 days Tyler was moved from the NICU to the intermediate nursery. He stayed in the hospital for a total of 7 days. When he came home, he was still not moving his left arm, and he tended to tilt his head to one side. His face was still a little bruised, but he was moving it symmetrically. The pediatrician told Leinani and Ivan to swaddle Tyler with his left arm across his chest. They were told that he should always be swaddled this way so the damaged nerves in his arm could rest and heal.

Tyler at Home

Tyler and his parents live with Ivan's aunt, cousin, and grandmother. The grandmother is elderly and all members of the household help to care for her. The family lives in a three-bedroom house in an outlying area of Honolulu. For the first few months they had no telephone, but Ivan carried a beeper and rode his bicycle to the shopping center a few blocks away to use the public phone to return calls. They have one car that breaks down occasionally, so they are sometimes forced to use the bus or borrow a car from relatives when they have important appointments. Leinani does not drive, and Ivan takes her to doctor and therapy appointments.

When Tyler was a few weeks old, his pediatrician suggested that he get physical therapy to help with his tight neck and weak arm. Although some improvement had occurred, Tyler was still not moving his arm much. He also kept his head cocked a little to the side, but this was not very noticeable to his parents, and they were not too concerned about it. They were very concerned about his arm, however. Ivan and Leinani called the therapist to set up an appointment for a day that Ivan was not working. They saw the therapist in the hospital once per week for 2 months. Table 6-1 presents a summary of the therapist's findings on first evaluating Tyler and when she discharged him 2 months later.

Summary of Physical Therapy Findings: Tyler

TABLE 6-1

	Initial findings	Discharge findings
Resting posture of head and neck	Right cervical rotation Left cervical lateral flexion	Neutral except when fatigued
Passive range of motion (cervical)	Full	Full
Passive range of motion (LUE)	Full	Full
Observations of movement	Left scapula winging	Scapulae symmetrical
Muscle tone	Decreased/flaccid (LUE)	Slightly decreased (LUE)
Strength (LUE)		
Shoulder flexion	Absent	Fair/good
Shoulder abduction	Absent	Fair/good
Elbow flexion	Poor	Good
Elbow extension	Poor	Good
Forearm pronation	Trace	Fair/good
Forearm supination	Poor	Good
Wrist flexion	Fair/good	Good
Wrist extension	Fair/good	Good
Finger flexion	Normal	Normal
Finger extension	Normal	Normal
Functional skills	• Can mouth right hand • Actively moves right shoulder • Moves right arm above head • No weight bearing through left arm in prone position	• Can mouth both hands • Moves both shoulders • Moves both arms above head • Weight bearing through left arm in prone

LUE, Left upper extremity.

Starting therapy was difficult at first for Leinani because she had to change the way she took care of Tyler. The therapist suggested more than exercises. She asked Leinani and Ivan to change the way they fed, burped, carried, and played with Tyler (Figure 6-3).

Leinani was pleased to have some specific things to do with him that would help him use his arm more, but it took a lot of attention to change how she handled him for all those different activities. She was able to make most of the changes, but when the therapist asked her to carry Tyler on her right shoulder, she just could not do it. Tyler was not used to turning his head to find her to the right, and Leinani was not used to holding him with her right arm. She tried but was never able to get used to carrying him on her right shoulder.

When the therapist saw Tyler in the clinic, she was able to monitor how Tyler was changing each week, monitor how his parents were doing their home program, and teach them how to modify their activities with Tyler as he got stronger. She was also able to do some deep stretching, including using myofacial release to help Tyler increase his range of motion. For a summary of the activities that his family does with Tyler, see Box 6-1.

Tyler is now 2½ months old. He has made very good progress during the past few months when his parents were doing his exercises with him several times per day. Now Tyler is lifting his left arm up above his head by himself. He is closing and opening his fist. Although he continues to use his left arm somewhat less than his right, his arms look significantly more symmetrical, and he has full active range of motion. He has learned to suck both thumbs

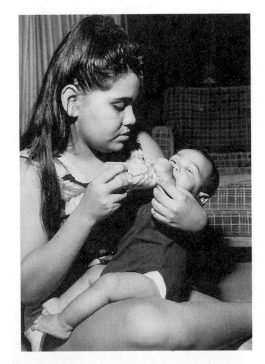

Figure 6-3 When Leinani feeds Tyler, she puts his left hand on the bottle. This gives Tyler tactile and temperature feedback through his left arm and hand, as well as visual feedback when he sees his hand on the bottle.

BOX 6-1   ## Home Activities for Tyler

1. Neck Stretch

While Tyler is on his back, bend his knees up toward his stomach, and put both of his hands on his knees. Holding his legs and lower trunk, gently rock him from side to side. When he is on his left side, lift up his legs and lower trunk so that he gets a stretch bending his neck sideways. Gently pull him toward you, holding him in this position. Repeat this activity at least four times each session, and do the routine at least three times every day.

2. Sensory Awareness

To help Tyler learn to become aware of his left arm, stroke it with a variety of textures. Use a terrycloth washcloth, soft cotton fabric such as his T-shirt, or your hand. Stroke from his shoulder down to his hand on the back of his arm and on the front of his arm. Do this several times a day.

3. Massage

Gently massage Tyler's left arm from his fingertips up to his shoulder. Roll his arm gently between your palms while moving from his hand to his shoulder. A good time to do this is when you are bathing him.

4. General Awareness

- To help Tyler become more aware of his left hand and arm, tie a small bell or rattle to his wrist so it will make noise when his hand or arm is moved. If he does not move his own arm, you can move it for him.
- Stroke his face and body with his left hand. Put his hands together. In this way he will get sensation through his left hand and arm as well as through his face and trunk.
- Place toys to his left side so he will need to turn his head to the left to see them.
- Place his crib so that he needs to turn his head to the left to see the door of the bedroom.

5. Neck Strengthening/Stretching

Place Tyler on your lap and hold him upright in a sitting position. Gently tilt him to the right and to the left, and help him hold his head up straight.

6. Feeding

Alternate the arm that you use to hold Tyler when you feed him. Place his left hand on the bottle, and hold it there as he drinks it. Encourage him to turn his head toward you.

7. Burping

Burp Tyler in a sitting position with his left arm across his body covered by the hand you are using to support him. Not only will he get a feeling of weight bearing through that arm; he will also feel the vibrations from you patting him on the back and his own burping.

8. Carrying: Alternate Positions

- Alternate carrying Tyler on your right and left shoulders so he will need to turn his head to both directions to face you. Hold his left arm up alongside his face when you carry him.
- Carry Tyler facing away from you against your body. Tilt him to the left so he will compensate by moving his head to the right. Support his left arm across his body.
- Carry Tyler facing you against your body, and tilt him to your right so he will tilt his head to his right. Support his left arm.
- Carry Tyler with his tummy straddling your forearm and your hand supporting his head/face. You can hold him across your body or facing outward. This is a good position to subtly monitor the position of his neck and modify your position. It is best done while he is awake and alert.

---

and prefers his left to his right. He usually holds his head in midline and has symmetrical passive range of motion in his neck. He can turn his head to both sides. He has been discharged from therapy. Tyler's parents continue to do the activities they were shown with him, and they will continue as long as they believe that he will benefit from them (Figures 6-4 through 6-6). They are pleased with his progress, although they believe that Tyler did most of the work to get better. They think that the activities and exercises that the therapist showed them helped a little.

Tyler has a fairly regular schedule now. He naps once in the morning and once in the afternoon for 2 hours each time. He sleeps 8 to 10 hours at night and has been sleeping straight through the night for a few weeks. Leinani stays at home and is a full-time mother. She has learned her son's temperament and needs and finds taking care of him easier than when he first came home from the hospital, when he seemed to cry all the time. She is able to go out with her friends sometimes when Ivan or Ivan's aunt watches Tyler for her, but she wants to be home for him

most of the time while he is an infant. Therefore she does not go out much.

Forty thousand dollars of unpaid hospital bills from both Leinani's and Tyler's stay in the hospital are still unpaid. Medicaid has promised to pay the bills, but the program has not officially accepted Leinani and Tyler yet. Leinani worries about the unpaid bills.

Leinani would like to take correspondence courses one day, perhaps to be a medical assistant. Through her experience with Tyler's birth and his subsequent problems, she has met different people in the medical professions. She believes that she would also like to help others.

When she looks at Tyler sleeping, Leinani remembers the Hawaiian name her aunt gave him. She whispers "E'ehupono" to him, remembering that it means "difficulty of coming into the world" combined with "power" and "righteousness." Leinani smiles at her small son. His broken wing has almost healed (Figure 6-7).

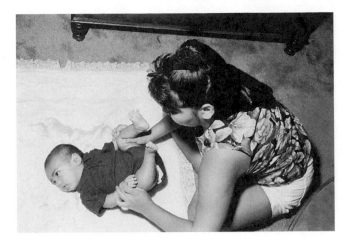

Figure 6-4 Leinani is doing Tyler's exercises. She puts his hands on his knees. Tyler gets sensory input through his hands, arms, shoulders, and trunk as he is rocked side to side.

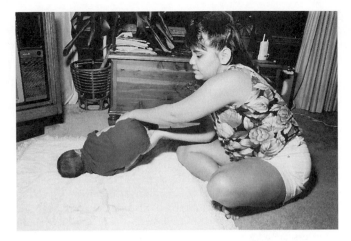

Figure 6-6 When Leinani lifts up on Tyler's pelvis, his neck is stretched into lateral flexion. She then slides him toward her, slowly increasing the stretch to his neck.

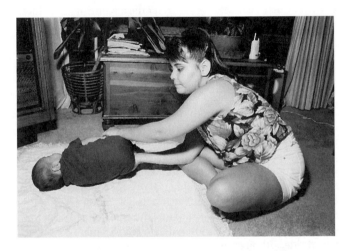

Figure 6-5 Rolling Tyler to his left side, Leinani keeps his hands on his knees. This gives him continued sensory input while he orients his head to his changing body position for strengthening.

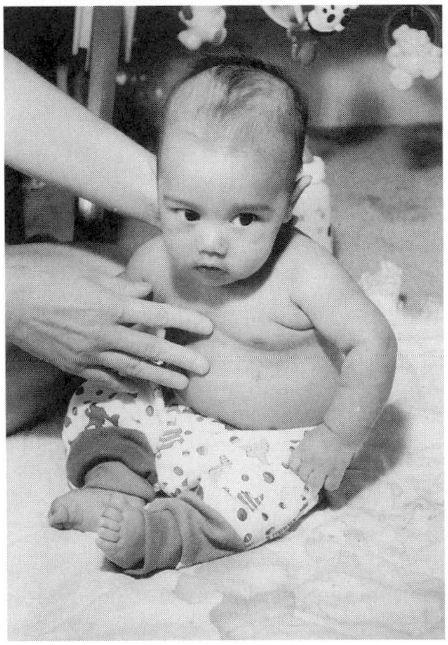

Figure 6-7 Although Tyler has full active range of motion at age 2½ months, he continues to let his arm fall into the "waiter's tip" position at times because of residual weakness.

BACKGROUND AND THEORY

Most of us have encountered orthopedic problems in our own lives, such as sprains or fractures. Perhaps some of these injuries affected us when we were children. Most orthopedic problems are transitory and heal completely in a few weeks or months. However, if our activities were curtailed by a musculoskeletal problem and we had to miss a dance recital or a baseball game in childhood, we usually remember the experience vividly into adulthood. Some orthopedic problems of childhood

have far-reaching consequences, especially those that occur in younger years or those that are more severe. Such problems that occur in infancy, particularly, have the potential for far-reaching developmental consequences.

Even minor anomalies of the musculoskeletal system in children can affect functional skills such as walking, running, climbing, or grasping. The adage that the "foot bone connects to the calf bone, and the calf bone connects to the thigh bone . . ." can help to remind us that an orthopedic disorder in one part of the body can affect the musculoskeletal system throughout the body. An example is the child with a clubfoot. The leg length discrepancy generated from the foot deformity can affect the spine, neck, and shoulders when the child learns to walk. Besides the global orthopedic repercussions of a musculoskeletal disorder, there are also developmental repercussions. Perhaps a new song can illustrate that "the bones are connected to the emotions, and the emotions are connected to the intellect. . . ." The child with an orthopedic deformity needs to contend with braces, splints, looking different, restricted activities, and other circumstances that can affect all areas of development.

Musculoskeletal disorders of childhood may range from congenital disorders, such as clubfoot, to disorders that may appear later in childhood, such as some forms of scoliosis, to acquired disorders, such as fractures or sprains. This wide range of problems in children can have developmental consequences with musculoskeletal, emotional, and intellectual implications. Physical therapy management ranges according to the diagnosis, but therapy providers must be aware of the far-ranging implications of the disorder that can sometimes outweigh the specific musculoskeletal problems being treated.

This chapter explores disorders that begin in infancy, including some foot and lower leg deformities, brachial plexus injuries, and torticollis. Scoliosis, a disorder that can develop in childhood, is also discussed, and acquired disorders, such as fractures and some sports injuries, are addressed. A Case Study of Tyler, an infant with torticollis and brachial plexus injury, demonstrates how these disorders can affect a family. An Applications section on splinting and orthotics for children provides an overview of this area.

The Child With Foot and Lower Leg Deformities

Foot deformities in infancy can be related to intrauterine positioning, neurological disorders such as myelomeningocele or cerebral palsy, and genetic disorders such as certain forms of arthrogryposis. Common foot disorders include deformities of the ankle and foot, usually called clubfoot, and those of the forefoot. Other, milder disorders include tibial torsion, which may not be evident until the child begins to stand.

Metatarsus Adductus

Some children are born with a positional deformity of the forefeet. The metatarsals are deviated medially, causing the toes to curve inward, and the child to appear to toe-in. The deformity is limited to the forefoot, however, and the heel is in correct alignment with the rest of the leg. The child has good range of the ankle, including dorsiflexion and plantar flexion. There are various grades of metatarsus adductus that range from mild to severe. In mild cases usually no treatment is indicated, and the

> ☀ To check the fit of an orthotic, have the parent put the device on the child 1 hour before the therapy session. You can remove it and check for redness at the beginning of your session and still have time to make modifications before the session is finished.

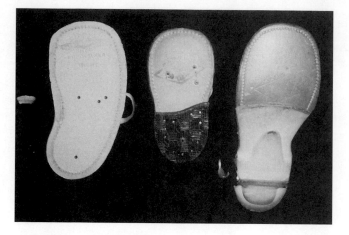

Figure 6-8 The straight-last shoe *(center)* has a forefoot-to-hindfoot alignment, which is straight, as opposed to a typical shoe *(right)* with the forefoot more adducted than the hindfoot. The reverse-last shoe *(left)* has the forefoot abducted in relation to the hindfoot. An easy alternative to expensive splints is to put the shoes on the opposite feet of a child. This creates the effect of a reverse-last shoe.

deviance corrects itself as the child grows. For moderate cases straight-last or reverse-last shoes may be used to correct the forefoot position (Figure 6-8). For severe cases progressive casting or surgery may be necessary to correct the alignment of the foot. Some physicians advocate no treatment at all until the child is walking and then surgery for those cases that do not correct with maturation.

Deformities of the Foot and Ankle

Deformities that involve both the ankle and the foot are usually called clubfoot. Technical names for the condition vary according to the actual deviance from typical alignment.

Talipes equinovarus. This is the classic form of clubfoot. It involves adduction of the forefoot, varus position of the hindfoot, and equinus at the ankle. In lay terms the forefoot is curved inward in relation to the heel, the heel is bent inward in relation to the leg, and the ankle is fixed in plantar flexion with the toes pointed down. The foot and ankle are usually small on the affected side, although 50% of the cases are bilateral (Cunningham & Albert, 1993). Twice as many boys as girls have clubfoot at birth, and it occurs in about 1 in every 1000 live births. Causes of clubfoot include positional deformities related to neurological disorders such as myelomeningocele or arthrogryposis, genetic predisposition, or positional deformities related to the size of the infant and the uterus. Many cases do not have easily identifiable causes.

Treatment usually involves manipulation, taping, stretching, bracing, serial casting (Figure 6-9), and/or surgery. The form of treatment may depend on related problems. For example, a protocol of stretching, taping, and splinting would be more appropriate for children with a lack of sensation than would serial casting, which has more potential for causing skin breakdown. Casting is most effective if started at birth, and it may be continued for several months as the child grows.

Surgery is usually indicated between 3 months and 1 year of age because it tends to provide a longer lasting correction than

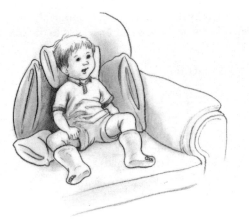

Figure 6-9 This child was born with bilateral clubfeet, in addition to other problems. He has both ankles casted to gently change the alignment of his ankle to a more typical one. The casts are changed every week to accommodate for his growth, and to continually re-mold to his changing alignment. Casting is most effective if started right at birth.

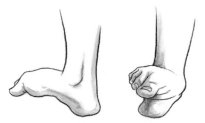

Figure 6-10 The foot with a calcaneovalgus deformity has dorsi-flexion of the ankle, valgus or eversion of the hindfoot, and abduction of the metatarsals.

the conservative measures. Some cases of clubfoot can be managed by casting alone, but most require surgery. The type of surgery varies according to how much soft tissue is released. Surgical intervention may also vary in relation to the cause of the disorder. For instance, children with no innervation to the muscles crossing the joint may require different surgical correction than those children with more typical innervation patterns. Extensive soft tissue releases are more effective in achieving a correction, but they may provide an overcorrection, causing a child to have resultant deformity in the opposite direction (Simons, 1985).

Physical therapy may be used to treat a child with only a club-foot, or it may be used for a child who has a clubfoot as part of a larger pattern of disability. Stretching, splinting, taping, monitoring casts, and teaching the parent appropriate developmental activities to promote typical sensory experience, motor skills, and developmental experiences all may be indicated. The physical therapist assistant (PTA) monitors casts, provides developmental intervention to promote typical skills, and assists in stretching and splinting.

Calcaneovalgus. Calcaneovalgus is sometimes classified as a form of clubfoot, but it is usually seen as a foot deformity distinctly different from clubfoot. The deformity involves dorsi-flexion of the foot, eversion or valgus deformity of the hindfoot, and abduction of the metatarsals (Figure 6-10). This deformity is

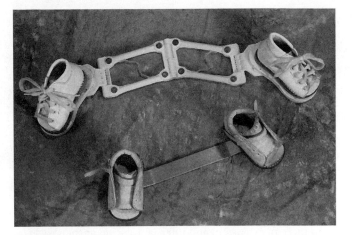

Figure 6-11 A child wears a Dennis Brown splint at night to reduce tibial torsion. The newer version of this splint allows some lower extremity movement. The straight-last shoes may also help correct metatarsus adductus.

common in individuals with cerebral palsy and other developmental disabilities such as spina bifida and arthrogryposis. Treatment is usually surgery in those who will benefit from a correction. Children with severe multiple disabilities who may never bear weight through their feet may not receive surgical correction because the risks of surgery outweigh any possible benefit.

Tibial Torsion

Torsion, or a rotation of the tibia in relation to the femur, can develop atypically for some children. All children have normal tibial torsion that changes from a medial rotation in infants (looks like toeing in) to a lateral rotation that develops as a child begins to walk (looks like toeing out). Torsion that is outside the typical ranges is difficult to see before a child is standing. Even when it is seen, unless one is skilled at this type of diagnosis, the condition can be difficult to differentiate from rotational differences, that are related to the hip. Many physicians treat differences in tibial torsion conservatively, recognizing that most cases resolve naturally. More active treatment includes braces with straps or cables that pull the lower leg into the opposite rotation. A Dennis Brown splint may be used for a young child to help correct tibial torsion (Figure 6-11). Braces or splints are most often worn at night. If abnormal tibial torsion causes functional difficulties for the child that cannot be resolved by conservative means, corrective surgery can be performed when the child is older.

The physical therapy provider works with the orthotist to fit and adjust braces and teaches parents how to provide appropriate developmental intervention for their child with a splint.

The Child With a Brachial Plexus Injury
Cause and Incidence

The brachial plexus is where nerve roots from the spinal cord come together and reorganize before they redistribute to innervate the muscles and skin of the arm. There are five roots involved in the plexus, which exits the thoracic cavity inferior to the clavicle by way of the axilla. During a difficult delivery the infant's shoulder may be forced into excessive abduction or flexion because of a breech position, the use of forceps, or a large infant trying to exit a small birth canal. This force can traumatize, stretch, or avulse (separate) the nerve roots, causing damage to the nerves themselves. Brachial plexus injuries occur in 0.4 to 2.5 of every 1000 deliveries (Eng, 1971; Jackson, 1988). Factors leading to brachial plexus injury include high infant birth weight, prolonged maternal labor, shoulder dystocia (too large for the birth canal), breech presentation, and forceps delivery.

Clinical Description

If the injury occurs to the upper nerve roots (C5 and C6), it is called Erb's palsy. This condition is also known as the "waiter's tip" palsy because of the characteristic posture of the child's arm in adduction, extension, and internal rotation at the shoulder, resulting from paralysis of the deltoid, elbow flexors, and brachioradialis muscles (Figure 6-12). Typical clinical signs are the absence of physiological flexion, and the absence of Moro and tonic neck reflexes on the side of injury. Erb's palsy is the most common type of brachial plexus injury, occurring in approximately 80% of injuries that take place during breech births (Geutjens, Gilbert, & Helsen, 1996).

If the injury occurs to the lower plexus (C8 and T1), the child's arm is generally moving well at the shoulder and elbow but has weakness in the wrist, hand, and fingers. This type of injury is called Klumpke's palsy; it is relatively rare, occurring in only one quarter of 1% of brachial plexus injuries. The third type of brachial plexus injury is a total injury, sometimes called Erb's-Klumpke palsy, in which the entire arm is involved. In such a case all the nerve roots are damaged.

Related problems that may occur with a brachial plexus injury include fractured clavicle or humerus, facial palsy, torticol-

lis, hemiparalysis of the diaphragm, and subluxation of the shoulder. All these problems may be related to trauma at birth.

Medical Treatment

Most mild brachial plexus injuries resolve during the first few weeks of life. For more severe injuries most functional return occurs during the first year of life, with some lesser return taking place during the second year. Because the initial cause of the injury is trauma that results in swelling and bruising affecting the function of the nerves, the initial treatment is rest. The infant's arm is usually swaddled in a position of adduction and internal rotation for 1 to 2 weeks to allow the swelling and bruising to decrease.

After the initial period of recovery, the arm may be moved in a gentle range of motion to decrease the risk of contracture and to promote functional use. Developmental activities are used to promote typical sensory input and motor output. Splinting may be used at night to prevent contractures, especially if weakness of the wrist and hand is evident. If significant nerve damage persists, tendon transfer surgery can be performed when the child is older to encourage more functional use of the extremity.

Physical Therapy Intervention

Direct therapy for the infant may occur, especially when the child is very young. Early parent teaching for swaddling, positioning, carrying, and providing range-of-motion exercises for their child is very important. Encouraging active motion of the arm for a very young infant is difficult because the infant has little voluntary control. Sensory input can encourage the return of motor skills and can help the infant become more aware of the extremity. Sensory input can be externally provided by stroking the arm with a towel or soft cloth, or it can be self-stimulated by stroking the infant with his or her own arm. Hand-over-hand assistance in bringing the hand to mouth or hand to feet can promote age-appropriate developmental skills. Approximation, or pressure through a joint, can provide another form of sensory input. This can be provided by manually placing pressure through a joint or by helping the infant bear weight through the joint.

If weakness persists in older infants, they can be encouraged to reach, grasp, and manipulate objects with both hands or only the involved side. Facilitated movement transitions from sitting to hands-and-knees position, from supine to sitting position, and from sitting to standing can encourage active use of a weak

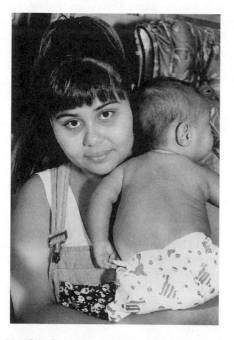

Figure 6-12 This classic posture of shoulder adduction, internal rotation, and extension—with elbow extension and forearm pronation—is characteristic of a child with an upper brachial plexus injury.

A small infant will sometimes calm down if you hold the infant away from your body in a "sitting" position, with the child's bottom on one of your hands and your other hand supporting the infant's trunk and head. Move the infant up and down (always supporting the head fully) at your face level or above, while talking to the child. The movement may help the infant organize behavior for a few more minutes of handling. Ultimately though, the crying child will need feeding, sleep, or a parent's touch.

extremity and foster age-appropriate developmental skills. For children who have persisting severe impairment, lack of sensory feedback from the arm can cause neglect. Teaching a child to be aware and careful of the arm can prevent injury as the child grows.

As the child with a severe injury grows older, teaching strategies to perform specific skills, such as tying shoelaces, shooting a basket, or driving a car, may be necessary. Assistive devices to help with activities of daily living, such as a shoelace holder, buttonhole device, book holder, page turner, or adapted steering wheel, may help the child participate more efficiently in daily activities. The child is usually resourceful in finding solutions for functional difficulties, but the experienced therapy provider may be able to share strategies learned from other children or to assist in solving problems. Range-of-motion exercises to prevent or minimize contractures may be necessary for the child's entire life. These skills can be learned and self-administered as the child becomes older.

Role of the PTA. The PTA may see the infant in the clinic or the home under the supervision of the physical therapist (PT) soon after birth. The PTA may also see the child with a moderate or severe injury later, during the school years. Parent teaching, range of motion, strengthening through developmental activities, and monitoring of range of motion and strength are all activities that the PTA may provide to the child during infancy. The same activities may be appropriate during the school years, with the addition of problem solving and direct teaching of the child to do self–range-of-motion exercises and strengthening and to use assistive devices.

The Child With a Congenital Torticollis
Incidence, Cause, and Clinical Description

Congenital cervical torticollis appears as a head tilt in a newborn. It may be noted immediately after birth or may not appear until the infant is 2 to 4 weeks of age. Contracture of the sternocleidomastoid muscle on one side causes lateral flexion to that side and rotation to the opposite side. One large study found the incidence of torticollis to be higher in boys than girls, with a 3:2 ratio. Sixty-two percent of the infants with torticollis had a difficult, breech, or cesarean delivery, and 6% had other congenital anomalies such as developmental dislocation of the hip or metatarsus adductus (Cheng & Au, 1994).

The cause of torticollis is unknown, but recent theories suggest a compartment syndrome occurring intrautero or perinatally (Davids, Wenger, & Mubarak, 1993). These authors found that birth position and the side affected by the contracture were associated. They postulate that head positioning in utero can selectively injure the sternocleidomastoid muscle, leading to the development of a compartment syndrome. Other theories relate birth trauma to specific trauma to the sternocleidomastoid muscle itself during the birth process.

Cheng and Au (1994) found that approximately one third of the cases they studied involved a fibrous tumor in the sternocleidomastoid muscle, one third included a postural torticollis with no abnormality in the muscle, and one third involved a muscular torticollis with no associated tumor. The presence of a tumor did not affect the outcome, and most tumors resolved spontaneously. Untreated torticollis may lead to facial asymmetries and upper spinal scoliosis caused by asymmetries of head and neck position. Early treatment can minimize or prevent these complications.

Medical Treatment

Conservative treatment has been shown to resolve symptoms in 70% to 97% of children with congenital torticollis (Cheng & Au, 1994; Porter & Blount, 1995). Conservative treatment consists of passive stretching, positioning, heat, and active stimulation. Surgical intervention for torticollis usually is not done until the child is 1 year of age to allow conservative measures time to be effective. Surgical release of the muscle at both the clavicular end and the mastoid end reduces the contracture. Children younger than 12 years have the best results with surgery, with only mild persistence of related problems (e.g., facial asymmetries and scoliosis); and in children older than 12, facial asymmetries and scoliosis usually persist into adulthood (Yu, Wang, Chin, & Lo, 1995).

Physical Therapy Intervention

Congenital torticollis can be treated very effectively with procedures and techniques used in physical therapy. Because of the high success rate of these methods, treating a child with congenital torticollis can be highly rewarding.

Positioning and stretching are essential in the early treatment of this problem. Because the therapy provider cannot be with the child every hour of every day, parent teaching is very important. Once the parents understand the benefits of handling and positioning in the treatment of their child's torticollis, they will usually be willing to comply with recommendations. Parents need to understand that, for optimal results, every position their child assumes, whether in the bassinet, infant seat, or in the parent's arms, needs to address the torticollis. The child should always be positioned so that the head turns toward the injured side (away from the contracture) for the child to see interesting things in the environment. To this end, attention to which end the child's head faces in the crib, the alignment of the infant seat in a room, and which side of the back seat the car seat is placed should all be considered.

When the child is being held, attention should be given to early righting reactions of the head and trunk to dictate the positions of choice. The child should be held so that he or she needs to turn to the appropriate side to see or nuzzle the parent. When bottle feeding, the child should be held so that the head needs to turn to the appropriate side to see the caregiver and root for the bottle.

Exercises that provide passive and active range of motion to the neck should be taught to the parents. It is both scary and difficult to move a small infant's head to provide stretching to the neck. Young infants do not usually tolerate this action well. It is easier to move the infant's trunk while the head is stabilized on the support surface, although care needs to be taken not to exercise with too much force. Parents can more easily encourage socialization and play when the activity is fun for both parent and child. The case study in this chapter elaborates on more exercises for passive and active range of motion for the infant with congenital torticollis.

Role of the PTA. The PTA will usually work under the direct supervision of the PT when working with small infants. To gain and maintain the trust of the infant and the parents, it is important that the therapy provider be very comfortable handling small infants.

Skills in consoling and handling a fussy infant will allow the maximal amount of direct therapy. Skills in relating to parents will encourage them to follow through on activities at home, thus providing the best overall services for the child.

Fractures in Children

Because children's bones are different from those of adults, they tend to sustain different types of injuries. Children's bones are more flexible, more porous, and lack the density of adult bones. This leads to different fracture patterns in children than are seen in adults. See Figure 6-13 for common fracture patterns in children. Children's periosteum is thicker and stronger than that of adults, leading to a better blood supply and therefore faster healing than adults. Ligaments and joint capsules are often stronger than bones in young children. Therefore sprains and strains are not as common as fractures.

Children's bones are growing, and they have active epiphyses (growth plates) that are vulnerable to injury from trauma. In growing bones the ephiphyses are weak and will respond to stress before the ligaments and joint capsules. Therefore fractures across the growth plate are not uncommon. Epiphysial injury can be serious in a child because the direction, symmetry, or amount of bone growth can be affected. Of skeletal injuries in children, 30% involve the epiphysis.

Fractures in children can occur from a variety of trauma. Motor vehicle accidents, falls, sports injuries, and abuse are only a few of the causes. Accidents on skateboards, rollerskates, bicycles, and trampolines cause many injuries in children. The cause of the injury and the direction and amount of force determine the type of fracture that will occur. Seventy-five percent of all fractures in children are located in the upper extremities, with 10% occurring in the elbow alone (Townsend & Bassett, 1996). The most common fracture in children occurs in the clavicle. Other common fracture sites in children include the humerus, radius, ulna, wrist, hand, and femur. Most upper extremity injuries are caused by falls that are "broken" by an outstretched hand.

Symptoms of fractures in children include swelling, redness, pain, deformity of the extremity, and muscle spasm or guarding. Very young children will not be able to verbalize what is wrong, but crying or refusal to use an extremity may be a major clue.

Treatment varies depending on the type of fracture and whether it requires a closed or open reduction. Most fractures require immobilization by splinting or casting for a specific period. Children heal in the same pattern as adults do but much faster. The younger the child, the faster the healing. Some pediatric fractures heal in just 2 or 3 weeks, whereas a typical adult fracture takes 6 to 8 weeks (Figure 6-14).

Physical Therapy Intervention

Physical therapy may be involved in teaching a child crutch-walking skills if a lower extremity injury was sustained. See Chapter 4 for more information about teaching a child to use crutches for mobility. If traction is required, bed exercises to maintain strength and mobility skills can be taught to the parent and child. After a sustained immobilization gentle range of motion or strengthening may be required to help the child regain functional skills such as walking. For children with typical gross motor skills and simple fractures, adequate rehabilitation usually occurs with normal daily activities.

Physical therapy may be working with a child who sustained

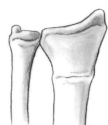
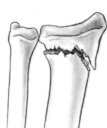

Buckle fracture   Epiphyseal fracture

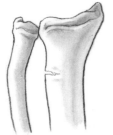
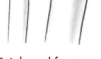
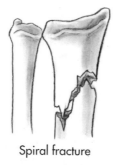

Greenstick (L) and   Spiral fracture
bending (R) fractures

Figure 6-13 Common fracture patterns for children.

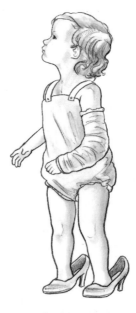

Figure 6-14 This 14-month-old child fell from a bench and sustained a buckle fracture of her left lateral condyle. She wore the splint for 3 weeks and was using her arm normally within 1 more week.

multiple fractures from a motor vehicle accident or other major trauma. Additional injuries may be present, such as a head injury or trauma to vital organs and soft tissue, and may complicate the rehabilitation process. Knowledge of the characteristics of pediatric fractures helps a therapy provider in determining and carrying out rehabilitation plans for a child with multiple traumas.

Excessive Spinal Curvature in Children

Each of us has normal curves in our spine that allow for flexibility, stability, movement, balance, and adaptation to directional forces. Normal spinal curves include lack of any lateral deviation of the spine, mild lordosis (or extension) at the cervical and lumbar levels of the spine, and mild kyphosis (or forward bending) in the thoracic region. Excessive spinal curves in any of these planes can occur as a result of neurologic, orthopedic, or idiopathic factors (Figure 6-15).

Excessive spinal curves can result in pain, respiratory difficulties, balance disturbances, deformity, and psychosocial problems. Depending on the cause, spinal curvature can occur at birth or may develop later during childhood or early adolescence. Scoliosis is a lateral curvature of the spine with or without a rotational component. Lordosis is an excessive extension of the spine, manifesting in a convex deformity. It usually occurs in areas where there is typically spinal extension such as the lumbar or cervical levels of the spine. Kyphosis is an excessive forward curvature or flexion of the spine, manifesting in a concave deformity, which usually occurs in the thoracic region. These disorders can occur singly or in combination with each other. If a person has two or more spinal curves, one may be compensating for the other. Treatment for excessive spinal curves ranges from observation and monitoring to bracing or surgery. Children with

abnormal spinal curves need to contend with a changing self-image as well as the sometimes invasive or pervasive treatment techniques that interfere with functional activities, recreation, and self-help skills.

Scoliosis

A lateral curvature of the spine, which may or may not include a rotational component, is called scoliosis (Figures 6-16).

Incidence and cause. Scoliosis can be caused by poor posture, congenital defects, orthopedic disorders, and neuromuscular disorders; however, in most cases the cause is unknown. The incidence of scoliosis may be as high as 1 in 10; however, the incidence of scoliosis that needs medical treatment to arrest the progress of the curve is much lower, about 2 in every 1000 (Bunnell, 1988). Scoliosis that is caused by neuromuscular disease or orthopedic impairment affects boys and girls equally. Most cases of scoliosis are classified as idiopathic, however, with no known cause. Idiopathic scoliosis affects girls more frequently than boys. There may be some genetic propensity for idiopathic scoliosis, but many children have no known history of the condition in their family.

Scoliosis can also be classified by age of onset and the number, vertebral level, and direction of the curves. The direction is classified as right or left, according to the direction of the apex of the curve. Some children have one major curve, and some have double curves, with one compensating for the other. The different types of scoliosis are summarized in Box 6-2.

The degree of scoliosis is measured on a radiograph by using the Cobb method. The beginning and end vertebrae of the curve are identified. Lines are drawn parallel to the end vertebrae, then additional lines are drawn perpendicular to these lines. The angle formed by the intersection of the perpendicular lines is defined as the degree of curvature (Figure 6-17).

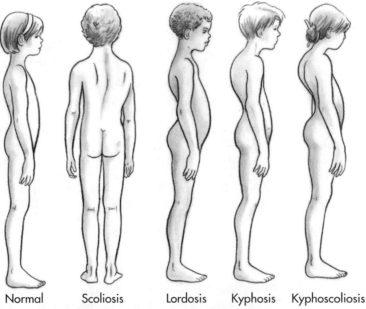

Normal   Scoliosis   Lordosis   Kyphosis   Kyphoscoliosis

Figure 6-15 Scoliosis, lordosis, and kyphosis occur with varying degrees in normal spines. Excessive curves can occur independently of each other or in combination.

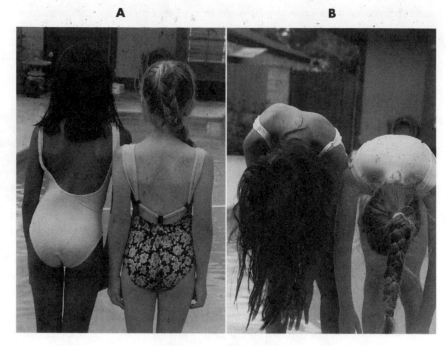

Figure 6-16 A, This 11-year-old girl *(at left)* has a significant right thoracic scoliosis with a rotational component, manifesting itself in a right rib hump. Her scoliosis developed and progressed suddenly within the last 6 months. Although the cause is unknown, she has other mild anomalies, including toe walking and weakness in some proximal muscles, leading to a theory of neuromuscular disease as a cause. **B,** Compare her spine with that of the child at the right.

BOX 6-2   Categorization of Scoliosis

A. Age of Onset

Congenital:	Birth to 3 years
Juvenile:	3 years to puberty
Adolescent:	During or after puberty

B. Magnitude of Curve

Mild:	0°-20°
Moderate:	20°-40°
Severe:	>40°

C. Direction, Location, Size, and Number of Curves

Direction:	Right or left apex
Location:	Cervical, cervicothoracic, thoracic, thoracolumbar, or lumbar curves
Size:	Minor or major curve
Number:	Single or double curve

D. Type and Etiology of Curve

Type of Curve	Etiology
Functional (also called postural, nonstructural) • No structural changes • Correctable with bending or postural correction	• May be related to poor posture • May be related to musculoskeletal anomalies
Structural • Changes in vertebrae and supporting tissues • Decreased flexibility • Usually rotation of vertebrae is present • Related changes to rib cage, pelvis, hips	*Congenital* • Malformation of vertebrae at 3 to 5 weeks of gestation *Neuromuscular (paralytic)* • Associated with neuromuscular diseases such as cerebral palsy, muscular dystrophy, or myelomeningocele. Diseases with orthopedic manifestations, such as arthrogryposis and osteogenesis imperfecta, can also be included here. *Idiopathic* • Cause is unknown • May be familial tendency for scoliosis • Prognosis varies with age of onset (variable) • Most common form of scoliosis *Traumatic onset* • Associated with spinal fractures, irradiation, tumors, or metabolic disorders (rickets)

Children who develop scoliosis before age 3 years are considered to have infantile scoliosis. If a curve develops between age of 3 years and the onset of puberty, it is considered to be a juvenile curve. If it develops during or around the onset of puberty, it is considered to be an adolescent curve. Infantile or juvenile curves occur in equal frequency in boys and girls, but girls more frequently than boys develop adolescent onset curves.

The time of development of the curve is significant in its prognosis. Most curves that develop in infancy, if not related to a neuromuscular disorder, resolve spontaneously. In contrast, those that develop in childhood have a high incidence of progression and usually require vigorous treatment. Three to nine percent of children who develop adolescent idiopathic curves progress beyond 10 degrees and require treatment. Girls are significantly more likely than

boys to have curves that progress beyond 10 degrees, and they are even more likely to have curves that progress beyond 20 degrees. Girls have the most serious curves by a factor of about 8 or 9 to 1.

Another factor in the prognosis of a scoliotic curve in children is the maturity of the skeletal system. The Risser sign, measured by a radiograph of the iliac crest, indicates the amount of ossification as it correlates to the level of skeletal maturity. Grades 0 to 5 indicate skeletal maturity levels starting with the absence of any ossification at grade 0 and ending with complete maturation and cessation of skeletal growth at grade 5.

School screening programs can be effective at identifying scoliosis in children. The optimal age to screen girls is just before the pubertal growth spurt at about 9 to 11 years. Because of the difference in initiation of puberty between boys and girls, the optimal ages to screen children for scoliosis may differ, with boys being more efficiently screened between 11 to 13 years of age. Schools usually screen children visually, using the bending test (see Box 6-3). Some researchers suggest that using more objective methods for screening, such as measuring the angle of trunk rotation, rib hump height, or Moire photography, may cut down on unnecessary referrals from school screenings (Pruijs, Keessen, van der Meer, & van Wieringen, 1995). However, these techniques take more equipment and more time. Because of funding issues, some school districts have cut their scoliosis screening programs entirely, relying instead on medical professionals to screen for scoliosis during routine examinations.

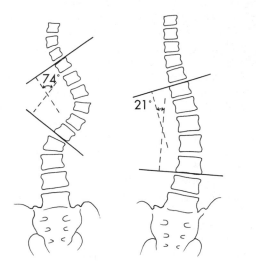

Figure 6-17 The Cobb method is used to determine the degree of curvature of the spine.

To screen for scoliosis, separate the boys from the girls. To ensure the best compliance, evaluate each child in a private location to avoid self-consciousness or embarrassment.

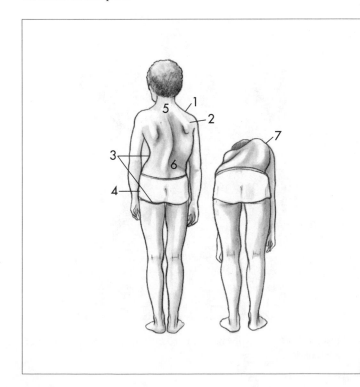

BOX 6-3 Screening for Scoliosis

Standing
The child is standing and facing away from examiner.
1. Assess symmetry of the shoulders. (Shoulder may be elevated on the convex side.)
2. Assess symmetry of scapulae and posterior rib cage. (Scapula may be high and rib cage may be prominent on the convex side of the curve.)
3. Assess symmetry of the waist and gluteal folds. (The waist may appear fuller on the convex side of the curve. Gluteal folds may be asymmetrical.)
4. Assess symmetry of the hips. (One hip may protrude.)
5. Drop plumb line from occiput to assess trunk alignment. (Plumb line may fall lateral to gluteal crease. If it falls over gluteal crease, check for a compensatory curve.)
6. Assess symmetry of spinous processes.

Bending Forward
The child bends forward from the waist as if to touch the ground. The arms should swing freely.
7. As the child bends forward, assess symmetry of the ribcage. (Rib hump may appear posteriorly on the convex side.)

Clinical features. Scoliosis can be characterized as either structural or functional. A functional, sometimes called postural, curve can be corrected with passive or active movement. No vertebral changes are seen on radiographical studies and correction can be obtained easily. This type of curve may be associated with poor posture, orthopedic anomalies, such as a mild discrepancy in a leg length, or weakness in supporting muscles, such as the gluteus medius on one side. A structural curve, on the other hand, cannot be corrected passively or actively. Structural changes to the vertebrae and connective tissue can be seen, and usually a rotation of some vertebrae is present, causing abnormalities in the rib cage, scapulae, or pelvis. Causes of structural curves include neuromuscular diseases, congenital abnormalities (e.g., congenitally wedged-shaped vertebrae) or idiopathic causes.

A child with a scoliosis may have asymmetrical gluteal folds, shoulder levels, or pelvic levels. Scapulae may be asymmetrical, with one side more posterior or more elevated than the other. Hanging a plumb line from the cervical spine may indicate asymmetry in the spine itself, with the line falling either laterally to the gluteal crease, or, if the curve is compensated, demonstrating a lack of symmetry between the plumb line and the spine. Parents may complain that the child's clothes hang "funny" or that the child walks or stands "funny."

Identification of the cause of the scoliosis, if possible, is important. Addressing an underlying cause, such as a leg length discrepancy or asymmetrical strength, may correct or prevent progression of a scoliosis. These interventions can be less invasive for a child than some treatments for scoliosis. Many causes, such as cerebral palsy, myelomeningocele, or congenitally wedged vertebrae, are not correctable, however, and in other cases the cause may not be identified.

A child with a severe curve of neuromuscular origin may have respiratory impairment, cardiac effects caused by pressure from an asymmetrical rib cage, and even spinal cord compression, causing weakness or paralysis. A commonly associated deformity is windswept hips; both legs are "swept" to one side in a structural deformity related to the asymmetry of the spine and the pelvis (Figure 6-18). This problem is especially pervasive when the child's posture and movements are dictated by the persistence of primitive reflexes, particularly the asymmetrical tonic neck reflex. Children with severe curves may have asymmetrical cervical range of motion, facial asymmetries, and rib cage deformities.

Curves of neuromuscular origin may progress differently from those of idiopathic origin. Aronsson, Stokes, Ronchetti, and Labelle (1994) found that children with cerebral palsy had more rotation of the spine into the convexity of the curve in relation to the amount of lateral deviation of the spine than children with adolescent idiopathic scoliosis or mild curves related to Friedreich's ataxia.

Treatment. Scoliosis can be categorized according to the degree of curvature. A mild curve has 20 degrees or less of lateral deviation. A moderate curve is between 20 and 40 degrees, and a severe curve is more than 40 degrees. Treatments vary according to the severity of the curve. A mild curve is usually treated with observation and monitoring through regular radiographs.

If the curve progresses to more than 20 degrees, bracing is usually indicated. The goal of orthotic treatment is to prevent the progression of the curve, but correction of the curve may not be possible. The Milwaukee brace is the most common orthotic used for idiopathic scoliosis (Figure 6-19), but other orthotics, including the thoracic, lumbar sacral orthosis (TLSO), may be used for a curve in the low thoracic or lumbar areas. Bracing used to be mandated for 23 hours per day, with 1 hour allowed out of the brace for bathing and exercise. More recently, however, bracing has been shown to be effective when used for fewer hours each day, usually up to 12 hours (Allington & Bowen, 1996).

Nighttime use of lateral electrical stimulation to promote a balance of muscle pull on the curve is used for some mild cases. This method is far less offensive to a child than wearing a brace. However, recent literature does not indicate any better results us-

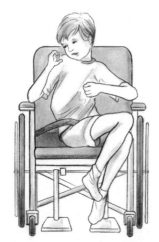

Figure 6-18 This child with a severe neuromuscular scoliosis has windswept lower extremities, rib asymmetries, and a severe thoracolumbar scoliosis.

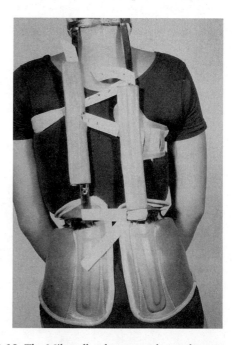

Figure 6-19 The Milwaulkee brace may be used to treat a moderate scoliosis.

ing electrical stimulation than are achieved through observation alone (Allington & Bowen, 1996; Nachemson & Peterson, 1995). Even part-time brace use was shown to be more effective in reducing the progression of the curve.

Another method of correcting posture and therefore of effecting a reduction in progression of scoliosis, is biofeedback. A child wears a device around the neck that beeps when the child's posture becomes asymmetrical. Research on the effectiveness of this device is not yet definitive.

Surgical intervention. If the curve progresses beyond 40 degrees, surgical intervention is usually indicated, not only to stop the progression, but also to provide correction. Several surgical procedures are used in different circumstances, some with an anterior approach and some with a posterior approach. Table 6-2 provides an overview of the most common surgical procedures used for treatment of scoliosis. Surgery performed to stabilize the spine is invasive, with an incision usually spanning the length of the segments being stabilized. Side effects include a long scar and decreased mobility in the segments stabilized. Metal instrumentation is left in place to align and stabilize the spinal segments. Approximately 1% of children undergoing spinal stabilization will have negative outcomes, including neurological damage, which may be temporary or permanent. Other risks involve the anesthesia and can include respiratory arrest, brain damage, and permanent disability. Risk

factors for neurologic damage include a major kyphosis, vertebral malformation, preoperative signs of neurological deficit, excessive correction, and accessing the spine both anteriorly and posteriorly (Carlioz & Ouaknine, 1994-5). Most children undergoing a spinal stabilization will have a good outcome (Figure 6-20).

Physical therapy intervention. A PT may be called on to help an orthotist fit a child for a brace. Checking the fit while the brace is being worn and communicating closely with the orthotist about areas of pressure or abrasions are essential to the success of this treatment. The therapy provider may also teach the child and family how to put on and remove the brace, what clothing is appropriate, and how to minimize the impact of the brace in social situations. Skills such as picking up objects from the floor, going up and down stairs, dressing, and getting in and out of bed may need to be relearned while the child is wearing the brace.

A child may be taught exercises to maintain trunk strength and flexibility during the course of treatment. Exercises are important to help the child maintain mobility and strength while wearing the brace, but they have not been shown to reduce the curve or to prevent its progression. Swimming is a particularly good exercise to maintain strength and flexibility while minimizing trauma to the spine. The use of a brace has not been shown to decrease bone density (Snyder et al., 1995), but it will

TABLE 6-2 — Common Surgical Procedures for Spinal Stabilization

Type of procedure	Description	Indication	Rehabilitation needs
Dwyer anterior fusion	Requires resection of a rib and cutting through diaphragm to expose vertebrae. Screws are applied to each vertebra with wires between them to stabilize spine.	Used only for low curves in thoracolumbar or lumbar areas.	All procedures use bony fusion of spine with instrumentation to stabilize fusion. Most require postsurgical orthosis. Newer procedures allow children to get up within first few days of surgery and increase their activities gradually over first year. Physical therapy input includes: • Teaching child and family to use postsurgical orthosis • Teaching child and family body mechanics and functional skills, including getting in and out of bed, transfers, dressing, and ambulation • Teaching general range-of-motion and strengthening exercises • Emphasizing importance of early ambulation • Monitoring fit and use of orthosis • Monitoring neurological signs and skin for stability of instrumentation
Zielke anterior fusion	Same as Dwyer but a newer procedure with better screws used with rods to stabilize segments.	Used only for low curves in thoracolumbar or lumbar areas.	
Harrington rod posterior instrumentation	Older procedure not often used. Two rods are attached by hooks to posterior spinal segments: distraction rod on concave side of curve and compression rod on convex side. Cannot control sagittal plane correction; always requires postsurgical immobilization of spine.	Formerly standard procedure for spinal stabilization. Currently infrequently used because of long rehabilitation time needed and poor correction in sagittal plane.	
Cotrel-Dubousset posterior instrumentation	Two rods with compression and distraction hooks are attached to pedicles or lamina of vertebrae. Normal spinal curves in sagittal plane can be obtained by contouring the rods. Children who have idiopathic scoliosis with good correction may not need spinal orthosis after surgery.	Commonly used for idiopathic scoliosis and neuromuscular scoliosis.	
Luque procedure (posterior)	Two L-shaped rods attach to each level with wiring. Provides good stabilization and allows for lumbar lordosis and pelvic stability.	Good for children with poor bone, skin, or muscle quality. Associated with higher risk for neurological damage.	

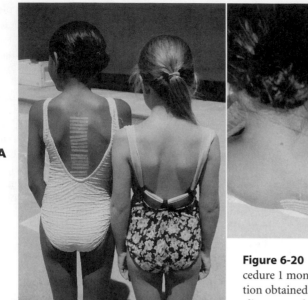

Figure 6-20 A, Child at left underwent a Cotrel-Dubousset procedure 1 month before the photograph was taken. Note the correction obtained, **B,** when compared with Figure 6-16. Note her spinal alignment when compared with the child on her right.

cause muscle weakness and even atrophy as a result of disuse. Individual exercises may be useful if the child has weakness in particular muscles or needs to develop specific skills while wearing the brace. If a child is exercising with peers, family members, or an organized group, compliance with the program may be easier to obtain. Use of a chart to document progress can help increase compliance. Exercises should be meaningful to the child. An example is customizing an exercise progression to a videotape or audiotape by using music that is chosen by the child. Adapting the physical education class curriculum may also be useful in helping the child continue participation with peers.

After surgery, depending on the procedure used, a child may need physical therapy intervention to redevelop mobility and self-help skills. Protocols for different surgical procedures vary and are summarized in Table 6-2.

Kyphosis

Incidence and cause. Kyphosis, sometimes called hunchback, occurs in about 4% of school-aged or adolescent children, with equal distribution between boys and girls (Renshaw, 1986). Kyphosis may be caused by genetic predisposition, neuromuscular abnormalities, such as myelomeningocele and spinal muscular atrophy, or postural anomalies.

Clinical features. Scheuermann's disease is a structural kyphosis characterized by a curve of 40 degrees or more. Although most common in the thoracic spine, Scheuermann's disease can also be seen in the lumbar or cervical spine, causing a flattening of the normal lordosis. Children with thoracic disease are unable to extend the spine to a neutral position. Posture is characterized by an excessive lumbar lordosis and a forward head, with an excessive cervical lordosis. Structural changes include anteriorly wedged vertebrae, narrowing of the intervertebral disk spaces, and irregular vertebral end plates. Thirty to forty percent of children have an associated scoliosis. The cause is usually ascribed to poor posture, but the condition has also been re-

ported to be transmitted by an autosomal dominant trait with an incidence of 0.4% to 8.3% (Tachdjian, 1990).

Congenital kyphosis results from abnormal formation of the vertebrae. The anterior portion forms incompletely, whereas the posterior portion forms normally, causing wedge-shaped deformities and a resulting kyphosis. This condition is progressive; the deformity increases as the child grows. Related problems include back pain, deformity, and neurological deficits. Complications can include compression of the spinal cord, leading to parasthesias and paralysis.

Neuromuscular kyphosis results from asymmetrical muscle pull on the spine caused by weakness, lack of innervation, or lack of control of certain muscle groups. Cerebral palsy, myelomeningocele, muscular dystrophy, and spinal muscular atrophy are a few of the neuromuscular diseases that can lead to a kyphotic deformity. Gravity may also affect a spine with inadequate muscle strength to maintain an erect posture against gravity.

Treatment. Exercises, bracing, or surgery are common treatments for kyphosis. Positioning may help a child with severe disabilities slow the progression of the deformity. The goal of treatment is to address the tight muscles that may lead to or result from the curve, resist the forces of gravity through positioning, arrest the progress of the curve, and correct the spinal deformity.

Exercises include stretching—for tight hamstrings, pectoral muscles, and abdominals—and strengthening for gluteal muscles, abdominals, and spinal extensor muscle groups. Passive spinal extension can stretch tight ligaments, and active spinal extension can strengthen weak muscles.

Orthotic management will usually includes a Milwaukee type of brace or a custom-molded body jacket called a thoracic lumbar sacral orthosis (TLSO). The Milwaukee brace has been shown to be more effective at initial management of a kyphosis than the TLSO, probably because the TLSO is more effective for lower curves.

Positioning to address a spinal kyphosis for a child with severe disabilities can be achieved by using gravity to assist the posture rather than fighting gravity to maintain an upright position.

Tilting or reclining the back surface of any adapted seating or wheelchair can achieve this goal. The trick is to maintain optimal pelvic positioning, and allow the child to access the environment visually while using gravity assisted positioning. To maintain good pelvic positioning, a tilt-in-space option for seating is usually more functional than a reclined back. A wedge behind the head or other positioning to keep the neck in some flexion allows the child to see forward rather than staring at the ceiling. Some children have strong flexor tone or strong righting reactions that cause them to pull into flexion, even when in a semi-reclined position. These responses will increase a kyphotic posture unless they can be controlled.

Lordosis

Many children have an excessive lordosis, sometimes called sway-back, during toddlerhood and early childhood. This condition usually resolves by age 8. Postural lordosis may be caused by obesity, pregnancy, or compensation for other curves, such as thoracic kyphosis. Lordosis may also be caused by neuromuscular deficits, including muscular dystrophy, cerebral palsy, and myelomeningocele. Treatment for lordosis is similar to that for scoliosis and kyphosis. Exercises may help to strengthen or stretch soft tissue, and bracing or surgery can arrest or correct a spinal curve.

Interventions for the Child With Severe Neuromuscular Disease and Scoliosis

It is important to note that children with neuromuscular diseases will generally have complications in addition to spinal deformities; these may include low or high muscle tone, weakness, persistence of primitive reflexes, soft tissue contractures, and behavioral, cognitive, or developmental issues. These related problems may affect the treatment protocol for the spinal deformity because of poor tolerance for a spinal orthosis, medical conditions that put the child at a high risk for surgery, or poor compliance potential with rehabilitation.

Positioning with adaptive equipment may be effective in slowing the progression of a spinal deformity. The use of a three-point trunk support for scoliosis, with pressure applied over the apex of the curve and the ribs at the cephalic and caudal end of the curve, can help a child with poor postural control maintain an upright position for functional activities (Figure 6-21). To maintain optimal alignment, custom-molded seating systems, gravity-assisted positioning, or trunk orthoses can all be effective alternatives to surgery, either singly or in combination. Attention to positioning in bed, on the mat, or in alternative positions can also affect the progress of a spinal deformity. Adaptive devices, such as the Vac-Pac (Olympic Medical), Versa Form Plus Positioning Pillows (Tumbleforms) or similar devices can provide custom positioning in sidelying, supine, prone, or sitting positions to support a spinal deformity (Figure 6-22).

Treatment protocol needs to be determined by a team of individuals, including the child, parents, teacher, physician, therapist, and others, who interact regularly with the child. The implications of long-term bracing, surgery, or lack of active treatment should be considered carefully before any decisions are made. The PTA should be aware of these and other related issues when planning and carrying out a treatment plan for a child with excessive spinal curvature.

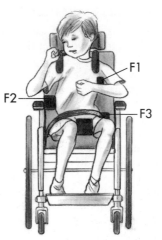

Figure 6-21 Postural correction has been achieved using the three-point method of trunk positioning for a child with scoliosis. Compare to Figure 6-18.

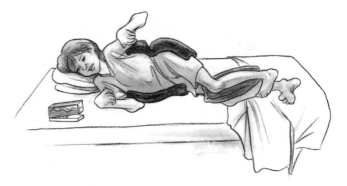

Figure 6-22 This child with a scoliosis uses a Vac-Pac for spinal positioning in sidelying.

The Child Athlete

Typically developing children and children with disabilities participate in sports every day. Team sports, such as baseball, football, and soccer, provide their own challenges to children, as do individual sports, such as running, swimming, and weight lifting. Although the number of children who are physically fit has been declining in recent years (Raunikar & Strong, 1991), approximately 50% of boys and 25% of girls between the ages of 8 and 16 years play competitive sports in the United States (Shaffer, 1980; Stanitski, 1989). Even more children participate in recreational sports, such as skiing, skateboarding, and bicycle riding.

This section addresses the ways in which children differ from adults and how these factors influence participation and injuries that children may incur. Children have different physiological capabilities than adults that can affect their participation in sports. Children are growing, which results in musculoskeletal, hormonal, and physiological changes that take place at a much faster pace than in adults. Because a child's musculoskeletal system is different from that of an adult, some of the orthopedic issues involved with children's sports are different from those of adults.

Team and Individual Sports and Recreation

Team sports occur in the context of school physical education classes, varsity and intramural competitions, and community-organized sports. These activities are generally physically demanding and may involve physical contact with other athletes. A coach, and sometimes an athletic trainer or PT, is usually directing the training and practices, as well as supervising rehabilitation from injuries, especially at the high school level. Coaches and instructors have varying levels of training regarding youth sports and sports injuries.

Individual sports for children include recreation activities, such as skateboarding or skiing, and training activities, such as running or swimming. These activities may be engaged in with or without the supervision of a coach. These sports are more conducive to overuse injuries or trauma related to falls. Protective equipment may not be used consistently or appropriately.

Family and community recreational activities, such as hiking, recreational swimming, or pick-up sports, constitute the third level of engagement. No trained supervision is usually present during these activities. Trauma or strain may result because of low training and fitness levels or inappropriate engagement in the activity.

Preparticipation physical examinations. Preparticipation physical examinations are generally required for all child athletes participating in organized sports. They are intended to ensure that the child is in adequate physical condition to participate in the activities required. A medical history, physical examination, and specialized tests for flexibility, strength, body composition, and visual acuity, as well as laboratory tests to assess urine and blood composition, may all be part of the examination. The physical examination may be conducted by the primary physician in a routine visit, or it may be conducted in a multistation model where all of the athletes are evaluated on the same day by a team of evaluators. This team may include a PT who can assess flexibility, strength, body composition, and vital signs. The preparticipation physical examination is intended to ensure the safety of the child by identifying contraindications for his or her participation and by preventing injury through proper assessment and education of the child athlete.

Protective equipment. Most sports have protective equipment, which can range from sunscreen for the swimmer or runner to thick body pads for ice hockey goalies and football players. Helmets for bicycling, wrist and knee pads for skateboarding, protective goggles for racquetball players, and sturdy shoes for runners are all intended to reduce injuries among participants. When used appropriately, this equipment can reduce injury rates. Frequently, however, the equipment does not fit properly, is not used as intended, or is not used at all. It is the responsibility of all involved individuals to ensure that children use protective equipment properly (Figure 6-23).

Competition. The school-aged child is beginning to understand competition in school and sports. When team sports are played competitively, children learn how to compete against others as a team and individually. Older children learn to compete against themselves to improve performance both academically and athletically. Some children thrive on competition, and others are not comfortable competing against others. These differences may relate to cultural background, individual temperament, past experiences, or environmental influences. Regardless of a child's preference, competition is a fact in competitive sports, such as soccer, baseball, football, competitive swimming, and running. Competition leads to injuries as children push themselves to win, and coaches, parents, and peers push them to try harder. Safety features (e.g., adequate protective equipment), proper training, and knowledge of or adherence to the rules may be ignored in the interest of winning. On the other hand, competition can spur a child to push harder to achieve more. This can lead to improved self-esteem and greater efforts in all areas (Figure 6-24).

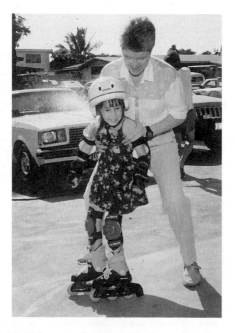

Figure 6-23 Helmets and other protective equipment can reduce injury in children.

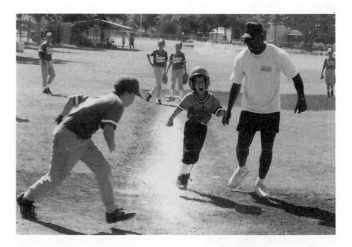

Figure 6-24 Athletic competition can lead to injuries but also to greater self-esteem and improved social and athletic skills.

The Athlete With a Disability

As inclusion gains momentum in schools and children with disabilities are more frequently being educated with their peers in integrated settings, sports and recreation are also being integrated. A young man with Down syndrome plays football with his high school team. A young boy with an upper extremity limb deficiency practices karate with his peers and is the pitcher on his baseball team. A young woman with cerebral palsy who uses a wheelchair is on the cheerleading squad for her high school. All these are true stories and there are many others like them. These athletes need adaptations to participate fully in their sports. The young man with Down syndrome playing football needs a radiograph of his cervical spine to rule out atlantoaxial instability, whereas his teammates do not. He may need extra help to learn the plays and more practice to develop his skills. He needs an exception to the age limits for playing with the team. The boy with a limb deficiency may need to be evaluated differently from his peers when he competes in karate tournaments because he is unable to complete some of the movements required. He needs to learn how to get his glove on and off his good hand quickly during the baseball game by using his mouth. The girl in the wheelchair needs modified cheerleading routines and must monitor the safety of her peers, who could injure themselves on her metal wheelchair.

Each of the athletes discussed here is at risk for many of the same injuries as his or her peers. Besides the specific needs they have because of their disabilities, they are engaging in competitive sports and risk overuse or traumatic injury. Their anatomical structure, physiology, or development may differ from that of their peers, and accommodations need to be made for treatment and rehabilitation of sports injuries.

Arenas also exist for athletes with disabilities to compete against other athletes with disabilities. The most well known include the Special Olympics and the Paralympics. In Special Olympics athletes 8 years of age or older who have mental retardation compete in multiple events, such as track and field, swimming, and bowling, on a community level. Many athletes have a physical disability as well as mental retardation. State championships lead to national competitions in Special Olympics. In these competitions winning is not emphasized. Each athlete is supported to participate as fully as he or she is able (Figure 6-25).

The International Paralympics are held every 4 years in concert with the Olympics. Athletes with disabilities compete in modified Olympic events against athletes with similar disabilities. Mental retardation is not a requirement for participation, and many athletes have physical disabilities, such as amputation or spinal cord injury. Competition is fierce with athletes training vigorously to be the best in their event. The quality of athletics is very high. Local winners compete against state and national champions to progress to the culminating event at the International Paralympics. These events are usually won by individuals with mature musculoskeletal systems, not by children. However, children with disabilities can begin training very young to develop their skills, just like other athletes.

Other opportunities to participate in sports include organized community recreation in which a child with a disability may be included and the creation of "challenger" teams in which children with disabilities play each other or rotate through the roster and play teams of children without disabilities. The thrill of participating in sports as part of a team can benefit a child with a disability in more ways than just physically (Figure 6-26). Improvements in cognitive skills (through learning the rules), social skills (through interacting appropriately with team members and competing teams), planning skills and motor skills are only some of the benefits. Coaches need training to address behavior issues, adaptations in rules and procedures for specific children, and ways to recognize and provide initial treatment to an injury received during the course of play.

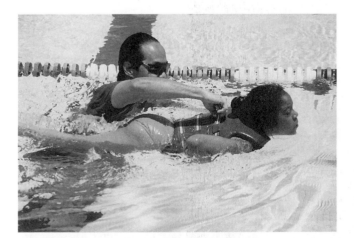

Figure 6-25 This young girl with cerebral palsy is competing in a swimming event in the Special Olympics. She needs individual support to participate.

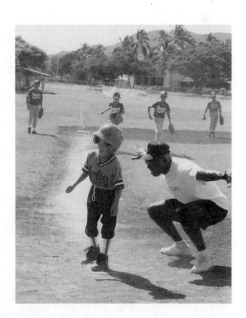

Figure 6-26 This young man is participating on a "Challenger" baseball team. Today his team is playing opposite a team of typically developing youngsters.

Pediatric Sports Injuries

Two primary types of orthopedic injuries occur in children while playing sports: the high-impact injury, such as a sprain or a fracture, and the overuse injury. These injuries are addressed in this section. Lacerations and abrasions may also occur and can be treated by medical means. Other types of injuries include traumatic brain injuries and spinal cord injuries, which are addressed in Chapter 9.

High-impact injuries. High-impact injuries occur as a result of contact between players or between the player and a solid surface, such as the ground. Sprains, strains, contusions (bruises), and fractures constitute the bulk of high-impact injuries. As in adults, sprains involve injury to the ligaments and can be categorized into three grades, depending on the extent of damage. Strains, which involve injury to the muscle and/or tendon, have three degrees of severity. Contusions can result in damage to muscle tissue, skin, and other soft tissues, with resulting hematomas. Pediatric fractures were discussed earlier in this chapter.

Treatment for high-impact injuries is similar to that for adults, except that for children the healing process occurs more quickly. Fractures and sprains should be seen by a physician immediately for evaluation on radiograph, confirmation of the diagnosis, and treatment through alignment and immobilization. Strains should be treated with initial immobilization, ice, and elevation to decrease swelling. Gentle active mobilization may be applied after the initial phase of healing to help maintain range of motion during the healing process. Children should not be allowed to continue playing after an acute injury to prevent chronic injury.

Contusions can be treated with ice and elevation. If the hematoma is deep, ultrasound may be used after the first 48 hours to help speed recovery. Ultrasound should be used carefully with children. It should not be used over any epiphysis, including the ends of long bones.

Overuse injuries. The epiphyseal growth centers and the sites of tendon insertion (apophyses) are the most common sites of traumatic sports injury in children (Risser, 1991). This is because these growth centers are most susceptible to injury.

Osgood-Schlatter disease. Osgood-Schlatter disease is an apophysitis (inflammation of the tendon insertion) of the tibial tubercle caused by chronic inflammation and microavulsion or slight tearing of the patellar tendon at its insertion point on the tibial tubercle. This condition occurs in girls from 8 to 13 years of age and in boys from 10 to 15 years. It is thought to be caused by rapid growth of the long bones coupled with stress on the patellar tendon from sports activities.

The clinical symptoms include pain, swelling, and prominence of the tibial tubercle. Treatment includes rest and analgesics for the pain. Ice may help to decrease the initial pain and swelling. The child should not return to active sports until the acute phase of the process has ended. This could take from months to several years. The child may have exacerbations until the age of 18 years, when most skeletal growth is completed. For severe cases immobilization of the knee into extension may be needed to reduce pressure through the patellar tendon and to allow healing to occur. The adolescent athlete will probably be unhappy at this turn of events, but it is important to protect the joint as healing occurs to prevent degenerative arthritis from occurring later in life. A child with Osgood-Schlatter disease will have difficulty kneeling on the affected knee because of pressure through the tubercle and may always have a prominent tibial tubercle on that side.

Physical therapy may be involved for modalities to relieve pain, and exercise may be used to preserve muscle strength of the quadriceps and to promote overall fitness during the recovery period. Isometrics of the quadriceps muscle with the knee in extension will not usually stress the insertion of the patellar tendon and will help to preserve muscle bulk; however, vigorous exercise of the quadriceps is contraindicated.

Sever disease. Sever disease is an apophysitis of the calcaneus. Its presentation is similar to that of Osgood-Schlatter disease, but it involves the heel.

Osteochondritis dessicans. The growing articular cartilage is susceptible to shear and other stress forces. Repetitive shear forces can cause microdegeneration of the articular cartilage, forming loose bodies that float around major joints. This condition is most common in the hip, knee, shoulder, and ankle. Treatment is symptomatic, with rest allowing eventual resorption of the loose body.

Other overuse syndromes. "Little League shoulder," a fracture of the proximal humeral growth plate common in young pitchers and catchers, is due to repetitive rotational stresses on the shoulder. "Little League elbow," also common in young pitchers, results in hypertrophy of the medial condyle of the elbow with pain and microavulsion of the condyle. Stress fractures are becoming more common in children. Rest, nonsteroidal antiinflammatory medication, and (sometimes) mild immobilization are the treatments of choice for all these conditions. Prevention of repetitive injuries by limiting the amount of pitching demanded of a young player, teaching proper throwing techniques, and early identification of problems is important to allow young athletes to continue their athletic careers. Little League and other community- and school-based athletic coaches need to be educated about young athletes to prevent injuries, and to address injuries once they occur. Many of these coaches are parents who volunteer, and they may not have the necessary training.

Pediatric Training

Children, as well as adults, can benefit from a training regimen to improve their strength, endurance, and skills to participate in a sport. There are significant differences between children and adults, however, that should be considered in planning a training regimen for a child. This information is important when designing or implementing a program to improve fitness or a program to rehabilitate a child with musculoskeletal, respiratory, or cardiac impairments.

The following information is applicable primarily to prepubescent and early-pubescent children. Once puberty is reached, children develop capabilities similar to those of adults to respond to training.

Thermoregulatory capability. A child has decreased cardiac output compared with an adult and a proportionately greater surface area. A child does not sweat like an adult. These factors combine to limit the child's ability to exercise in conditions of high humidity or heat. A child also cannot maintain body heat as well as an adult in cold conditions, particularly in water. Although a child's cardiorespiratory improvement with training is limited compared with that of an adult, training has been shown to improve strength, endurance, and skills.

Cardiovascular training. A prepubescent child does not increase his or her maximum oxygen uptake significantly with training. Therefore a child does not appear to benefit from aerobic training. In fact, however, the child's performance in running long distances improves with low-intensity, long-duration training. Short intense workouts, such as interval training, have not been shown to improve performance in children.

Strength training. Because prepubescent children lack the androgens to build muscle bulk, it was formerly thought that they could not benefit from weight training. Research has shown that children can, indeed, benefit from weight training by increasing their muscle bulk and strength (Sewall & Micheli, 1986; Sailors & Berg, 1987). Concern remains, however, about the fragility of children's growing bodies. Recommendations re-

garding prepubescent children's weight training by several groups include requirements that all children have a preparticipation physical, adequate supervision, and proper warm-up and cooldown to avoid injury. Weight training should be a part of a comprehensive program designed to improve motor skills and overall fitness. No child should attempt a maximal lift or compete in weight lifting. Training should occur two to three times per week for 20 to 30 minutes, and no resistance should be used until proper form is demonstrated. Weight should be increased in small increments (1 to 3 pounds) only after the child is able to do 15 repetitions at the previous weight level (Duda, 1986).

Other considerations. Nutrition, the ratio between height and weight, a level of maturity indicating ability to follow directions and accept supervision, stage of growth, and overall health should all be assessed and taken into consideration when designing or implementing a training program for a child.

APPLICATIONS Use of Splints and Orthoses With Children

GAY M. NAGANUMA

PTs who work with children frequently use splints and orthoses as an adjunct to the therapy program. An appropriately designed, well-fitting orthosis or splint can serve many purposes. It can act as an extra pair of hands, allowing the therapist to provide support or alignment at more proximal joints while the splint supports a more distal joint. It can duplicate or approximate the support or sensory input provided during therapy. In this way an orthosis can help maintain skills learned during therapy and can reinforce correct movement patterns between therapy sessions. An orthosis or splint can be useful in minimizing joint contractures, as well as in maximizing strength and functional skills through improving joint stability.

A splinting system can enhance a consistent, well-directed therapeutic exercise program if the orthotic treatment and the therapy program address the same therapeutic goal. When orthoses are used in therapy, the therapist needs to consider which activities should be performed with the orthoses and which ones should be done without them. For example, a child with cerebral palsy who is able to stand independently with good alignment might perform standing balance activities in bare feet. The same child might need to wear orthoses during gait training when the postural challenge increases. The orthoses can be removed as the child's active control of the joint improves. One goal of an orthotic program is to minimize the client's dependence on the device (Huber, 1995).

The splints and orthoses described in this section represent those appliances most commonly used with children. An extensive overview of all the upper and lower extremity orthoses that are used with children is beyond the scope of this section. Tables 6-3 and 6-4 summarize the information about specific splints and orthoses presented.

The term *orthosis* refers to a device used to support, position, or immobilize a part; to correct deformities; to assist weak muscles and restore function; or to modify tone (Trombly, 1989). There exists considerable variability in the literature regarding the use of the term *splint*. Splints are sometimes considered to be more temporary devices than orthoses and are used solely as a

means to apply corrective forces to a joint (Fess & Philips, 1987). Splints are generally fabricated by therapists, whereas orthoses are fabricated by an orthotist. This section uses the term *splint* to refer to an upper extremity orthosis (Trombly, 1989) or a lower extremity device that is used for alignment purposes only.

Hand Splints

Because of the importance of hand use to global development, therapists who work with children place the remediation of hand dysfunction high on the list of therapy priorities. Traditional intervention strategies used in the treatment of hand dysfunction may include passive or active range-of-motion exercises, strengthening exercises that use muscle facilitation techniques or progressive resistance, sensory awareness activities, reflex inhibition, weight-bearing activities, functional play or activities of daily living, and surgical or orthopedic correction of deformity. Such intervention strategies are frequently augmented by the use of hand splints. When muscle activity or joint stability is inadequate, the external force of a splint can be helpful to maintain the joint in an optimal position for function and to prevent development or progression of joint and soft tissue contractures (Figure 6-27).

Use

In general, hand splints are used to maintain mobility and alignment for functional movement and neuromuscular reeducation of the extremity. Box 6-4 contains detailed information regarding splint use and precautions.

Types

Static splints. Static splints have no movable parts. They provide external support to maintain a prescribed functional joint position. Static splints limit joint activity to provide physiological

TABLE 6-3 Overview of Hand Splints

Splints	Materials	Indications	Benefits	Precautions
Static				
Dorsal resting hand splint Volar resting hand splint	Low-temperature thermoplastics	Cerebral palsy Head injury Arthrogryposis Limb deficiency Juvenile rheumatoid arthritis Burns Trauma	Low cost Lightweight Durable Attractive Comfortable Broad contact area (decreased pressure) Can be easily remolded	Splint fit must be monitored as child grows to prevent skin breakdown. Prolonged use can produce joint stiffness.
Static thumb index webspace splint	Low-temperature thermoplastics	Cerebral palsy Head injury Spasticity Fisted thumb	Inhibits spastic muscles Maintains range for thumb opposition Places thumb in a functional position	Monitor splint edges around thumb because this can be area of increased pressure.
Semidynamic				
Sof-Splint Joe Cool thumb splint Good Samaritan splint Neoprene webspace splint Benik Corporation thumb abduction splint	Neoprene Neoplush	Marked thumb adduction Cerebral palsy Webspace tightness Increased tone in hand Limited active use of thumb Excessive thumb joint mobility	Allows controlled arc of motion Stable and functional position of thumb Quick and easy to fabricate Inexpensive Allows sensory exposure of hand Elasticity prevents too much pressure	Not to be used with fixed deformity, bony changes, or strong flexion pattern at wrist. With Neoprene webspace splint, skin needs to be monitored closely because it has poor ventilation.
Dynamic				
Orthokinetic wrist splint MacKinnon splint	Low-temperature thermoplastics Dowel Straps Latex tubing	Spastic cerebral palsy Hemiplegia with fixed posture of upper extremity	Inhibits spastic flexor muscles Facilitates extensor muscles Encourages bilateral hand use	Not recommended for children with fisted hands, cortical thumb, or severe radial or ulnar deviation.

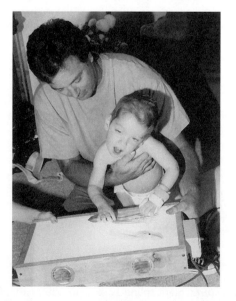

Figure 6-27 Volar resting splints help Ian use his hands to play with bright fishing lures illuminated by a light box.

rest for painful or injured structures and to prevent movement that might interfere with the process of tissue repair. They can be used by children experiencing an active inflammatory phase of rheumatoid arthritis or immediately after surgical correction of a nerve or tendon injury. In addition, static splints are used in the treatment of contractures caused by soft tissue scarring, resulting from burns, trauma, or infection and to prevent development of deformity secondary to abnormal forces of muscle imbalance, soft tissue shortening, pain, or spasticity. By limiting motion or by altering the direction of stress on a joint, static splints can relieve pain caused by overstretching of soft tissue, abnormal motion at a joint, and compression of neural structures.

Static splints can be used to maintain range and alignment obtained during therapy sessions. Range of motion can be increased by using a series of static splints that gradually and successively position the joint nearer to the desired limits. Finally, static splints can stabilize one or more joints, enabling other joints to function correctly. For example, a girl with spastic cerebral palsy who displays a flexed wrist posture would be unable to grasp a juice-filled cup with sufficient power to get the cup to her mouth. A wrist

TABLE 6-4   Overview of Lower Extremity Orthotics and Splints

Splints	Materials	Indications	Benefits	Precautions
Orthotics				
Dynamic ankle-foot orthotics (DAFO)	Polypropylene	Neuromuscular disorder	Contoured to produce even pressure distribution Varying degrees of ankle support Holds forefoot and hindfoot in alignment	Splint fit must be monitored as child grows to prevent skin breakdown.
DAFO with free plantarflexion	Polypropylene	Mild or severe abnormal lower extremity tone	Allows dorsiflexion and plantar flexion Allows maximal lower leg contact during crawling Does not interfere with balance reactions	Splint fit must be monitored as child grows to prevent skin breakdown.
Solid-backed DAFO	Polypropylene	Inability to place voluntary foot flat during stance	May eliminate hyperextension of knee Keeps heel down in splint Can prevent shortening of calf muscles	Observe for redness and poor skin tolerance.
Floor reaction brace	Polypropylene	Crouch gait caused by weakness (myelodysplasia)	Blocks ankle dorsiflexion Easy donning and doffing Encourages hip and knee extension	Poor intrinsic foot control. Does not work well for children with crouch gait because of high tone (spastic diplegia).
Splints				
Resting splints	Low temperature Thermoplastics Polypropylene	Plantar flexion contracture not managed by daytime splinting	Prolonged stretch on soft tissues Worn at night Static standing	Not for ambulation.
Foot orthotics	Polyethylene foam Polypropylene	Hypotonicity Hypermobility of feet with good control of muscle activity	Support weight-bearing surface of foot Help with balance Improve mild discrepancy in alignment	Does not control spastic foot. Does not help with foot that fixes into a poorly aligned position.

BOX 6-4   Use of Splints

Purpose

Splints are used to:
- Prevent joint stress caused by excess motion
- Prevent or correct contractures and deformity
- Maintain range-of-motion gains achieved by casting, manipulation, or surgery
- Rule out undesirable joint motion
- Support joints in optimal functional position
- Simplify patterns of coordination
- Facilitate muscle activity
- Decrease agonist spasticity

Precautions

When splints are used, avoid:
- Unnecessary restriction of movement
- Interference with sensory input
- Pressure/friction over bony prominences or at splint edges
- Nerve compression
- Incorrect angle of pull
- Misalignment between movable splint axis and actual joint axis
- Improper size of splint

Observe patient for:
- Stressing or overstretching of a joint
- Developing stiffness in a splinted joint
- Impaired circulation
- Weakening muscles

cock-up splint would position her wrist in extension and place her finger flexors in a position of greater mechanical advantage so that she could grasp the cup more effectively.

How a static splint might be used is illustrated through the case study of Camila, a 5-year-old with polyarticular juvenile rheumatoid arthritis. Camila wears a volar resting splint at night to position her wrist and fingers in slight extension. The splinting material extends to her fingertips to maintain the length of her long finger flexors. The splints were fabricated by her therapist using a low-temperature thermoplastic material.

A number of static thumb-index webspace splints have been designed to prevent webspace contracture (Figure 6-28). An opposable thumb has great functional impact on manual dexterity and pinch/grasp effectiveness. In addition to maintaining the range-of-motion necessary for thumb opposition, static thumb abduction splints may have an inhibitory effect on a spastic hand by reversing the most distal component of a total synergy of upper extremity flexion. For example, by reducing the fisted thumb position of a child with cerebral palsy, thumb abduction splints may improve a reaching pattern by helping to break up total patterns of abnormal movement (Naganuma & Billingsley, 1990).

Semidynamic splints. Semidynamic splints have no moving parts. They position joints in a manner that encourages functional movement of the extremity. They maintain a desired joint position while allowing a controlled arc of motion at the splinted joint without actually producing forces for movement.

A semidynamic thumb abduction splint called the Sof-splint was developed to inhibit marked thumb adduction in children with cerebral palsy (Reymann, 1985). It consists of two straps that can be adjusted to grade the amount and direction of pull on the thumb. One strap is a wrist band. The other strap loops

around the thumb to hold it out of the palm. Thumb-loop splints are made of a semielastic material, such as neoprene or Neoplush, a neoprene-like material with nylon lining on one side and a Velcro loop pile on the other. The elasticity provides dynamic properties that allow active movement of the thumb while maintaining a more stable and functional position of thumb abduction and opposition. The splint can then be used during functional fine motor tasks or daily living activities. A commercially available splint, similar in design to the Sof-splint, is the Joe Cool Thumb Splint.*

Therapists at the Good Samaritan Hospital in Puyallup, Washington, have developed a neoprene webspace splint pattern that consists of a thumb sleeve that attaches to a wrist strap in a graded manner to allow positioning of the thumb out of the palm. The splint is used to (1) provide therapy carryover and maintain the decreased tone and increased functional hand position achieved during a treatment session, (2) supply stability for joint integrity and active movement, (3) maintain functional webspace mobility while not restricting joint movement, (4) decrease tone and inhibit upper extremity flexor synergy, (5) preserve arches and natural curves of the hand, (6) provide an open hand position for increased function and sensory input, and (7) provide a cost-effective alternative to more expensive and complicated hand splints.

Commercially made neoprene thumb abduction splints that use a similar design are available from the Benik Corporation.† They fabricate a variety of neoprene thumb splints, many of which include proximal control from a wrist sleeve or distal control from an index finger sleeve.

Dynamic splints. Dynamic splints use moving levers in the form of springs, wires, rubberbands, or other elastic materials to compensate for muscle weakness or imbalance while permitting continued activity of unaffected muscle groups. This enables normal muscles to maintain their function and power while encouraging weak muscles to strengthen. Dynamic splints are useful with children who have some voluntary movement by providing supplemental power or guidance to the active movement. Movement of the involved joint prevents the complications of immobilization sometimes associated with prolonged static splinting: adhesions, joint stiffness, muscle atrophy, decreased circulation, and edema. Dynamic splints allow active exercise while maintaining proper joint alignment. Provision of dynamic support can prevent dysfunctional compensations made by the child to alleviate pain, spasm, or weakness. The orthokinetic wrist splint (Hill, 1988) and the MacKinnon splint (MacKinnon, Sanderson, & Buchanon, 1975) are two examples of dynamic splints and are described in Table 6-3.

Lower Extremity Orthoses

Until the mid-1970s, steel or aluminum braces with adjustable ankle joints were used for children with lower extremity weakness, paralysis, or orthopedic deformity. Similar to the braces used with adult clients, these heavy, bulky, and rigid braces were

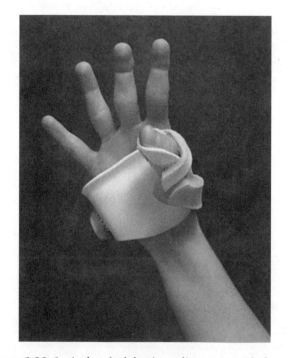

Figure 6-28 Static thumb abduction splints assist with the open hand posture needed for functional hand use. (From Coppard, B.M., & Lohman, H. [1996]. *Introduction to splinting* [p. 269]. St. Louis: Mosby.)

*For information, call 1-800-233-3556; 404 N. 4th St., Olathe, CO 81425.
†For information, call 1-800-442-8910; 9465 Provost Rd NW #204, Silverdale, WA 98383.

often attached to stiff orthopedic shoes. Polypropylene (a high-temperature thermoplastic material) orthoses were first introduced in the 1960s but not used commonly with children until the mid to late 1970s. Early designs using polypropylene included a fixed ankle and a flat soleplate. These orthoses offered the advantages of improved appearance, lighter weight, increased flexibility of design, and improved pressure distribution caused by increased contact area.

By the early 1980s, polypropylene orthoses were being molded with features designed to hold the subtalar joint in neutral and to inhibit spasticity. This concept was developed through the use of inhibitive casts to reduce lower extremity tone (Hinderer, 1988). When therapists began noting decreased lower extremity tone with serial casts, they proceeded to bivalve the casts and build up the footplate for weight bearing. These casts met with good success during therapy sessions but were too heavy and bulky for prolonged use. The casts were used to fabricate splints of high-temperature thermoplastics that incorporated the same features as the inhibitive casts. Because of their effect on lower extremity muscle tone, these splints have been referred to as inhibitive orthoses. It was originally thought that changes in tone were produced by inhibition of foot reflexes and spasticity through pressure and positioning. Newer theories promote optimal biomechanical alignment as causing the changes in tone. The alignment and support provided by ankle-foot orthoses are believed to place lower extremity musculature in a position of maximal mechanical advantage and to result in improved control of posture and movement (Buethorn, 1995) (Figure 6-29).

Use

Lower extremity orthoses may be used to prevent a deformity that has not yet occurred or to minimize one that would progress without treatment. An orthosis protects cartilaginous and soft tissues from the deforming effects of inappropriate weight bearing and tensile strains. For example, the biomechanical support of an orthotic can help a child with spastic diplegia experience the emotional and physiological benefits of standing and walking without foot deformation. Orthoses can also be used after surgery or serial casting to maintain newly achieved correction.

A specific application of this principle is night splinting. A reduction in muscle tone often occurs during sleep and allows an orthosis to apply greater stretch to a joint than would be possible during the day. Some children tolerate night splints well, and others, not at all. Camila's mother (see Case Study, Chapter 5), for instance, applies her night splints after Camila is asleep, so Camila will not remove them. Orthoses can sometimes be used to correct a deformity by applying corrective forces to the joints over a prolonged period, thereby affecting tissue modeling during growth. Orthoses support optimal joint alignment and mechanics. Joint axes must be aligned properly to respond appropriately to direction and degree of force applied by muscles and weight bearing. Support of structural alignment in the foot promotes an improved balance of muscle power and tone.

By providing variable range-of-motion, a well-designed orthosis offers as many normal movement options as possible while providing structural support for optimal biomechanical alignment. Selective restriction of range-of-motion is often necessary to assist weak muscles, oppose spastic muscles, or protect certain soft tissues postsurgically. When splints are used to minimize excessive motion, they should not completely block movement that the child is learning to control. While stabilization from splinting can allow improved function, too much immobilization prevents the child from gaining control over a specific arc of motion. The amount of support provided by the splint can be reduced gradually as the child gains active control. The use of low-temperature thermoplastics can be helpful in minimizing the cost of frequent adaptations or refabrication. Splint-

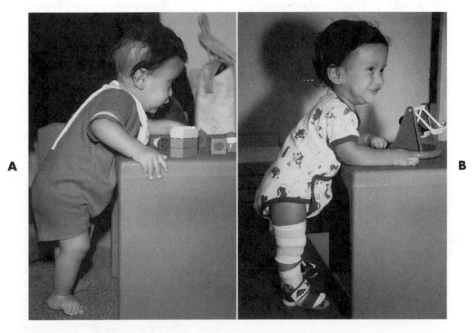

Figure 6-29 Foot and ankle alignment (**A**) of Ronnie, a child with spina bifida, is greatly improved when he is wearing dynamic ankle-foot orthoses (**B**).

ing materials, such as Aquaplast, are easy and inexpensive to use and do not require the assistance of an orthotist, as is the case with high-temperature thermoplastics (Cusick, 1990).

The optimal joint alignment provided by lower extremity orthoses provides accurate and usable sensory feedback. For example, an ankle-foot orthosis with a plantar flexion stop strap prevents excessive plantar flexion in stance and allows weight bearing through the heel in stance. This proprioceptive input reinforces standing alignment with a foot-flat position. The stable and consistent proprioceptive feedback information that occurs as a result of splinting provides more helpful and reliable information for balance and postural control.

Types

Dynamic ankle-foot orthoses. The most common orthotic used with children who have a neuromuscular disorder is a dynamic ankle-foot orthotic (DAFO). It consists of a shell that fits the contours of the foot and holds the heel and forefoot in correct relationship to each other. Made of custom-molded polypropylene, the DAFO provides total contact and distributes pressure more evenly throughout the brace, reducing the tendency for skin breakdown. Made of thin and flexible plastic, the orthotic can be wrapped completely and comfortably around the foot and still is easy to put on and take off. DAFOs have varying proximal trimlines of the polypropylene to provide different degrees of support to the ankle. The product of cooperative teamwork with pediatric therapists, these DAFO designs combine the features of what works well from a therapeutic perspective with progressive orthotic technology. Characteristics of the various orthotics and splints are summarized in Table 6-4.

A custom-contoured soleplate supports the dynamic arches of the foot and places structures in a position of maximal mechanical advantage. This type of soleplate is a characteristic that differentiates dynamic AFOs from standard AFOs. The soleplate, or footplate, stabilizes the foot in corrected alignment and maintains optimal functional positioning.

A DAFO with free plantar flexion provides good forefoot and hindfoot control while allowing motion into dorsiflexion and plantarflexion. This permits the child to practice emerging control of ankle motion in the sagittal plane while the foot is maintained in optimal biomechanical alignment. The DAFO with free plantarflexion can be appropriate for children with severe to mild abnormal lower extremity tone (Figure 6-30). The posterior cutout that allows plantarflexion makes this a good splint for children who are making the transition between crawling and walking. Because it does not hold the ankles at 90 degrees of dorsiflexion, but allows some dorsiflexion and plantar flexion, this splint does not interfere with balance responses as do more static splints.

Solid-backed dynamic ankle-foot orthoses. Solid-backed DAFOs block plantar flexion and allow free dorsiflexion (Figure 6-31). They are used for children who are not able to get voluntary footflat during stance or those who exhibit excessive muscle fixation as a result of any lower extremity muscle activation. The wrap-around design of the plastic encloses the dorsum of the foot. This anterior closure, combined with a 45-degree angle instep strap, gives good control of heelrise within the splint. Stabilizing the heel helps the child to keep the heel down in stance and to practice dorsiflexion during walking. Heel contact can

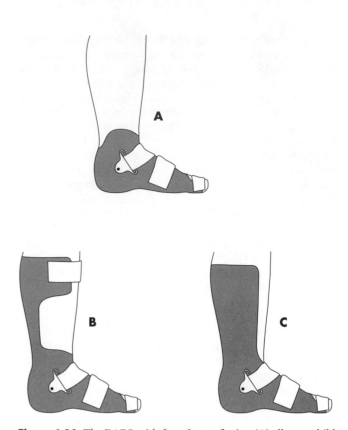

Figure 6-30 The DAFO with free plantar flexion (**A**) allows a child to move in the sagittal plane yet maintain good foot and ankle integrity. The resist plantar flexion (**B**) and stop plantar flexion (**C**) DAFOs provide increasingly rigid plantar flexion resistance.

prevent shortening of the calf muscle and may eliminate hyperextension of the knee that can be caused by too much tone in the calf muscle.

The use of a solid-backed DAFO can be illustrated by the case study of Andrew, a 5-year-old boy who has cerebral palsy (see Chapter 7). Andrew has low trunk tone and increased extremity tone. He tends to move in total patterns of flexion and extension. His posture and movement are influenced by persistence of the tonic labyrinthine reflex, symmetrical tonic neck reflex, positive support reflex, and plantar grasp reflex.

Andrew can roll across the floor, using a total extension pattern, and needs support to sit because he tends to throw his trunk backward into extension. Andrew loves to stand but does so with stiffly extended legs and a strong equinovarus position of his foot. When supported, Andrew can take steps forward, but he uses a reflex gait pattern with excessive hip adduction during the swing phase.

Andrew recently received a pair of DAFOs, and the alignment and stability they provide improves his ability to take steps in his Rifton walker. With an improved base of support, Andrew's total body alignment in his prone stander is improved. Andrew's position in his bolster chair is also improved because the DAFOs help him keep his legs and feet relaxed so he does not push into an extensor thrust while in his chair.

Floor-reaction orthoses. A floor-reaction orthosis is designed to block ankle dorsiflexion and encourage hip and knee

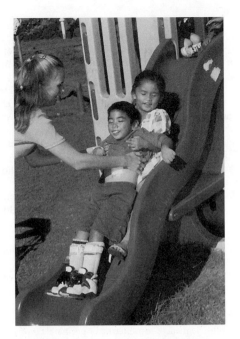

Figure 6-31 DAFOs provide Joshua with the lower extremity support he needs for independent mobility at home and school.

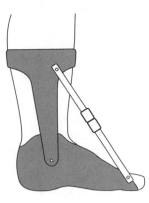

Figure 6-32 An adjustable night splint controls foot alignment to prevent overstretching of the midfoot.

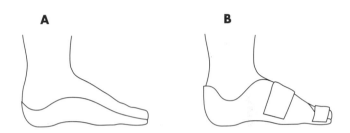

Figure 6-33 A, Foot orthoses can be used for feet that lack stability because of excess motion. **B,** Maximal support foot orthoses wrap higher up on the foot to provide additional support.

extension. It works well for children who exhibit a crouched gait caused by plantar flexion weakness (e.g., children with myelodysplasia), but not so well for children who are crouched caused of high muscle tone (e.g., children with spastic diplegia). The splint design is open in the back to allow for easy donning and doffing, but the lack of heel stabilization limits intrinsic foot control. The plastic is closed over the dorsum of the foot and about two thirds of the way up the front of the lower leg.

Lower Extremity Splints

Resting splints. Resting splints are generally not used for ambulation. They provide good prolonged positioning for night wear, sitting, prone standing, and transfers. An adjustable night splint may have a diagonal strap from the tibia to the forefoot that can be adjusted to change the dorsiflexion angle of the splint (Figure 6-32). Such a splint must provide hindfoot control to hold the heel down and back in the splint so the stretching action of the straps affects the talocrural joint rather than the midfoot. This splint is effective for a wide variety of individuals who exhibit plantar flexion contracture if daytime management alone does not sufficiently control loss of range-of-motion.

Foot orthoses. Foot orthoses are designed for the child who has fairly good graded control of muscle activity in the lower extremities (Figure 6-33, *A*). They are intended to support the weight-bearing surfaces of the foot to help with mild discrepancies in alignment and subtle balance impairments. Foot orthoses can be fabricated out of soft closed-cell polyethylene foam and may be reinforced with polypropylene plastic to provide greater mechanical support.

The use of foot orthoses can be illustrated by the case study of Camila, a 5-year-old girl with polyarticular juvenile rheumatoid arthritis (see Chapter 5). Camila wears maximal control foot orthoses inside her shoes to maintain her foot in a position that

will protect the joints from overstretching or injury. Having her feet feel more stable has helped Camila's balance, and her walking has lost some of its stiff-legged quality.

Maximal support foot orthosis. Higher trimlines characterize the maximal support foot orthosis. The orthosis wraps up and over the dorsum of the foot, providing greater external support and sensory feedback for proper alignment (Figure 6-33, *B*). This foot orthosis is good for hypotonic, or hypermobile, feet, which exhibit excessive motion and lack of midline stability. Because support is relatively flexible and does not cross the ankle, foot orthoses are not good for controlling a spastic foot or a foot that fixes into poorly aligned positions.

Summary

The literature on splinting and orthoses for children with neuromuscular disorders presents a great deal of variability regarding selection of materials, design, and wearing schedule and the mechanism of splint effect on muscle tone and function. Despite this lack of agreement, the use of splints and orthoses remains a common form of treatment for movement dysfunction. Therapists continually develop innovative ways of applying splinting principles to meet the individual needs of their patients. Splints and orthoses can be effective in encouraging a child's progress toward more normal movement, posture, tone, and function.

EXERCISES

1. Find a group of 2- and 3-year-old children (a preschool setting is the most likely place to find such a group), and look at the variation in alignment of their legs and feet. Note what normal alignment is for children of different ages, and note normal variation.

2. Using a doll, teach a peer how to do activities with a young infant with congenital torticollis. How and when might you use a doll to teach parents activities to do with a young child?

3. Heat some low-temperature thermoplastic material in a pan of warm water. Manipulate the material to see what it can do. Make a rudimentary upper extremity splint for a doll. Make a rudimentary resting splint for a doll's foot. What happens when the material gets too thin? What can you do to correct your splint if it hardens in the wrong shape?

4. There is likely at least one person in your class who has a protruding tibial tubercle from Osgood-Schlatter disease during adolescence. This person can describe his or her experience with the disease for the class.

5. Perform scoliosis screening on your peers. At least one person in your class will likely have a scoliosis with a structural component that may or may not have been identified during adolescence.

QUESTIONS TO PONDER

1. Some states are funding athletic trainers or PTs to work in high schools with student athletes. Would one professional be better than the other? What are the specific skills that each might bring to this situation?

2. Is it important for a child athlete with an injury to be seen by a therapist with specific pediatric skills? What information is needed by a therapist or a PTA who is working with children with orthopedic injuries? How are children different from adults?

3. Funding is sometimes difficult to obtain for pediatric orthotics. Are these devices important for children? Why? Can you justify to a third-party funding agency why they should pay for an orthotic for a child with cerebral palsy?

Annotated Bibliography

TeamRehab Report. Malibu, CA: Miramar Communications.

This monthly magazine reviews both new technology and new uses for old technology. It incorporates case studies, written by therapists and rehabilitation engineers, about children and adults with complex rehabilitation technology needs. Seating and positioning, augmentative communication, play, adaptive self-help skills, and environmental controls are all addressed in articles that are practical and timely. Advertisers promote new products, and legislation related to technology is reviewed here regularly. If you work with children who need assistive technology, this magazine is a great way to stay up to date with the newest technology. A subscription to this magazine can be obtained free if the subscriber meets the publication's guidelines. Otherwise, a subscription costs $36.00 per year in the United States. For more information, write to TeamRehab Report, P. O. Box 16778, North Hollywoood, CA 91615-6778.

References

Allington, N. J., & Bowen, J. R. (1996). Adolescent idiopathic scoliosis: Treatment with the Wilmington brace. A comparison of full-time and part-time use. *Journal of Bone and Joint Surgery (Am.), 7*(78), 1056-1072.

Aronsson, D. D., Stokes, I. A., Ronchetti, P. J., & Labelle, H. B. (1994). Comparison of curve shape between children with cerebral palsy, Friedreich's ataxia, and adolescent idiopathic scoliosis. *Developmental Medicine and Child Neurology, 36,* 412-418.

Buethorn, D. (1995). *Dynamic splinting workshop manual.* Bellingham, WA: Cascade Prosthetics and Orthotics.

Bunnell, W. P. (1988). The natural history of idiopathic scoliosis. *Clinical Orthopaedics and Related Research, 229,* 20-25.

Carlioz, H., & Ouaknine, M. (1994-1995). Neurologic complications of surgery of the spine in children. *Chirurgie, 11*(120), 26-30.

Cheng, J. C., & Au, A. W. (1994). Infantile torticollis: A review of 624 cases. *Journal of Pediatric Orthopedics, 6*(14), 802-808.

Cunningham, S. M., & Albert, M. C. (1993). Congenital clubfoot. *Today's OR Nurse, 6*(15), 31-34.

Cusick, B. D. (1990) *Progressive casting and splinting for lower extremity deformities in children with neuromuscular dysfunction.* Tucson: Therapy Skill Builders.

Davids, J. R., Wenger, D. R., & Mubarak, S. J. (1993). Congenital muscular torticollis: Sequela of intrauterine or perinatal compartment syndrome. *Journal of Pediatric Orthopedics, 2*(13), 141-147.

Duda, M. (1986). Prepubescent strength training gains support. *Physician and Sportsmedicine, 14*(2), 157-161.

Eng, G. D. (1971). Brachial plexus palsy in newborn infants. *Pediatrics, 48,*18.

Fess, E. E., & Philips, C. A. (1987). *Handsplinting: Principles and methods.* St. Louis: Mosby.

Geutjens, G., Gilbert, A., & Helsen, K. (1996). Obstetric brachial plexus palsy associated with breech delivery: A different pattern of injury. *Journal of Bone and Joint Surgery (Br.), 2*(78),303-306.

Hill, S. G. (1988). Current trends in upper extremity splinting, In R. Boehme (Ed.), *Improving upper body control.* Tucson: Therapy Skill Builders.

Hinderer, K. A., et al. (1988). Effects of "tone-reducing" vs. standard plaster-casts on gait improvement of children with cerebral palsy. *Developmental Medicine and Child Neurology, 30,* 370.

Huber, S. R. (1995). Therapeutic application of orthotics. In D. A. Umphred (Ed.), *Neurological rehabilitation (3rd ed.),* St. Louis: Mosby.

Jackson, S. T., Hoffer, M. M., & Parish, N. (1988). Brachial-plexus palsy in the newborn. *Journal of Bone and Joint Surgery, 70A,* 1217-1220.

MacKinnon, J., Sanderson, E., & Buchanan, J. (1975). The MacKinnon splint—A functional hand splint. *Canadian Journal of Occupational Therapy, 42*(4), 157-158.

Nachemson, A. L., & Peterson, L. E. (1995). The effectiveness of treatment with a brace in girls who have adolescent idiopathic scoliosis. A prospective, controlled study based on data from the Brace Study of the Scoliosis Research Society. *Journal of Bone and Joint Surgery (Am.), 6*(77), 815-822.

Naganuma, G. M., & Billingsley, F. F. (1990). Use of hand splints with the neurologically involved child. *Critical Reviews in Physical and Rehabilitation Medicine, 2,* 87.

Porter, S. B., & Blount, B. W. (1995). Pseudotumor of infancy and congenital muscular torticollis. *American Family Physician, 6*(52), 1731-1736.

Pruijs, J. E., Keessen, W., van der Meer, R., & van Wieringen, J. C. (1995). School screening for scoliosis: The value of quantitative measurement. *European Spine Journal, 4*(4),226-230.

Raunikar, R. A., & Strong, W. B. (1991). The status of adolescent physical fitness. *Adolescent Medicine State of the Art Reviews, 2,*65-75.

Renshaw, T. (1986). *Pediatric Orthopedics.* Philadelphia: WB Saunders.

Reymann, J. (1985). The Sof-splint. *Developmental Disabilities Special Interest Section Newsletter, 8,* 1.

Risser, W. L. (1991). Epidemiology of sport injuries in adolescents. *Adolescent Medicine State of the Art Reviews, 2,* 109-124.

Sailors, M., & Berg, K. (1987). Comparison of response to weight training in pubescent boys and men. *Journal of Sports Medicine and Physical Fitness, 27,* 30-37.

Sewall, L., & Micheli, L. J. (1986). Strength training for children. *Journal of Pediatric Orthopedics, 6,* 143-146.

Shaffer, T. E. (1980). The uniqueness of the young athlete: Introductory remarks. *American Journal of Sports Medicine, 8,*370.

Simons, G. W. (1985). Complete subtalar release in club feet. Part 1: A preliminary report. *Journal of Bone and Joint Surgery (Am), 7*(67), 1044-1055.

Snyder, B. D., Zaltz, I., Breitenback, M. A., Kido, T. H., Myers, E. R., & Emans, J. B. (1995). Does bracing affect bone density in adolescent scoliosis? *Spine, 14*(20),1554-1560.

Stanitski, C. (1989). Common injuries in preadolescent athletes. *Sports Medicine, 7,* 32-41.

Tachdjian, M. O. (1990). *Pediatric orthopedics* (2nd ed.). Philadelphia: WB Saunders.

Townsend, D. J., & Bassett, G. S. (1996). Common elbow fractures in children. *American Family Physician, 6*(53), 2031-2041.

Trombly, C. A. (1987). *Occupational Therapy for Physical Dysfunction (3rd ed.).* Baltimore: Williams & Wilkins.

Yu, S. W., Wang, N. H., Chin, L. S., & Lo, W. H. (1995). Surgical correction of muscular torticollis in older children. *Chung hua I hwueh tsa chih (Taipei), 2*(55), 168-171.

PART THREE

Neurological and Muscular Disorders of Childhood

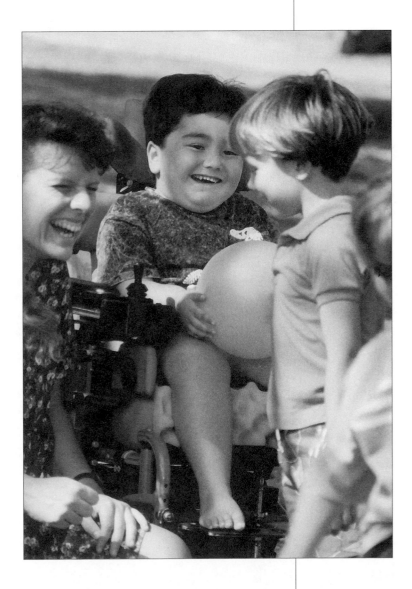

Cerebral Palsy

7

KEY TERMS

cerebral palsy
hypotonia
hypertonia
spasticity
athetosis
ataxia
severe multiple impairments
  (SMIs)
hemiplegia
diplegia
quadriplegia
sensory integration (SI)
neurodevelopmental treatment
assistive technology
computers
augmentative communication
switch access

CASE STUDY — Andrew, A Boy With Cerebral Palsy

Andrew's respite provider, Mrs. Soriano, adjusted the sunshade over his stroller to block the afternoon sun. They walked the several blocks to town. When they reached the ice cream store, the teenaged girl behind the counter saw Andrew through the open door and called, "Hi, Andrew!" Mrs. Soriano waved, looked at Andrew, and said, "Andrew, say 'hi' to Louise."

Andrew tilted his head back and to the side and looked into the shop. "Ahh." Mrs. Soriano wiped his mouth with a washcloth she kept in his stroller bag, waved again to Louise, and walked on. When they reached the dry goods shop, they turned into the store. "Hi, Charley, do you have any of that green fabric left?"

"Sure, it's right over here." The shop owner directed her to a table loaded with fabric scraps and then turned to Andrew. "Hiya, Andrew! I've been saving something for you." He reached behind the counter and brought out a bright-red cowboy hat. He put it gently on Andrew's head and stood back with an appraising look. "It fits pretty well."

Mrs. Soriano turned and saw the hat. "Oh, Charley, you shouldn't give him that!" She laughed. "He looks great though. Andrew, what do you think?" Andrew lifted his head and met her eyes. One of his eyes was covered by the hat. Mrs. Soriano laughed and wiped his mouth again. She turned to the owner. "Are you sure you want to give him this? I don't know what his parents would say."

"It's his. I've been saving it for him." He turned to Andrew. "You take it home now, Andrew. Don't listen to anyone else."

When they walked by the ice cream store on the way home, Louise shouted out, "Andrew, I love your hat!" Andrew lifted his head and grinned.

Developmental History

Andrew was born prematurely in a rural hospital at 30 weeks of gestation. His mother had undergone surgery for an ectopic pregnancy of Andrew's twin at 6 weeks of gestation, but Andrew remained a viable fetus at that time. His mother was admitted to the hospital in premature labor at 30 weeks and was given terbutaline to stop her contractions. When the contractions continued, the terbutaline was stopped and her water was broken to allow the infant to be born. Unfortunately, then labor stopped and had to be augmented by pitocin.

Andrew weighed 1470 g, or a little over 3 pounds, at birth. Because he was not breathing well, a tube attached to a ventilator had to be put down his trachea to help him breathe. Within hours of his birth, Andrew was rushed to the neonatal intensive care unit (NICU) at Children's Hospital by medical transport plane.

Andrew is the second child of Ann and Will Stevens. Their older son, John, was 5 years old when Andrew was born. Ann is a certified public accountant who was working for a construction company when she gave birth to Andrew. Will works as a caretaker for a large estate in their neighborhood.

Ann remembers lying in the hospital alone after Andrew had been flown to Children's Hospital. The woman in the next bed had her infant with her. She explained to Ann that she had not known that she was pregnant and had given birth into the toilet, thinking she was having a bowel movement. Yet her infant was healthy and full term. Ann remembers thinking that it was not fair. She had taken the utmost care during her pregnancy, watching the food she ate, exercising, and going regularly to the doctor to monitor Andrew's development. But it was her infant who had been born prematurely and sick.

It was not until the next day that Andrew's parents could join him because Ann had to recover from Andrew's birth, and they needed to arrange care for John while they were gone. Although they had been in telephone contact with the staff at the hospital, they were shocked when they finally saw their newborn son. He was very small and attached to many tubes. The nurses and doctors were efficient and explained what each of the tubes meant and what procedures Andrew needed since his admittance to the NICU, but no one was able to tell them whether Andrew would live or what he would be like after his premature birth. Ann felt that it was difficult for her to bond with Andrew. Some of the nurses who were taking care of Andrew let her hold him, but some would not even let her touch or stroke him.

Ann and Will spent hours at their son's bedside, watching him and listening to the beeps and bustle of the NICU. They began to feel they had no choices about what interventions would be given to Andrew. Although he was breathing on his own shortly after arrival at the hospital, the oxygen levels had to be increased. Another line needed to be started. Andrew had to begin yet another medication. When he was 11 days old, an ultrasound of his head showed that he had periventricular leukomalacia, or less dense areas of his brain, and cysts or pus-filled areas around his ventricles. He also had moderate hydrocephalus, or swelling of the ventricles in his brain. His parents wondered whether they had done the right thing in letting the medical staff bring Andrew to this large medical center. Perhaps it would have been better if they had let him die naturally if it was so hard for him to survive. They began to understand that their son had been damaged by the events surrounding his early birth.

As the weeks passed, Andrew did not die but became stronger. His parents traveled back and forth from their home, staying several days or a week at a time in the city. It was a very stressful time for them. Finally, when Andrew was 3 weeks old, his parents felt that he could go home with them. The doctors did not agree, feeling that Andrew needed more time to feed and grow in the safe environment of the NICU. Ann and Will became insistent. Andrew was their son, and they wanted to care for him in their home. They loved him and wanted the best for him, and they wanted to be able to take him home. If he was going to die, they wanted it to be at home. If he was going to live, they wanted that to be at home, too. Ann and Will learned how to wrap Andrew so that he could maintain his body temperature, how to gavage feed him by putting a tube down his throat when he got too tired from taking his mother's breast milk from a bottle, and how to dress and bathe him.

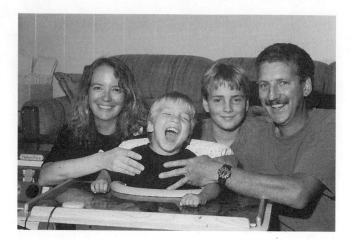

Figure 7-1 Family portrait.

Reluctantly, the doctors, realizing the depth of the family's feelings, agreed. When Andrew was 3 weeks old, still 7 weeks before his expected birth date, he went home.

Andrew was followed medically and developmentally every 6 months by the NICU follow-up clinic in the city. There was a developmental pediatrician, a social worker, and a developmental physical therapist (PT) on the team. His regular care was provided by a local pediatrician. Andrew thrived at home, and his family felt less disrupted after they got him home (Figure 7-1). After the rush of the first few months of caring for Andrew, Ann, who had quit her job to stay home with him, started to look to community resources for help. She called state agencies that she found in the telephone directory to see what services they offered.

It was apparent right away that Andrew was not moving the way his brother had moved when he was an infant. Andrew was a floppy infant at first. He would arch his whole body when he tried to move. When he started moving his arms and legs, his movements were stiff, and he did not move much. He was unable to hold his head up, sit up, or stand with his feet flat when his parents held him. He looked at his family members but did not follow them with his eyes. He developed a wonderful smile that lit up his whole face. It was this smile that kept Ann on the phone, looking for more resources for her son.

Ann found a local state-run infant development program that offered physical, occupational, and speech-language therapy for free. She took him there once a week for services and started to meet other families who had children with atypical development. An Individual Family Support Plan (IFSP) was developed for Andrew that included goals for equipment use in the home for positioning and exercise.

At his 9-month follow-up visit with the NICU follow-up clinic, Andrew was diagnosed with cerebral palsy. Over the months Ann and Will became resourceful advocates for Andrew. Once Ann saw a mother with a child in a wheelchair on the sidewalk. She chased after them on foot, introduced herself, and asked questions about how and where this mother obtained services for her child. It was this chance encounter that introduced her to a special state Medicaid program that would provide funding for equipment and services for Andrew. She applied for the program and Andrew was accepted.

When Andrew was 3 years old, his developmental services

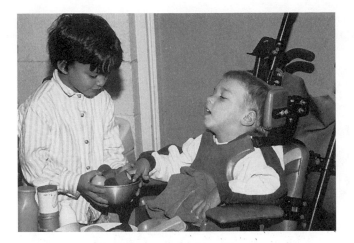

Figure 7-2 Andrew at school interacting with a peer in the regular kindergarten class.

shifted from the infant program to a preschool program run by the Department of Education. He attended every day. An IEP was developed for him and included goals for feeding, independent mobility, and positioning. Andrew received direct physical and occupational therapy once weekly. Ann enlisted the help of therapists at the preschool to determine which equipment Andrew could best use at home. By the time he was 4 years old, she was able to get a bolster chair with a lap tray, a prone stander, a mobile walker, and a feeder seat through the special state Medicaid program. She was also able to get respite care every afternoon for 4 hours when Andrew came home from school, which allowed her to work in her new freelance bookkeeping business.

Andrew's family had received approval from Medicaid to purchase a wheelchair for him, and they worked through a local durable medical equipment vendor to order a pediatric wheelchair. When the wheelchair came, they found that it was too heavy, did not fit into the family car, and did not provide good support for Andrew. They returned it, and Ann decided to find someone who specialized in seating for children to help her find the right wheelchair. By attending a conference on assistive technology and following up with some of the presenters at the conference, she found an assistive technology center at a state institution in the city that was willing to evaluate Andrew for his assistive technology needs at no charge. Ann took a day off work to bring the whole family to the city for a combined speech-language and mobility evaluation to assess which assistive technologies would be best for Andrew. They were seen by a PT and speech-language pathologist who did a combined evaluation. They were able to try several wheelchairs and communication devices with Andrew and decide which one they liked best. They were even able to practice folding the wheelchairs to see which one fit most easily into their car.

Ann filled out all the paperwork and did all the measurements to order the wheelchair with the help of the therapist from the assistive technology center. She communicated with the mainland company that manufactured the wheelchair and made decisions about color and hardware, based on the recommendations from the assistive technology center. When Andrew got his wheelchair at 4 years old, it was just what they expected (Figure 7-2). When parts subsequently broke or needed to be replaced because of Andrew's growth, Ann was able to follow up with the manufacturer to get the right replacement parts. She trained the local vender about this type of wheelchair so that Medicaid payments could be made locally and the vender could follow up in the future.

Andrew at School

Andrew is now 5 years old and attends kindergarten at his local elementary school, which is four blocks from his house. Before beginning kindergarten, he received a physical therapy evaluation. See Box 7-1 for a summary of the findings.

Andrew is picked up at 7:30 AM and brought to school by 8:00 AM in a small yellow school bus that has an electric lift for his wheelchair. He is met at the bus by Mrs. Tong, his special education teacher, who greets him warmly and wheels him to his fully self-contained classroom. Andrew is the only child in his classroom who uses a wheelchair.

He starts out the day lying on a mat on the floor with some toys near him. Andrew likes to play near the other children, so he arches his back and neck to roll over and off the mat. It takes him about 5 minutes, but he is finally able to reach the other children who are playing a few feet away. His friend Matthew puts some Legos near Andrew and sits close to him, piling toys on Andrew's chest. Andrew grins and Matthew giggles.

Mrs. Tong holds Andrew under his arms as she helps him "walk" into the bathroom to get his diaper changed. He takes high, scissored, stereotyped steps but enjoys his ability to walk with help.

During storytime Mrs. Tong positions Andrew in a Tumble-form seat on a mobile base and rolls him to the reading corner. Other children sit around him on the floor to hear Mr. Smith, a classroom aide, read a story with a main character named Andrew. Andrew grins every time his name is read. He reaches his hand over to Matthew and puts it on Matthew's shoulder. Matthew takes Andrew's hand and holds it for a minute.

When the recess bell rings, Mr. Smith lifts Andrew into his Rifton walker, snugs his ankle straps, and pushes him out into the open hallway. Andrew says "I go" and pushes stiffly with his legs. Mr. Smith encourages him to take steps and move toward the playground at the other end of the school (Figure 7-3). Andrew's head is down. He takes high patterned steps but is prevented from too much scissoring by the straps around his ankles. It takes energy, concentration, and most of the recess period to get to the playground. Mr. Smith follows along, encouraging him. Other adults stop to talk to Andrew as they walk by. Andrew lifts his head and smiles at passersby. When he reaches the playground, the bell rings. It is time to turn around and walk back to the classroom again.

At lunchtime, all the children from Andrew's classroom sit together at a table in the cafeteria. Andrew sits in his wheelchair and is assisted to eat by Mrs. Tong. He has brought his lunch from home. Because his family is vegetarian, Andrew's teachers enjoy seeing what interesting foods his mother packs for him each day. Today he has soft food made of brown rice and cooked minced vegetables and tofu mixed together with split pea soup. In a separate container he has applesauce. Part way through the meal, Andrew's occupational therapist (OT), Mrs. Blemmon, comes in to help with feeding. Using hand-over-hand assistance, she helps Andrew scoop food onto his spoon and then bring the spoon up to his mouth. He has a hard time holding his head up,

BOX 7-1   Physical Therapy Evaluation Summary: Andrew

Social and Medical History
Addressed in the Case Study.

Range of Motion
All within normal limits except for limitations in the following areas:

Elbow extension: −20 degrees on right, −25 degrees on left
Hip extension: −10 degrees bilaterally
Hip external rotation: 40 degrees bilaterally
Knee extension: −25 degrees on right, −30 degrees on left
Ankle dorsiflexion: Neutral bilaterally
Spine: Functional kyphosis, absent lumber lordosis, posterior pelvis

Muscle Strength, Tone, and Bulk
Andrew has significant low proximal tone with compensatory increased tone with effort, especially distally. He tends to use extension patterns of gross movement but has some voluntary control of his arms in gross movements. His attempts at movement tend to elicit associated reactions in his trunk and other extremities. His strength is difficult to measure because of the overlay of abnormal muscle tone, but grossly it tends to be in the poor ranges. He is able to use some of his hypertonicity functionally for trunk extension against gravity and patterned walking movements. Muscle bulk is on the low side of normal overall.

Reflexes and Developmental Reactions
Andrew continues to exhibit an obligatory asymmetrical tonic neck reflex to both sides but is able to hold his head in midline for many tasks. A symmetrical tonic neck reflex does not appear to influence his functional skills. Head righting is limited by lack of cervical and trunk strength. Andrew has no balance skills in sitting or standing nor any protective extension.

Mobility Skills
Andrew can roll from supine to prone position and back by using trunk and cervical flexion and extension. He is able to scoot on his back up to 10 feet with an extension pattern of his trunk and neck. He is dependent in wheelchair mobility and transfers. When Andrew was 4 years old, he tried a power wheelchair with a right joystick over a period of several months. He was able to start and stop on command by grabbing and letting go of the joystick but was not able to functionally direct the chair. He appeared to understand cognitively how to move the joystick but

was limited by lack of motor ability, even when he was positioned with adequate trunk support in the chair. The decision was made to address power mobility again in a few years.

Transfers
Andrew is dependent for all transfers. His parents usually pick him up from the front, holding him under his arms.

Functional Positions
Andrew has several functional positions. He is able to use his arms when positioned in his wheelchair to manipulate toys to a degree. He can also manipulate objects or hit a large switch when in the prone stander or bolster chair with a lap tray. He is most mobile when on the floor when he can roll or scoot on his back. Other positions that he is in during the day include sitting on an adult's lap or in a Tumbleform seat.

Adaptive Equipment
- Scott Spectrum wheelchair with Scott seating components in a stroller base configuration. Seating components include a contoured back, hip guides, lateral trunk supports, anterior chest panel, three-piece adjustable head rest, and a pelvic belt.
- Prone stander (at home and at school)
- Rifton gait trainer (at home and at school)
- Tumbleform seat (at home and at school)
- Plastic inflatable pillow for the bathtub
- Speakeasy communication device with dual switch holder and two buddy button switches
- Adapted tape recorder with a buddy button switch activator

Activities of Daily Living
- Andrew is dependent in most skills.
- Bathing: Addressed in the Case Study
- Eating: Addressed in the Case Study
- Toileting: Diaper
- Oral Care: Andrew needs assistance to brush his teeth

Recreation and Leisure
Andrew attends a hippotherapy program on Saturdays. He enjoys music and can strum a ukulele. He tries to blow into his father's flute but cannot make sound yet. He enjoys sandbox play and going to the beach with his family. He enjoys attending John's baseball games with his family.

so she helps by standing behind him and putting her arm around his head, supporting his chin. She reminds Andrew not to bite on the spoon but to use his lips to get the food off the spoon. She prompts him by putting her fingers over his lips and helping him remove the food from the spoon. Mrs. Blemmon teaches Mrs. Tong how to help Andrew eat because she cannot be there every day. She writes a note home to Ann in Andrew's communication book to praise the consistency of his food. The thick food stays on the spoon easily and is easier for Andrew to move around in his mouth and swallow.

After lunch Andrew is positioned on his prone stander. Standing is important to keep the muscles in his legs stretched, maintain the strength of his long bones, and help his efficiency in breathing and digestion. While Andrew is standing, Mrs. Tong sets up a tape recorder with a switch activation system for him to activate. Andrew enjoys playing his favorite tape, which is marching music by Souza!

After 30 minutes of standing, Andrew has his diaper changed again. The standing position sometimes facilitates both his bowel and bladder to move. The teachers and his mother feel that

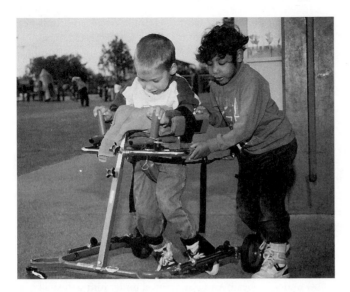

Figure 7-3 Andrew walking to recess with his friend, Matthew. Andrew is using a Rifton gait trainer.

standing helps Andrew's chronic constipation. He is positioned back into his wheelchair for the last hour of the day when he joins Mrs. Cooper's regular kindergarten classroom. When Mrs. Tong wheels Andrew into the classroom, the children are working hard at tables, cutting and gluing to make valentines. Because Andrew cannot fit at a kindergarten-height table with his wheelchair, Mrs. Cooper brings her chair up to him to help him make his valentine on his lap tray. She puts his fingers into the holes in the scissors and helps him cut red paper in a heart shape.

After the valentines are put away, the children spread out across the floor to work on individual and group activities during free play. Mrs. Tong wheels Andrew to the house corner to participate with the children who are playing there. Several children bring plastic food over for Andrew to see and touch. When the last bell rings, all the children rush to clean up their materials and line up. Mrs. Tong pushes Andrew back to his classroom and gathers his things to take home. Then she pushes him outside to wait for his bus.

Andrew gets direct physical, occupational, and speech therapy every other week for 1 hour each. Ann is concerned that the professionals are not working together to develop an integrated program for Andrew. She asks that they meet with her and Andrew's teacher before his next IEP meeting to discuss his needs and to develop an integrated plan. At their first meeting they identify some of Andrew's needs as follows:

1. Andrew needs access to the kindergarten-height tables in the regular kindergarten room so he will not be isolated when working on projects.
2. Andrew needs to move independently.
3. Andrew needs opportunity for social interaction. Currently he loses out on social activities because it takes him the entire recess period to walk to the playground.
4. Andrew needs playground equipment that is accessible for him.
5. Andrew needs more direct play and interaction with other children. Their attempts at interaction are usually brief because Andrew cannot respond.

6. Andrew needs to express his wants and needs.
7. Andrew needs to participate in group activities as an active, rather than a passive, observer.
8. Andrew needs to be able to express whether or not he understands the academic concepts presented to him.
9. Andrew needs to be able to manipulate the kindergarten level activities such as wooden blocks, shapes, and color swatches that are used in the classroom so he can have access to the same kinesthetic learning as his peers.

Together they brainstormed and came up with some ideas, including the use of assistive technology to address Andrew's identified needs. They planned to try some of the ideas before his annual IEP meeting to assess what would work effectively with Andrew. See Box 7-2 (p. 169) after you have thought about how you might address these barriers.

At the IEP meeting 1 month later, Andrew's parents, teachers, and therapists met again to develop an IEP for him based on their knowledge of Andrew and their work with him over the past month. They wrote objectives that integrate his physical, social, emotional, and educational goals.

Think about how you would write goals that integrate Andrew's physical needs, social needs, and educational curriculum. Then check Box 7-3 (p. 170) to see some sample objectives.

Andrew at Home

After school the bus drops Andrew at home at about 2:30 PM. Mrs. Soriano, a respite worker who is paid by Medicaid, is waiting for him. She has been taking care of him after school every day for a year, and she and Andrew have a special relationship. Andrew's mother has developed a schedule for him after school, and Mrs. Soriano and Andrew are busy for a few hours with a diaper change, range of motion, snack, and finally standing on the prone stander at home. Andrew eats a snack of homemade pudding while sitting in the Tumbleform seat. Mrs. Soriano takes his Speakeasy communication device out of his school backpack and sets it up so that he can access it. The device has been modified with a red and a green switch on a dual-switch holder. When Andrew chooses the green switch, his mother's preprogrammed voice says "yes." When he hits the red switch, the voice says "no." Mrs. Soriano asks, "Do you want more pudding?" Andrew is consistent with "yes" and "no" responses, but the switches need to be placed just right for him to be able to reach them.

When he is standing on the prone stander, Mrs. Soriano sets up the Speakeasy again for him with the switches on the tray of the prone stander. She asks him, "Do you want to play catch or play with blocks? Catch?" Andrew hits the green switch, "Yes." Mrs. Soriano asks, to confirm, "Blocks?" Andrew hits the red switch, "No." She sits on the floor in front of the stander and gives Andrew an 8-inch ball. The tray of the stander tilts down toward Mrs. Soriano, so when Andrew lets go of the ball, it rolls off the tray to her. She catches it and lightly tosses it back to him so he can trap it under his arms. Andrew grins. This is his favorite game. After 30 minutes of standing, Mrs. Soriano transfers Andrew to his wheelchair again, and they go for their daily walk through the center of town (Figure 7-4).

At 5:30 PM Will and John come home from John's baseball practice, which Will coaches, and Mrs. Soriano goes home. John disappears into his room to play and to do his homework. He is now 10 years old. Andrew is happy to see his dad. Will sits with Andrew on his lap for awhile, talking to him. While talking, Will absentmindedly bends and straightens Andrew's legs and arms and holds him in such a way that Andrew must hold his own head up for short periods (Figure 7-5). Then Will positions Andrew in his bolster chair with some switch toys on the tray, while he starts making dinner.

Ann comes home late from meeting a client and finds her family sitting on the floor eating together. John is talking about a new computer program he wants, Andrew is in his Tumbleform seat, and Will is hand-feeding him soft green beans, clumps of rice, and squares of tofu in between bites of his own dinner. When Andrew does not want any more, he lets his dad know by turning his head away. If his dad is persistent, Andrew vocalizes loudly in protest. Ann mixes some of the rice with applesauce and helps Andrew eat with a spoon. He is able to get the spoon to his mouth if she helps him scoop the food from his plate. He has eaten enough and complains loudly that he does not want any more. Ann brings over the Speakeasy and asks Andrew if he wants more dinner. Andrew's hand goes directly to the red button, "No, no, no, no," as he hits it many times. Ann laughs and takes his plate to the kitchen.

Ann and Will sit in the bathroom together to talk about some of the events of their day while Andrew plays in the tub. Andrew enjoys lying in about 6 inches of water with a plastic inflatable pillow under his head. Ann puts a towel under him so he will not slip easily on the slick surface. Andrew can splash the water with his hands but has not mastered kicking yet. Ann wishes that she could find a seat or positioning device that would allow Andrew to sit up in the tub because she believes that he would be able to play better and that he would be safer. When he was smaller, Andrew sat in a baby bath ring and enjoyed being able to splash more effectively.

Ann brings up the subject of surgery, which had been recommended by an orthopedic surgeon at Shriners Hospital for Children. She and Will talk quietly so Andrew does not hear. Because Andrew has such tight muscles, his hips are at risk for dislocation later in life if his muscles are not surgically released soon. The surgeons recommend having the surgery performed between 4 and 6 years of age. A triple release of his hamstrings, adductors,

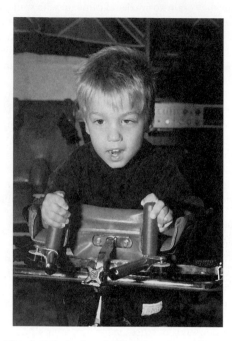

Figure 7-4 Andrew in his gait trainer at home.

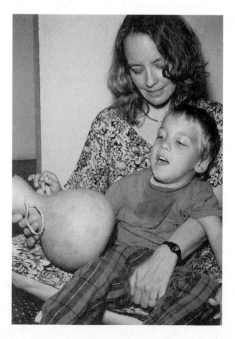

Figure 7-5 Andrew playing a Hawaiian instrument with his mother.

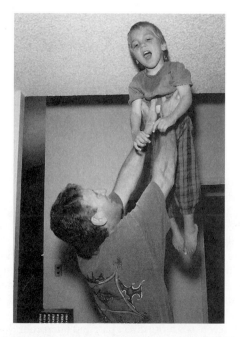

Figure 7-6 Andrew rough-housing with his dad.

and heel cords on both sides was recommended. Ann and Will are very reluctant to allow surgery on Andrew. Even though they have been reassured that the surgery is fairly safe, they worry that he may have an adverse reaction to the anesthetic or that he will lose function as a result of releasing his muscles. They understand the risk of hip dislocation if they do not do the muscle releases now, which would necessitate a far more invasive surgery later. During the day Ann talked with the school PT, who recommended going ahead with the surgery. The PT thought that Andrew had potential to improve his function as a result of the

muscle releases. At the very least he would probably be more comfortable, be able to sit better, and potentially avoid pain and more invasive surgery on his hips later. Ann and Will reluctantly decided to schedule the surgery, which has a 4-month wait, as they continued to explore their feelings about this step.

Andrew gets wrapped in a fluffy towel and is carried over his father's shoulder into his bedroom (Figure 7-6). He shrieks with delight and arches his body stiffly as he tries to balance in this precarious position. Giggles are heard by his mother as Andrew and his dad disappear around the doorway. Ann straightens up

---

BOX 7-2   ## Proposed Solutions to Identified Needs in Andrew's Education

1. Andrew needs access to the kindergarten-height tables in the regular kindergarten room so he will not be isolated when working on projects.
   - Consider putting bricks under the four legs of one work table when Andrew is participating in the activity. He will be able to access the table where the other children are working.
2. Andrew needs to move independently.
   - Power mobility has been explored recently for Andrew with the result that he was unable to use a joystick functionally because of lack of motor control. Other options for controlling the power chair should be explored over the next year or two, including a micro joystick, a five-switch array, head control, and sip and puff. Funding limitations will limit the exploration of technology for wheelchair access for Andrew until he can develop more consistent skills. In the meantime Andrew can use a joystick to operate toys, including Nintendo, to develop his motor skills. The team will explore the development of a switch-activated rocking chair with adaptive seating for Andrew to elicit vestibular stimulation for himself.
3. Andrew needs opportunity for social interaction. Currently he loses out on social activities because it takes him the entire recess period to walk to the playground.
   - Andrew should begin walking to the playground before the recess bell rings so he has enough time to play after he arrives. Consider getting regular education peer volunteers to walk with him to the playground.
4. Andrew needs playground equipment that is accessible for him.
   - The team will explore adaptive seating for the sandbox, so that Andrew can sit in the sandbox and play with his peers. Adaptive seating for swings will also be explored, although the school is considering removing all swings because too many children are getting hurt on them.
5. Andrew needs more direct play and interaction with other children. Their attempts at interaction are usually short-lived because Andrew cannot respond.
   - Develop an awareness/education program for his peers in kindergarten. Andrew can participate in several short presentations by his parents, teachers, or therapists about what cerebral palsy is, what he is able to do, and what he needs help with, demonstrations of how to play and communicate with him, how to push his wheelchair or help him walk in his walker, and what to be careful of with him. A "circle of

friends" can be developed to include peers who are interested in being friends with Andrew. They can take turns helping him become integrated in kindergarten and school activities.
6. Andrew needs to express his wants and needs.
   - Andrew does not currently use his Speakeasy communication device consistently at school. The speech pathologist will consult with his teacher and classroom aides on how to position the device and have it accessible for Andrew. Several scenarios throughout the day will be identified as opportunities to use the Speakeasy for yes-and-no answers. Andrew will be progressed to different statements that are applicable in the context of school as he learns how to use the device in a scan mode.
7. Andrew needs to participate in group activities as an active, rather than a passive, observer.
   - The team will develop large group activities that have opportunities for Andrew to actively participate. Examples of activities include: marching or dancing activities where Andrew can turn the music on and off, purchasing a bowling ramp that Andrew can push balls down as the pitcher in a game of kickball, purchasing or borrowing a pitching machine that can be adapted to use a switch access so Andrew can pitch for other ball activities. Care would need to be taken that he was out of the line of the ball to avoid injury.
8. Andrew needs to be able to express whether or not he understands the academic concepts presented to him.
   - The teacher and classroom aides will use the Speakeasy more consistently during academic instruction and encourage Andrew to respond to yes-and-no questions.
9. Andrew needs to be able to manipulate the kindergarten-level activities such as wooden blocks, shapes, and color swatches that are used in the classroom so he can have access to kinesthetic learning tools.
   - Andrew will use a computer at least twice per week to encourage learning and manipulation of shapes, colors, and objects on the computer screen with a trackball. Computer software will be researched by the computer teacher that will allow Andrew access to these kinesthetic tools on the computer screen. Andrew does not have the motor skill to manipulate objects precisely, but he needs to experience holding these objects in his hands and moving them around on a table in front of him. These experiences will be provided to him.

BOX 7-3 Sample Integrated Individualized Education Program Objectives

In 1 year Andrew will perform the following activities:

1. During free play, when asked by a peer, Andrew will indicate his play preference by using a switch activated yes/no communication device for 7 consecutive school days.
2. During structured learning, Andrew will use a switch-activated communication device to respond correctly in three out of five trials to questions about beginning number concepts (e.g. matching numbers to groups of objects or understanding larger and smaller) for 7 consecutive school days.
3. During mealtimes Andrew will indicate food preferences among four choices by using either his electronic communication device or manual signs to express yes or no for 7 consecutive school days.
4. By using a manual or electronic pitching device, Andrew will participate actively as a pitcher in a school or class kickball game for at least 10 innings during the year.
5. During free play Andrew will take turns using switch-activated toys with one to two of his peers three to five times per week for 2 consecutive weeks.

6. By using appropriate positioning for a given activity, Andrew will participate daily in the normal routines of the school day and after school program. Suggested positions include the following:

Positioning device	Activity
Prone on scooter board	Obstacle course
Stander	Water and sand play
Bolster chair	Music
Wheelchair	Lawn bowling, kickball, field activities
Prone on wedge	Carpet/floor play and art
Adapted seat	Sandbox play
Rocking chair	Story time

7. Andrew will participate in classroom storytelling activities by pointing to pictures and sounds on a four to eight choice board to sequence a story, choosing story characters, sound effects for story characters, or other story elements for 5 consecutive sessions.
8. Andrew will correctly activate a switch when he agrees with a peer in picture identification five out of five times.

from the tub, rubbing her back, and wonders what will happen as Andrew grows.

Andrew is dressed in his pajamas, and Ann comes in to read him a bedtime story. Andrew lies in his twin bed with rails and padded rail bumpers all around. Ann remembers when he got his foot caught in the rail one night and he screamed until she was able to get there to release it. She checks the ties on the bumpers carefully before kissing him goodnight and turning off the light. She notices a red cowboy hat on the chair in the corner of his room and wonders how it got there.

CASE STUDY Cyril, A Teenager With Cerebral Palsy

Cyril looked beseechingly at Mrs. Moore. Then he slowly typed a word into the augmentative communication device on his lap tray. It spoke: "GUITAR." Mrs. Moore smiled and got up from the table. "Okay, Cyril. We can go listen to the boys play today." Cyril smiled as Mrs. Moore gathered his lunch things. She moved around the other stragglers in the cafeteria to put his trash into the rubbish can and his tray onto the lunch counter. She had eaten her lunch earlier, while Cyril was in art class.

Mrs. Moore released Cyril's wheel locks on his wheelchair and pushed him through the thinning crowd of intermediate school students to the courtyard outside the cafeteria. A group of boys was gathered around one of the cement picnic tables. Two boys were sitting on the table top and playing guitars. They looked up as Cyril and Mrs. Moore approached but returned to their playing without acknowledging them. Several of the boys standing near also had instruments but were not playing them. Some girls hovered around the periphery of the group in twos and threes. The sound of the guitars could be heard above the laughter and voices of the crowd. Cyril and Mrs. Moore sat nearby watching and listening. Cyril smiled but was too shy to try to catch anyone's eye. When the bell sounded to end the lunch period, the crowd dispersed noisily. Mrs. Moore pushed Cyril in his wheelchair to his next class.

Developmental History

Cyril's adoptive father, a minister, was attending a seminar about 200 miles from where the family lived in the Philippines. At the house where the father stayed, he saw two very small infants, and he inquired as to who they were. "Oh, they are not ours. We are just taking care of the two infant boys because their mothers cannot," the family responded. "Would you like to take one?" Cyril's father was overjoyed. He and his wife had two teenage daughters but no sons. He wanted a son to carry on his work as a minister.

The father went home to confer with his family, and they all decided that they would like to have a new baby. He brought his wife back with him, and they took one of the boys home. The infant had no birth certificate or other papers, and the adoption was informal (Figure 7-7).

Within the next few months it became apparent that Cyril's development was not normal. His family loved him and coped the best they could. His mother hired a PT to come to the house and teach her exercises to do with Cyril. When Cyril was 3 years old, his father had the opportunity to move to Hawaii to become the minister of a church. He moved his family to Hawaii, but, because Cyril had no birth certificate or adoption papers, the family was unable to take Cyril with them. It took 5 years before

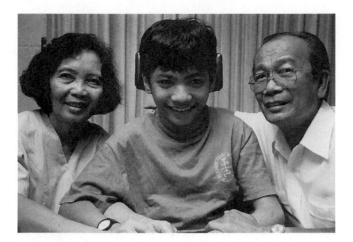

Figure 7-7 Family portrait.

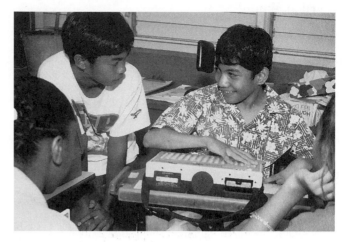

Figure 7-8 Cyril participates in a group study session in social studies class.

the paperwork could be completed to get Cyril to Hawaii with his family. In the meantime he lived with his grandparents and then his aunts in the Philippines. They had the assistance of housekeepers to help with Cyril's care. His mother returned to the Philippines for 3 months each year to reassure Cyril that she still cared for him and to plan for his care over the coming year. She arranged for Cyril to have a tutor in the home, and a PT continued to come to his home to provide services.

When Cyril was 8 years old, the legal hurdles were resolved, and he was finally able to come to Hawaii to live with his adopting family. His older sisters were grown. One sister was in college, and the other was married and lived with her husband and daughter in California. Cyril and his parents lived in a three-bedroom apartment, which was on the ground floor of a house in a residential area. When Cyril came from the Philippines, he had no wheelchair, and his parents carried him wherever he needed to go. It had been 5 years since they had lived together, and they needed to relearn how to take care of Cyril. His parents hoped that they would be able to find some services for Cyril in Hawaii so that he would be better off than he was in the Philippines.

His parents enrolled Cyril in third grade at the local elementary school. Cyril was in a fully self-contained special education classroom with three other children with severe disabilities. He used a borrowed wheelchair until he could get one of his own. His father supported the family on his salary as a minister, which was not large, but he had health insurance for his wife and Cyril.

Cyril was obviously intelligent. He started third grade in Hawaii, having never attended school before. He did not speak or understand English but learned very quickly at school. His parents spoke English and helped Cyril learn English at home, too. Cyril was not able to speak well, but his family could understand some of what he said. He was more comfortable speaking in Tagalog than English. A speech-language pathologist at the elementary school took an interest in Cyril. She believed that he had the potential to communicate by using augmentative communication. She started him out on a cardboard communication board on his lap tray. Cyril could use one arm fairly well and was able to point to pictures. It soon became apparent that

a picture board was not enough. Cyril wanted to say increasingly complicated sentences and needed a more sophisticated method to express himself.

Cyril also received physical therapy in school. His therapist worked with him on range of motion, standing activities using a supine stander, and self-propulsion in his wheelchair.

After his arrival in the United States, Cyril became enrolled in Shriners Hospital for Children, where he received his first wheelchair. The orthopedic team was concerned about his hips, which were subluxing, and performed several surgeries to release his adductors, hamstrings, and heelcords. Finally, when Cyril was 11 years old, they performed a derotation osteotomy on his right hip and constructed an acetabular ridge to extend his acetabulum. He had an internal plate on his right femur. He was casted in hip and knee flexion. After his spica cast was removed, Cyril had a right-knee flexion contracture of 35 degrees and a right hip flexion contracture of 20 degrees. Standing activities were much more difficult for him.

When Cyril moved from elementary to intermediate school, the emphasis shifted away from classroom positioning to academic activities, and he was included in more regular education classes. His standing program was discontinued. His mother is convinced that the contractures are a result of the position of flexion in which he was casted. She also believes that his language skills deteriorated after the surgery and that Cyril is unable to remember as well since the surgery. She refuses to allow any more surgeries.

When Cyril was in sixth grade, he got a new manual wheelchair with a one-arm drive propulsion, which was financed through his father's health insurance. The balance was paid by Shriners Hospital for Children. The wheelchair was recommended at Shriners by their seating clinic team with some input from his PT at school. Cyril had a custom linear seating system, with lateral trunk supports, head support, hip guides, and an abductor pommel. When he was in seventh grade, Cyril began using a Liberator augmentative communication device, which was owned by the school and loaned to him. Both his speech-language pathologist and his special education teacher worked hard with Cyril to help him learn to use the Liberator (Figure 7-8).

Cyril at School

Cyril is now 13 years old and in his last year at the intermediate school. Next year he will move up to ninth grade at the high school. His current school-based services are provided by a special education teacher, a full-time educational assistant, a speech-language pathologist, a PT, an OT, and several regular education teachers. He receives a full reevaluation only every 3 years, but the team is gathering information to ensure that his transition to the high school is a positive experience for Cyril and that the supports he needs are in place (Figure 7-9). A summary of key findings in his physical therapy evaluation is shown in Box 7-4.

Cyril comes to school daily on a yellow school bus with an electric lift. It picks him up daily at home at 6:30 AM and delivers him to school by 7:30 AM. A foster grandparent volunteer is waiting for him and pushes him to a tree-shaded area to wait until his teacher arrives. Other special education students gather around the benches to wait for school to start. As 8:00 AM approaches, a crush of intermediate school students pushes by Cyril, not looking at him but forging ahead to their classrooms. Finally, Mrs. Batangan arrives and greets Cyril warmly. She pushes him to his homeroom class.

Cyril's special education teacher is the homeroom teacher for an eighth grade class. As she gives the students information and school announcements that they need for the day, Cyril types the date and sequence of classes for the day into his Liberator. When Mrs. Batangan asks him, he pushes a button and his Liberator speaks the information for the other students.

After the bell to end homeroom rings and the other students have gone to their first-period classes, Cyril and his friend Mimi, who is the only other student in the special education class with Mrs. Batangan, begin their lessons for reading, English, and math. Mimi also has cerebral palsy and uses an augmentative communication device to communicate. Mrs. Batangan works with Cyril on reading skills, while Mrs. Moore, the educational

assistant, works with Mimi on her math skills. Cyril is using a new color laptop computer that was recently purchased for the special education department. He reads a book out loud in a soft voice as Mrs. Batangan holds it. Some of the words are recognizable, and most are approximated, but it is clear that he is actually reading the words. He uses word prediction software as he answers content questions from Mrs. Batangan on the computer. The word prediction software allows him to use only 2 to 3 keystrokes to type a longer word and saves significant time. The word processing program he is using reads his sentences out loud as he types them. His reading and spelling skills are at about the third grade level.

When the bell rings to announce recess, Cyril and Mimi eat a snack in the classroom. Mrs. Moore helps them get their snacks out of their backpacks. Mimi types, "Can I have a cookie?" on her Touch Talker. Cyril catches her eye and laughs as he hands her one of his cookies (Figure 7-10).

After his snack Cyril is taken to the bathroom by Mrs. Moore. He uses the special education bathroom, which is locked so other students cannot use it. This bathroom has grab bars and a wheelchair accessible stall. Cyril is transferred to the toilet by Mrs. Moore, who uses a dependent manual lift. When he was in the fifth and sixth grades, Cyril had to use diapers because his teacher and aide thought that he was too heavy to transfer. Mrs. Moore was instructed by the PT in how to do a safe transfer with Cyril. She is comfortable with his transfer and is glad that Cyril can have the independence to use the bathroom, even though he needs help to transfer to and from the toilet.

After recess Cyril goes to shop class. He is pushed through the covered walkways of the school by Mrs. Moore, who sits with him in shop and assists him with papers and materials he needs to manipulate. Cyril wistfully watches as the other students measure and cut wood for their projects. Other students do not talk with

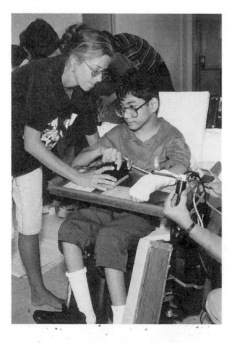

Figure 7-9 Cyril tries out a power wheelchair in school. He was able to drive well but could not get his own chair because of funding and access issues.

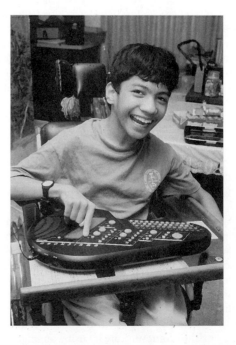

Figure 7-10 Music is an important part of Cyril's life. He can play this electronic instrument by himself.

BOX 7-4 Physical Therapy Evaluation Summary: Cyril

Social and Medical History

Addressed in the Case Study.

Range of Motion

All within normal limits except for limitations in the following areas:

Hip extension: −20 degrees on right, −5 degrees on left, hard end feel bilaterally

Hip flexion: 75 degrees on right, 85 degrees on left, hard-end feel bilaterally, loud pop heard and felt with passive flexion on right; x-rays confirm that hip is sliding in and out of socket and popping over acetabular shelf

Knees: −35 degrees extension on right, within normal limits on left

Ankles: Hypermobile bilaterally into dorsiflexion

Upper extremities: Grossly within normal limits except for −15 degrees of wrist extension on the left, −20 degrees of elbow extension on the left, and −60 degrees of shoulder flexion and abduction on the left

Spine: Mild right structural thoracic scoliosis with a mild right rib hump

Muscle Strength, Tone, and Bulk

Cyril has low tone proximally with compensatory increased tone distally. He has functional use of his right upper extremity and tends to use flexion patterns rather than extension patterns of gross movement. His strength is difficult to measure because of abnormal muscle tone but grossly tends to be in the poor/fair ranges in his trunk and neck, fair/good ranges in his right upper extremity, and is overlaid with tone in his other extremities. Muscle bulk is on the low side of normal overall.

Reflexes and Developmental Reactions

Primitive reactions do not appear to interfere with Cyril's movements. His balance reactions are not functional in sitting or in standing. He is aware of his position in space and can right his head in supported sitting for a few minutes at a time. Head righting is limited by lack of cervical and trunk strength.

Mobility Skills

Cyril has minimal independent mobility in any position. He can roll from supine to prone position using a full flexor pattern of movement. He can roll from prone to supine position using cervical extension. His most functional mobility skill at present is wheelchair propulsion using a right one-arm drive wheelchair. He is able to go about 15 feet in 3 to 5 minutes. Cyril has tried a power wheelchair and is able to control a joystick with a T adapter. He can follow directions to stop, go forward, back, right, and left when he is positioned with adequate trunk support in the chair. Funding is not available currently for him to obtain his own power wheelchair.

Transfers

Cyril is dependent for all transfers. He is able to assist by holding on with his right arm but requires maximum assist to transfer. He can take moderate weight briefly through his left lower extremity when doing a pivot transfer with maximum assistance but is unable to take any weight through his right leg. His parents usually pick him up from the side under his arms and hips.

Functional Positions

Cyril is most functional in his wheelchair, although his positioning is not optimal. In his wheelchair he tends to sacral sit with a kyphotic trunk leaning to the left. The wheelchair is where he spends most of his day. Other positions he assumes are sitting propped on the couch at home and lying on a foam futon on the floor.

Adaptive Equipment

- Everest and Jennings Hot Wheels upright right one-arm drive manual wheelchair.
- Scotty linear seating system with antithrust seat, flip-down abductor pommel, hip guides, I back, lateral trunk supports, three-piece adjustable head support, anterior chest panel with four-point restraint, pelvic belt.
- Left wrist splint to maintain wrist range for night wear.
- Liberator augmentative communication device from Prentke Romich Company. This is owned by the school district, but Cyril is allowed to take it home at night and on weekends to assist with his homework.
- Color laptop computer with trackball. This is owned by the school district and Cyril is allowed to use it in school only.
- U-shaped wooden table for safety when on the toilet for use at home.

Activities of Daily Living

- Cyril is independent in some skills and needs assistance for others.
- Bathing: Addressed in the Case Study.
- Eating: Cyril can use a fork or spoon independently in his right hand. He needs assistance to cut up food or occasionally to stabilize his plate. He can drink by using his right hand to hold a cup but spills occasionally.
- Toileting: Cyril can inform others when he needs to use the bathroom. He requires stabilization to sit on the toilet safely.
- Oral Care: Cyril needs assistance to complete his tooth-brushing.

Recreation and Leisure

Addressed in the Case Study.

him or try to include him in their projects. A young girl smiles at him as she walks by his wheelchair, and Cyril smiles back.

Later, when the students gather to discuss shop rules, the shop teacher asks Cyril a question. Everyone waits while he types the answer into his Liberator. He answers it correctly and grins. His shop teacher, as well as other teachers are finding it a real challenge to include Cyril in their classes. They would like him to participate more but are not sure what he can do or how to give him opportunities to join in activities. Mrs. Batangan and Mrs. Moore are also fairly new to inclusion and are not sure how to help Cyril to be more integrated with his peers.

After shop is art class. Mrs. Moore pushes Cyril to art class, unlocking the elevator to get to the second floor of the building. She leaves him in art and goes to lunch. His art teacher has divided the class into groups and has instructed Cyril's group how to help him. Today they are making coil pots out of clay. Cyril is able to roll his coil with a flat hand but needs some help from another student to form the coil into a base for his pot. Different students in his group take turns helping him, letting him do as much as he can for himself (Figure 7-11). The art room is bright and cheerful with colorful posters covering the walls. This is only the second day of art class because the spring semester has just begun, so the students do not know each other well yet. They are attentive and quiet as they work, and bursts of laughter erupt from the various groups working around the room. The teacher circulates, helping here and there. She helps Cyril hold a scoring tool more securely so that he can score his coils. When it is time to clean up, Cyril's group members efficiently clear the table. Cyril helps by gathering up the newspaper and crumpling it to be thrown away. When the bell rings, Mrs. Moore is there to take Cyril to lunch.

After lunch Cyril has social studies. He is pushed into a regular eighth-grade classroom by Mrs. Moore, who stays to assist him. Today the class is studying maps. The students form cooperative learning groups to quiz each other on the shapes of the states in the United States by using flash cards that they draw themselves. Cyril's group holds up flash cards for him, and he types his responses into his Liberator, which speaks them for him. He watches as the other students draw their flash cards.

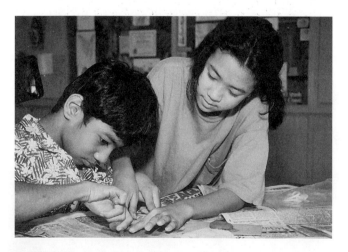

Figure 7-11 Cyril's friend, Maryanne, helps him roll out clay in art class.

Near the end of social studies, Cyril asks Mrs. Moore to reposition him. He complains that his abductor pommel is hurting him. He gestures toward his lap to indicate that it hurts. Mrs. Moore repositions him in his chair and loosens the pommel. Cyril slides down so that his groin is resting on the pommel again, but he says that it helped. He has difficulty typing from this position, however.

Guidance class is the last class of the day. There is a substitute teacher who gives the class a worksheet. Mrs. Moore works quietly with Cyril in the corner of the room, assisting him to do the worksheet on definitions. Cyril is able to type his answers into his Liberator, which prints them out. The printout can be attached to the worksheet and turned in to the teacher.

The bus comes a little early to pick up Cyril, and he needs to leave class a few minutes early. The bus driver comes on campus to pull Cyril out of class and push him to the bus. Cyril does not have time to say good bye to Mrs. Moore or Mrs. Batangan and is rushed onto the waiting bus. There are other students to pick up and take home from other schools.

Cyril's speech-language pathologist and PT spent time with him and his teachers in school to identify needs for his successful transition to the high school, as well as needs to meet his own long-term goals of eventually working and becoming more independent in his self-care skills. The following is a list of needs that were discussed:

1. Cyril needs independent mobility.
2. Cyril needs better social integration with the other students at school.
3. Cyril needs independence from adult assistance during the day.
4. Cyril needs more friends at school.
5. Cyril needs a way to participate in after-school activities.
6. Cyril needs to be included in class discussions.
7. Cyril needs improved comfort in his wheelchair.
8. Cyril needs better positioning in his wheelchair so he can access his Liberator, laptop computer, or other materials on his lap tray, even after repositioning.
9. Cyril needs more independence in toileting at home and school.

In consultation with his teachers, parents, OT, and educational assistant, remedies were proposed to address the identified barriers. See Box 7-5 (p. 176) after you have thought about how you might address these barriers.

In the spring the team of people working with Cyril developed an Individualized Education Program (IEP) for him, as well as a transition plan for moving from intermediate school to high school. Objectives that integrated his physical, social, emotional, and educational goals were specified with specific criteria for meeting each objective. Think about how you would write goals that integrate his physical needs with his educational curriculum. Then check Box 7-6 (p. 177) to see some sample objectives.

Cyril at Home

Cyril lives with his mother and father in a three-bedroom apartment, which is half of the bottom floor of a large house. There is a small step into the entryway that is shared with the other downstairs neighbors. When the apartment is entered, there is a living room on the left and a smaller dining room and kitchen on the right. A narrow hallway leads to the back of the house where the bedrooms and bathroom are located. There is a sharp corner in the hallway that makes it impossible for Cyril's wheelchair to maneuver. The bathroom is long and narrow, with the tub at the far end. The bedrooms are at the end of the hallway.

Cyril's parents believe that this apartment is a very good deal for them financially. They are not willing to ask the landlord to make adaptations so that the apartment will be more accessible for Cyril, and they are not willing to move because they fear they would have to pay more for an apartment that may be less accessible to his father's job.

Because Cyril's wheelchair cannot fit into the back hallway of the house, his parents need to carry him from the living room to the bathroom (Figure 7-12). He sleeps on the floor of the living room on a foam mattress, which is put away during the day. They believe that sleeping on the floor is beneficial for Cyril, the hard floor is good for his back. Cyril's parents are both in their early sixties now, and both have had significant back injuries from lifting their son. Cyril's mother, a small woman, can no longer lift him into the bathtub, so the job of bathing him falls to his father. Because his father frequently gets home late, bath time is usually in the morning. Cyril's mother gets everyone up at 4:30 AM on bath days because the school bus comes at 6:30 AM. His father carries him to the tub and gets in with him. After he is bathed, Cyril is dried and dressed, then positioned in his wheelchair for breakfast. This procedure exhausts everyone. Cyril is bathed twice per week, but his mother sponge bathes him and washes his hair when he does not take a bath. His mother made the decision not to enroll him in summer school between seventh and eighth grades to give her husband a rest from getting up so early.

His mother is home alone with Cyril from the time he arrives home from school at 2:30 PM until his father arrives after dinner. She does not drive and cannot take him out. The neighborhood is residential with no stores within easy walking distance. When Cyril gets home, he works on his homework with his Liberator and watches TV. He has made wonderful progress in learning how to use the Liberator from these long hours of working with it. Frequently he complains to his mother that the abductor pommel is painful. In fact, his mother wonders whether the pain and discomfort may actually trigger mild seizures. When Cyril is particularly uncomfortable, sometimes she cannot rouse him for minutes at a time and describes him as having a vacant look on his face. She is interested in learning how to position him out of the wheelchair but is limited by having no positioning equipment at home, no room for equipment, and limited physical ability to transfer him.

Cyril used to play with several children in the neighborhood when he was younger, but now that they have grown older, the neighborhood children are not as interested in spending time with him. His mother reports that it is hard for them to spend the time and effort to communicate with him.

On the suggestion from Cyril's speech-language pathologist, his mother enrolled him in an after-school club for a short time. He was to be transported home by the handicapped van service run by the city. Because the van was 2 hours late in picking him up on the first day and Cyril did not get home until after dark, his mother was very worried and refused to let him go again. Cyril continues to be very lonely because he has very few peer relationships or opportunities to develop them.

When Cyril needs to use the bathroom at home, his mother must carry him from the living room to the bathroom. She had a friend make a wooden U-shaped table that she pulls around Cyril when he is sitting on the toilet for support and safety (Figure 7-13). His mother complains that Cyril takes a long time to "evacuate" because he sits all day long and becomes constipated. His constipation worries her.

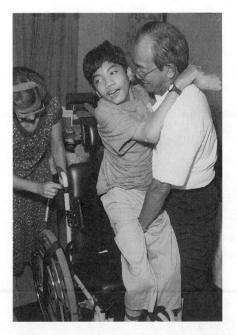

Figure 7-12 Mr. Rivera is having back problems and has trouble transferring Cyril.

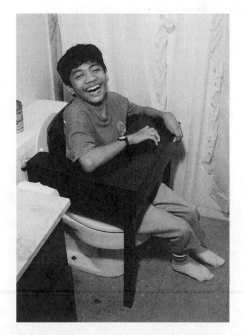

Figure 7-13 Mrs. Rivera had a friend make this table to help Cyril be safe on the toilet.

BOX 7-5   Proposed Solutions to Identified Barriers to Cyril's Education

1. Cyril needs independent mobility.
   - Cyril will be referred to Shriners Hospital for Children for a power mobility evaluation. The school PT will assist in writing a letter of justification for a power wheelchair add-on kit for his current wheelchair. An add-on kit is necessary so that the family can transport the wheelchair. In the meantime efforts will be made to find a power chair for Cyril to borrow so that he can develop his driving skills in school.
2. Cyril needs better social integration with the other students at school.
   - A meeting will be held with all the teachers who are involved with Cyril, including his regular and special education teachers and his educational assistant. Also present will be his related service providers, including PT, occupational therapist (OT), speech language pathologist, and his parents. The district special education resource teacher will facilitate the meeting to brainstorm strategies that might help Cyril become more integrated in the school. Some proposed solutions could include peer support systems in and out of class so that Cyril is paired with peers either one on one or in small groups for particular tasks, educational programs for his classmates to teach them about Cyril and how to interact with him, teaching Cyril social skills so that he is better prepared to participate on a social plane with the other students, and helping Cyril become more independent in mobility and other life skills so that he does not always have an adult with him.
3. Cyril needs independence from adult assistance during the day.
   - Work with students in his peer group who would be willing to push Cyril from class to class, help him with his work in class, and include him in student activities. Help Cyril become more independent in mobility and other self-help skills.
4. Cyril needs more friends at school.
   - The above solutions may address this problem somewhat. Participation in after-school and social activities also need to be addressed for Cyril.
5. Cyril needs a way to participate in after-school activities.
   - The IEP team will meet to discuss this problem and brainstorm solutions. Some possible solutions include the following: Work with school authorities to fund a later bus so that Cyril and other students are able to participate in after-school activities. Find parents of other students who partic-

ipate who might be willing to transport Cyril home. Find funding to pay for private transportation by taxi or Handi-Cab for Cyril. Research weekend activities where Cyril's parents may be able to transport him. Talk with Cyril's mother to see whether she might be willing to have scouts or another group meet at her home.
6. Cyril needs to be included in class discussions.
   - Cyril's special education teacher will work with the other teachers to develop questions for Cyril before the day of class. In this way Cyril can preprogram answers into his Liberator and be ready to answer when the question is asked. In addition, the teacher will work with Cyril to develop certain generic answers that will always be preprogrammed into his Liberator.
7. Cyril needs improved comfort in his wheelchair.
   - Address his wheelchair positioning immediately. If Shriners Hospital for Children is unable to see Cyril in their seating clinic within the next month, take Cyril to another local seating clinic that specializes in seating for the developmentally disabled. The PT will make Cyril custom foam inserts for his wheelchair seat and back that will position him more comfortably and allow for better wheelchair positioning so that he can access his Liberator and laptop computer easily.
8. Cyril needs better positioning in his wheelchair so he can access his Liberator, laptop computer, or other materials on his lap tray, even after repositioning.
   - See number 7.
9. Cyril needs to be more independent in toileting at home and school.
   - Work with Cyril on using a urinal in the wheelchair at school and at home. Obtain a commode chair from Shriners or through medical insurance to which Cyril could be transferred in the living room at home, and wheeled into the bathroom.

Make adaptations as appropriate for positioning and safety. An additional need identified through his home evaluation is that of bathing in a manner that is easier for his parents. A bath bench with chest strap and armrest will be borrowed and assessed to see if his parents can to use it safely. If use of the bath bench improves safety and function in bathing for Cyril, funding by his health insurance will be pursued. If not, other alternatives will be explored.

Cyril's parents have requested respite services to help them in caring for their son. They now receive 4 hours per week respite services. His parents are required to find their own respite care, pay for it out of pocket, and then submit a claim for reimbursement. Cyril's mother has a hard time finding anyone who is willing to commit to only 4 hours per week. She prefers to save her respite time so that she and her husband can sometimes take a trip back to the Philippines.

Because she and her husband are having such a hard time caring for Cyril, they are seriously considering sending him back to the Philippines to be cared for by other relatives who are younger. They love him very much but think that, as they get older, they

will be able to do less and less for him. Although they think that the resources for Cyril are much better in Hawaii than in the Philippines, they do not believe that they have any alternatives.

The primary agencies working with Cyril are the Shriners Hospital, the school, and the Developmental Disabilities Division of the Department of Health. No agency sees Cyril's problems at home as its responsibility. Cyril's school-based IEP team is aware of the family's concerns, however, and is attempting to access community resources to address some of the problems. They are concerned that Cyril will not be able to attend school if they cannot help the family solve some of the problems regarding transfers, toileting, and bathing at home.

BOX 7-6 Sample Integrated Individual Education Program Objectives

IEP objectives that use technology are usually phrased specifically regarding the criteria for meeting the objective, but generally when the equipment used to accomplish the goal is being described. The reason for this is that the IEP is a legal document and the school is legally obligated to provide the equipment specifically stated in the IEP. Although Cyril currently has the use of a Liberator and a color laptop computer, when he moves to a different school, different technology might be available to help him that would accomplish the same goal. For instance, a computer station might be available in each classroom to replace the portable computer that he currently takes with him. Therefore wording is intentionally nonspecific in identification, yet specific in function of the equipment.

Objectives should be written to express integration of functional skills. Too frequently, isolated specific objectives are written; for example: Cyril will be positioned well in his wheelchair, Cyril will maintain his hip flexion range at least 85 degrees on the right, and Cyril will use his augmentative communication device to communicate in class. A functional objective integrating the previous three objectives might be: Cyril will maintain an adequate position in his wheelchair to access his communication device for class participation. This is more appropriate. To write an integrated objective, include the educational or social context for using the skill.

Although all the objectives listed here do not relate specifically to Cyril's gross motor goals, a PT or PTA should be able to contribute to the formulation of all of the objectives, based on an overall knowledge of Cyril and his long-term goals.

In 1 year Cyril will do the following:

1. Use a computer to write a paragraph about a topic in European history with complete sentences and appropriate grammar.
2. Read a book of at least 40 pages and, with an augmentative communication device or a computer, answer written questions about the content using complete sentences.
3. Use an augmentative communication device to do three 5-minute presentations in front of the class on educationally relevant topics.
4. Use a math program on the computer to calculate long division problems to at least the fourth decimal place.
5. Use an augmentative communication device or another means of communication to initiate conversations with a classmate or ask a question in class at least 10 times.
6. Use an augmentative communication device to make at least three phone calls to his mother, or someone else, from school.
7. Use an augmentative communication device to describe the layout of the high school and how to move from one end of the campus to the other.
8. Use a power wheelchair to consistently and independently drive himself between classrooms on the high school campus.
9. Maintain an adequate position in his wheelchair to access his communication device for class participation throughout the day.
10. Use an augmentative communication device to teach someone how to assist him in taking care of his power wheelchair.
11. Use an augmentative communication device or computer to assist in the creation of written diagrams and/or verbal descriptions that would instruct someone on how to transfer him from his wheelchair to the toilet, tub, or floor at home or at school.

BACKGROUND AND THEORY

The functions of the brain are sometimes mysterious and unfathomable. The process of writing this paragraph uses my brain in many ways, including sensory tasks of visually obtaining information from the books piled around me, retrieving other information stored deep in my brain, processing and organizing the information, and sending messages to my fingers to type words on the keyboard. I must also sit upright in my chair, hold my head upright, and balance while I move my arms to turn the pages in the books. Through studying disorders of the brain, scientists have been able to discover where in the brain many of these activities take place. Disturbances in any of the areas that affect my eyesight, memory, motor skills, or balance can impair my ability to write this paragraph.

I have a mature brain that is relatively static in its functions, but an infant's brain is developing and organizing itself very quickly during gestation and the first few years of life. An infant's brain is particularly vulnerable to many negative influences in the environment such as toxins, infections, or trauma. An insult to the developing brain can occur prenatally, during birth, or within the first few years after birth when the brain continues to develop very quickly. Any insult to the developing brain that causes permanent and nonprogressive damage that affects posture or movement of the child is called cerebral palsy. There is an array of types and manifestations of disturbances to the developing brain, which can result in various motor dysfunctions in the child. Figure 7-14 presents a diagram of the developing brain with areas of damage related to these types of motor dysfunctions. Attempts have been made to classify these dysfunctions, and, although imprecise, classifications can help to organize treatments and predict outcomes.

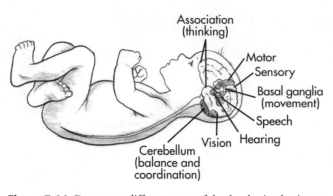

Figure 7-14 Damage to different areas of the developing brain can lead to different types of motor dysfunctions.

Overview

This chapter discusses the causes of cerebral palsy, classifications of this condition, and treatments. Medical treatments, both orthopedic and neurological, are explored, as well as different therapeutic approaches that have been developed over the past half century. Finally, a functional treatment approach for children with cerebral palsy, which uses elements from many of the therapeutic approaches discussed, is presented and applied to children with different manifestations of cerebral palsy.

A case study of Andrew, a young child with severe cerebral palsy, highlights the important role of the family as advocate for young children. Andrew is seen in the context of his family and kindergarten classroom. His premature birth is typical of many children with cerebral palsy. Andrew's developing ability for mobility and communication is fostered by his family and the team of individuals at school who are assisting him to be as functional as possible.

A case study of Cyril, a teenager with cerebral palsy, is presented to highlight the role of the school and the family in helping an older child with severe motor disability develop the necessary skills and resources to succeed. The role of the therapist will change as children mature. In many families, including Cyril's, cultural awareness and consideration is important because the family's reactions, actions, and language are influenced by their belief systems, family structure, and methods of interacting that may be different from those of the therapist or the school.

An Applications section on Assistive Technologies for Learning is presented on p. 208. The world of technology is changing fast and is providing opportunities to access information and skills that children of decades past could not even imagine. Technology can provide opportunities for children with motor or intellectual impairments to participate in school, family, and recreation activities that were not possible a few years ago. It is important for therapists to be aware of these recent advances in technology to be able to help children and families access this information. The cost of technology and third-party reimbursement are important factors in choices related to assistive devices. It is essential to work as a team with teachers, other therapists, medical personnel, insurance companies, and families so that efforts, knowledge, and resources can be coordinated to provide the most appropriate technology to children with cerebral palsy and other disorders.

Prevalence, Causes, and Classification of Cerebral Palsy

Incidence

Cerebral palsy is difficult to diagnose in young infancy because the developing infant changes so quickly. Transitory motor problems may occur and resolve without permanent effects. In severe cases cerebral palsy can be diagnosed before 6 months of age, and in moderate cases it is usually diagnosed by 1 year of age. Mild cases may be diagnosed by the time the child is walking. The prevalence of cerebral palsy is the same in most Western countries, about 2 per 1000 live births (Paneth & Kiely, 1984; Hagberg, 1978).

Etiology

For the developing brain there are two significant time periods when different influences can be important. Congenital cerebral palsy results when the insult to the developing brain occurs during gestation or the birth process. Eighty-five percent of cases can be attributed to influences during these critical times. The remaining 15% of cases of cerebral palsy can be attributed to influences that occur after the birth of the child but during the first few years of life, when the brain is still developing quickly (Perlstein, 1952). This is called an acquired deficit. A more recent study indicated that only 12% of children with cerebral palsy had an acquired deficit (Niswander & Gordon, 1972).

Although care of premature infants is improving daily, the percentage of children with cerebral palsy is not changing. Some researchers believe that the ratio of children with different types of cerebral palsy is changing; for example, there are fewer children with athetoid cerebral palsy because of better treatment of Rh factor incompatibility between mother and infant, but there are more cases of children with spastic diplegia today because of the improved survival of premature infants.

Researchers today are reluctant to attribute causes to individual cases of cerebral palsy, believing that in most cases several causative factors may be relevant. In particular, the role of perinatal asphyxia is decreasing as an attributed single cause of cerebral palsy. Researchers are realizing that many children with significant perinatal asphyxia recover completely (Ellenberg & Nelson, 1979; Churchill, 1958; Davies & Tizard, 1975). The factors that allow one child to recover completely from perinatal asphyxia and another to have severe cerebral palsy are unknown, but researchers assume that other influences on the child, including genetic predisposition, prenatal effects, and environmental influences, are affecting the outcome. Up to 25% of children with congenital cerebral palsy have a normal birth with no attributable etiologic factors (Bleck, 1987).

Prenatal influences. Prenatally, environmental influences play a strong role. Certain viruses that may be contracted by a woman during pregnancy may have only mild effects on her, belying their potentially stronger effects on the developing fetus. Cytomegalovirus, herpes, and rubella can cause damage to the motor centers and other areas of the developing fetal brain. Environmentally borne bacteria such as toxoplasmosis, which can be carried in cat feces, can also result in deleterious effects on the unborn child (Figure 7-15).

Prematurity and low birth weight have been shown to be significant predictors in the development of cerebral palsy. Bleck

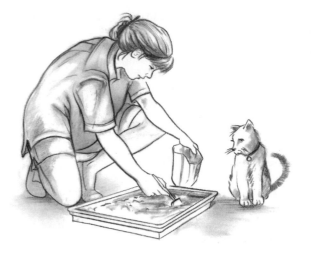

Figure 7-15 Seemingly benign environmental influences, such as cleaning the cat litterbox, can have devastating effects on the unborn fetus.

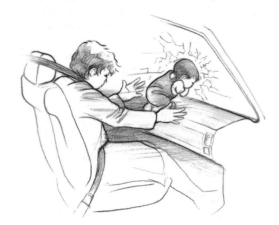

Figure 7-16 Trauma is a leading cause of acquired cerebral palsy.

BOX 7-7 Selected Known Causes of Cerebral Palsy

Prenatal	Perinatal	Postnatal
Genetic	Prematurity	Infection
Viruses	Low birth weight	Trauma
Herpes	Severe jaundice	Motor vehicle accident
Cytomegalovirus	Intraventricular hemorrhage	Child abuse
Rubella	Poor nutrition	Shaken baby syndrome
Infections	Asphyxia	Asphyxia
Toxoplasmosis	Prolonged labor	Head injury
Drugs	Breech birth	Near-drowning
Alcohol	Prolapsed cord	Cardiac arrest
Prescription and nonprescription drugs with teratogen effects		Cerebral vascular accident
		Brain tumor
		Lead exposure
		Thrombosis
		Sickle cell anemia

(1987) estimates that 43% of the children he sees with cerebral palsy were born prematurely. Scherzer and Tscharnuter (1982) are more conservative, and, after a review of the literature, they estimated that at least 30% of children with cerebral palsy are born prematurely. The related problems of prematurity may include severe jaundice, bleeding in the brain, and poor nutrition. It is unclear which problems are significant in the development of brain damage. Questions arise about the nature of the infant who is born prematurely and whether or not preexisting conditions that dispose the infant to cerebral palsy may influence the premature birth in some cases.

Genetic causes. Familial genetic causes of several types of cerebral palsy have been identified, but these are extremely rare. Congenital ataxia is an autosomal recessive trait, requiring carrier genes from both parents to manifest in a child. Familial spastic paraplegia is an autosomal dominant trait, needing only one parent who manifests the disease to pass it to the child.

Perinatal causes. Events surrounding the birth of a child may also contribute to cerebral palsy. Risk factors include pro-

longed labor, breech birth, prolapsed umbilical cord, and birth trauma. Other risk factors include lack of oxygen to the infant for a prolonged period and Rh incompatibility between the mother and the fetus (kernicterus).

Postnatal causes. Although acquired cerebral palsy has several different causes, postnatal infection such as meningitis or encephalitis is responsible for approximately 60% of the cases (Stanley & Blair, 1984; Bleck, 1987). Head injury or trauma accounts for 20% of the cases (Bleck, 1987), with near-drowning, cardiac arrest during surgery, cerebral vascular accidents, tumors, lead exposure, and thromboses from sickle cell anemia responsible for most other cases (Figure 7-16).

The incidence of causes vary according to the geographical location and availability of medical care. For instance, in Micronesia most cerebral palsy is acquired through meningitis infections. Infants born prematurely do not usually survive in Micronesia.

See Box 7-7 for a summary of the influences on a child that can cause cerebral palsy.

Classification

Cerebral palsy has been classified according to the quality of muscle tone or movement, pattern of motor involvement, and sometimes by severity. For example, a child may have a diagnosis of severe spastic diplegia.

Muscle tone. Muscle tone has been defined as the "passive resistance to stretch offered by a muscle group to external manipulation" (Gans & Glenn, 1990, p. 2). Muscle tone is dynamic and can be influenced by body and head position, emotional factors such as anger or depression, systemic factors such as illness or fatigue, environmental factors such as temperature or type of supporting surface, and behavioral factors including effort. Because it is subjectively measured and can change as a result of influences outside the muscle itself, muscle tone is controversial as an objective tool to document clinical observations. Clinicians continue to use quality of muscle tone to describe subjective and objective impressions of posture and quality of movement, however, because muscle tone reflects central nervous system dysfunction in characteristic ways. Qualities of muscle tone seen in cerebral palsy include spasticity or hypertonus, hypotonus, fluctuating tone or athetosis, and rigidity.

Spasticity. Spasticity can be defined as hypertonia (increased resistance to passive stretch that may be velocity dependent), hypersensitivity to sensory stimuli, clonus, hyperactive deep tendon reflexes, and abnormal posturing or movement of the extremities (Haley & Inacio, 1990). Children with spasticity may exhibit abnormal synergies of movement including associated reactions and extensor or flexor patterns of movement with effort. They may adapt poorly to movement, which leads to poor balance, less initiation of movement, and less speed of movement compared with their peers without spasticity. They may have less postural stability, which leads to decreased strength, balance, and skill in activities of daily life. Their mobility or gait may be impaired, and

they may develop contractures and deformity in their spine and extremities. Spasticity related to cerebral palsy is usually a result of a fixed lesion in the motor cortex of the brain. Different lesions produce different distributions of spasticity and are discussed further in this chapter. Over 50% of children with cerebral palsy have a spastic type (Scherzer & Tscharnuter, 1982).

Hypotonus. Children with hypotonus or low tone may have floppy joints, poor definition of muscles, hypermobility of joints, and decreased strength and endurance. They can be characterized as floppy rag dolls. Deep tendon reflexes and response to sensory input may be decreased. Children with hypotonicity tend to lie or sit passively and may have trouble moving against gravity (Figure 7-17). The condition of hypotonicity can be a precursor to either spasticity or athetosis.

Athetosis. A child with athetosis is characterized by having fluctuating muscle tone throughout the body, including the face. The child tends to have involuntary movements and moves between one extreme of range of motion to the other using a writhing pattern of movement. Difficulty in maintaining postural stability in midranges and a general need to "fix" or stabilize the extremities by wrapping an arm or a leg around a stable surface are characteristic of the child with athetosis (Figure 7-18). Athetosis may develop after a hypotonic infancy. Athetosis may be accompanied by involuntary, unpredictable small movements of the distal parts of the extremities (choreoathetoid movements). It may be characterized as "tension athetosis," in which increased muscle tone blocks some of the involuntary movements. Another type of athetosis, called dystonic athetosis, is characterized by abnormal positioning of limbs, head, and trunk with unpredictable tone (Wilson, 1984). A child with athetoid cerebral palsy generally has a strong persistence of obligatory abnormal reflexes.

Athetosis is usually the result of a lesion in the basal ganglia of

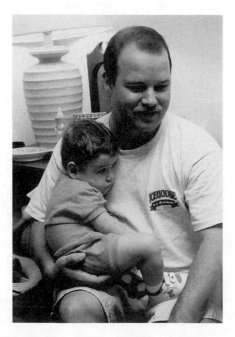

Figure 7-17 Matthew, a child with hypotonic cerebral palsy, is being cuddled by his dad.

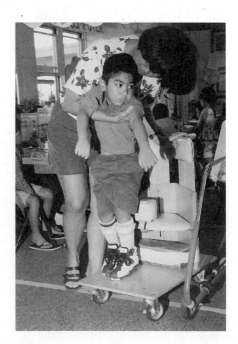

Figure 7-18 Joshua, a boy with athetoid cerebral palsy, is helped by his therapist to get into his corner chair in the classroom.

the brain. Franco and Andrews (1977) noted that formerly 30% of children with cerebral palsy had an athetoid type but, because of improved treatment of neonatal hyperbilirubinemia (jaundice) and improved care of premature infants, this has been reduced to 10% or less.

Rigidity. A child with rigidity tends to have severe and pervasive brain damage, especially at the brainstem level, which affects the communication between the cortex and central areas of the brain such as the reticular formation, the basal ganglia, and the thalamus. A child with a decerebrate lesion of the brain postures with all extremities in extension because of disinhibition of the reticular formation. The excitatory postural impulses from the reticular formation to the motor neurons are not opposed by higher centers in the brain. The extensor muscles of all extremities have a uniform resistance to passive movement throughout the range of motion. Unlike spasticity, this resistance does not depend on the speed of the movement and is the same throughout the range.

A child with a decorticate lesion may posture with flexion of the arms and extension of the legs. The regulatory influences of the cortex on the basal ganglia and thalamus have been removed, and a child cannot move voluntarily or with purpose.

A third type of rigidity involves muscles on both sides of a joint and can lead to a "cog wheeling" effect in which the joint may release and catch intermittently and consistently when passively moved throughout the range. A child with rigidity has involuntary increased muscle tone throughout the range with little voluntary movement and a high risk of developing contractures (Figure 7-19).

Ataxia. Although ataxia is not directly related to muscle tone but to balance reactions, it is sometimes used as a descriptive term for classifying cerebral palsy. The child with ataxia is almost always hypotonic. A child with ataxic cerebral palsy demonstrates unsteadiness of movement. The ataxia may be classified as truncal, which means having an unstable trunk, or general. An ataxic child walks with a wide base of support, usually holding the upper extremities in abduction and retraction of the shoulders, with elbow flexion (high guard) to assist in balance. A child with ataxia has difficulty with precise movements and demonstrates tremors or overshooting when reaching with a hand or foot. Ataxia is a result of a lesion in the cerebellum that monitors and fine tunes the position of muscles for precision and balance (Figure 7-20).

Mixed. Many children demonstrate changing patterns of muscle tone as they grow, or several different patterns at the same time. An example of a changing pattern is the infant with hypotonicity who develops athetoid movements at the age of 3. Many children who later develop spastic cerebral palsy start out with hypotonic muscles as infants. Most children with spastic cerebral palsy have hypotonicity in their trunk and proximal musculature to some degree with hypertonicity in their extremities. Other children may demonstrate both spasticity and athetosis at the same time. The athetosis may be more apparent in their upper extremities as they try to use them functionally, whereas the spasticity may be more apparent in their lower extremities as they exert effort to use their arms functionally. Although there are characteristic features of muscle tone in cerebral palsy, it is important to realize that every child is unique. See Table 7-1 for a comparison of clinical signs for children with different tone manifestations in cerebral palsy.

Patterns of motor involvement. Most children with ataxic, rigid, athetoid, or hypotonic cerebral palsy have motor impairment throughout their entire body. Children with spastic cerebral palsy, however, show characteristic patterns of spasticity, depending on where the lesion in the motor cortex occurred. Although the pattern is usually described by the number and position of the limbs involved, it is important to remember that the trunk is also frequently involved and deficits in trunk stability, strength, and symmetry need to be addressed. See Figure 7-21 for a schematic representation of common patterns of motor involvement for a child with spastic cerebral palsy.

Spastic monoplegia. The child with spastic monoplegia demonstrates spasticity in one extremity. If taxed by running,

Singing is a great technique that has multiple therapeutic applications. Singing quietly can calm a child, and singing vigorously can stimulate a child. Singing incorporates rhythm, language, social skills, and movement (dancing). Best of all, it is a tool that you can always access.

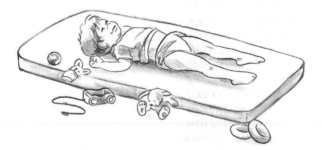

Figure 7-19 Jennifer, a child with rigid cerebral palsy.

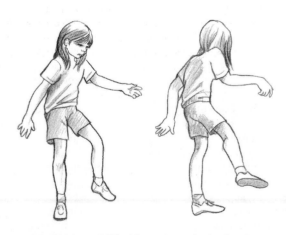

Figure 7-20 Megan, a child with ataxic cerebral palsy, demonstrates a typical ataxic gait pattern.

Comparison of Clinical Signs for Hypotonic, Hypertonic (Spastic), and Athetoid Cerebral Palsy

TABLE 7-1

	Hypotonicity	Hypertonicity	Athetoid
Characteristics	Low tone, floppy, "rag doll"	High tone—spastic, stiff, or rigid	Fluctuating tone, writhing, constantly moving
Distribution	Generalized, symmetrical	Generalized, often asymmetrical	Generalized, can be asymmetrical
Range of motion	Excessive, too much joint movement, stiffness caused by lack of movement in older children	Limited, contractures developing with age	Full range of motion resulting from constantly moving through range
Risk for contractures and deformities	Risk of dislocation (jaw, hip, atlantoaxial joint), risk for contractures caused by lack of movement in older children	Risks for contractures (flexor), dislocation (hip) and deformities (scoliosis, kyphosis)	Risk for deformities (scoliosis, lordosis), risk for joint contractures if spasticity present in addition to athetosis
Deep tendon reflexes	Weak	Abnormally strong	Abnormally strong
Integration of primitive reflexes	Weak display of reflexes, sometimes delayed integration	Often delayed integration, reflexes may be obligatory	Often delayed integration, reflexes may be obligatory
Achievement of motor milestones	Delayed (amount of delay correlates with severity of hypotonicity)	Delayed (amount of delay correlates with severity of hypertonicity)	Delayed (amount of delay correlates with severity of tone deviations)
Influence of body position	Tone remains the same	Tone fluctuates with change in body position	Tone fluctuates with change in body position
Consistency of muscles	Soft, doughy	Hard, rocklike	Stringy and elastic
Respiratory problems	Shallow breathing, choking because of weakness in pharyngeal muscles	Decreased thoracic mobility, limited inspiration and expiration	Decreased thoracic mobility and shallow breathing related to poor control of respiratory muscles
Speech problems	Shallow breathing, difficulty with sustaining voice sounds	Dysarthria secondary to hypertonicity in oral muscles	Dysarthria secondary to poor motor control in oral muscles
Feeding problems	Weak gag reflex, open mouth and protruding tongue, poor coordination of swallowing and breathing	Abnormally strong gag reflex, tongue thrust, bite reflex, rooting reflex	Abnormally strong gag reflex, tongue thrust, poor coordination of oral muscles for chewing and swallowing

Modified from Naganuma, G. M., Harris, S. R., & Tada, W. L. (1995). *Genetic disorders*. In D.A. Umphred (Ed.), *Neurological rehabilitation* (3rd ed., p. 298). St. Louis: Mosby.

jumping, or another difficult motor task, the child with an apparent monoplegia of a lower extremity will sometimes demonstrate involvement of the upper extremity on the same side of the body. A true hemiplegic involvement then becomes apparent. A child with a mild motor impairment who is just beginning to walk may demonstrate pronation, or toeing in, of one foot during gait. It is important to assess the involvement of the arm on the same side to prevent overlooking upper extremity motor impairment that could impact on school performance. The child with monoplegic cerebral palsy may also have motor impairment of one upper extremity.

A child with motor involvement in one lower extremity may have difficulties with gait. Advanced gait activities such as climbing stairs, running, and jumping may be problematic. A child with involvement of an upper extremity may have difficulty with bimanual fine or gross motor activities such as dressing, crawling, climbing or recreational activities such as baseball or dance. The child may have difficulty with balance and a higher than normal risk for developing a scoliosis caused by asymmetrical muscle pull on the spine.

Spastic hemiplegia. This is the most common type of cerebral palsy (Wilson, 1984). The child with spastic hemiplegia has

difficulty using the arm and leg on the same side of the body. This disorder may appear in infancy when the child responds asymmetrically in a Moro response or startle reaction. The older infant may reach for toys with only one arm. Milder cases may become apparent when the child begins to walk and motor problems are evident. The arm is frequently more involved than the leg. The child with a hemiplegic pattern of motor involvement has generally had an insult to one side of the motor cortex in the brain that causes motor impairment to the opposite side of the body. A frequent cause of hemiplegia is a bleed into or around one of the ventricles of the brain. Some children have strokes similar to those of adults. The brain of a child is more adaptable than that of an adult, so the manifestations of the stroke may be different than in an adult. The child's developing brain can recover some of the functions of damaged neurons through development and maturation. The child with a hemiplegia will have many of the same problems as the child with a monoplegia. These can include difficulties with fine motor coordination, gait, advanced gait activities, and balance, and a risk for scoliosis. Characteristic posture and gait deviations include shoulder adduction and internal rotation, elbow and wrist flexion, and pos-

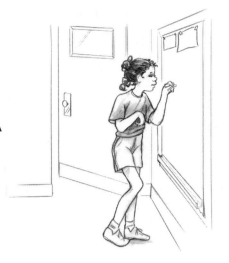

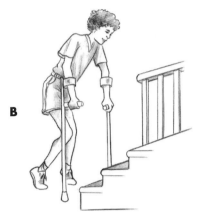

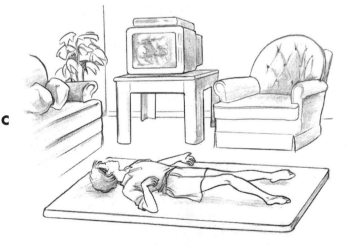

Figure 7-21 Schematic representation of different patterns of motor involvement for children with spastic cerebral palsy. **A,** Hemiplegia. **B,** Diplegia. **C,** Quadriplegia.

sible fisting of the hand in the involved upper extremity, especially with effort. The lower extremity, on the other hand, tends to turn into internal rotation at the hip and either extension at the knee with ankle plantar flexion or flexion at the knee with

ankle plantar flexion. Gait is characterized by asymmetry, decreased step length and stride on the involved side, poor pelvic and shoulder girdle rotation with retraction on the involved side, and absence of heel strike on the involved side.

Spastic diplegia/paraplegia. Spastic diplegia is the most common type of cerebral palsy to be seen in premature infants. It is generally caused by a condition called periventricular-intraventricular hemorrhage, or bleeding in and around the third ventricle of the brain. A related condition called periventricular leukomalacia (PVL) is manifested by lesions in the white matter of the brain around the ventricle. In about 25% of cases of PVL, bleeding is seen, but the causal relationship between the two conditions is not known (Armstrong, Sauls, & Goddard-Finegold, 1987). It is clear that premature infants have a fragile circulatory system and events leading to bleeding or lack of oxygen to the brain may include respiratory distress.

Children with mild forms of spastic diplegia are sometimes diagnosed with spastic paraplegia. These children have motor involvement in their legs only. Most children with spastic diplegia have some motor impairment in their upper extremities as well, although it is milder in the upper extremities than the lower ones. Most children have significant weakness in the trunk and spasticity of the extremities. The primary functional problem includes difficulty with mobility and posture, ranging from needing a wheelchair for mobility, to the use of walkers or crutches, to mild gait disturbances in otherwise independent walkers. For children with milder motor involvement, advanced gait activities such as running, climbing, jumping, and skipping may be impaired. Other problems include postural deviations, including inability to sit without support, inability to stand, and difficulty with movement transitions. Upper extremity weakness and incoordination can lead to school-related problems and dependence in self-care activities such as eating or brushing teeth. Standing posture is characterized by flexion, adduction and internal rotation of the hips, flexed knees, and bilateral equinus feet. Gait is usually crouched because of weakness in the hip and knee extensor muscles, with contractures subsequently developing in the flexor groups.

Spastic triplegia. The child with spastic triplegia has spasticity in three extremities. Frequently the spared limb is an upper extremity, which allows the child some upper extremity function. The child with triplegia may walk with assistive devices, but, because of the motor impairment of one upper extremity, frequently uses a wheelchair for mobility. The cause of triplegia is unclear and may be varied. It may be a combination of spastic diplegia and hemiplegia or an asymmetrical quadriplegia.

Spastic quadriplegia. A child with spastic quadriplegia has spasticity in all four extremities, with significant trunk involvement as well. The spasticity tends to overpower significant underlying weakness in the trunk, sometimes called underlying hypotonicity. Usually an extensor pattern of spasticity predominates, with the lower extremities tending to move into internal rotation, adduction, and extension with effort and the upper extremities also moving into extension, internal rotation, and adduction. If a child has a flexor pattern of movement, the hips and knees will tend to flex with hip abduction and ankle dorsiflexion. The upper extremities will also tend to move into shoulder abduction or adduction and elbow and wrist flexion. Each child is an individual, however, and exhibits unique patterns of movement. An important factor influencing the posture and movement of a child with severe cerebral palsy is the position of the body and head, which stimulates persistent primitive reflexes. Other factors, such as temperature, external postural support, emotions, and sensory input, can influence muscle tone.

Severity. Cerebral palsy can also be classified into levels of severity according to motor distribution and type of movement that the child exhibits. Severity can be applied to the functional capabilities of the child, with decreased functional skills correlating with increased severity of the disease. There are many standardized and nonstandardized tests that measure functional skills from gait to self-care skills (see Applications, Chapter 3), but none have been universally used to classify cerebral palsy. Other types of classifications include the use of cinematography, electromyography, or tests of oxygen consumption to quantify the extent of gait deviations and abnormal muscle firing or effort. Although these tests are helpful in classifying some of the related problems of cerebral palsy, they are not used universally to classify the overall severity of cerebral palsy. Russell and Gage (1989) developed a classification system to document the severity of cerebral palsy, which is convenient and simple. It is reproduced in Table 7-2. The classification system uses only three levels of severity—mild, moderate and severe—and applies them to the functional areas of fine motor, gross motor, IQ, and speech. Although this system is not yet used universally, it reflects the common-sense classification that many physicians and other health practitioners apply subjectively.

Other classification strategies. Gage (1991) prefers to classify cerebral palsy by the method of central control in the brain—selective or automatic. Selective control relates to the pyramidal tracts of neurons in the brain; damage to these tracts

causes spasticity. The pyramidal tracts control voluntary muscles. Automatic control relates to the extrapyramidal tracts, and damage to them causes athetosis or ataxia. Extrapyramidal tracts control postural muscles. A mixed disorder (spastic athetoid) involves damage to both kinds of neurons. Physicians may classify cerebral palsy according to pyramidal or extrapyramidal types as designated here.

Milani-Comparetti and Gidoni (1967, 1980) classified cerebral palsy into three syndromes: regression, defect, and disharmony. Regression syndromes are characterized by patterns of movement like those seen in early fetal stages. Defect syndromes are characterized by lack of postural control. Disharmony syndromes are characterized by disorganized movement. The authors of these studies believed that these classifications provide for a more reliable prognosis of development than the traditional classification schemes. These types of classifications are rarely used by physicians in diagnosing cerebral palsy but may be used by therapists. Table 7-3 provides a summary of the major methods of classification of cerebral palsy.

Influence of Developmental Reflexes

Developmental reflexes, which would normally be integrated into mature movement patterns, may persist in children with cerebral palsy. In addition, a delay in the development of normal postural reflexes can have a profound effect on the motor development and experiences of a child with cerebral palsy. Persistent developmental reflexes can limit the acquisition of skills such as rolling, reaching, and eating solid foods. Delay in the development of postural reflexes can result in the inability to roll,

---

TABLE 7-2   Severity of Cerebral Palsy

Severity	Gross motor	Fine motor	IQ	Speech	Overall
Mild	Independent walker	Unlimited function	>70	>2 words	Independent function
Moderate	Crawl or supported walk	Limited function	50-70	Single words	Needs assistance
Severe	No locomotion	No function	<50	Severely impaired	Total care

From Russman, B. S., & Gage, J. R. (1989). Cerebral palsy. *Current problems in pediatrics, 29,* 75.

TABLE 7-3   Classifications of Cerebral Palsy

Quality of muscle tone	Pattern of motor expression	Area of brain involvement	Severity
Hypotonic	Whole body involvement	Generalized	Mild
Rigid			or
Ataxic		Extrapyramidal Cerebellar	Moderate
			or
Fluctuating tone/athetoid/dystonic		Extrapyramidal Basal ganglia	Severe
Spastic/hypertonic	Monoplegia	Pyramidal Motor tracts	
	Diplegia/paraplegia		
	Hemiplegia		
	Triplegia		
	Quadriplegia		
Mixed		Multiple areas	

sit up, or crawl. Because of the lack of reinforcement from individuals and things in the environment, which can be a powerful motivating force, a child with persistent developmental reflexes may be dependent and passive in interacting with the world. This further limits the child's ability to learn and socialize. Some of the most common and debilitating persistent reflexes in cerebral palsy are explained in the following sections.

Asymmetrical tonic neck reflex. The asymmetrical tonic neck reflex (ATNR) is stimulated by the position of the head and neck. When the head is turned to the side, the arm and leg on the face side are extended and the arm and leg on the scalp side are flexed. The ATNR is usually present from birth to 6 months of age. The child with normal reflex development will move in and out of the ATNR posture, but the movements of a child with cerebral palsy may be dictated by this reflex. The persistence of an obligatory ATNR prevents or delays the child from learning to roll, reach out for toys, bring toys or food to the mouth, and progress to sitting and creeping on hands and knees. Some children with cerebral palsy are able to move in and out of the ATNR position when their head is turned to the side, but most who have persistence of this reflex are obli-gated to move into the reflex position when their head is turned. The persistence of this reflex can have profound implications on positioning, carrying, and handling the child with cerebral palsy. Some children learn to use this reflex functionally as they grow older. For instance, they may look at food to reach for it and look away to get it to their mouth to eat (Figure 7-22).

Symmetrical tonic neck reflex. The symmetrical tonic neck reflex (STNR) is stimulated by the position of the neck in flexion or extension. When the child's neck is in flexion, the upper ex-tremities tend to move into flexion and the lower extremities tend to move into extension. When the child's neck is in extension, the upper extremities tend to move into extension, and the lower extremities tend to move into flexion. The reflex is elicitable in children between the ages of 4 to 12 months but, again, is never in the typically developing child. The persistence or obligatory nature of this reflex is first apparent when the child with cerebral palsy is trying to maintain a hands-and-knees position. It is difficult to maintain this position with the head either extended or flexed (Figure 7-23). The persistence of the STNR has a profound influence on a child's ability to walk. To keep the legs extended, a child with a persistent STNR positions the head forward in flexion. The child also extends the neck in order to extend the arms to reach out for objects but will be unable to remain standing when reaching because of flexion of the hips and knees.

Tonic labyrinthine: prone and supine. The tonic labyrinthine reflex (TLR) is stimulated by the position of the body in space. The supine position stimulates the tonic labyrinthine response in supine. The trunk, arms, and legs are rigid in extension, with the head unable to be flexed against gravity. This response can be elicited in typically developing children before 5 months of age but is not obligatory. The TLR limits the ability to come up to a sitting position, to lift the head up to begin rolling, and to use the arms and legs functionally in the supine position. When the body is in prone, the response is one of total body flexion. The arms and legs tend to be flexed under the body, and the head is flexed downward. When influenced by the TLR, a child cannot lift the head up against gravity or reach with the arms; the child has great difficulty moving up against gravity into a hands-and-knees position, tall kneel, or pulling to stand (Figure 7-24).

Startle and Moro reflexes. The startle reflex is elicited by a sharp noise and results in an abduction and flexion of the upper extremities, opening of the mouth, and sometimes a cry (Figure 7-25). It is frequently confused with the Moro reflex in which a similar response is elicited when the head drops back in relation to the body. In both responses the arms slowly come back to midline again in a movement sometimes equated to an embrace. This response is normal before 6 months of age. Persistence of the startle reflex can occur in parallel with a hypersensitivity to

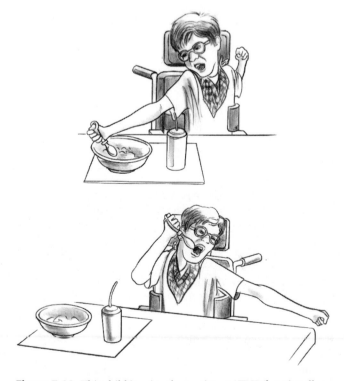

Figure 7-22 This child is using the persistent ATNR functionally to eat.

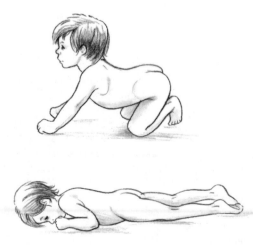

Figure 7-23 A child with a persistent STNR has difficulty maintaining a hands-and-knees position.

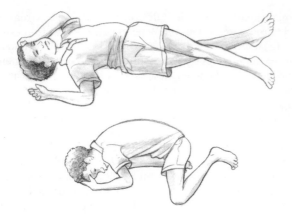

Figure 7-24 The tonic labyrinthine reflex in prone and supine positions.

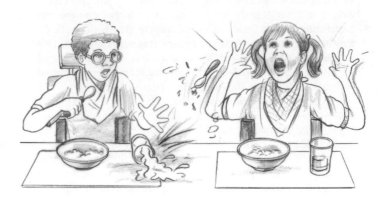

Figure 7-25 The startle reflex can impede attention, socialization, and learning.

noise. Persistence of the Moro reflex can point out again the importance of head positioning and support. Frequent startle responses can impair a child's ability to pay attention and may be confused with seizures.

Related Disorders

Mental retardation. Mental retardation is a common related disorder among children with cerebral palsy. In 1953 Hohman found that 75% of children with cerebral palsy have some degree of mental retardation. In 1978 Nelson and Ellenberg noted that 50% to 65% of children with cerebral palsy had mental retardation. It is clear that some distributions of cerebral palsy have a higher incidence of mental retardation. The groups of children who are the most likely to have normal or above normal intelligence are those with spastic hemiplegia and those with ataxia. Children with athetoid cerebral palsy are also more likely to have normal or above normal intelligence (Bleck, 1982). The group most likely to exhibit mental retardation are those children with spastic quadriplegia, rigidity, and atonia, or lack of muscle tone (Molnar, 1985).

Seizures. Nelson and Ellenberg (1978) also found that 30% of children with cerebral palsy had seizures, with the most common group to have seizures being children with mental retardation and spastic quadriplegia. Children who had acquired cerebral palsy were also more likely to have seizures. Other authors (Gersh, 1991; Molnar, 1985) stated that 50% of children with cerebral palsy had seizures, with the most likely group being those with quadriplegia or hemiplegia. See Chapter 12 for a more thorough discussion of seizures.

Hearing impairment. Approximately 10% of children with cerebral palsy will have problems with their hearing (Robinson, 1973). Children with athetoid cerebral palsy are more likely to have deafness or hearing impairment than children with other types of cerebral palsy. Children who were exposed to maternal rubella may also have a higher incidence of hearing loss, although this condition is much less common than in past decades because of better awareness and prevention of maternal rubella during pregnancy.

Vision impairment. About 50% of children with cerebral palsy have problems with their vision (Gage, 1991). Problems include motor problems of the eye muscles such as squinting or

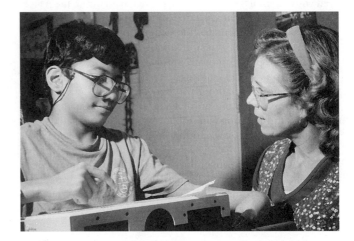

Figure 7-26 Cyril can see much better after glasses are prescribed for him.

strabismus. Premature infants are prone to retrolental fibroplasia, also called retinopathy of prematurity, in which abnormal growth of the blood vessels occurs in the premature retina, which is stimulated by too much oxygen. Retinopathy of prematurity can cause blindness. This disease is decreasing in frequency as physicians learn to control respiratory needs in premature infants with lower doses of oxygen. Nystagmus, in which the eye repeatedly moves quickly laterally and then slowly returns to its normal central position, is common, especially in children with ataxia. Other vision problems include cortical blindness, from damage to the visual cortex in the brain, and hemianopsia and tunnel vision, which are visual field deficits (Figure 7-26).

Sensory deficits. Children with damage to the motor cortex can also sustain damage to the sensory cortex, which is in close proximity. Besides specific sensory deficits such as poor stereognosis or temperature sensation, children with cerebral palsy may have poor integration of their sensory systems. This problem can manifest itself in several ways. The child may be hypersensitive to sensory input, startling or withdrawing from light touch or cold, for instance. The child may have poor organization of movements, speech, and behaviors caused by poor integration of sensory stimuli, which is unrelated to motor deficits (Ayres, 1979).

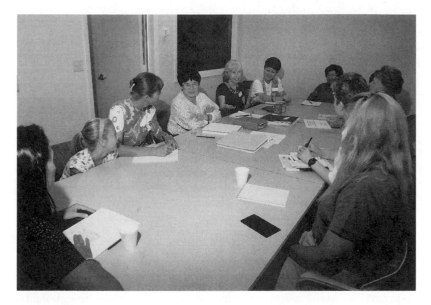

Figure 7-27 A team meets regularly to plan services and programs for a child.

Sensory integration as an evaluation and treatment approach is discussed in more detail later in the chapter.

Speech deficits. A speech or language deficit is present in almost 50% of children with cerebral palsy (Bleck & Nagel, 1982). Motor impairments may cause speech deficits, including dysarthria from paralysis or incoordination of the speech musculature. Other children may have dyspraxia or an inability to organize and select speech.

Visual-motor and perceptual disorders. Children may have difficulty finding hidden shapes in pictures, copying shapes, or seeing relationships between visual stimuli. It is unclear in some children with cerebral palsy whether the perceptual problems are due to poor visual-motor performance or whether there is true underlying perceptual dysfunction. Nelson (1995) believed that children with poor head control accumulate distorted visual input that leads to an inadequate perceptual base for later learning. Bleck and Nagel (1982) found that children with spastic types of cerebral palsy have more perceptual problems than children with athetoid types. Children with spastic hemiplegia are particularly prone to this disorder, and the visual-perceptual deficits are not correlated with the extent of motor impairment. Visual perceptual problems may lead to specific or more generalized learning disorders.

Oral-motor disorders. The child with cerebral palsy may have difficulty with coordination of oral musculature, leading to poor swallowing, excessive drooling, and teeth grinding. Consequences of poor oral-motor control could include respiratory infections from aspirating liquids, and dental caries. Skin problems including rash and ulcers around the mouth can result from excessive drooling.

Behavior disorders. Some children with cerebral palsy may have behavior disorders directly related to nonmotor areas of brain dysfunction. In other children behavior problems are related to emotional components such as frustration at lack of motor control or communication difficulties. Family dynamics related to the child's dependency may either contribute to behavior problems or alleviate potential problems through effective communication and management.

Orthopedic disorders. Because of the motor problems, orthopedic disorders are common in children with cerebral palsy.

Conditions such as joint contractures, hip subluxation or dislocation, and deformities such as scoliosis, rib hump, clubfoot, equinovarus, and tibial torsion are common, especially in the child with spastic muscles. These conditions and their management are discussed later in the chapter.

Management of Cerebral Palsy

Management of cerebral palsy includes management of the related disorders, as well as the central motor disturbance. In the model of a medical home in which the physician acts as a care coordinator, he or she may refer the family to agencies or professionals who can address the individual needs of the child. In cases where the physician does not assume this role, a social worker or public health nurse may make the referrals. Frequently, however, it is the family who learns to access resources in the community. Sometimes the family learns by trial and error. Other times they are good researchers and find the resources they need through multiple telephone calls, networking with other families, and persistence. It is always the role of professionals to give the family access to resources that can help their child. The family is ultimately responsible for their child. Becoming an advocate and learning to access needed resources are very important functions for the family of a child with disabilities.

Services that a child with cerebral palsy needs may include primary medical care, nutrition, seizure management, orthopedic management, education, behavior management, therapy (occupational, physical, speech), and recreation. The individuals who may provide these services include a pediatrician, nutritionist, neurologist, neurosurgeon, orthopedic surgeon, early childhood educator, special educator, teacher, psychologist, OT, PT, speech-language pathologist, and recreation therapist. Others who may be involved with the child and family include the orthotist, adapted physical education teacher, and assistive technology specialist, among others. The group of individuals providing services to the child and the family are considered the child's team (Figure 7-27). Depending on the way the members work together, they could be a multidisciplinary, interdisciplinary, or transdisciplinary team. The role of team members is discussed more explicitly in Chapter 1. It is important that team members communicate with and respect one another and that the child's welfare directs the actions of the team. Although the physician may not be as actively involved in the day-to-day activities of the child as those associated with the educational arena, he or she remains a key team member because the physician's signature and approval are frequently needed for third-party payment for services and equipment.

Medical Management

Pharmaceuticals. The child with cerebral palsy may be medicated for a variety of reasons. Seizures are commonly treated with drugs that can cause severe side effects, such as swollen gums and decreased alertness. Some drugs used to treat seizures include phenytoin (Dilantin), carbamazepine (Tegretol), phenobarbitol, and valproic acid (Depakene).

Other medications may address spasticity. Valium (Diazepam) can be used to induce relaxation of muscles. Side effects include respiratory depression, and some families have reported that this drug interferes with ability to learn in school (Bleck, 1987). This drug is usually given orally, with intravenous administration also effective. Baclofen is another muscle relaxant that is gaining popularity in use with children with cerebral palsy. It is usually given orally, but problems with cycling periods of effectiveness, caused by the drug wearing off between doses, have prompted physicians to experiment with intrathecal administration. A child wears a pump that administers the drug constantly through a catheter inserted into the lower spinal canal. The benefits of this method of administration for children with cerebral palsy are still being studied.

Orthopedic surgery. Children with spasticity may need orthopedic surgery to (1) prevent deformity and pain, (2) correct deformity, (3) improve comfort, and (4) improve function. The orthopedic surgeon frequently works closely with the PT to observe and to monitor the child's function in sitting, walking, and other functional activities. The orthopedic surgeon may also address problems with hand and upper extremity use. Most severe pain that affects comfort and function of the person with cerebral palsy does not appear until adulthood because of lifelong joint degeneration and deformity. Surgery applied to the child is frequently an effort to prevent this pain and dysfunction in adulthood.

Common soft tissue surgeries performed in children with cerebral palsy are muscle lengthening and tendon releases of spastic muscle groups, including hamstrings, adductors, and gastrocsoleus muscles. Muscle lengthening involves partially cutting the tendon to allow the muscle to lengthen. The cut is frequently done in a Z-shape and may be called a Z-plasty. This weakens the muscle but preserves some function. In a tenotomy the surgeon will completely sever the tendon and allow the muscle belly to retract. Neurectomies to denervate spastic muscles are frequently performed in conjunction with lengthening and releases of nearby muscles. In the past multiple surgeries were performed separately to allow the child to recover between them. Currently it is clear that the muscle groups of the lower extremities are interdependent in their function, so neurectomies, muscle lengthening, and tendon releases are performed concurrently. Doing the surgeries concurrently also allows for reduced recovery time and involves less trauma to the child and family. The most com-

mon age to perform soft tissue surgery is in a young school-aged child from 5 to 7 years old (Bleck, 1987).

If surgery is contemplated to improve gait, gait laboratories can help the therapist and the surgeon determine the extent and quality of gait deviation in the child with cerebral palsy. Usually gait analysis is performed when the child's gait is mature, between 6 and 10 years of age (Gage, 1991). The child is observed from the front, the back, and the side during gait. Supplementary aids to direct observation may include videography, computerized video analysis, and electromyography (EMG), in which individual muscle electrical output is measured by surface or needle electrodes. The results of these tests can help the surgeon determine which surgery may improve gait and evaluate the effectiveness of surgery to improve gait. Temporary nerve blocks can be used in older children to mimic the effects and to evaluate potential surgical procedures.

A child who has soft tissue releases is usually placed in a spica cast or bilateral long leg casts, with a bar between to maintain abduction, for 6 to 8 weeks. The casts are heavy and bulky and create unique problems for transferring, positioning, mobility, and bowel and bladder care (Figure 7-28). The therapist needs to be directly involved to plan for seating and mobility in the casts and to teach family and classroom staff how to move and position the child safely. Physical therapy input is necessary after the casts are removed to encourage mobility and function, to maximize range of motion, and to help strengthen muscles that have been weakened by immobility.

In a child with soft tissue spasticity that has not been addressed or has caused bony deformity nonetheless, hip surgery for subluxed or dislocated hips may be indicated. This surgery is not usually performed until the child reaches skeletal maturity in adolescence or early adulthood. The benefits of reseating hips that are subluxing or dislocated include preserving joint integrity, which can reduce pain and dysfunction in later adulthood. Another benefit is reducing deformity to allow better positioning in a wheelchair or easier perineal care. The surgeon may need to reconstruct the acetabulum, create a shelf above the acetabulum to increase its depth, or change the angle or rotation of the femoral neck to the shaft of the femur. In all cases the goal

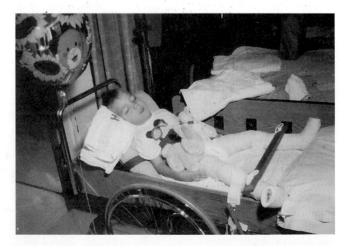

Figure 7-28 Orthopedic surgery can disrupt routines for a while.

is for the femoral head to be seated securely in the acetabulum. In severe cases of adults with intractable hip pain, the head of the femur is removed completely. This procedure is performed only in nonambulatory adults who are awakened at night with severe pain.

Other corrective surgeries that may be performed include tendon transfers and joint arthrodesis. The transfer of a tendon can change the pull of the muscle on the bone to improve function or position by replacing a spastic or weak muscle. One example is the transfer of the peroneus brevis tendon from the lateral foot to the posterior tibial tendon medially on the foot. This procedure changes the function of the peroneus brevis from abduction and pronation of the ankle to ankle adduction and supination. Tendon transfers are not often performed on children. Arthrodesis is the fusing of a joint and is a common procedure to correct a valgus deformity of the ankle in children. In arthrodesis, sometimes called the Grice procedure, the subtalar joint is fused exterior to the articular surfaces to preserve bone growth.

Spinal deformities require surgery to reduce scoliosis, kyphosis, and lordosis to preserve posture and respiratory function. Several different types of surgeries are performed, usually during adolescence. See Chapter 6 for a more complete description of treatment for scoliosis.

Dorsal rhizotomy. Peacock, Arens, and Berman (1987) advocated the use of selective cutting of the dorsal roots in the spinal cord to decrease spasticity in children with cerebral palsy. This surgery is recommended for children in two categories: (1) those who are ambulatory and have sufficient strength, cognitive skills, and voluntary control to maintain and improve their functional abilities; and (2) those who are nonambulatory and whose spasticity interferes with their sitting, positioning, and functional activities, including daily care (Styer-Acevedo, 1994). Children are usually between 4 and 5 years of age and have not had any orthopedic surgeries. During the surgery the spinal cord in the lumbar area is exposed, and dorsal roots are dissected. Through testing, the roots that have the most influence on spasticity are identified and cut (Figure 7-29). Children who receive dorsal rhizotomy need intensive physical therapy for at least 6 to

12 months after the surgery to optimize strength, range of motion, and functional skills. Different protocols for physical therapy after dorsal rhizotomy are available, but most emphasize strengthening the muscles that have been affected, stretching to optimize range of motion, and muscle reeducation to improve movement and coordination skills. After the rehabilitation period is over, any necessary orthopedic surgeries can be performed.

Other neurosurgical strategies. The spinal cord stimulator uses implanted electrodes in the cervical spine to reduce spasticity in individuals with athetosis and dystonia (Waltz & Davis, 1983; Waltz, Andreeson, & Hunt, 1985; Hugenholtz, Humphreys, McIntyre, Sparof & Steele, 1988). This approach is not widely used and is controversial because the application parameters are not yet uniform and results are not yet clear. A child who receives optimal results from the spinal cord stimulator needs intense physical therapy to strengthen weakened muscles, reeducate muscles into functional patterns of movement, and help the child develop functional skills.

Cerebellar stimulation has been more widely used, but the evidence is still unclear as to its effectiveness (Davis, Barolat-Romana, & Engle, 1980; Whittaker, 1980). Stimulation of the anterior cerebellum through activating a self-controlled stimulator, which is implanted on the surface of the cerebellum, has been touted to decrease extensor hypertonia.

Therapeutic Management Systems

Various techniques and schools of thought have developed over the past half century in Europe and the United States with regard to therapeutic management of children with disabilities. Systems of treatment have focused on coordination of motor output, facilitation of righting and equilibrium responses, control of sensory input, and development of functional skills, among other approaches. Although most therapists use an eclectic technique to work with children, taking what is useful from individual therapy approaches, a brief review of some of the more visible therapeutic approaches is given here. The variety of theories behind the different approaches is illuminating and serves to illustrate the concept that there is no right answer.

Doman-Delacato system. Sometimes called patterning, this system of vigorous motor training for rehabilitation developed out of theories that were originally expounded by Temple Fay. Fay believed that movement sequences paralleled evolutionary movements and that a child with brain damage could begin to learn appropriate patterns of movement by making movements similar to those of amphibians and reptiles. Doman and Delacato, who expanded on this theory, believe that the stimulation of highly systematic movement and sensory input can promote sensory and motor integration in undamaged brain cells. Therefore in the Doman-Delacato system the child's limbs are passively moved through patterns of flexion and extension by family members or volunteers for several hours each day. This approach to treatment was popular among some families in the United States during the 1970s who hoped to cure their children of cerebral palsy; however, it has lost support as families burned out from working so intensively with their child. It never had the support of the medical or therapy community but has been featured in popular media as an item of interest. Therefore many

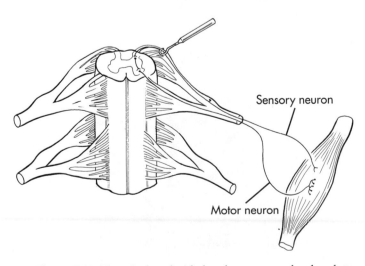

Figure 7-29 The spinal cord with dorsal roots exposed and ready to be cut during dorsal rhizotomy surgery.

Sensory neuron

Motor neuron

individuals have been exposed to it. Today families are usually discouraged from pursuing this treatment regime because it removes the child from the mainstream of life rather than facilitating inclusion in the home and community, as well as putting onerous burdens on the family. Patterning is mentioned here because it is still practiced in enclaves around the country, and therapists should be familiar with it.

Conductive education. Conductive education was developed in Hungary beginning in 1945 by Professor Peto. Its popularity spread to other areas of Europe and it is beginning to be seen in this country. The basic premise of conductive education is that the child's day can be integrated in a unified approach that combines treatment, education, self-help skills, and social skills. It is a holistic approach in which a motor disorder is seen as a learning difficulty rather than a condition to be treated. The child attends a program with other children of similar ages, who have similar needs, and abilities. The group of children is led by a "conductor" who uses daily routines to facilitate purposeful, functional activity. Language is used through repetitive inner and outer speech to guide intention. This is called rhythmical intention. Task series are created from the children's goals, which are broken down into individual steps. The conductor assists children to accomplish the steps by learning and practicing motor skills. Practice in social skills, functional skills, language, cognitive skills, and motor skills are all integrated into the structure of the day by the conductor who uses group activities to reach individual goals. Conductive education appeals to many parents who may see it as an intensive approach to address their child's needs for integrated learning and functioning. Members of the therapy and medical community may have reservations about conductive education because of (1) prohibitive cost, (2) lack of outcome data beyond anecdotal that supports the program, (3) lack of community and social integration in the program, (4) reliance on conductors who do not have specific medical, educational, or therapeutic training, and (5) reliance on the child's ability to change to the exclusion of modern technological supports.

Rood system. Margaret Rood was an American OT and PT . She believed that motor patterns can be modified through sensory stimuli. She developed an approach to treatment of the neurologically involved child that focused on the use of sensory stimulation to normalize tone. After tone has been normalized, the child can bear weight through the affected extremity, and can begin to move through developmental sequences of movement. Rood believed that repetition of movement is important for learning sensorimotor control and that facilitation and inhibition techniques should be used within the movement sequences. Typical Rood techniques include stimulation of the skin, such as slow stroking, fast brushing, and ice, and joint compression techniques, such as tapping, deep pressure over a broad surface, and weight bearing. The sensory stimulation, limited to only 3 seconds in one place, will either facilitate or inhibit muscle tone so that movement is possible (Figure 7-30). In the United States Rood techniques are frequently used in conjunction with other treatment methods.

Proprioceptive neuromuscular facilitation. Techniques of proprioceptive neuromuscular facilitation (PNF) were developed by Kabot, Voss, and Knott in the late 1940s to treat children with poliomyelitis. Their premise is that muscles are more efficient when working in patterns and that functional movement occurs in diagonal planes rather than in straight planes. By facilitating movements in diagonal patterns and using different sensory and behavioral techniques, including stretch, manual contact, joint position, verbal stimulus, timing, reinforcement, and maximal resistance, therapists can facilitate either increased range of motion or increased strength in affected limbs. PNF has been criticized as requiring a high level of cooperation and intellectual understanding by the child or adult receiving services. It also has been criticized as reinforcing spasticity in individuals with neurological deficits rather than developing functional movement patterns. It has been found effective in working with children with spina bifida and athetosis and is another treatment modality to consider (Eckersley & King, 1993).

Sensory integration. A. Jean Ayres, an OT, recognized that some children with neurological disorders had difficulties with tasks other than motor coordination. They had difficulties with attention, behavior, and visual perception that were not being addressed with traditional therapy. She believed that these problems were related to a dysfunction of sensory integration (SI). According to Ayres (1979), "The brain is not processing or organizing the flow of sensory impulses in a manner that gives the individual good, precise information about himself or his world" (p. 51). Dysfunction in integrating sensory stimuli can lead to aberrant behavior, learning problems, poor self-esteem, distractibility, delayed speech development, poor muscle tone and coordination, learning problems, and teenage problems. Ayres believed that all learning disabilities are related to sensory integrative dysfunction, although not all children with SI dysfunction have learning disabilities.

According to Ayres (1979), "therapy involving sensory stimulation and responses to stimulation is often more effective than drugs, mental analysis, or rewards and punishments in helping the dysfunctional brain to correct itself" (p. 135). By directing and controlling the environment, especially influences on the vestibular system, muscles and joints, and skin, the therapist can

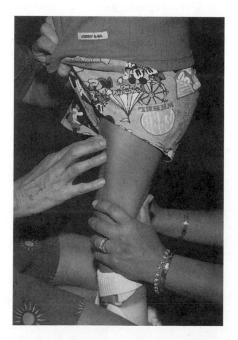

Figure 7-30 Sensory techniques originated by Margaret Rood can influence muscle tone.

assist the child to form adaptive responses spontaneously to integrate the sensations. Each child has specific needs that can be identified through evaluation by a therapist trained in sensory integrative techniques.

Techniques used by the SI-trained therapist include brushing or rubbing the skin either lightly or vigorously. Deep pressure is sometimes applied by wrapping a child up in a mat and making a "sandwich." Joint compression or traction is used in the context of play. Vibration to various parts of the body can be applied using a handheld vibrator or a vibrating board. The sense of smell can be stimulated by using strong odors such as oil of wintergreen. Vestibular stimulation is probably the hallmark of SI therapy, with the bolster swing and the scooterboard key pieces of equipment (Figure 7-31). Each of the sensory systems has connections throughout the brain and stimulating one system can help the brain process other sensory input. The vestibular system has the most connections throughout the brain and is stimulated most frequently by the SI therapist.

Ayres stresses the continual evaluation by the therapist of the child's response to sensory stimulation. It is this response that determines the effectiveness of the therapeutic technique and the direction of the therapy. She also emphasizes the importance of having the child direct the activities within the context of the environment set up by the therapist.

Neurodevelopmental treatment. Berta Bobath, a PT, and her husband Karl, a physician, developed neurodevelopmental treatment (NDT) in England in the 1940s as a response to their clinical observations of children and adults with neurological deficits. The approach has become very popular throughout the world for treating both children with cerebral palsy and adults with hemiplegia.

Although it emphasizes all aspects of a child's development, the NDT approach concentrates on the effects of disturbed postural reactions and abnormal reflexes, which are present in many people with neurological deficits and can affect functional skills. One premise of the NDT approach is that everyone has automatic postural mechanisms that help maintain an upright position against gravity and keep a predictable orientation to the world. In children with cerebral palsy these postural mechanisms are faulty, causing them to develop compensatory and inefficient ways of moving and maintaining themselves against gravity. The vestibular, visual, tactile, somatosensory, and proprioceptive sensory systems are also seen as having an important effect on posture. Sensory feedback helps an infant organize posture, as well as learn to anticipate postural disturbances, by making postural adjustments. An example of a postural adjustment is the automatic tightening of an infant's abdominal muscles before being picked up by an adult.

The therapist trained in NDT techniques can help a child experience active movement with correct alignment and more efficient movement patterns, as well as anticipate changes in posture. By experiencing active, appropriate movement repeatedly in various positions, a child may learn to move more efficiently without assistance. The NDT therapist may work through the developmental sequence to help the child learn to move more efficiently. The NDT therapist addresses functional goals for the child such as sitting independently, reaching for toys, and independent mobility.

Skills developed by the therapist trained in NDT emphasize handling. Through handling a child, the therapist can assist the child to unlearn inefficient motor patterns so they can be replaced with more normal patterns of movement. As Eckersley and King (1993) state, "During treatment sessions, the physiotherapist becomes part of the sensory input system of the child, and handling is a constant interplay between the therapist and the reactions of the child" (p. 335).

Other methods that the NDT therapist uses include inhibition of abnormal responses and positions through reflex inhibiting postures (RIPs), with key points of control, facilitation of normal movements, and use of movement sequences to develop functional skills (Figure 7-32). RIPs are postures that re-

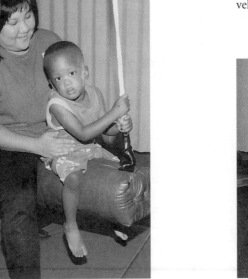

Figure 7-31 Sensory integration uses sensory input to affect motor output.

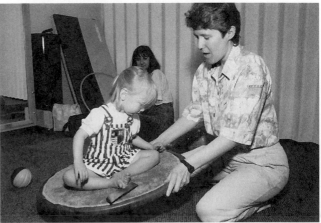

Figure 7-32 Neurodevelopmental treatment is sometimes seen as essential training for therapists working with children. Zandra is working on her equilibrium reactions on the tilt board.

duce abnormal reflex activity, which stimulates abnormal muscle tone. By reducing abnormal motor responses to position (reflexes), more normal movements are allowed to occur. Examples include keeping the child's head in midline to reduce the effects of the asymmetrical tonic neck reflex, bending the child's knees and hips to reduce the effects of the tonic labyrinthine reflex in the supine position, and rotating the pelvis and trunk to reduce extensor spasms. Key points of control are usually proximal, such as the shoulders or the pelvis, and are points where facilitation of normal movement can occur. It is important that the skills the child learns in therapy lead to functional behavior.

Many parents who have been exposed to NDT and have seen the sometimes dramatic effects in their child's functional skills are convinced that it is the best method of therapy. They may request an NDT-trained therapist when they change treatment providers or schools. Detractors, however, believe that, with the constant hands-on help of therapists, the child will not learn to do things independently. Research studies have pointed out the lack of evidence that NDT improves the functional outcomes of children with cerebral palsy. NDT-trained therapists counter by explaining that it is primarily the quality of movement that is improved and that this cannot be measured adequately with functional tests. The theory behind NDT continues to evolve as better research is applied to posture, movement, and development of functional skills for children with cerebral palsy.

The MOVE Program.   Linda Blair, now executive director of MOVE International, was a special education teacher in Bakersfield, California, when she noticed that many children with severe disabilities lost mobility skills as they got older. She began addressing this problem in the early 1980s by developing standing and mobility equipment, which was appropriate for children of many ages and abilities, especially those with severe disabilities. She has also been involved in developing a curriculum to integrate learning mobility skills with education and forming MOVE International, an organization promoting mobility for all children.* The theory is that children who can move will develop greater skills and independence than children who are dependent in mobility skills. Specific mobility equipment has been developed for children, much of which is manufactured by Rifton Equipment.†

The repercussions of this program include many classrooms throughout the country purchasing mobility equipment for children previously thought not to have much potential for independent movement. The equipment and training have provided new opportunities for children to develop new skills through movement. MOVE International supports the curriculum that this organization developed through a training and certification program. Although the program emphasizes functional mobility and other skills acquired through education for children, there is potential for misuse if improperly trained people try to apply curriculum components or use the equipment without proper knowledge of the needs of children with disabilities. The equipment can be costly and should be prescribed carefully by therapists or others familiar with the children and their potential. Physical therapy can play an important role in supporting teachers to help students develop mobility skills in a safe and functional manner.

*1300 17th St., City Centre, Bakersfield, CA 93301-4533; 805-636-4561.
†P.O. Box 901, Rifton, NY 12471-1901.

Commonalities to treatment approaches.   Many treatment approaches for the child with cerebral palsy have common themes. Some of these include the importance of early intervention, the central role of the child and family in all aspects of treatment, the use of sensory stimuli to effect motor outcomes, and the importance of functional goals and age appropriate activities, including play during therapy.

More controversial are treatments that emphasize handling and sensory integration, purely orthopedic approaches, and those approaches that require many hours of family and volunteer time. Because cerebral palsy affects all aspects of a child's life, taking a narrow approach to treatment is not usually as effective in improving function as working with a team of providers who address the functional needs of a child in the school, home, and community. Many therapists are trained in a medical model, where they treat specific deficits in range of motion, strength, or skills. A shift in perception is frequently required to look at the overall functional needs of a child in the context of the activities and settings of the child's life.

Functional Approach to Treatment of the Child With Cerebral Palsy

An eclectic approach to therapy, beginning with the needs of the child and family, can help to design an effective treatment program. Most therapists use aspects of many different approaches to address the unique needs of each child. The provision of therapy to children has changed over the past few decades, and most therapists who work with children are recognizing that therapy is most effective if it is given in the context of the child's day. This means that rather than seeing a child for a half an hour in a small therapy room twice per week, the therapist goes into the home, preschool or school classroom, or community site to provide support for the child, parent, teacher, or aide. Therapy is provided in context on the playground, in the gym, sitting at the desk, or climbing the stairs on the way to lunch. There are exceptions to this rule, of course, such as the adolescent who wants to learn a particular skill out of the sight of peers. Tools from the treatment approaches discussed here can be very helpful in addressing functional needs of the child and family.

Working with the child with hypotonia.   The child who will develop cerebral palsy may exhibit hypotonicity in infancy. This is particularly true of the child who will develop ataxic or athetoid cerebral palsy but may also be true of infants who will develop spastic types (Figure 7-33). Children with disorders other than cerebral palsy, such as specific genetic disorders or general developmental delay, may also have hypotonia.

The following description is of a typical child with severe hypotonia, and some of the elements may not be true of all children with hypotonia. As an infant, the child with hypotonia may move less than the average child, especially moving against gravity. Posture will be gravity dependent. In the supine position the child will lie with hips in a frogged position, and arms will be held in external rotation and abduction. The child will feel limp when handled, and parents may have difficulty finding stable positions in which to carry, feed, or burp the child.

The child with hypotonia may have trouble feeding because of weak suck and swallow reflexes. Because of weak facial muscles, which leads to a decrease in facial expressions, the child may have limited nonverbal communication. This may lead to difficulty in parent-child interaction and may be mistaken as a sign of cognitive deficits.

Lifting the head in the prone position or prone support on forearms may be difficult for the child with hypotonia. There will be a head lag and poor head and trunk control in supported sitting. Typically the child will sit with a rounded trunk and either a flopped forward head or a head balanced on a hyperextended neck. The child will not take weight or will be inconsistent at taking weight through the legs in supported standing and through the arms in propped sitting or prone on forearms. The child with hypotonicity will have difficulty moving in a controlled way because of poor postural tone and weakness. Therefore movements may occur through gross patterns of extension or flexion, such as arching or curling up. Weakness of the respiratory muscles may cause shallow breathing. Because of difficulty accessing the environment—visually because of poor head control, tactually because of poor motor control and weakness, or through voice—the child with hypotonicity may develop a passive personality. This may cause problems with learning and motivation later.

The older child with hypotonicity may develop joint contractures resulting from lack of movement. The contractures will typically be into directions where the child tends to remain posturally, such as shoulder abduction, elbow flexion, hip abduc-

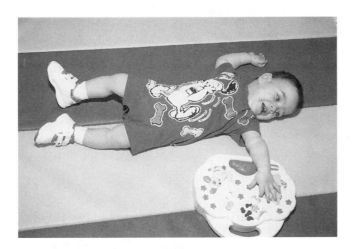

Figure 7-33 When lying on his back, Matthew cannot lift his head or arms against gravity. His posture is influenced by his persistent ATNR, seen in his upper extremities and more subtly in his lower extremities and trunk.

A round plastic (usually colorful) hoop, sometimes called a hula hoop, is a simple toy with many applications. It can be used as a fairly sturdy support for the child learning to walk (with you also holding the hoop). It can stimulate advanced gait activities, including side stepping, jumping, and stepping over. All children can be included in activities with the hoop.

tion, hip and knee flexion, and ankle plantar flexion. Children with hypotonicity are also at risk for subluxation at the hip and other joints because of joint laxity. Scoliosis may occur as a result of constant leaning because of poor postural stability or asymmetrical muscle pull.

The child with hypotonicity tends to develop slowly and shows delays in gross motor skills. Sitting and walking skills may develop late, if at all, depending on the extent of the hypotonicity. Some children can "outgrow" their hypotonicity, whereas others develop different tone patterns as they grow, including spasticity and fluctuating tone. The following are some examples of activities and treatment approaches that could be used during therapy of a child with hypotonia. See Table 7-4 for a sample of long- and short-term goals for a child with hypotonia at different ages. Suggested activities to address the goals are also listed.

Positioning and adapted equipment. Physical therapy will focus on positioning to maximize function. Teaching parents to handle and carry their child to protect lax joints and to maximize access to the world is paramount. The infant's arms should not be allowed to fall to the side but should be kept near the body. Legs should be kept aligned in neutral to prevent frog-legged deformities. The trunk and head should be aligned in midline so the child can look around (Figure 7-34). Traditional infant positioning devices such as infant seats, car seats, strollers, and front or back packs can be used as is or can be modified with towel rolls, foam, or cardboard to provide support for a child with hypotonia. The child should have a variety of positions to provide a variety of perspectives on the world to enhance cognitive development, encourage interactions with others, and minimize the possibility of developing joint contractures.

Parents should be taught about the safety considerations of using a child walker for any child (nationally a high percentage of visits to the emergency department is due to accidents involving child walkers). The use of walkers or bouncy seats for a child with hypotonia is generally contraindicated because of poor trunk and head control. Many therapists also believe that the full extensor tone required of a child with atypical muscle tone to bounce or propel a walker precludes or delays the learning of more appropriate graded movement control for later development of independent walking skills. Parents frequently see that the child using a walker gains independence by being able to move without assistance, but they do not see the long-term view of the appropriate development of motor control. Because independent movement is important developmentally to promote cognitive skills, therapists frequently compromise and advise the parents to limit using the walker to between 30 minutes and 1 hour daily for those children who have adequate trunk and head control to sit in it. Positioning aids such as towel rolls or foam can help the child sit in a better midline position. A good time to use the walker is during dinner preparation when the parent can use the freedom to work in the kitchen yet closely monitor the child.

The older ambulatory child may use adaptive devices, such as walkers, crutches, and braces. Posterior walkers have been demonstrated to assist a child improve postural extension better than anterior walkers, which they tend to lean into. Crutches are generally aluminum Lofstrand or forearm style, which are lighter, more comfortable, and easier to use than the traditional wooden axillary crutches. Foot and ankle braces have evolved to

TABLE 7-4   Sample Developmental Goals: Child With Hypotonia

Family or child long-term goal	Physical therapy short-term objectives	Activities to address long-term goals and short-term objectives
Infant		
Child will roll at least 5 feet for mobility.	1. Child will roll supine to prone position without assistance.	• Encourage child to reach for toys in a diagonal pattern across the child's body.
		• Place the child on a wedge or inclined surface to facilitate rolling.
	2. Child will roll prone to supine position without assistance.	• Swing child in a "hammock" sheet or towel to encourage awareness of position in space.
	3. Child will notice and make approaching movements toward toys that are at least 5 feet away.	• Use music boxes and toys with bright colors and movement to get the attention of the child.
		• Start the session with toys close to the child, and gradually move them away up to 5 feet.
Toddler		
Child will walk independently.	1. Child will pull to standing at the furniture by using a half-kneel intermediate position.	• Work with the child on trunk and hip stability through facilitated movement transitions on the mat. Put toys on a low surface such as the seat of a cube chair and help the child move from prone or supine position to kneeling and sitting to reach the toys.
		• Work with the child on the therapy ball in prone, supine, sitting, and movement transitions to develop balance, trunk co-contraction, and endurance. Work in front of a mirror and sing for rhythm and entertainment.
		• Have the child stand at a waist-high surface to play. Put toys on the floor or on an intermediate height surface that the child can squat or bend to reach.
	2. Child will "cruise" along the furniture at least 3 steps in either direction.	• Move some toys just out of reach so the child will need to take a step to get them. Make sure of success so the child will not get frustrated or discouraged.
		• Walk around the clinic/house with the child holding one or two hands. Give support as needed for good lower extremity positioning.
		• Coordinate obtaining lightweight ankle-foot orthoses for the child to support feet and ankles in a neutral position in standing, if needed.
Preschooler		
Child will dance.	1. Child can jump with two feet.	• Work with child using a small mat that is 1 inch off the carpet/floor. Encourage the child through games to move on and off the mat to improve balance in standing.
		• Facilitate jumping on a trampoline. Use approximation through the pelvis with a quick stretch to facilitate a burst of muscle activity for jumping.
		• When you are sitting on a chair, have the child stand with one foot on each of your knees. Gently bounce your knees to challenge balance and give the feeling of jumping while you support the child as needed.
		• Encourage the child to go up onto tiptoes through reaching for toys, playing follow the leader, and playing imaginary games.

TABLE 7-4   Sample Developmental Goals: Child With Hypotonia—cont'd

Family or child long-term goal	Physical therapy short-term objectives	Activites to address long-term goals and short-term objectives
Preschooler—cont'd	2. Child will balance on one foot for 3 to 5 seconds.	• Incorporate motor skills of balancing into singing games of London Bridge, Ring Around the Rosy, and other songs. • Have child hold a hula hoop with both hands while playing Simon Says. You are also holding the hula hoop and can vary the amount of support you are giving child. • Play ball games where the child needs to stand on one foot to kick the ball. Give support as needed.
School-aged child Child will participate in regular physical education classes.	1. Child will catch an 8-inch ball five out of seven times.	• Roll ball back and forth to child when sitting on the ground. • Play basketball with lowered nets during therapy. Child must catch the ball before it can be placed into the net. • Play modified 4-square in which child must catch ball after one bounce.
	2. Child will throw an 8-inch ball within 2 feet of a target that is 6 feet away.	• Play basketball as above. • During recess facilitate a game of catch on the playground, supporting the child to participate with peers.
Adolescent Child will walk between classes independently.	1. Child will walk 500 feet without assistance.	• Build endurance and strength through training for Special Olympics walking races or basketball after school. • Child will join after school water aerobics class where there is volunteer assistance.

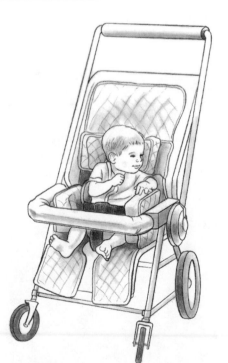

Figure 7-34 Infant seats and strollers can be adapted to provide adequate support to a child with hypotonicity.

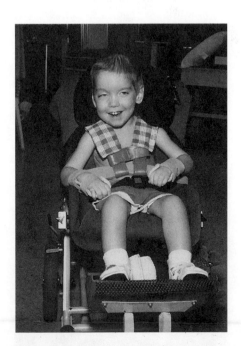

Figure 7-35 A wheelchair tilted slightly in space can provide enough postural support to minimize or avoid anterior straps for a child with hypotonicity.

be lightweight and plastic, as opposed to the heavy metal braces of years past. A well-fitting, high-temperature plastic ankle foot orthosis can assist a child in foot positioning and offers lateral and some anterior and posterior support for the ankle. These elements can improve a child's sense of balance and security in the upright position.

For a nonambulatory older child, positioning is very important to promote appropriate sensory experiences, normal alignment in space, and optimal access to the environment. A well-fitting wheelchair is important to provide good positioning and mobility. The child with hypotonia may tend to slump forward out of the seating system. A slightly tilted back seating system is preferable to straps to hold the child upright (Figure 7-35). The child also needs alternate positions for different circumstances. A floor sitter is necessary for a young child in a daycare or preschool situation, where the children are sitting on the floor. These are manufactured by a number of companies and should have enough adjustability to allow the child to sit in midline with good trunk and head alignment. A child with hypotonia may need a sitter with a recline or tilt feature to allow for full trunk

extension. For an older child an adaptable chair can help provide an alternate support in the classroom. Depending on the child's needs, this can range from an armchair that reclines to a custom-adapted wooden chair with lateral trunk and head supports. For children who have very little postural tone, a sidelyer, prone wedge, and a supine stander might provide appropriate alternative supports.

Optimizing postural tone for functional skills. Physical therapy goals include the development of postural tone to allow the child to move and to sit alone. Because the child with hypotonia tends to sink into support surfaces, including the therapists hands, light touch and guidance is often used to facilitate movements. This needs to be done in the context of an engaging activity, such as reaching for a toy. Other times the therapist may support the child proximally to encourage movements distally. For instance, an infant can be encouraged to play with hands and feet together or hands or feet to the mouth. Support the limb proximally to encourage movement against gravity. All that may need to be done in this case is to put a roll under the infant's pelvis in the supine position (Figure 7-36). To support the trunk in prone extension or supported sitting, the therapist's support is gradually lowered down the trunk as the child gains control. This encourages the child to develop cocontraction of the trunk muscles for greater independent postural control (Figure 7-37).

Weight bearing through the trunk or extremities in various positions also stimulates postural tone. For instance, in the prone position the child can be positioned to bear weight through the elbows. Facilitated weight shifting will help the child develop cocontraction around proximal joints so independent weight shift can be accomplished (Figure 7-38). Another example is weight bearing through the feet in a supported sitting position. The child's weight could gradually be shifted forward to get more active weight bearing, even to the point of coming to stand. A sidelying position can provide different sensory input and encourage the child to lift the head laterally.

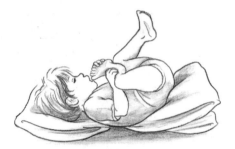

Figure 7-36 Infants with hypotonicity can learn to play with their feet with just a little help.

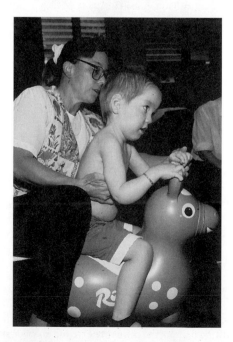

Figure 7-37 Support at the trunk can be lowered to encourage children to use their own postural tone to stay upright.

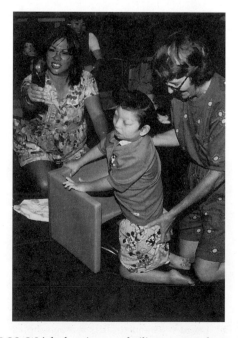

Figure 7-38 Weight bearing can facilitate postural tone in many positions.

Sensory input to improve functional skills. Graded sensory input can help children experience sensations that they are not able to obtain through their own movements. A child with typical movement patterns rolls, creeps, drags, rubs, bangs, and mouths objects and surfaces with the mouth and whole body. This helps the child develop a sense of the boundaries of his or her own body. A child with limited movement options needs help to experience these sensations. Objects with different textures can be rubbed on the extremities, trunk, and face. Deep pressure can be applied through rolling a large therapy ball over the child, folding the child up in a mat or carpet, pressing the child's limbs against the mat or carpet, or laying parts of your body or limbs on top of the child's body or limbs. These sensations can be used on parts of the body such as hands, feet, or arms until the child is comfortable with the whole body being involved.

Sometimes vigorous sensory input can stimulate stronger motor output. This can take the form of vestibular input through swinging the child in a hammock or sheet, playing airplane, holding the child and spinning, or putting the child on a platform swing to spin or swing. Helping the child jump on a trampoline can also provide vigorous vestibular and proprioceptive input. Tapping muscles can provide sensory input to help the child activate the muscle. Facilitated foot stomping, hand banging, or whole body rolling can promote recruitment of more motor units, leading to increased strength or control of postural and voluntary muscles.

Progressing through developmental positions. Infants progress through certain positions as they gain motor control through maturation. As we learned in Chapter 3, the sequence of development of gross motor skills is based on the development of certain skills in the young child. Control usually develops from the head and progresses down the trunk. It also develops proximally and progresses distally. Because this pattern does not always hold in children with neuromuscular disorders, they will need to develop control proximally before they can develop control and functional skills distally. Just as infants with typical development practice and refine skills through attainment of developmental positions, so can children with cerebral palsy. Developmental positions are developmentally and functionally appropriate as therapeutic tools. The attainment of positions with more or less support can be functional goals for children as well.

Although some therapists may still think that a child cannot progress to a more advanced developmental position, such as standing, until the earlier developmental positions, such as sitting, are mastered, most therapists work with multiple positions for the child. Developing shoulder stability, for instance, is important for prone on elbows, propped sitting, hands and knees, pulling to stand, and standing with support. Therefore all these positions can be used to help the child develop shoulder stability. Movement between these positions can also help to develop stability in the shoulder. To build up to more difficult tasks, therapists frequently work in lower positions first and progress to more advanced positions during the therapy session. This is a convenient way to structure the therapy session, but it is important to start where the child is. If the child wants to stand first, the therapist should take advantage of that. Later the child may be willing to play in a sitting position.

Role of the PTA. The physical therapist assistant (PTA) may be working in an infant and toddler development program or a school system. The PTA may be asked to see children for individual therapy or to work with the child in the context of the classroom. Either way, the therapy session needs to be structured according to the goals of the child and the needs of the classroom or home. If work is being done individually with a younger child, it is likely that the parent will be present during the session. This is a good opportunity to discuss with the parent what has been happening at home, including any problems or concerns they may be having. If working in a regular preschool or kindergarten classroom, the PTA may have leeway to design a movement program for the whole class that could incorporate the needs of the child with cerebral palsy. There may also be opportunities to work with the child in the context of existing class activities, such as sitting on the floor during circle time. If working with an older child in a more typical classroom, hands-on therapy may be most appropriate at recess time. The PTA can be available to consult with the student, teacher, aide, or family regarding mobility, positioning, or other needs at school. If the child is in a self-contained classroom, there may be more opportunity to work directly with the child in the classroom along side the teacher and aide.

Working with the child with spasticity. The child with spasticity may have hypotonia, hypertonia, or normal tone early in life that will change as the child matures. Muscle tone and the child's ability to move in a graded way to perform voluntary actions will change throughout infancy and childhood because of the many anatomical, physiological, and environmental effects on the child. As the child with spasticity grows in size, muscle growth does not keep pace with bone growth, causing a tightening of the muscles and an appearance of greater spasticity (Bleck, 1987). The stretch reflex is hypersensitive in spastic muscles, causing a further shortening of the muscles. Environmental effects may temper these anatomical and physiological changes. For example, the child may learn to move in a more coordinated fashion, drugs can reduce the spasticity, and serial casting can stretch the shortened muscles. The effects of spasticity are not static. The variety of manifestations of spasticity in cerebral palsy have been described earlier in the chapter and are dependent on the area of damage inflicted on the developing brain.

The child with spasticity almost always has poor balance and equilibrium caused by poor postural reflexes. In other words, the child may find it difficult to lift the head or trunk up against gravity when sitting or being held. The child may have difficulty finding the upright direction with the head or trunk. The child with spasticity also has difficulty relaxing to conform to the lap of a parent, the floor, a swing, or a carseat. The child feels stiff and cannot subtly modify a position to accommodate to changes in how support is given, as does a child with more normal muscle tone. The child with severe spasticity will have only a few positions that can be regularly assumed without help.

Movements of the child with spasticity are frequently ruled by persistent reflex patterns that have not been integrated into more mature patterns of movement. It is therefore important for the therapist to know the stimuli for these reflex patterns of movement so these stimuli can be modified for the child.

Spastic muscles may be weak underneath the spasticity. In other words, the muscle must be activated in a spastic pattern with other muscles in the pattern also being activated and cannot move efficiently by itself. An example is children who are able to walk with support and use a stepping, patterned gait but are too weak to sit up without support. As another example of underlying weakness, children who have had dorsal rhizotomies and have had the spastic nerve roots cut have significant weakness in the affected muscles. Sometimes spasticity is characterized as "fixing" distally to compensate for weakness proximally. Children with weak postural muscles may recruit tone in their distal muscles to help them achieve a gross motor task, such as sitting up without support. An example is the child who can sit up briefly with arms in a high-guard position and legs curled around the legs of a chair. This child may be able to sit up briefly without support but cannot do anything functional in this position because all muscle groups are engaged in maintaining the sitting position.

The child with spastic hemiplegia. The child with spastic hemiplegia has difficulty with balance because of poor muscle control in the arm and leg on one side of the body. Protective responses of catching oneself when falling toward the involved side can be impaired. The trunk may also be affected, causing even more problems with balance. Scoliosis may become a problem because of asymmetrical muscle pull on the spine, as well as postural asymmetries in sitting and standing. Other problems may include leg length discrepancies, decreased sensation on the involved side, and visual field deficits.

The child with hemiplegia usually learns to walk. Bleck (1987) reports that children with hemiplegia whom he studied all walked between 18 and 21 months of age. Gait deviations and asymmetries can cause functional problems such as tripping, falling, and difficulty walking on uneven surfaces and stairs. Characteristic gait deviations include retraction of the pelvis and shoulder on the involved side, decreased step length on the involved side, and pronation or plantar flexion of the foot on the involved side (Figure 7-39). During walking, the child's involved arm may assume a characteristic posture of adduction and internal rotation at the shoulder, elbow flexion, forearm pronation, wrist flexion, and fisting of the hand. Advanced gait skills, such as running, jumping, skipping, and hopping may be delayed or absent. Other possible problems include poor use of the involved hand for functional skills, such as playing, writing, eating, and self-care skills. The noninvolved arm and hand can usually serve to compensate in most of these activities, with the involved hand serving as a "helper hand" for two-handed activities. Table 7-5 presents a summary of the long-term goals and short-term objectives for a child with spastic hemiplegia of different ages. Sample activities to address the objectives are also included.

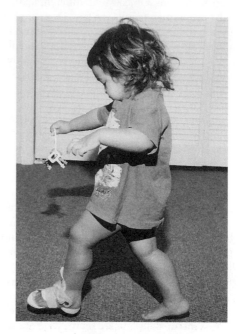

Figure 7-39 Krystalyn has an asymmetrical gait caused by her hemiplegia. The ankle-foot orthosis helps her to bring her left leg through during the swing phase of gait. Note that she has retraction of her left shoulder and hip.

TABLE 7-5   Sample Developmental Goals: Child With Spastic Hemiplegia

Family or child long-term goal	Physical therapy short-term objectives	Activities to address long-term goals and short-term objectives
Infant		
Child will play with toy using both hands.	1. Child will reach past midline for a toy with the involved upper extremity in supported sitting or supine position.	• Encourage child to play with toys that are light and big to encourage bilateral play (4-inch red plastic ring, stuffed animals, infant toys at least 4–inches wide. • Glue strip of hooked fabric onto toy or bottle. Put mitten with strip of loop sewn on palm to encourage hand to object, awareness of hand in space, and bimanual activities. • Advise family to use a bottle with a divided trunk so the child can hold with both hands after involved hand is placed. • Use switches to activate toys and encourage use of involved hand. Switch can be vibrating to give tactile feedback. Move switch slowly to and past midline as child gains skill.
	2. Child will prop on both forearms.	• Use a towel roll under child's chest to help support weight and position both forearms. Make sure toys are within reach and will make noise or light when touched. • Lie in supine position with your head on a pillow and place the child prone on your chest. Facilitate a forearm propping position of the child while you talk and make eye contact.

TABLE 7-5 Sample Developmental Goals: Child With Spastic Hemiplegia—cont'd

Family or child long-term goal	Physical therapy short-term objectives	Activities to address long-term goals and short-term objectives
Toddler Child will walk up and down stairs while holding on with one hand.	1. Child will climb ladder to slide with guarding only.	• Facilitate gait with equal swing through on both sides while playing games with mother or sibling during therapy. • Create obstacle course and assist child to climb up stools, creep up incline mat, and crawl through tunnel. • Assist the child to ascend the slide. Grade the assistance as the child gains more confidence and skill.
	2. Child will walk without assistance between rooms of the house with a 3-inch level difference.	• Give the child experience walking over uneven surfaces including sand, gravel, and grass. • Assist the child to walk with one foot on the balance beam. This may initially need to be the uninvolved foot, but progress to having the involved foot on the balance beam. • Walk in the parking lot, going up and down the curb cut, and stepping up and down the curb with assistance as needed.
Preschooler Child will ride tricycle without assistance.	1. Child can hold and direct handlebar on tricycle.	• Work with child on wheelbarrow games where the child "walks" on hands while you are holding trunk and lower extremities off the ground. Later the child can shift weight in this position to pick up toys, wave to mom, and so on. • Play child golf game in which the child must hold plastic golf club with both hands to hit the ball. • Support the child on the tricycle and push it so the child has only to steer. Assist as needed.
	2. Child will pedal the tricycle with both legs.	• Play ball games, encouraging the child to kick the ball with both legs. • During group activities, have children march, touch their knees to their elbows, and stamp on paper footsteps or "monsters" with both feet. • Adapt tricycle so that the child's feet can be secured to pedals. This can be done by bolting an old pair of shoes to the pedals so the child's feet can be tied into the shoes or by securing straps and footplates to the pedals.
School-aged child Child will play baseball in Little League.	1. Child will swing the bat and hit the ball.	• Practice bimanual activities, including holding a baton and "directing music," swinging a golf club, and swinging a jump rope with two hands. • Adapt hand position on bat to allow for the greatest power during swing. • Practice swinging bat and hitting ball during therapy to develop eye-hand coordination and increase skill.
	2. Child will run 100 feet in 2 minutes.	• Work with child during therapy on gait during running activities. • Use a cuff weight around involved ankle for increased awareness while practicing. • Develop a training schedule for the child to do at home. Rewards can be built in for intermediate successes.
Adolescent Child will drive a car.	1. Child will steer with involved upper extremity.	• Use a simulation program on computer to develop skills in driving/steering with involved upper extremity. • Consider using a car with automatic transmission to decrease level of fine and gross motor skills needed for task.

The child with spastic diplegia. Spastic diplegia has more variation in its expression than spastic hemiplegia. The expression may vary from a mild gait disturbance, including in turning toes and a mildly crouched gait, to a child who cannot walk or sit up alone. Most children with milder forms of spastic diplegia learn to walk. Several studies show that motor performance in children with spastic diplegia plateaus at 7 years of age (Bleck, 1987; Crothers & Paine, 1959; Beals, 1966). If children are not walking by the time they are 7 years, they probably will not walk at all. In Bleck's study (1987), most children with spastic diplegia were walking by the time they reached 4 years old. Bleck found that nonwalking was closely correlated with the persistence of infant reflexes beyond infancy and the absence of normal postural reflexes at 12 months of age.

Problems of a child with spastic diplegia may include lack of postural reflexes (leading to no independent sitting or standing), gait deviations, poor balance in sitting and standing, impairment of protective responses, and impaired use of upper extremities for functional tasks such as eating, writing, typing, and self-care activities. In children who are ambulatory, gait is usually characterized by a crouching posture caused by weakness in the hip and trunk extensor muscles and possible contractures in the hip flexor muscles. A lumbar lordosis may be caused by hip flexion contractures, and the child may have plantar flexion contractures, leading to toe-walking. There is usually poor dissociation of the legs from each other and from the pelvis and of the pelvis from the trunk. This means that the legs tend to move together rather than independently. A characteristic mobility strategy for the child with spastic diplegia on all fours is the bunny hop, in which the legs move together to propel the child across the floor in a hopping motion (Figure 7-40). The child is unable to move the legs individually for a reciprocal creeping movement. During bunny hopping (and also during upright gait) the pelvis and the trunk move with the legs, causing a lack of rotation at the pelvis and trunk. Therefore the child with spastic diplegia tends to rotate the entire body when walking. If the child is not using both arms to hold an aid for balance, such as crutches or a walker, a high guard of the arms is usually held for balance. A characteristic sitting posture for the child with spastic diplegia to gain stability without using trunk rotation is the W-sit.

Other less common problems for a child with spastic diplegia are feeding and speech difficulties caused by poor control of oral-motor muscles. See Table 7-6 for a sample of long- and

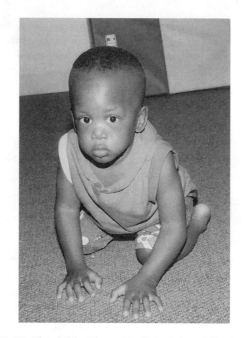

Figure 7-40 The child with spastic diplegia has difficulty rotating his trunk to creep on hands and knees or sit. He uses a bunny hop for mobility and a W-sitting position for stability in sitting.

TABLE 7-6	Sample Developmental Goals: Child With Spastic Diplegia	
Family or child long-term goal	**Physical therapy short-term objectives**	**Activities to address long-term goals and short-term objectives**
Infant		
Child will pull to standing.	1. Child will assume tall kneeling position while holding onto furniture.	• Place the child quadruped over a bolster to play. This will give abdominal support while encouraging weight bearing through extended upper extremities and through knees. • Develop trunk strength and control through facilitated coming to sitting, transitioning to hands and knees, and to tall kneeling during play. • Play at a table with the child supported between your legs in a tall kneeling position. Grade your support to allow the child to develop control.
	2. Child will use half-kneel intermediate position to pull to stand.	• Encourage reciprocal kicking through developing isolated control in each leg. With the child in supine position, hold one leg still either in full flexion or full extension while encouraging the child to kick with the other. • Place the child in a half-kneel position over your leg while playing at a table. Facilitate weight shifts forward and back while playing with the child.

TABLE 7-6	Sample Developmental Goals: Child With Spastic Diplegia—cont'd	
Family or child long-term goal	Physical therapy short-term objectives	Activities to address long-term goals and short-term objectives
Toddler Child will walk with a walker.	1. Child will "cruise" at the furniture.	• Consider external support for the foot and ankle such as dynamic ankle foot orthoses. • While the child is playing at a table, facilitate hip and knee extension by directing manual input through your hands from the child's hips to the knees and from the child's knees to the feet. The direction of force is into the base of support (the feet). • Have the child play baseball while standing in an upright static stander. Work on trunk control by having the child reach for toys to the side, diagonally, and forward and backward while standing in the stander.
	2. Child will walk with two hands held.	• Give the child assistance to shift weight diagonally while walking holding onto both of your hands. • Assist the child to walk while facilitating gait from the pelvis to give the child a feeling of walking with pelvic rotation, lower extremity dissociation, and weight shift from the pelvis. • Help the child to walk in the parallel bars.
Preschooler Child will climb jungle gym without assistance.	1. Child will lift body weight through arms.	• Help the child do press-ups on parallel bars and walker. • Play "Tarzan," swinging the child who is dangling from a baton or dowel that is held by a parent and you. Encourage the child to pull up to see over the bar. • Have child push up on blocks in sitting to let animals or bugs walk underneath the child.
	2. Child will climb up 12 inches with upper extremity support.	• Create an obstacle course in which the child must climb up and over objects and through and around them. Use chairs, mats, wedges, sheets, stools, and other objects to create the course.
	3. Child will extend legs and trunk to reach above head to grasp toys.	• While the child is in the prone, supine, and sitting positions, have the child kick objects suspended from your hand or furniture. Give the child a reward for each success (hug, sticker, tickle). • Have the child help hang holiday ornaments from a tree, the wall, or a doorway. The child must reach to hang the ornament.
School-aged child Child will participate fully in a regular education class.	1. Child will sit upright comfortably at a desk for up to 45 minutes.	• Adapt a classroom chair to provide lateral trunk support, good foot support, and the correct height of the desk to allow for optimal upper extremity function. • Provide a soft sitting surface because the child cannot effectively weight shift in chair.
	2. Child will walk between classes.	• Provide a peer buddy to ensure safety and inclusion while walking between classes using posterior walker. • Build motivation for improving walking endurance by creating a chart that documents how far the child walked each week. • Enroll the child in an after-school swim program to develop strength and endurance.
Adolescent Child will have independent mobility between classes on high school campus.	1. Child will propel a three-wheeled scooter independently.	• Develop a training program with basic and advanced skills that the child must learn before being allowed to use a scooter independently. Use a chart to document progress.
	2. Child will maintain scooter without assistance.	• Child will develop (with help) a maintenance manual for the scooter, including how and when to charge it, how to break it down for transport, and how to provide basic maintenance. • Child will teach at least one other person how to maintain the scooter (parent, sibling, friend).

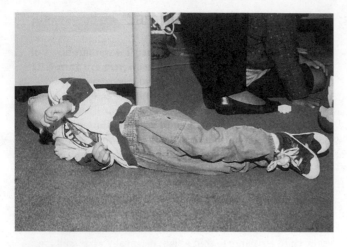

Figure 7-41 Andrew uses full body extension, called an extensor thrust, to try to roll to his friends in the classroom.

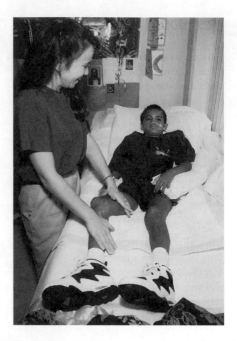

Figure 7-42 When muscle tone is strong, external rotation of the extremities can sometimes "break" the pattern of tone to obtain a more functional position.

short-term goals for a child with spastic diplegia at different ages, along with suggested activities to address the goals.

The child with spastic quadriplegia. The child with spastic quadriplegia usually demonstrates movement and functional problems before children with more mild forms of cerebral palsy are diagnosed. Sometimes, rather than spastic quadriplegia, children are classified as having "whole body involvement." Because all four limbs and the trunk are involved, the prognosis is not as good for independence in mobility and functional skills as for children with other forms of cerebral palsy. Assistive technology, however, can make a big difference in the lives of children with spastic quadriplegia.

Children with whole body involvement tend to move in patterns. A common pattern of movement is a full extension spasm. In what is sometimes called an extensor thrust, affected children arch their back and neck, with associated reactions of their arms and legs, into extension when they are trying to move or express themselves (Figure 7-41). They may also exhibit this pattern of movement when they are startled or have a seizure. It is common for them to arch to try to reach for an object, roll, or adjust their posture. Some children are so limited to this type of movement that they may not have any other options available to them. These children may get stuck in a hyperextended posture called an opisthotonic posture. Less frequently, affected children may move in flexion patterns. When they try to move, their legs will pull up into flexion and abduction and their arms may move into abduction and flexion at the shoulder. They may either extend their trunk or bend forward into flexion with effort. Some children are able to move between these two patterns. Other children may have more variety of movement available to them.

Positioning and adapted equipment. Positioning is important to maximize functional skills and interaction with others and to minimize contractures for children who need postural support. Children with more mild forms of spastic cerebral palsy, such as hemiplegia or diplegia will not have as many positioning needs as the child with spastic quadriplegia. Positioning can help children maintain their head in midline to avoid stimulating the asymmetrical tonic neck reflex. It can provide flexion at the neck, hips, and knees to avoid stimulating the tonic labyrinthine re-

flex. These are called reflex-inhibiting postures. Proper positioning can also help a child perform functional skills, such as eating, schoolwork, and social activity. Alternate positioning can help a child stay healthy by stimulating the lungs, bladder, and bowels to work more efficiently. Positioning should be functional for a child and should be tailored to the activity and the needs of the child and family.

Positioning and mobility can be achieved by using adapted equipment. This can range from adapted infant seats and high chairs to forearm crutches, walkers, and wheelchairs. See the Applications sections in Chapters 8 and 9 for more thorough descriptions of handling and positioning, and seating and wheelchairs for children.

Optimizing postural tone. Just as with a child with low tone, it is important to help a child with hypertonicity to overcome the effects of tone to use muscles more effectively. Strategies for assisting the child include positioning to avoid the abnormal movements related to persistent reflexes as discussed above. Helping the child learn to relax can also assist in recruiting more muscle control. Relaxation can be achieved through handling, gentle rocking, rhythmic movements, and external influences such as music or warm water. A child's muscle tone can be so strong that it is difficult to position the child in a seat or provide perineal care.

The classic position of a child with spastic cerebral palsy who is excited or upset is extension and adduction of the legs. A simple technique to relax limbs that are strongly extending (upper or lower) is to use patterns of movement that are outside the typical pattern of movement for those limbs. For example, if the legs are thrust into adduction and extension, they can be rotated laterally. Place your flat hands, palm down, on the inner thigh of the near leg of the child, and roll the leg toward you. You may need to put one hand on the child's pelvis to stabilize it. As you feel the leg start to roll toward you, you can begin to move the knee and hip into flexion to "break" the pattern. You may be able to do this on one leg at a time, or you may need to roll both legs outward at the same time (Figure 7-42). Although this is a simple technique, it is important to remember to respect the modesty of children, especially adolescents, who may resent this kind of handling. In particular, some children who have been sexually abused have trouble with being touched and moved in this way. Discuss what you will be doing with the child and gain the child's cooperation if possible. If you are trying to modify the movement pattern of extended upper extremities, your hand position will be on the inner aspect of the upper arm and you will roll it into external rotation. This can be a convenient method of assisting a child with range of motion, positioning, dressing, or perineal care.

Sensory input to improve functional skills. Sensory input can be effective to help the child with high tone relax to develop functional skills just as it is effective to help a child with low tone increase strength and function. The sensory experiences are different, however. Warm water can help a child to relax. This can be provided in a bathtub, whirlpool, or heated swimming pool. A swimming pool is a wonderful medium for providing therapy. Once a child is used to the water and the feeling of being surrounded by water, he or she may be willing to bear weight through the legs to stand and walk with support. Working in a pool can entice nondisabled peers, parents, teachers, or even administrators to participate and can promote integration of groups in the school.

Other sensory inputs may include deep pressure to promote awareness of where the limb is in space. This can be provided manually or by rolling a ball or mat over the child's limbs and trunk. It is important to enlist the child's cooperation and to watch carefully for signs of fear or distress when doing this activity. The use of firm, sustained pressure is the best method of moving the limb of a child with spasticity through range of motion. Fast, rough motions can cause muscle spasms, but soft, gentle movements may be ineffective.

Gentle rocking and rhythmic movement lying across a therapy ball or sitting on a swing can help a child to relax. These movements can also aid the child in learning to adapt the head and body position in space. If the child has a poor sense of self in space or does not trust the therapy environment, any of these activities may increase, rather than decrease, atypical muscle tone. It is important to monitor the child closely to assess the effects of what you are doing. It is also essential to direct the activities toward functional skills for the child. Improved muscle tone is helpful to the child only if it is used functionally. For example, if a child can become relaxed while sitting on a therapist's lap so that muscle spasms decrease, turning his or her head to a sound, reaching out for toys, holding the trunk upright against gravity, or weight bearing through the feet in preparation for standing are the next functional tasks to accomplish. Relaxation is not a functional goal in itself.

Progressing through developmental positions. For a child with high tone, it is probably important to progress from early developmental positions, such as prone or supine, to later positions, such as hands and knees, tall kneeling, and standing. A child with hypertonicity needs help to become aware of increasing muscle control and to develop trust in the therapist before progressing to more difficult positions. The hands-and-knees, tall-kneeling, half-kneeling, and standing positions require more postural control than do the lower positions of prone, supine, and supported sitting. It is the development of this postural control that can occur when working in the prone, supine, and sitting positions, as well as independence in transitions between these positions. A solid base of support allows the child to develop stability in other positions. Of course, the capabilities and goals of the child should dictate what you do during therapy. A toddler with hemiplegia will not tolerate working in the supine position for very long, if at all! You should always work from where the child is and in positions the child prefers. See Table 7-7 for a sample of long- and short-term goals for a child with spastic quadriplegia at different ages, along with suggested activities to address the goals.

Role of the PTA with the child with hypertonicity. The PTA works with the child with spasticity in the home, infant program,

TABLE 7-7 Sample Developmental Goals: Child With Spastic Quadriplegia

Family or child long-term goal	Physical therapy short-term objectives	Activities to address long-term goals and short-term objectives
Infant		
Child will have access to the environment.	1. Child will have appropriate positioning devices to allow optimum environmental access. 2. Child will hold head up in supported sitting at least 30 seconds when presented with an interesting toy.	• Adapt the infant seat, stroller, and high chair to provide postural support for child. Use wood, foam, towel rolls, or cardboard. • Sit the child on your lap as you are in a semireclined position on the floor. The child should be leaning back against your bent knees with the child's head supported laterally between your knees. Gradually increase the angle of your knees to sit the child up higher as you talk to the child. Use the social interaction between you and the child to encourage improved head control. • When the child is in a supported sitting position, encourage head turning to follow an object or sound. • Gently rock the child in a sitting position to encourage righting reactions to hold the head upright. Sing or talk to the child to encourage eye contact during the activity.

Continued

Sample Developmental Goals: Child With Spastic Quadriplegia—cont'd

TABLE 7-7		
Family or child long-term goal	**Physical therapy short-term objectives**	**Activities to address long-term goals and short-term objectives**
Toddler		
Child will play with toys.	1. Child will grasp a toy.	• Choose toys that have handles and parts that can be grasped by small hands. • Place a toy which has a sound component (rattle, bell) in the child's hand so that when the hand moves, the toy will attract the child's attention. • Place toys in front of the child on a table or tray within reach. If the child does not yet have a functional grasp, try a hook and loop mitt that can snag toys when swiped near them. • Assist the child to reach for toys by facilitating at the shoulder or elbow. Help the child open the hand by stroking on the back of the hand or tapping on the forearm extensor muscles.
	2. Child will bring toy to the mouth.	• Position the child in prone position on forearms (with support if necessary) with toys placed between hands on the floor/mat. Assist the child to grasp toys and bring to the mouth.
Preschooler		
Child will have mobility in classroom.	1. Child will scoot on back purposefully at least 10 feet.	• Provide opportunities for child to bear weight through feet by kicking, stomping, marching, and "jumping" in the supine position. The weight bearing surface can be the floor, your body, or a tactile board. You may need to facilitate the movements. • Place the child on a slippery surface such as a wood floor or on a blanket on a wood floor. Provide resistance to the child's feet in supine position so that when the child pushes, movement will occur. Teach the child to isolate the movement so a full extensor pattern is not elicited each time. • Position the child in a chair or seat with a wheeled base that is low to the floor. The child's feet should touch the floor. Encourage the child to push to move the chair. Supervise closely to prevent accidents.
	2. Child will direct a switch-operated car or cart.	• Work with the child on accessing switches through trying different types and configurations of switches that are attached to toys. • Ensure that the child is positioned well in the device and can access the switch. • Teach the child to stop, go, turn, and so on. • Supervise closely to prevent accidents.
School-aged child		
Child will access computer for learning.	1. Child will have good positioning to access computer.	• Ensure that the child is positioned well in a wheelchair or adapted classroom chair that will be used when working on the computer. Consult with vendor or therapist who has expertise or experience in adapted positioning if necessary.
	2. Child will access keyboard.	• Work with team to determine the best method of access to computer for the child. Consider different keyboards, placement of keyboard, single or multiple switches, placement of switches, among other options.
Adolescent		
Child will have good peer relations.	1. Child will have friends at school.	• Work with teachers and other school personnel to develop a "circle of friends" for the child. This is a group of peers who care about child and are willing to learn how to interact and support the child. • Assist peers in interacting with the child. Teach them appropriate methods of communication, touching, and moving the child.
	2. Child will be active in the community.	• Assist the family in finding appropriate after-school and weekend recreation activities for child. Work with community groups to help them include the child.

preschool, or school. The PTA is responsible for carrying out many of the direct therapy sessions, including facilitating developmental positions and milestones, such as sitting without support, pulling to stand, and standing without support. They provide gait training to those children who are developing walking skills and consult with teachers and parents regarding appropriate activities for the child at home and in the classroom. The PTA most likely is the primary point of contact for the child and physical therapy and may need to collaborate with other professionals regarding seating and positioning, activity-based programming, and integration into physical education and other classes at school. It is important to communicate regularly with the PT to reevaluate goals and to obtain support for the many challenges in working with a child with spasticity.

The child with fluctuating tone (athetosis). The child with athetosis may evolve from the hypotonic infant. Although a typical "pure" athetoid pattern of movement can be described, most children with athetosis today have a mixture of spasticity and athetosis. Muscles on both sides of joints cannot be coordinated to stabilize the joints. Therefore the child cannot stabilize in the middle ranges, and tends to move from one extreme of range to the other. A semblance of stability may be obtained in one extreme of asymmetry, such as trunk rotation to the right, cervical rotation to the left, upper extremity wrapped around a supporting surface such as the push handle of a wheelchair, and the lower extremities wrapped around chair legs or the front rigging of a wheelchair (Figure 7-43). The child may develop a feeling of comfort and stability in an extreme of asymmetry such as this and may tend to take this position when any stability is wanted. Thus deformities can develop, most likely as a scoliosis with rotation in the trunk and flexion contractures of the elbows, knees, and hips. Because a child may move through all extremes of motion, deformities do not always occur. They are more likely when spasticity is mixed with the athetosis. Persistence of early reflexes

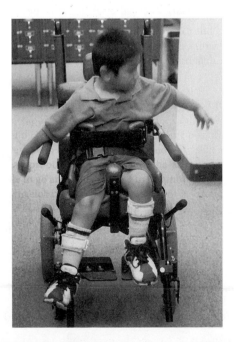

Figure 7-43 A child with athetosis gets external stability any way he can.

is almost always seen in a child with athetosis. The asymmetrical tonic neck reflex is the most dominant force affecting movement and adds to asymmetries in posture.

The child with athetosis usually has difficulty in achieving stability of facial muscles as well as the trunk and extremities. This causes problems with eating, drinking, and speaking. Fluctuating tone in the face causes what appears to be facial grimacing and drooling. Children may use a tongue thrust, exaggerated jaw opening and closing, and pursed lips to try to gain some stability in the face. Breathing is also affected, with irregular breaths caused by the fluctuating muscle tone. Children with athetosis usually have impaired expressive communication resulting from poor control of respiration and muscles of speech. Some may speak with significant difficulty and may be difficult to understand. They usually have normal cognition, however, and can be greatly frustrated by their inability to speak and move the way they would like.

Children with athetosis are usually very thin. This is because of their difficulty in eating and their huge energy expenditures in motor output. A child with athetosis is usually very motivated to find ways to do what he or she wants. A therapist can capitalize on this by using the child's ingenuity to help find solutions to barriers and problems. The development of functional skills is more important than "normalizing" muscle tone. This may mean letting a child use the asymmetrical tonic neck reflex for function such as eating or reaching.

Positioning and adaptive equipment. Infants who develop athetosis need to be evaluated individually for positioning needs. Support in midline is very important so that the child can optimize functional and social skills and so the visual system will develop normally. Feeding is often a problem because of fluctuating muscle tone, and positioning can help to align the child for more efficient and safer feeding.

Some children with athetosis can learn to walk, particularly if there is an element of spasticity that might help them gain some stability in their hips. Their gait is usually slow and labored, and it is likely that they will need the help of assistive devices, such as a walker or forearm crutches, to help with balance. They require extra room to walk because their gait is wide based, and they use many extraneous movements during gait. Walking skills develop later than in other children with cerebral palsy, and some affected children do not walk until their teen years.

Many children with athetosis learn to drive manual or power wheelchairs. To propel a manual wheelchair, the child's common posture of choice is sitting rotated in the chair with one foot propelling the chair backward, the opposite arm wrapped around the push handle, and the neck craned backward to see where he or she is going. This position, although awkward looking, provides the child with stability through maximal rotation. Usually the child prefers to sit in a chair with a sling seat, which has little support and little to impede the child's fully rotated posture. Once children with athetosis discover for themselves this method of wheelchair propulsion, it is very difficult to get them to change to a more conventional method. The problem involved in propelling the wheelchair with so much rotation is that deformities are likely to develop. Moving to a power wheelchair can solve some of these problems. The joystick can be placed in a more neutral position, and the child can be positioned more in midline. This allows for greater function of the upper extremities when sitting in the wheelchair. Several drawbacks to a power wheelchair are that many homes are not acces-

> Make a videotape of a child you are having difficulty with, and share the tape with peers—who may have ideas that will help you. (Get consent from the family first.)

sible, the chair is heavy and difficult to transport, and the chair needs constant maintenance. The power wheelchair may break down frequently and could be gone for long periods for repair.

Older children with athetosis are usually very aware of what positions and equipment work well for them. It is important that the therapist provide these children with options, suggestions, opportunities to try new equipment, and positions or strategies that may help them be more functional. The therapist can make suggestions, but the individual needs to make the final decision.

Optimizing postural tone for functional skills. Because the child with athetosis has poor joint stability, hands-on therapy is usually directed toward assisting the child to develop midline control for functional skills. Slow and steady movements of the therapist can help the child regulate movements in a more controlled way. For a young child, swaddling or holding the child with legs and arms bent and close to the body can help organize movements. With the child in this position, the therapist can facilitate hand-to-mouth or hand-to-toy movements. Family members can do this also. An older child with cerebral palsy can assist you if you explain what you are doing. Using a slow and rhythmic voice pattern can help the child readjust the speed and rhythm of personal movements. Use of techniques such as sustained joint compression through the spine, shoulders, and hips can aid in stimulating some joint cocontraction. Facilitated slow, controlled movements from sitting to standing astride a bolster or the therapist's leg can help to develop postural control during movement transitions.

Sensory input to improve functional skills. The child with athetosis has a difficult time organizing and responding to sensory input. Firm, controlled pressure through the spine and other joints can help to provide central stability. Broad touch, as

with the palmar surface of the hands, can be more effective than fingertip touch. Firm touch can be more effective than light touch.

Using developmental positions to facilitate motor skills. Developmental positions provide a good starting place for the development of motor skills for the child with athetosis. Transitions between positions can help to develop stability and strength. The therapist needs to be cognizant of the age of the child and focus energies on age-appropriate activities. Creeping on hands and knees may not be appropriate for a preteenager, although learning to sit independently on the floor may still be appropriate. The child will probably have strong views on what he or she wants to learn to do. It is very important to listen and to respond to the child's expressed desires. As the child grows, there comes a point when he or she must do things the way that is most efficient. The therapist can provide input and advice, but the child needs to learn to live with the body he or she has and to make adult decisions. Therapists need to encourage this adaptation.

Table 7-8 presents a sample of long- and short-term goals for a child with athetosis at different ages, along with suggested activities to address the goals.

The child with severe multiple impairments. Some children are born with severe multiple impairments (SMIs), which may include cerebral palsy, blindness, deafness, mental retardation, seizures, microcephaly, metabolic disorders, cleft lip and palate, and others. They may have other significant problems, including difficulty feeding and poor nutrition, absence of speech and language, poor skin integrity, severe respiratory problems, and orthopedic problems, such as dislocated hip(s) or severe scoliosis. These are children who are usually identified at birth as having early intervention needs (Figure 7-44). They are all individuals with unique personalities and characteristics. Most parents are willing and able to take on the care of their child with significant disabilities. When this is not possible, children may be placed in foster care. School is a respite for these parents and foster caregivers. It allows them to work as well as providing teaching, physical therapy, occupational therapy, speech-language therapy, nursing, and other interventions for their children.

TABLE 7-8   Sample Developmental Goals: Child With Athetosis

Family or child long-term goal	Physical therapy short-term objectives	Activities to address long-term goals and short-term objectives
Infant		
Child will interact appropriately with individuals and toys.	1. Child will have appropriate positioning devices to allow postural stability and midline orientation.	• Work with family to adapt infant carrying devices such as the infant seat, car seat, stroller, and backpack. • Teach caregivers appropriate carrying techniques.
	2. Child will reach for and grasp toys.	• Sit the child on your lap facing away from you. The child should be leaning back against your trunk with your arms providing lateral support. Use a coffee table or the seat of a child-height chair as a surface for toys. Use your trunk and arms to stabilize the child and encourage active reaching. • Position the child in a prone position over a small wedge to provide trunk support. Place toys on the floor in front of the child. • Use toys that are attractive and can be easily grasped such as those with handles.

Sample Developmental Goals: Child With Athetosis—cont'd

TABLE 7-8		
Family or child long-term goal	**Physical therapy short-term objectives**	**Activities to address long-term goals and short-term objectives**
Toddler Child will have independent floor mobility.	1. Child will roll independently	• Work with the child on rolling downhill with a wedge or inclined mat. • Promote both log rolling and segmental rolling by facilitating at the pelvis and shoulder girdle. • Lay the child on a blanket and lift up one side to facilitate rolling with trunk flexion. • Use music and rhythm to help the child organize motor activity.
	2. Child will propel a floor-level cart.	• While the child is seated and properly aligned, encourage the use of arms to propel the wheels forward or backward. • Discourage the use of feet to propel if the child tends to push into a full body extension pattern when propelling backward.
Preschooler Child will have independent upright mobility.	1. Child will walk using walker.	• Assist the child to stand using a static prone or supine stander. In this way the child can experience weight bearing through properly aligned limbs and can begin to use trunk co-contraction to stay upright. • Adjust upper extremity support to minimize extraneous movements in standing and walking. This may include forearm support, platform support with straps, or adjustment of the height of the support. • Use ankle-foot orthoses to maximize stability of lower extremities. • Facilitate gait through the pelvis using diagonal weight shifts to allow the child to bring each step through motion.
	2. Child will drive a joystick-operated power wheelchair.	• Use computer simulator games to teach the child how to use a joystick. • Place a dowel in soft clay, and encourage the child to "drive" a wheeled chair with you providing the power. • Experiment with different joystick placements until the child has maximal control.
School-aged child Child will participate in after-school activities.	1. Child will have access augmentative communication device.	• Ensure that the child is positioned well in a wheelchair or adapted classroom chair when using the device. Consultation with the vendor or a therapist who has expertise or experience in adapted positioning may be necessary. • Work with the teacher, speech-language pathologist, and other team members to position and mount the device.
	2. Child will swim using a flotation device.	• Provide therapy services in the context of a community swimming class or activity to help the child be included.
Adolescent Child will have an after-school volunteer or paid job.	1. Child will use public transportation.	• Use community-based instruction to problem-solve and practice skills of using the public bus, handicapped-accessible van service, or a taxi. • Use peer supports to help a child use public transportation.
	2. Child will operate power wheelchair safely in public areas.	• Use community-based instruction to identify accessible routes of travel. Problem-solve how to open and traverse doorways and obstacles and how to maneuver in crowded areas.

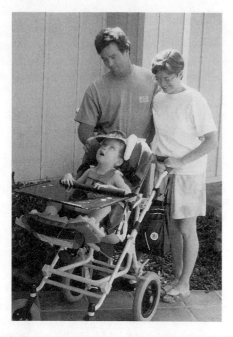

Figure 7-44 The child with severe and multiple disabilities can benefit from good positioning to access the environment.

When the children reach adulthood and "age out" of school, daily programs are much less likely to be available to them. Parents must then face the issues of custodial care or continued training for their children.

Children with multiple disabilities were formerly placed in institutions for custodial care. Today institutional care is seen as creating dependencies in both staff and individuals with disabilities who learn to function in an institutional "culture." The institutional culture is not seen as "normative" and does not allow the individuals placed there to experience and benefit from normal interactions. It is also very expensive. For both philosophical and financial reasons, large institutions are being downsized or phased out completely.

Role of physical therapy for children with SMIs. A therapy provider working with a child who has so many problems and may be medically fragile will sometimes feel overwhelmed. It is important to view the child as a person. To do this, spend time with the child and the teacher, aide, or parent who knows the child well. Find out what the child likes or dislikes. Get to know some of the child's facial expressions, gestures, or movements and what they mean. Find out what the child is capable of doing, and believe that more is possible.

Take an active role in the team process of setting integrated goals and objectives for the child. Help the team look at many aspects of the child's development, including toilet training, visual regard and attention, communication, recreation (including arts and sports), education, and independent skills of eating, dressing, moving, and self-care. Goals may be very limited for children with multiple disabilities and might include moving the eyes to look toward a sound, moving the arm far enough to draw on a piece of paper with a crayon taped to the hand, or urinating according to a schedule. Explore the role that assistive technology can play in the development of skills, play, and social interaction for a child with significant disabilities. Switches to activate battery-operated toys, computers with touch screens or head pointers, adaptive positioning equipment, and simple or complex communication systems can help the child with significant disabilities participate more fully in all aspects of school, home, and community.

APPLICATIONS Assistive Technologies for Learning

JAMES R. SKOUGE

This is a very exciting time to be a professional who is supporting children with disabilities to learn and socialize in school and at home. A true technological revolution is underway that permits children with even the most severe disabilities to play and learn with other children by using toys, appliances, and computers that are now accessible through emerging technologies, such as switches and scanning, trackballs and other pointing devices, enlarged keyboards, augmentative communication devices, and multimedia software.

It is important for the physical therapy provider to understand these new assistive technologies because the key to accessing new technologies for children with physical challenges is often appropriate seating and positioning. When seating and positioning is inappropriate, the opportunities for play and learning remain out of reach and the child is passive. However, when a child is seated and positioned appropriately to access toys, "talkers," and computers, an exciting world of possibilities opens. The child gains control and becomes an active participant in community life.

The therapy provider needs to be familiar with technologies for learning so he or she can participate as a full member of the team around a child with a disability. Understanding the learning and play tasks of a child can direct seating and positioning. Familiarity with computers, software, augmentative communication, and adapted toys allows the therapy provider to see possibilities for children and to be creative in implementing therapy plans and approaches.

To introduce technologies for learning, assistive technology supports for four of the children included as case studies in this textbook are explored: Andrew, a kindergartner with cerebral palsy (Chapter 7); Rik, a kindergartner with generalized muscle weakness (Chapter 8); Luke, a sixth grader with autism (Chapter 10); and Cyril, an eighth grader with cerebral palsy (Chapter 7). Each child presents creative challenges to the educational inclusion team. For example, within mainstream classrooms, how do we:

- Include young children who cannot manipulate toys, game pieces, scissors, glue sticks, paint brushes, and plasticene?
- Promote a love for the language arts among children who cannot grasp pencils or turn the pages of books?
- Celebrate the power of spoken language with children who either do not understand what they hear or cannot speak aloud their intentions and ideas?

These are challenging questions. They include issues related to the very life of the school: play, socialization, academic learning, and communication. These questions can best be addressed through the creative collaboration of teachers, therapists, technologists, parents, and other committed citizens. The four case examples that follow are intended to stimulate your imagination and enthusiasm for assistive technology supports.

Andrew

Andrew is a bright little boy with an involved case of cerebral palsy. Reliably moving any part of his body comes with great difficulty. He giggles, laughs, and smiles—but does not speak. He is a beautiful boy in a difficult situation.

Recently, however, a powerful event occurred in Andrew's 5-year-old life. Andrew began to reliably click two jellybean switches attached to the lap tray of his wheelchair—a red switch and a green one. The switches were mounted 1-inch apart, with hook-and-loop technology, to a square of indoor-outdoor carpeting that had been cut and fitted to his lap tray. By stabilizing his wrist between the two switches, Andrew learned to roll his hand to the left to click the green switch and to the right to click the red one. Andrew's discovery did not come easily. It took experimentation, patience, and faith on the part of his team—and so much practice from Andrew!

In the spring Medicaid authorized the purchase of a Speak Easy for Andrew—a little electronic "talker" that could be controlled with his two switches. It arrived parcel post with a videotape that showed his parents, Will and Ann, how to charge its battery and program its messages. Within 2 hours of the delivery, for the first time in Andrew's young life, he clearly and consistently shouted "yes" and "no" to the world.

"Is this your sock, Andrew?" Ann asked, as she dangled his tennis shoe within his line of vision. Hunched over his lap tray, Andrew lifted his head, stared at the mislabeled item, looked back at his switches, and ever so slowly and painstakingly rolled his wrist to the red switch.

"No," he shouted.

"Is it your shirt?" Ann asked amid tears of joy and expectation.

"No!" again, Andrew shouted, after great, deliberate effort.

"Is it your tennie?" Ann breathed.

And after what seemed an eternity, Andrew rolled to green.

"Now, everyone will know that Andrew is a smart boy!" Ann tearfully exclaimed. "I always knew it. But now everybody else will know!"

Soon the "talker" was a permanent part of the backpack that hung on Andrew's stroller. "Want to go for a walk, Andrew?"

"Yes!"

"Want to go to the pet store and pet the puppies."

"Yes!"

Andrew's mastery of reliable access to two switches represents a very important milestone in his life. It means that he can now learn to use one switch to scan to a "choice item" and the other switch to select or activate it. This is called step-scanning. Step-scanning will empower Andrew both to communicate and to activate toys, appliances, and computers. One day through step-scanning Andrew will be able to write essays, program his VCR, telephone his friends, and cruise the Internet. Realistically, however, for this to happen, Andrew's inclusion team will have many new skills to learn themselves because these are emerging technologies that are new to all of us.

What follows are imaginary examples of inclusion possibilities for Andrew. As you read through them, imagine yourself as part of Andrew's inclusion team. What new skills would you need to learn, and where would you go to learn them? How could Andrew's assistive technology be paid for? We face a daunting challenge: Although our resources appear limited, Andrew's possibilities seem unlimited. Can we imagine the possibilities and make them realities?

Life at Home: Andrew's Dare-to-Dream Vignette 1

Using a laptop computer, Ann learned to create computer screens of pictures that talked and played music when clicked by Andrew. Andrew's red and green switches were plugged into the computer, and he learned to use his red switch to step from picture to picture and his green switch to make his selection talk or sing. This was very exciting because now Ann could design "talking" picture screens that allowed Andrew to initiate communication.

For example, Ann created a "Simon Says" picture board on the Macintosh computer so that Andrew could direct a game at his birthday party. He stepped to the picture of choice with his red switch and then made "Simon" speak with the green one. With the computer connected to the amplified speakers of the stereo in the living room, when Andrew clicked his switch, Simon boomed. When Simon said, "Put your hands on your head and turn around five times," all the kids at Andrew's party did just as they were told.

Ann also created a breakfast picture board on the computer so that Andrew could say the blessing, ask for more milk and cereal, sing a wake up song ("It's time to get up. It's time to get up. It's time to get up in the morning."), and tell a new bit of exciting news. The portable computer sits on the kitchen table out of harm's way. The red and green switches stay mounted on his lap tray—right where Andrew can get to them.

Ann created a picture board that illustrated the steps of going shopping with Andrew. A sequence of eight pictures on the computer screen illustrate getting into the car, stopping at the store, finding specific food items, paying at the cash register, and coming home. Will (Andrew's father) recorded his own voice on the computer to annotate the pictures. Ann and Andrew together step through the pictures to visualize the trip before they leave.

The family's laptop computer came complete with a CD-ROM player so that everyone, including Andrew's older brother, could enjoy the terrific multimedia software that is now commercially available. Andrew loves "Just Grandma and Me," a computer-based "book" that permits children to listen to a story, turn the "pages," and animate hundreds of objects in the illustrations to make them say and do funny things—all by pointing and clicking with a mouse, trackball, or touch window.

These very popular Living Books are marketed for typical children who, unlike Andrew, can use the standard mouse or trackball to navigate and click. Because of very powerful software called Click It! and Overlay Maker, the Intellitools company now makes the Living Books accessible to Andrew. With his red switch, Andrew "step scans" past the umbrella and the starfish until he gets to Grandma, snoozing on the sand; then with the green switch he entices a little critter to tickle her toes. "Awesome, Andrew! You made it happen! You tickled Grandma!"

Life at School: Andrew's Dare-to-Dream Vignette 2

Ever since Andrew was a toddler, his parents and teachers explored simple cause-and-effect, switch-activated battery toys and appliances. Initially, switches, a switch-latch timer, and battery interrupters were borrowed from Andrew's infant development center. Once the jellybean switch was identified as the switch of choice, four were purchased—two for school and two for home. Andrew especially enjoys turning on toys that play music and rhythms (Figure 7-45).

When Andrew was included in his regular kindergarten classroom, quite naturally his classmates wanted to play with him. But because Andrew did not speak, walk, or manipulate objects, the creative challenge was to discover ways to genuinely engage him with his peer group. Recently his teachers discovered the Powerlink from Ablenet. This device has everyone excited because now Andrew can use his switches to control any plug-in electrical appliance (tape recorder, blender, popcorn popper, hair dryer, pitching machine, fan, and lights). Andrew can click his switch to toss Nerf balls for his classmates to catch. This is perfect for "T-ball" because now Andrew can bat. He pulls up to the plate, activates the pitching machine with a remote controlled switch, and heads for first (a peer providing the power). "Go, Andrew, go!"

In addition Andrew controls the music on the tape recorder when the children play musical chairs. He also activates the paint spinner in the art corner.

A local pharmacy has donated film to a photographer in town who volunteers to make slides of beautifully illustrated children's stories that the teacher reads to the group daily after lunch. The remote control of a Carousel Kodak slide projector was adapted by a volunteer senior citizen (a retired engineer) so that Andrew's red and green switches can move back and forth through the slides. Now Andrew "turns the pages" of the projector during story time. Everyone loves it because the slides make the book larger than life. Andrew's classmates walk up to the pictures in

the darkened room to point and talk. "Turn the page, Andrew. Make it happen, buddy."

The newest switch to challenge everyone's imagination is a wireless switch that transmits a radio signal to any battery toy or plug-in appliance. This means that Andrew no longer needs to be tethered by wires to the toys and appliances he activates. Andrew's teacher is now budgeting for a battery-operated train to be set up on a track in the manipulative play area so that Andrew can conduct the train through the fantasy world of Legos and action figures created by his classmates. The train will be a transporter for building materials and figurines. Perhaps best of all, Andrew's red and green switches plug right into this wireless switch. Andrew does not need to relearn any new access strategies.

With his new wireless switches, Andrew can squirt the battery-powered squirt gun to help wash the chalkboards from anywhere in the room. He can make the tape recorder play the Star Spangled Banner during the opening circle.

Andrew's classroom has a color Macintosh computer with CD-ROM. Through an inservice training program, his teacher was introduced to the products from the Intellitools Company, including Intellikeys, Intellipics, Intellitalk, Overlay Maker, and Click It! She is using Intellipics and Click It! to create simple activities that reinforce the basic concepts of number, color, size, and motion. All the children love the software, especially now that their teacher can take their photographs with a digital camera and include their voices and pictures in the programs. Perhaps greatest of all, Andrew can enjoy the software too. Mrs. Ching pairs him with his friend Billy. The two children take turns. Billy uses the trackball for his turn. Andrew step-scans for his. "Make three red 'Billy's slip and slide." "Make 10 blue 'Andrew's hop and hop."

Andrew's Assistive Technology Supports

Jellybean Switches and Velcro

Switches come in all sizes and shapes, but they all function identically: either they turn toys or appliances "on" and "off" or, when a computer is used, they send a keyboard or mouse function such as "click" or "double click." Andrew learned to use two brightly colored "jellybean" switches, each about the size of his small fists. The switches were mounted to his lap tray with the "hook" part of hook and loop technology and a piece of indoor-outdoor carpeting to stand in for the "loop."

Ablenet, Inc. 1-800-322-0956

Wireless Radio Switch

This is a very exciting development for children, like Andrew, who play with switch toys in cooperative learning groups. This switch is larger than the "jellybean," but instead of being "wired" to a toy, appliance, or computer, it emits a radio signal that activates a receiver that in turn performs the desired function. It sits on Andrew's lap tray and activates toys, tape recorders, and software without the wires that get in the way of children at play.

Ablenet, Inc. 1-800-322-0956

Power Link II

For Andrew to activate the blender, tape recorder, hair dryer, vacuum cleaner, popcorn popper, lamp, electric train, or other "on/off" appliances, each is plugged into a switch interface box called the Power Link II, which in turn is plugged into the wall outlet. This allows Andrew's "jellybean" switch or "wireless radio switch" to control the appliances. It is a quick and easy solution for activating all of our "home conveniences."

Ablenet, Inc. 1-800-322-0956

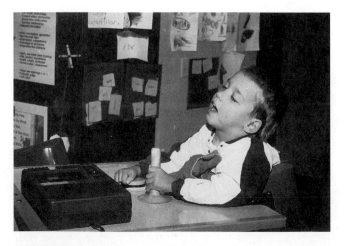

Figure 7-45 Andrew can sing along with music he makes by using a switch-activated tape player.

SpeakEasy

There are many different augmentative communication devices or "talkers." This is a relatively inexpensive one that holds up to 8 messages, each of which can be activated via Andrew's "jellybean" switches. Like a tape recorder, his parents or teachers record messages that are appropriate to Andrew's interests and routines. Messages can be easily and quickly changed.

Ablenet, Inc. 1-800-322-0956

Desktop computer with CD-ROM player

The new multimedia computers with 8 megabytes of RAM, color monitor, and CD-ROM player provide powerful supports for Andrew, his family, and his classroom. They can be programmed with customized talking picture boards that can be activated with Andrew's "jellybean" switches. They also offer exciting children's software, all of which is now accessible using switches.

Consumer Electronics Outlets: $1800-$3500

Intellikeys

This is an exciting programmable "keyboard" that can serve as a talking word board for Andrew. It attaches to Macintosh computers or PCs and provides "plug-ins" for Andrew's "jellybean" and radio remote switches so that he can activate all commercial software. The keyboard is portable and can be transported between home and school.

Intellitools 1-800-899-6687

Speaking Dynamically and Boardmaker

This software allows Andrew's inclusion team to design talking picture boards that include line drawings, color pictures, and photographs—it will grow with Andrew. Since he can use his "jellybean" switches to step-scan, Andrew will learn through this software to communicate thousands of messages created to fit his interests and needs.

Mayer-Johnson Company 1-619-550-0084

Living Books

These are fun-filled, animated children's stories on computer, and they are perfect for children like Andrew, who are using step-scanning and switches. Using Click It!, Andrew can explore and animate hundreds of little critters on the screen and then turn the pages of the book all by himself. These are commercial, off-the-shelf electronic books that are made switch-accessible through "instant access overlays." These books are fun for persons of all ages and provide exciting opportunities for reading and language growth.

Broderbund Software, Inc. 1-800-521-6263

Click It!, Overlay Maker, Intellipics, and Intellitalk

These are very reasonably priced software packages that add enhanced functionality to the Intellikeys keyboard. They permit switch access to any commercial software and the "authoring" of multimedia programs that will allow Andrew to participate in classroom activities actively, including storybook discussions and show-and-tell.

Intellitools 1-800-899-6687

Rik

Rik is an active 6-year-old with a great sense of humor, a terrific curiosity about the world, and an imagination populated with Power Rangers and Ninja Turtles. Unlike Andrew, Rik can speak for himself and get around everywhere with his hot-pink powered wheelchair. Rik is fully included in a first-grade classroom. Not surprisingly, his favorite time is recess, when he and his buddies chase and hide, race and fly to all the distant corners of the playground and the imagination. Rik has a little use of his arms and hands, and he can turn his head and talk, whisper, giggle, and laugh. Other than that, most of his control comes through the joystick of his wheelchair. Rik is always moving. His hand is always on the joystick. Just like any 6-year-old, Rik does not stand still.

Rik's independent mobility has been of some concern. His chair is heavy, and Rik goes as fast as he can. He has turned it over once and has emerged, so far, unscathed. Some of the sidewalks at school are raised several inches above the play yard. Rik needs to be careful—that he does not fall off the edge when on the sidewalk and that he does not ram the edge when cruising on the play yard. When Rik's chair hits something and abruptly stops, his head flops forward and he cannot lift it up. Fortunately, his friends lift it for him. Usually, there are four or five kids running at his side, which is great but a little risky, too. Rik has driven over one child's foot. The bones were not broken, but everyone had a good scare. When the children line up to walk to recess or lunchroom, Rik is careful to drive defensively. "No tailgating, Rik!"

During the spring of Rik's kindergarten year, his parents and teachers became acutely aware that Rik would need computer support to learn his 3-Rs. Up until that time, Rik's "educational assistant," Mrs. McQuillan, functioned as his scribe and secretary. Usually she would grip a crayon, hand-over-hand, with Rik, and the two of them would copy letters and shapes, and complete the worksheets that supplemented Mrs. Chin's curriculum. Sometimes Rik would dictate stories to Mrs. McQuillan, who would write them in Rik's notebook. During free reading Rik would indicate to her when to turn the pages of his books. The problem, of course, was that Rik was not independent. It was too easy to allow Mrs. McQuillan to do it for him. Rik was not learning his letters and numbers; nor was he learning independent study habits.

What follows is a hypothetical example of an assistive technology intervention strategy for Rik. As you read through this scenario, imagine yourself as part of Rik's inclusion team. What new skills would you need to learn, and where would you go to learn them? How might Rik's assistive technology be paid for? As with Andrew, we face a very real challenge. Although our resources appear limited, Rik's possibilities seem unlimited. Can we imagine the possibilities and make them realities? Dare to dream.

Bridging Home and School: Rik's Dare-to-Dream Vignette

An educational technologist evaluated Rik for computer access. Just as he could handle the joystick on his powered wheelchair, so could he manipulate a trackball—rolling the ball to point and then clicking to activate (Figure 7-46). Because of the weakness in Rik's arms, he became too tired pecking with his fingers at the keys of a standard keyboard. A Tash Mini-keyboard was borrowed from the Alliance for Technology Access demonstration center. This tiny keyboard (about the size of an outstretched hand) was perfect for Rik's range of motion, but the keys were difficult for him to push. What to do?

The computer teacher at Rik's school came up with the perfect solution. She found an on-screen keyboard called "Screendoors" that presented a small keyboard right on the computer

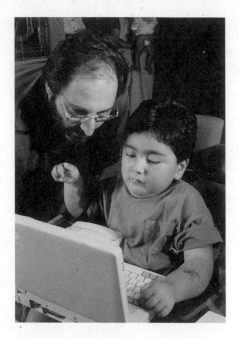

Figure 7-46 Rik's dad helps him learn a new software program so he can do his homework.

screen, so that Rik could roll the trackball with his index finger and then click on the letters and numbers of choice. This tiny "virtual keyboard" in combination with a word processing software called "Intellitalk" was an instant hit! Rik could type letters and words, which the computer in its squeaky, whiny voice could read aloud. Soon Rik was in great demand in the classroom to be everyone's scribe. "Make it say the words, Rik."

The first-grade year is presenting many new challenges for Rik's inclusion team. A color Macintosh, moved in from the computer lab, contains a growing number of software programs that support the math, language arts, and science curriculum. These multimedia programs that are enjoyable for all the children in the classroom include award-winning titles, such as Bailey's Book House, Millie's Math House, Sammie's Science House, and the Living Books Series. Rik's first-grade teacher is excited because these programs are new to her, too. They offer exciting possibilities for her to enrich the curriculum for all her children. Already she groups the children for computer activities and plans for cooperative learning. She looks forward to a computer projector so that she can also use the computer for large group instruction.

There is a scanner in the administration office that is now being used to scan worksheets and storybooks onto disk. Using Kid Pix, Rik is learning to complete the scanned worksheets on his computer. He uses the line tool to connect pictures and words, underline, and cross out. It is so much easier than using a pencil, and he can even use the Kid Pix "stamps" to adorn his work.

Homework is a serious consideration. The school is Macintosh based. Rik's parents, on the other hand, use a PC. Although it is becoming easier to identify software that works on Mac and Windows platforms, the situation is not ideal. Yet to be decided is whether Rik requires a laptop computer that can go home.

This can be an expensive decision and needs to be considered carefully by Rik's IEP team.

Rik's Assistive Technologies for Learning

Laptop computer with CD-ROM player

A laptop computer may be the computer of choice for Rik because it is small enough to be positioned on his lap tray and, in turn, to be transported home. In the classroom the computer can be attached to a standard-sized color monitor so that other children and the teacher can participate.

Trackball

Rik uses a large trackball about the size of a billiard ball. The trackball is positioned in the center of his lap tray so that Rik can use the fingers of both of his tiny hands to roll it. The "Easy Access" control panel on the Macintosh allowed the mouse speed to be slowed way down. With the "Biggy" software the pointer/cursor on the screen was made quite large so that Rik could see it easily.

Don Johnston, Inc. 1-800-999-4660

Scanner

Once a week Rik's educational assistant uses an inexpensive, single-sheet scanner to digitize the upcoming homework worksheets. The worksheets are created as "pict" files and then opened into Kid Pix so that Rik has many "kid-friendly" painting and text tools available for his work.

Screen Doors

This is an on-screen "virtual" keyboard that Rik uses with his trackball. Screen Doors works even with Kid Pix when Rik uses the built-in mini–word processor accessible with the text tool.

Madenta Communications 1-800-661-8406

Kid Pix

This is a powerful children's "painting" program with many motivating "tools" for children, including stamps. For Rik this is particularly fun because he cannot easily manipulate many "real toys." With "Screen Doors" Rik can make the stamps large. Kid Pix also contains a word processor that can be learned through reading the manual (option-shift-text tool).

Broderbund Software Inc. 1-800-521-6263

Bailey's Bookhouse, Millie's Math House, Sammy's Science House

This is exciting software that "extends" the kindergarten and first-grade curriculum in language arts, math, and science by using multimedia. The software is accessible through trackball, touch-window, and scanning so that children with physical disabilities can participate.

Edmark Corporation 1-800-426-0856

Luke

Luke is 12 years old and has autism. He is likable, handsome, and bright, but he does not activate or initiate very much in his world. He imitates sounds and sentences but may not understand the power of language for communication. Luke watches television. He hums and sings to himself. He rarely initiates interactions with others; he does not draw or play with manipulative toys or engage in sociodramatic play. A train set, Lego blocks, or action figurines fail to capture Luke's attention. He will sit and hum and perhaps walk away.

Three years ago Luke's father brought home from work a color IBM computer and a Walt Disney reading program with Mickey Mouse. The program required Luke to select cartoon characters, actions, and locations to tell Mickey what to do, with whom, and where. Once Luke's selections were made, the computer would highlight the words, read aloud, and make little Mickey do just exactly what he was told. Luke, a passive little boy who was not used to telling anybody what to do, was about to enter the world of "take charge."

Luke was introduced to Mickey Mouse by way of that ubiquitous little thing that is attached to every computer—the mouse. Ever so warily Luke clicked on "walk," "telephone," "living room," and "Goofy" and then the magic began. Mickey got up out of chair, walked into the living room, and picked up the phone. "Goofy, hello, this is Mick. Want to come over for dinner tonight?" Ever so cautiously, Luke picked the same four words again, and again, and again, and again. And each time Mickey phoned his friend, and Luke smiled and then laughed aloud. Luke had never asked anything of anybody, and here Mickey did it time and again. "Magic, Luke!"

Luke fell in love with computers. By the time he was in sixth grade, there were three computers in the house with CD-ROM and including three different sound cards! For 6 months Luke played with Mickey for 3 or 4 hours per day. Luke memorized every sentence, written and spoken. Skeptics within the family and the neighborhood wondered if this was an example of "autistic perseveration" in which Luke was "rote learning" rather than thinking and generalizing information. These doubts came to a halt when his mother, Camilla, who read to Luke everyday, noticed that Luke was beginning to read the words with her with increasing animation and enthusiasm. Luke was learning to read.

One day, after months with Mickey Mouse, Luke indicated that he was done with the program and ready for something new. He loved anything with sound, animation, surprise, humor, text, and voice. In succeeding months he memorized all the Living Books and many natural science CD-ROMs, especially ones dealing with sharks. He also mastered many drill and practice programs for spelling, reading, and math. In 3 years Luke became a reader, progressing from "nonreader and uninterested" to "fourth-grade reader with enthusiasm." Luke now picks up books and requests that they be read with him.

During one of Camilla's many forays to the computer software store, she identified a software package called "Kidworks II," which included a talking word processor that would read the letters, words, and sentences as they were typed (using a rather growling voice). It also printed the compositions in a large, inviting, primary font. Camilla initiated a daily regimen of letter writing with Luke, in which at first she would handwrite three sentences to his grandparents and then ask him (1) to copy the sentences on the computer, (2) check for accuracy by listening to the computer read, and then (3) print and mail the letter. As Luke's spelling skills progressed, the procedure evolved into sentence dictation, in which she and Luke would think of a sentence together and then Luke would type it without benefit of a handwritten model. As always, Luke would read aloud with the computer as it read his work. Camilla's dream is that one day Luke will initiate written composition. This has not yet happened. Will Luke ever sit down to write a letter to a loved one?

People with autism by definition have trouble socializing. This is true for Luke—on or off the computer. He appears to enjoy being with his friends at the computer—awaiting his turn if they take over the mouse or keyboard. But, when it is his turn, it is as if he enters a Magic Kingdom in which his friends are uninvited. No one knows yet what to do about that, either.

Building a Communication System: Luke's Augmentative Communication Dare-to-Dream Vignette

In an attempt to build a social function for the computer, Luke's teachers have become interested in augmentative communication software produced by Words Plus and Mayer-Johnson. Much like the multimedia software mentioned earlier for Andrew, Luke's inclusion team can learn to create computer-based picture boards that speak. If Luke is hungry, for example, he can click on a picture of food, which, in turn, displays pictures of breakfast, lunch, dinner, and fast foods. If, then, Luke clicks on "fast foods," the computer displays his favorites, such as McDonald's, Burger King, Taco Bell, and Subway. When he clicks on "McDonald's," graphics of Big Macs, vanilla shakes, fries, and so forth are displayed. These are referred to as dynamic picture displays because new picture menus become available at every level of choice. Each of the pictures, in turn, can be programmed to speak, with a voice that is appropriate for Luke—either computer synthesized voice or a recorded human voice.

Receptive language is also difficult for Luke. Luke appears not to be able to visualize or remember what is described to him. If Camilla tells Luke that they are going to go to the beach and that he needs to get a towel, swimsuit, snorkel, and fins, he may not comprehend that message. With the above-described software, Camilla or Luke's teachers or therapists can create talking picture boards that go through each step of the trip to the beach with familiar pictures attached to a familiar recorded voice. In this way Luke can hear, see, and rehearse the routine as many times as needed. In turn, the picture boards can be printed, placed in plastic paper protectors, and taken on the trip for review.

It is too early to tell if these types of augmentative communication supports can help to make the world more comprehensible to Luke. Luke's inclusion team is excited about the possibilities because computer-based activities are obviously so important and powerful to Luke.

Luke's Assistive Technologies for Communication

KidWorks II

An integrated software package that includes a "talking word/icon processor," paint program, and storybook reader. Many nouns, verbs, adjectives, and adverbs can be displayed either as icon symbols or text—making it an exciting program for beginning writers or readers.

Davidson and Associates, Inc. 1-800-545-7677

Write Outloud

This is a premier talking word processor and storybook text reader. It is ideal for Luke because he can listen to words, sentences, and stories at his own pace and under his own control. With the click of a button, he can listen to his stories one word or sentence or paragraph at a time—and then choose to proceed or repeat. This fits Luke's learning style, which values repetition and self-determined pacing.

Don Johnston, Inc. 1-800-999-4660

Talking Screen

This very exciting program allows the creation of "hyper-linked" talking picture boards. The software includes 3500 graphics that can be edited and customized. Photographs, graphics, and even video clips can be "imported" into the program. Pictures can speak with recorded human voices or a wide choice of computer synthesized voices. This may be ideal for Luke to review his life routines and to communicate within specific activities at home or school.

Words+, Inc. 1-800-869-8521

Cyril

Cyril is 14 years old, in the eighth grade, likable, sociable, good looking, and lonely. He has cerebral palsy. Cyril speaks through a Liberator, writes his lessons on a Macintosh Powerbook, and is just learning to make music through an electronic music synthesizer. He loves sports and music and would like to go to college.

Although Cyril has quadriplegia, he has limited use of his right arm and hand. He "pecks" at a keyboard slowly but accurately with his right index finger, without needing a key guard. He also accurately manipulates a trackball. This means that Cyril can access anything on a computer, but slowly. Cyril is very bright. With all these skills there is no technological reason to hold Cyril back from academic excellence, although he needs ongoing support from his teachers, therapists, parents, and peers.

Cyril arrived from the Philippines 5 years ago and was immediately enrolled in an intimate, supportive, segregated special education program. The program was headed by a very enthusiastic speech therapist, Mrs. Lee, who recognized Cyril's potential and worked tirelessly to equip him with augmentative communication and computer supports. In his first year, just as soon as he learned rudimentary spelling, Cyril graduated from an IntroTalker (limited to 32 pictures with recorded voices) to a TouchTalker, which permitted Cyril to compose his own messages, encode them with Minspeak symbols, and "speak" them efficiently with two or three keystrokes to activate the TouchTalker's voice synthesizer.

Although the TouchTalker sounded robotic and "funny," it permitted Cyril to accumulate hundreds of messages that he could access and "speak" in relatively short periods of time—usually 15 to 20 seconds. His teachers were patient. Cyril's communication skills grew, and his teachers were delighted with his progress. When Cyril was in sixth grade, he was introduced to a Liberator, which further enhanced his power to communicate (Figure 7-47). Mrs. Lee also introduced him to a Macintosh Powerbook and two pieces of cutting-edge software: Write Out-Loud and Co-Writer. This computer system was exciting on a number of counts:

- The computer fit easily on Cyril's lap tray and had a screen that could be adjusted for easy viewing.
- The Write OutLoud program functioned both as a screen reader and a talking word processor. Cyril could listen to stories that were scanned and "pasted" into the program,

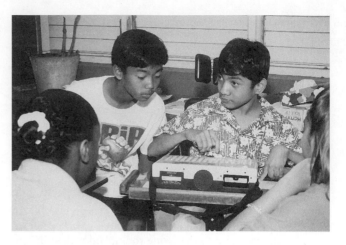

Figure 7-47 Cyril's Liberator allows him to communicate with his classmates.

and he could also compose and print stories that in turn he could "read" aloud.

- The Co-Writer program provided word prediction, which allowed Cyril to type more quickly because he no longer needed to type all the letters of any given word, but Cyril's typing speed was still painstakingly slow—perhaps two or three words per minute.

When Cyril graduated to junior high school, he began to face an entirely new set of assistive technology barriers and issues—perhaps more "human" than "technological." The protective and supportive environment of elementary school dissipated into the frenetic, chaotic life of junior high. Cyril was assigned to a new special education teacher for two daily academic periods, math and language arts; he was mainstreamed for industrial arts, social studies, art, music, and physical education. Cyril's life was not the same on many counts.

Perhaps most significant, Mrs. Lee, Cyril's long-time advocate and therapist, could no longer visit on a regular basis because the junior high was not her home school. When she did visit, it was in the capacity of consultant to Mrs. Batangan, his new special education teacher. Mrs. Batangan knew nothing about computers or augmentative communication devices. She was willing to learn, but she needed more support than Mrs. Lee was able to provide. Little things began going wrong: software files would be lost, programs would crash, and things would fail to print. Further, the small LCD screen on the Powerbook was difficult for Mrs. Batangan to see, and the voice on the Write OutLoud software was hard for her to hear and understand. What she did not know was that an external speaker could have made the voices louder and an external monitor could have made the screen larger. In short, Mrs. Batangan needed learning supports that were unavailable. Cyril paid the price.

Cyril spent most of the day out on the campus in regular classes. Because his family could not afford a powered wheelchair, he was pushed from class to class by a paraprofessional who was assigned as his full-time educational assistant. Cyril felt self-conscious. It simply was not "cool" to be pushed around by an adult in junior high school. Kids stared. "Is that boy sick or what?"

Because the laptop computer and the Liberator would not fit simultaneously on Cyril's lap tray, Mrs. Batangan encouraged him to leave the laptop in the special education room while taking the Liberator with him to regular classes. This seemed appropriate because the Liberator was more than a "talker," it also had its own small printer so that Cyril could both speak and compose typed assignments. Sadly enough, after some months Cyril began refusing to take the Liberator to class. Although some of his classmates were interested and supportive of him, others thought that the robotic voice sounded funny, and they even pressured Cyril to enter four-letter words and "off-color" phrases, which got him and others into trouble. Finally, one day Cyril refused to use the Liberator altogether.

To compound Cyril's sense of isolation, he was unable to participate in any before- or after-school social activities. The wheelchair accessible van delivered him to school just minutes before the ringing of the homeroom bell and then whisked him back home before the final period had even ended. Every day, 5-minutes before the final bell, Cyril was in the van and heading home. There was no time to hang out or say good-bye.

Cyril arrived home daily at 3 o'clock. He remained in the living room watching television, typing assignments on the Liberator, and strumming music on a Suzuki Omnichord.

Cyril had always loved listening to his mother's singing and to music on the television and radio, but he had never been able to produce music himself—that is, until the discovery of a remarkable electronic keyboard loaned to him by faculty at the university. With the Omnichord, Cyril pushed buttons, one at a time, to select and change chords, tempos, and instrument sounds; he then gently rubbed his finger on a touch-sensitive pad to strum the octaves. His parents became enthusiastic about the instrument because they had never seen Cyril so involved and happy. They wished they could afford to purchase one themselves, but it cost nearly $300.

Of increasing concern to Cyril's teachers and therapists was the fact that he did not immerse himself in reading. Cyril was at the age where he should have been celebrating the world of children's literature by living inside the world of books. Cyril's poor reading habits were attributed to the fact that it was impossible for him to turn the pages of most books and magazines. He simply did not have the manual dexterity to do so. He could not quite get one page to turn at a time. There are, of course, many alternative strategies available, including:

- Reading aloud with peers every day
- Listening to books on tape (including free equipment loans from the Library for the Blind)
- Reading books on CD-ROM with the laptop
- Reading stories that have been scanned onto disk and "pasted" into his Write OutLoud text-to-speech program

All these strategies can make books and stories accessible to Cyril. The challenge is to provide the necessary organizational and technology supports, which currently the school simply cannot seem to muster.

Cyril's situation illustrates both the empowering possibilities of assistive technology and the very real human barriers and frustrations that must be faced. For Cyril to feel good about learning, he needs to be accepted by his peer group and become a part of the social life of his school and community. His peers can be trained to push his wheelchair, assist him with his computer and "talker," and enjoy learning with him. To make this possible, however, Cyril's teachers need ongoing training, support, and enthusiastic encouragement—factors that are just as important as all the hardware and software that has been acquired.

As expressed by a classmate in his art class, "Cyril can't walk, talk, or use his hands very well, but he's got a wheelchair and a talker, so that shouldn't have to be a problem." Cyril's classmate is right. It should not have to be a problem. Recently, when this writer asked Cyril how he was doing, Cyril thought for a minute, smiled wistfully, and then slowly and painstakingly typed a message: "I am lonely. I want to play football. I want friends." Cyril, you deserve it.

Cyril's Assistive Technologies for Learning and Communication

Liberator

The Prentke-Romich Company produces an extensive line of "dedicated" augmentative communication devices, with the Liberator at the top. With a Min-Speak mnemonic structure, users can access unlimited numbers of prestored messages, and produce novel, spontaneous utterances. The device includes a small built-in printer to permit written communication. It can also function as an input device for commercial computers. The company provides excellent customer support in accessing funding resources.

Prentke Romich Company 1-800-262-1984

Co-Writer Word Prediction Software

Even under optimal circumstances, word processing is very slow for Cyril. He is able to access the laptop computer's keyboard with his right index finger, but his "hunt and peck" style takes time. The Co-Writer software reduces the number of required keystrokes to type words. With each letter that Cyril types, the software displays a "prediction list" of the words it thinks Cyril may be trying to type. The list becomes more refined with each additional letter Cyril types. Usually the software can "predict" his word within 2 or 3 keystrokes.

Don Johnston, Inc. 1-800-999-4660

Internet Connection

Given Cyril's difficulties in accessing printed information, an Internet connection for him would be very appropriate. Using the World Wide Web, Cyril can research his reports, save and edit pictures and text, and in this way benefit from the "global library" like everyone else. It would also permit him to develop electronic pen pals via e-mail to compensate for some of the many hours he spends home alone. Unlimited Internet connectivity costs approximately $20 per month.

Omnichord

The Omnichord is a powerful "strum" instrument that can be fully accessed with a single switch and/or button pushes and light-touch pressure on a membrane pad. It is ideal for Cyril, given his severely restricted hand and finger movement. The instrument is portable and comes with a hard carrying case. It is even appropriate for Cyril's participation in orchestra, band, or music classes.

Suzuki Corporation 1-619-566-9710

Talking Book Player

Many teachers and parents are unaware that the "talking books" and "recordings for the blind" are available to anyone who has a print-related disability. Cyril qualifies because he is unable to turn the pages of books. This national service provides tape players and unlimited access to recorded books at no charge. It provides a wonderful opportunity for Cyril to fall in love with children's literature during those hours that he now spends in front of the television.

Contact your local library for details

Resources, Training, and Financial Issues

Andrew, Rik, Luke, and Cyril present many challenges to their inclusion teams. Each requires a broad range of assistive technology supports for play, learning, socialization, and communication. Their teams require ongoing inservice training and consultation supports. If one or several members of the team are already computer literate, a 2-day inservice training with monthly follow-ups may be adequate. Who will provide the training, and how will it be paid for? This must be discussed and written into each child's IEP. Perhaps the training can be provided by a district level inservice training team or a local university. Whatever the case, it is essential that all team members actively participate—PT and PTA, speech therapist, inclusion specialist, mainstream teacher and educational assistant, school technology resource teacher, and, of course, the parents.

There is also the issue of funding. How will we pay for training, equipment, and software? Can creative arrangements be designed that allow for cost-sharing across agencies, community groups, insurance carriers, and families? We are in a society that is not accustomed to cost-sharing. Often we hear, "If it is in the IEP, then the school must pay," or "Wheelchairs are covered only by insurance," or "Home computers are the family's responsibility." This restrictive form of thinking stifles creative problem solving.

In 1988 Congress passed the Technology Related Assistance Act for Individuals with Disabilities, typically known as the "Tech Act." The rationale for this legislation was a growing national recognition that technology is making a significant impact on everyone's lives and may be making particular impact on the lives of persons with disabilities. If we do not make a concerted national effort to identify and make available technologies for individuals with disabilities, many will never have access. This legislation has resulted in "Tech Act" projects in every state providing technology information and support.

Several years ago the Apple Corporation sponsored development of nonprofit organizations across the United States to support persons with disabilities and their families to find computer solutions for leisure, learning, and communication. These organizations are now known as the Alliance for Technology Access (ATA). They currently function independently of Apple and, in fact, are supported by a broad spectrum of computer software and hardware industries. ATA centers exist in every state. They typically provide hands-on opportunities for demonstration and loan of equipment. Individuals can borrow computers and software to try in their homes before purchasing. Some of the centers also loan switch toys.

Other resources for technology include the Council for Exceptional Children (CEC), which has a division on technology and media (TAM). TAM publishes a journal on technology and media that provides essential information to teachers and administrators. RESNA is a national organization of people interested in promoting technology for people with disabilities. By contacting any one of these groups, an interested person can find out about all of them.

The goal is not just finding a "technology fix" but creatively looking at individual situations and seeing what possibilities exist, especially given the new and changing technologies. Start by assuming that what children really need can be acquired, if an appropriate support team is mobilized. Begin by contacting your local Alliance for Technology Access Center (1-415-455-4575) and your lead office of the Tech Act (1-703-524-6686). Both of these organizations can provide creative suggestions for assistive technology assessment, funding, training, and consultation.

Conclusions and Reflections

Assistive technologies are opening doors of great opportunities and possibilities. Even 5 years ago, most of what we have considered in this section would have been unattainable and perhaps even unimaginable.

As members of inclusion teams, we must understand that we are all embarking on a course of lifelong learning. If computers, for example, open great opportunities for individuals with disabilities, then we as providers and parents must learn to imagine those possibilities and acquire the skills to make them realities—even if it means weekend workshops, summer courses at the university, Internet dialogues, or, reading technical manuals.

We must collaborate as team members. Children play, communicate, learn, and grow through many diverse activities. Although the new technologies offer great possibilities, they also require creative problem solving, so that children can get on with the natural process of childhood.

Ultimately the issue comes down to opening ourselves to technological change. We now are immersed in the "information society." Fortunately for persons with differing abilities, much of this cyber society can be made "accessible" regardless of physical, emotional, or cognitive differences. We are limited only by our imaginations.

EXERCISES

1. Research local agencies that assist programs and families with assistive technology. What services do they provide (help with funding, loan bank, assessment, information and referral, etc.)? What technologies do they address?
2. Andrew wants to sit in the sandbox to play with his peers. Develop three different activities to address this goal during therapy. Share your ideas with classmates.

QUESTIONS TO PONDER

1. A parent questions you about the prognosis for walking for her 2-year-old child with severe spastic diplegia. How will you respond? What should your role as a PTA be in responding to parent concerns such as this?
2. What should be the role of the school system in paying for computers and augmentative communication devices for school-aged children who need them? What about power wheelchairs?

Annotated Bibliography

Finnie, N. R. (1975). *Handling the young cerebral palsied child at home.* New York: Dutton-Sunrise.

Although more than 20 years old, this book is still a fountain of information. In a friendly manner it presents activities of daily living for children with cerebral palsy. Simple line drawings illustrate carrying and positioning techniques, construction of adapted equipment from available materials, and ways of feeding, bathing, and playing with children who have cerebral palsy. Many therapists have "grown up" on this book and still find the information useful and timely.

Alliance for Technology Access (1996). *Computer resources for people with disabilities: A guide to exploring today's assistive technology.* Alameda, CA: Hunter House.

This is an indispensable guide to assistive technology possibilities and resources for home, school, and workplace. This book can make a tremendous difference. It describes problem-solving strategies and lists helpful resources and references, including the following:

- Alliance for Technology Access Centers
- State Tech Act Programs
- Americans with Disabilities Act
- Assistive Technology Organizations
- National Conferences
- Publications
- Telecommunications Resources
- Technology Vendors

This guide is available from Hunter House Inc., P.O. Box 2914, Alameda, CA 94501-0914 (1-800-266-5592) for $17.95.

References

Armstrong, P. L., Sauls, C. D., & Goddard-Finegold, J. (1987). Neuropathologic findings in short-term survivors of intraventricular hemorrhage. *American Journal of Diseases of Children, 147,* 617-621.

Ayres, A. J. (1979). *Sensory integration and the child.* Los Angeles: Western Psychological Services.

Beals, R. K. (1966). Spastic paraplegia and diplegia: An evaluation of non-surgical and surgical factors influencing the prognosis for ambulation. *Journal of Bone and Joint Surgery, 48a,* 827-846.

Bleck, E. E. (1987). *Orthopaedic management in cerebral palsy.* Clinics in Developmental Medicine No. 99/100. Suffolk, Great Britain: Mac Keith Press.

Bleck, E. E., & Nagel, D. A. (1982). *Physically handicapped children: A medical atlas for teachers* (2nd ed.) New York: Grune & Stratton.

Churchill, J. (1958). The relationship of Little's disease to premature birth. *American Journal of Diseases of Children. 96,* 32.

Crothers, B., & Paine, R. S. (1959). *Natural history of cerebral palsy.* Cambridge: Harvard University Press.

Davies, P., & Tizard, J. (1975). Very low birth weight and subsequent neurological defect. *Developmental Medicine and the Child 17,* 3.

Davis, R., Barolat-Romana, G., & Engle, H. (1980). Chronic cerebellar stimulation for cerebral palsy—5 year study. *Acta Neurochirurgica, supplement 30,* 317-322.

Eckersley, P. M., & King, L. (1993). Treatment systems. In P. M. Eckersley, *Elements of paediatric physiotherapy* (pp. 323-341). Edinburgh: Churchill Livingstone.

Ellenberg, J. H., & Nelson, K. B. (1979). Birthweight and gestational age in children with cerebral palsy or seizure disorders. *American Journal of Diseases of Children, 133,* 1044-1048.

Franco, S., & Andrews, B. (1977). Reduction of cerebral palsy by neonatal intensive care. *Pediatric Clinics of North America 24,* 639.

Gage, J. R. (1991). *Clinics in developmental medicine No. 121: Gait analysis in cerebral palsy.* New York: Mac Keith Press.

Gans, B. M., & Glenn, M. B. (1990). Introduction. In M. B. Glenn & J. Whyte (Eds.), *The practical management of spasticity in children and adults.* Philadelphia: Lea & Febiger.

Gersh, E. S. (1991). Medical concerns and treatments. In E. Geralis (Ed.), *Children with cerebral palsy: A parent's guide.* Bethesda, MD: Woodbine House.

Hagberg, B. (1978). The epidemiological panorama of major neuropediatric handicaps in Sweden. In J. Apley (Ed.), *Care of the handicapped child. Clinics in developmental medicine, No. 67.* Philadelphia: J. B. Lippincott.

Haley, S. M., & Inacio, C. A. (1990). Evaluation of spasticity and its effect on motor function. In M. B. Glenn & J. Whyte (Eds.), *The practical management of spasticity in children and adults* (pp. 70-96). Philadelphia: Lea & Febiger.

Hohman, L. B. (1953). Intelligence levels in cerebral palsied children. *American Journal of Physical Medicine, 32,* 282-290.

Hugenholtz, H., Humphreys, P., McIntyre, W. M., Sparof, R. A., & Steel, K. (1988). Cervical spinal cord stimulation for spasticity in cerebral palsy. *Neurosurgery, 22,* 707-714.

Milani-Comparetti, A. (1980). Pattern analysis of normal and abnormal development: The fetus, the newborn, the child. In D. Slaton (Ed.), *Development of movement in infancy.* Chapel Hill, NC: University of North Carolina.

Milani-Comparetti, A., & Gidoni, E. A. (1967). Pattern analysis of motor development and its disorder. *Developmental medicine and child neurology, 9,* 625.

Molnar, G. E. (Ed.). (1985). *Pediatric rehabilitation.* Baltimore: Williams & Wilkins.

Nelson, C. A. (1995). Cerebral palsy. In D. A. Umphred (Ed.), *Neurological rehabilitation* (3rd ed), St. Louis: Mosby.

Nelson, K. B., & Ellenberg, J. H. (1978). Epidemiology of cerebral palsy. In B. S. Schoenberg (Ed.), *Advances in neurology* (Vol. 19, pp. 421-435). New York: Raven Press.

Niswander, K. R., & Gordon, M. (1972). The collaborative perinatal project. *The women and their pregnancies,* (DHEW Publication No. 73-379). Washington, DC: U.S. Government Printing Office.

Paneth, N., & Kiely, J. (1984). The frequency of cerebral palsy: A review of population studies in industrialized nations since 1950. In F. Stanley & E. Alberman (Eds.), *The epidemiology of the cerebral palsies. Clinics in developmental medicine No. 87* (pp. 46-56). Philadelphia: Lippincott.

Peacock, W. J., Arens, L. J., & Berman, B. (1987). Cerebral palsy spasticity: Selective dorsal rhizotomy. *Pediatric Neuroscience, 13.* 61-66.

Perlstein, M. (1952). Infantile cerebral palsy: Classification and clinical observations. *JAMA, 149:*30

Robinson, R. O. (1973). The frequency of other handicaps in children with cerebral palsy. *Developmental Medicine and Child Neurology, 15,* 305.

Russman, B. S., & Gage, J. R. (1989). Cerebral palsy. *Current Problems in Pediatrics, 29,* 75.

Scherzer, A. L., & Tscharnuter, I. (1982). *Early diagnosis and therapy in cerebral palsy.* New York: Marcel Dekker.

Stanley, F., & Blair, E. (1984). Postnatal risk factors in the cerebral palsies. In F. Stanley & E. Alberman (Eds.), *The epidemiology of the cerebral palsies: Clinics in developmental medicine No. 87* (pp. 135-149). Philadelphia: J.B. Lippincott.

Styer-Acevedo, J. (1994). Physical therapy for the child with cerebral palsy. In J. S. Tecklin (Ed.), *Pediatric physical therapy* (2nd ed, pp. 89-134). Philadelphia: J. B. Lippincott.

Waltz, J. M., Andreeson, W. H., & Hunt, D. P. (1987). Spinal cord stimulation and motor disorders. *Pace-pac Clinical Electrophysiology, 10,* 180-204.

Waltz, J. M., & Davis, J. A. (1983). Cervical cord stimulation in the treatment of athetosis and dystonia. *Advances in Neurology, 37,* 225-237.

Whittaker, C. K. (1980). Cerebellar stimulation in cerebral palsy. *Journal of Neurosurgery, 52,* 648-653.

Wilson, J. M. (1984). Cerebral palsy. In S. K. Campbell (Ed.), *Clinics in physical therapy: Pediatric neurologic physical therapy* (pp. 353-413). New York: Churchill Livingstone.

Genetic Disorders

KEY TERMS

genetic disorders
school-based therapy
inclusion
integrated goals
integrated therapy
Down syndrome
spinal muscular atrophy
Duchenne muscular dystrophy
Prader-Willi syndrome
osteogenesis imperfecta
back care
transfer
mechanical lift
handling
positioning
adaptive equipment

8

CASE STUDY   Rik, A Boy With Spinal Muscular Atrophy

Rik leaned toward his friend Michael, a sparkle in his eye and a black felt-tipped pen balanced in his right hand. He was careful not to lean too far so he would not fall, but the black pen moved closer and closer to Michael's clean white shirt. Michael tucked his chin close to his chest to watch the drama unfold, and when a solid black dot appeared on his chest, both boys sat back, caught each other's eye, and laughed. Children milled around them, busy with their own tasks. The teacher, Mrs. Chin, and the teacher's aide, Mrs. Young, were busy helping children with their writing assignments and setting up the various center-based play

areas. Rik leaned precariously toward Michael with his pen raised toward Michael's face. Michael, even more interested in the game now, leaned closer to Rik to help get his face close enough. When he felt the cold prick of the pen touch his cheek, he pulled away and looked at Rik's face to see if they had been successful. Rik grinned widely, and Michael doubled over in glee. The boys slowly, as in a dance, leaned toward each other to repeat their game. The teacher's aide noticed what they were doing and rushed over, taking the pen away. She separated the boys and focused Michael's energy toward the white worksheet in front of him. It had a large "B" on it. Michael was supposed to trace the "B" and copy it multiple times on the paper.

Mrs. Young then sat down beside Rik and set up a Toshiba laptop computer. She opened up a program called KIDPIX and had Rik use the mouse to choose the "B." Using the mouse, he could then stamp "B" all over the screen, just like Michael was doing on his paper.

Developmental History

Rik was the firstborn child of his Japanese-American mother, Jenny, and Jewish-American father, Ben (Figure 8-1). Both parents are highly educated professionals. Rik weighed 7 pounds, 7 ounces, and was born by natural childbirth in a hospital in New York City. He received only breast milk until he was 8 months old and was a charming infant. It was not until he was 6 months old that anything was noted to be abnormal in his development. His mother had noticed that he was not rolling, but thought that it was due to his being a chubby infant. At his 6-month checkup, the pediatrician was concerned about Rik's delay in gross motor development, absence of deep tendon reflexes, and low muscle tone, and referred the family to a pediatric neurologist.

At 8 months of age, Rik finally was able to see the neurologist. His mother remembers another mother in the waiting room asking her, "What's wrong with your baby?" At that point, she was still unsure that anything was really wrong, and replied, "Nothing." The neurologist soon put to rest any hopes that Rik might escape problems with a firm list of possible diagnoses. The one his parents feared the most was spinal muscular atrophy. The neurologist said that this was only a slim possibility but that the disease was fatal. After blood tests, an electromyogram, then a muscle biopsy, and several weeks of living with increasing anxiety, Rik's parents were informed that he indeed had spinal muscular atropy, type II. They were told that children with type II spinal muscular atrophy generally live until adolescence and frequently die from respiratory complications.

Rik was referred to a state-run infant development program near their home. As his primary caregiver, his mother took him

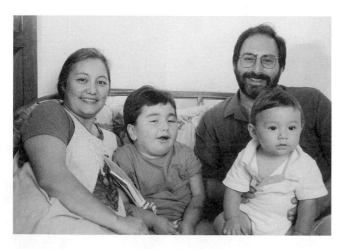

Figure 8-1 Rik's Power Ranger sword figures prominently in a family portrait. He also has temporary Power Ranger tattoos on both arms.

there one to two times per week and he received multiple services from a team of professionals. Services included physical therapy, occupational therapy, speech language pathology, and education. An individualized family service plan (IFSP) was written for Rik, emphasizing goals that his family thought were important for him. Jenny was instructed how to position Rik, how to carry him, what types of equipment might allow him to sit up, and how to encourage his development in many ways. She became comfortable with the staff and believed that they had Rik's and the family's best interests in mind. Rik also received services from Shriners Hospital for Children. Shriners addresses orthopedic problems in children through surgery, rehabilitation from the surgery, and mobility equipment needs. They helped Rik by supplying him with an Orlau walker when he was 3 years old and encouraging his standing. They also followed his orthopedic needs. The Muscular Dystrophy Association supplied a stander for Rik when he outgrew the Orlau walker. When Rik was 4 years old, the othopedic surgeon at Shriners thought that, because of subluxation of both hips, standing might cause future joint erosion and subsequent pain, so his standing program was discontinued.

When Rik turned 3 years old, he was no longer able to be served by the infant development program. He was referred to the Department of Education (DOE), which provides services to children from 3 to 5 years old under Public Law 94-457. His family did not want him in a special education preschool, however. They thought that Rik would do better in a private Montessori program near their home. A special grant-funded project at the local university assisted in working with the preschool and the DOE to accommodate Rik in the Montessori program. It was while in the preschool situation that Rik finally began to talk. Once he started, he found he had a lot to say! Because Rik was not able to manipulate his environment manually, he found power in his voice.

During his preschool years, many strides were made in his functional skills through the use of assistive technology. He was introduced to the computer and found he could manipulate a mouse control. Rik tried and passed the test for using a power wheelchair at Shriners when he was only 2½ years old. Unfortunately, it took longer for funding to be obtained to purchase him his own wheelchair. His medical insurance company refused to pay, although they agreed to pay for a manual wheelchair. Their rationalization was that his condition was fatal. When Rik was 4 years old, after a year and a half of frustration and repeated denials from his medical insurance, Shriners agreed to purchase him his own power wheelchair .

Getting the power chair was even more of an adjustment for his parents than when Rik learned to talk! All of a sudden he could leave the room by himself. Suddenly, they had to teach him what "NO" meant! Rik learned very quickly, but had no fear. When he was 4 years old, Rik drove himself off some steps and landed upside down with the wheelchair on top of him. Luckily, neither he nor the wheelchair were hurt, except for a few superficial scrapes. He learned a healthy respect for gravity, however.

When Rik started kindergarten, his parents were certain that they wanted him in a fully included classroom. They wanted him attending school with other children of all abilities. The preschool transition program at the university again assisted in helping him get the support he needed to be a member of the kindergarten class at his home school.

Rik at School

Rik received the services of a team of professionals through the DOE. His team members included (1) Rik, (2) his parents, (3) his teacher, (4) a psychologist, (5) a physical therapist (PT), (6) an occupational therapist (OT), (7) a speech-language pathologist, (8) a nurse, (9) an educational assistant, and others including the principal and other members of the school staff. He received a comprehensive evaluation on being admitted into the DOE. A summary of key findings in his physical therapy evaluation can be found in Box 8-1.

Rik's physical and occupational therapists provided consultative services to his teacher and educational aide. Their job was to support his educational goals. They came into the classroom to observe how Rik fit into the flow of the day. Sometimes they came together so that they could discuss ideas and adaptations with each other and the teacher before making any decisions. They consulted his teacher at the beginning of the school year to help troubleshoot any problems that were immediately apparent, and again after a month or two of school. They also were available whenever the educational assistant or teacher asked for their help.

Rik "walks" to school accompanied by his mother or a nanny

BOX 8-1   ## Physical Therapy Evaluation Summary: Rik

Social and Medical History
Addressed in the Case Study.

Range of Motion
All within normal limits except for limitations in the following:
   Cervical rotation: 45 degrees to right, 40 degrees to left, both limited by pain, soft end feel
   Elbow flexion: −25 degrees on right, −20 degrees on left, hard end feel bilaterally
   Knee flexion: −45 degrees bilaterally, hard end feel
   Ankle plantar flexion: −10 degrees bilaterally, resilient end feel
   Hip internal rotation: Normal range but soft end feel is limited by pain bilaterally
   Hip external rotation: Hypermobile bilaterally
   Spine: Functional kyphosis in thoracic spine with lack of lumbar lordosis, structural right thoracic scoliosis with mild right rib hump

Muscle Strength
Grossly, strength is in the poor ranges with some distribution to trace and fair minus in some muscle groups. In general muscles in his right upper extremity are stronger than his left, and muscles in his left lower extremity are stronger than his right. Functional strength assessed through observation follows:
   Fair minus (moves partial range against gravity) strength: Cervical rotation (bilateral), cervical lateral flexion (bilateral), shoulder internal and external rotation (left), elbow flexion (left), forearm supination and pronation (left), ankle plantar flexion and dorsiflexion (right, plantar flexion only on left), knee extension (right).
   Poor (moves through partial range, but not against gravity): Cervical flexion, cervical extension, elbow flexion (right), forearm pronation and supination (right), wrist flexion and extension (left), finger flexion and extension (left).
All other groups are absent, trace, or poor minus—not functional strength for Rik.

Muscle Tone and Bulk
Muscle tone is flaccid or extremely hypotonic throughout. Muscle bulk is difficult to ascertain as muscles are difficult or impossible to palpate.

Reflexes and Developmental Reactions
Deep tendon reflexes are absent, or unpalpable. Primitive reflexes appear appropriately integrated and do not influence movement. Balance reactions are limited by lack of strength. Balance reactions are present minimally in sitting, Rik can identify neutral and maintain his head and trunk in a balanced position until jostled or fatigued. He is unable to right his head or trunk against gravity. Balance reactions in any other position are not tested. He has no protective responses.

Mobility Skills
Rik is dependent in all mobility when in bed, in a seating device, or on the floor. He cannot roll or sit up without maximum assistance. When in his power wheelchair, however, he is independent in his mobility. He can turn the power on and off and change the level of speed without assistance. He can negotiate narrow doorways, obstacles, and uneven surfaces well. He has run over classmates' feet several times when they were standing very close to his wheelchair because of being unable to see them, but, when informed of obstacles near him or behind his chair, he demonstrates good judgment. He has developed a technique to facilitate head righting in his wheelchair. When his head flops forward (usually after going over a bump or uneven ground), he will accelerate the wheelchair, using the momentum to right his head.

Transfers
Rik is dependent in all transfers. The method used by his parents and home caregivers, which was taught to his educational assistant at school by his mother, is as follows. The caregiver stands in front of Rik and turns off the power to his chair. His pelvic belt is undone, and the caregiver grasps Rik under his arms with her hands. Rik is then lifted up and out of the wheelchair and laid carefully against the caregiver, shifting her arms to his bottom. His head leans over her shoulder. He is carried in this way to where they need to go (the bathroom, the bed, an alternate seating device). When he is put down again, the caregiver moves one arm behind Rik's back to support his back and head as he is put down.

Functional Positions
Addressed in the Case Study.

Continued

BOX 8-1   ## Physical Therapy Evaluation Summary: Rik—cont'd

Adaptive Equipment

Adaptive equipment used by Rik includes:

- Quickie P5000 power wheelchair with planar seating components: I back, lateral trunk supports, hip guides, lap tray, one-piece foot support, 3-piece angled head support.
- Padded wooden adjustable chair with arm support for use in classroom. No head, trunk, or foot support.
- Television pillow for use during floor activities in the classroom. Another pillow is at home.
- Jogging stroller for use at the beach.
- Lap desk for eating when propped in the corner of the couch.
- Toshiba laptop computer with attachable trackball (attaches to side of keyboard). This goes back and forth to school with Rik.
- PVC-type adjustable bath chair.
- Commercially available plastic lawn chair used as a shower chair and as a beach chair.
- Commercially available folding plastic lawn chair for alternative seating at home.
- Custom-made table for wheelchair access. This is currently stored at home but was made for Rik's use in preschool.
- Custom, removable wooden ramps for access between levels in the home and into the back door.
- Motorcycle ramps that were cut shorter and are used to put Rik's wheelchair in and out of the family minivan.
- Toddler safety seatbelt stabilizer for use in the front seat of the family van.
- Light plastic cup with built-in straw.

Activities of Daily Living

Rik can assist with some skills of daily living.

- Bathing: Rik uses a PVC pipe bath chair with webbing support in the bathtub. It has a reclining back feature to allow his hair to be washed. He prefers to use it in a more upright position so he can play in the water. He also uses a plastic lawn chair to shower.
- Eating: Rik is able to use a spoon or fork but prefers to eat finger foods that he can pick up more easily. He can feed himself unless the food is more complicated or there is a time constraint. He drinks from a commercially available plastic cup with a built-in straw.
- Toileting: Rik informs adults around him when he needs to use the bathroom. He is dependent in undressing, transferring to the toilet, and wiping himself. He can assist in maintaining his balance on the toilet if provided with a stable base of support but needs close supervision to prevent falls.
- Dressing: Rik is dependent in all dressing skills.
- Oral Care: Rik can assist in brushing his teeth but needs help to do a thorough job.
- Respiratory Care: Rik can hold the funnel for his aerosol treatments and can breathe the steam independently.

Recreation and Leisure

Addressed in the Case Study.

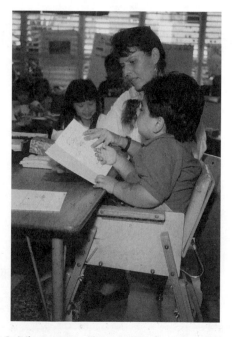

Figure 8-2 Rik sits in an adapted chair that allows him to be the same height as his classmates so he can sit at the kindergarten-height tables. Rik's full-time educational assistant helps him manipulate his work materials.

in the mornings. He drives himself to the classroom in low gear because of the concern about colliding with other children on the busy walkways in the morning. He is assisted in the classroom by Mrs. Young, his educational assistant, who spends all day with him. When Rik sits at the group table with three other children, he is transferred into a padded wooden adaptive chair, which can be pulled up to the table (Figure 8-2). The table serves as his upper extremity support, and a foam block plus a large book are used under his feet to support his legs. Mrs. Young helps Rik use the laptop computer that he brings from home for academic activities. He has a trackball that is attached to the side of the computer, but it is difficult for him to move his arm far enough to the side to easily access the trackball.

Rik uses a soft, weighted television pillow when he sits on the floor with the other children to listen to his teacher, Mrs. Chin. The pillow has to be propped up with his wooden chair behind it so it will not slide on the floor, and therefore he sits slightly behind all the other children. He usually listens attentively but frequently slides sideways on the pillow and has to be repositioned by Mrs. Young.

During center-based activities, Rik frequently chooses large-sized Legos, because he can manipulate these himself and build wonderful, fanciful creations such as a "Ninja Star." He is transferred back into his wheelchair, so he can use his lap tray to support his activities with the Legos. Other children are in different centers around the room including the painting center, where two easels are set up side by side; the household center with a

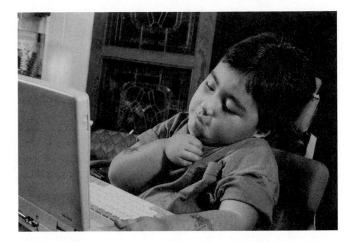

Figure 8-3 Rik uses a laptop computer to accomplish some curriculum objectives. He can sit in his wheelchair and have the computer positioned on his lap tray. He uses a trackball to move the cursor around the screen and to access an on-screen keyboard because he has difficulty reaching all corners of the keyboard efficiently.

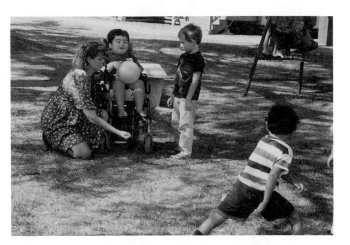

Figure 8-4 An adapted physical education teacher helped to develop this game that Rik can play at recess with his classmates. When Rik rolls the ball off his lap, Mrs. Young hits it up into the air so his classmates can chase and retrieve it.

cash register, plastic food, and dress up clothes; the block center; book corner; and finger painting center. Rik works alone on his lap tray, but other children stop and talk to him or admire his Legos creation as they walk by (Figure 8-3).

At recess, Rik lines up with the other children, files out to the playground, and eats his snack from home in the shade of the trees on the edge of the playground. Mrs. Young or a friend helps him to open his snack. When the food is gone, Rik shifts into high gear and takes off across the playground, bouncing between groups of children and talking to everyone. His friend Steven keeps pace with him, running to keep up. Rik has a creative method of righting his head. When he goes over bumps on the uneven ground, his head frequently bounces too far beyond his balance point to keep it upright and it falls forward. Rik simply accelerates and uses the momentum to right his head. Once, when he ran into a wall because he did not stop soon enough, his head fell forward and he could not right it. Steven helped him right his head and helped him get his hand back on the joystick. Then Rik was off again, Steven loping beside him.

After recess, while the rest of the class sits on the floor to listen to a lesson from Mrs. Chin, Rik goes to the bathroom. He is allowed to drive in high gear to the bathroom because the other children are in their classrooms and not on the walkways. Mrs. Young goes with him to help. She transfers him to a padded wooden table in the corner of the boys bathroom to remove his pants, and then carries him to the toilet. The stall is small enough that Rik can prop himself on the toilet, but he needs help to wipe. Then he is transferred back to the table, his pants are put back on, and he is repositioned in his wheelchair. He drives at high speed back to the classroom with Mrs. Young trailing behind him.

At lunch time, Rik lines up with his class to go to the cafeteria. He goes through the line with Mrs. Young holding his tray. He sits at the head of his class's lunch table with Mrs. Young next to him to help him eat. At naptime after lunch, Mrs. Young transfers him to his own thick denim sleeping mat on the hard linoleum floor of the classroom. First he wants to be on his side,

but after a few minutes he asks to be moved onto his back. In comparison to the squirming children lying all over the floor, Rik lies very still.

At afternoon recess Mrs. Chin gives the children a special treat, letting them go out to the playground immediately outside their classroom. Mrs. Young helps organize a ball game. Rik, the center of the game, pushes the ball off his lap and Mrs. Young hits it with her hand so that it rises high in the air over the children. They run shrieking to catch or retrieve it and rush back to lay it on Rik's lap again (Figure 8-4). Other children play on the monkey bars or the slide.

At the end of the school day Mrs. Chin plays music and lets the children dance around the classroom. Rik moves his joystick back and forth to the music, dancing in his chair. The other children dance around Rik but leave him room so they will not get their toes run over! The closing song at the end of the day is sung by all just before the bell rings.

After the first few months of school, during her consultation visit to the classroom, the physical therapist identified the following barriers to Rik's education:

1. The wooden adaptive chair was not providing adequate foot, trunk, or head support for Rik in the classroom.
2. The television pillow was not providing adequate lateral trunk or head support.
3. The television pillow was not stable enough to allow Rik to be positioned within the larger group of children.
4. Rik worked alone when sitting in his wheelchair without opportunities to interact with the other children who were working in groups at tables or on the floor.
5. The current method of transferring Rik was difficult for his educational assistant and was potentially traumatizing his shoulder girdle.
6. Rik has lost range of motion, particularly in his knees, elbows, and ankles, which impacts his ability to assume alternate positions. He is developing a scoliosis and his current wheelchair does not adequately support his spine.

7. Rik was uncomfortable when positioned on the floor for naptime.
8. When Rik was in his wheelchair, because of the size of his chair, he could not be part of the group of children sitting on the floor but had to stay behind the group.
9. Rik lost class time when using the bathroom.

In consultation with his teacher, parents, and educational assistant, remedies were proposed to address the identified barriers. See Box 8-3 (p. 226) after you have thought about how you might address these barriers.

In the fall, the team of people working with Rik developed an individualized education program (IEP) for him. Objectives that integrated his physical, social, emotional, and educational goals were specified with specific criteria for meeting each objective. Think about how you would write goals that integrate his physical needs with his educational curriculum. Then check Box 8-4 at the end of this Case Study (p. 227) to see some sample objectives.

Rik at Home

The family's one-story, rented, three-bedroom home is arranged to accommodate Rik's mobility needs. There are homemade wooden ramps connecting the various one-step level changes in the house. The family areas have large open spaces, so Rik can have access with his wheelchair. Furniture is grouped at the sides of the rooms. Some walls and doorways have gouges from Rik's foot plates when he was in a hurry or misjudged the distance. There is a small pool in the backyard that is used by Rik and his dad when the weather and the water are warm enough. The driveway is a wide expanse of asphalt that provides an accessible play area.

Piled in the corner of the family room, beside the box of Power Ranger weapons, are several adapted high chairs, infant seats, and adapted child-sized chairs, which no longer fit Rik. Next to them sits another high chair for Rik's 10-month-old brother Sean. On the back patio is a baby jogger with large wheels that the family uses to take Rik to the beach, and a back pack for Sean. Next to them is a child-sized plastic lounge chair, which has a tall reclined back and built-in arms and can be buried in the sand for stability. This chair is also used as a shower chair for Rik, although he has almost outgrown it. In the bathroom behind the door is stored a blue mesh and PVC pipe bath chair, with adjustable seat and back angle. In front of the toilet, a low stool leans against the wall, ready to be pulled down to provide a seat for Rik's mother or father as they guard him on the toilet. In Rik's room, his toys are neatly arranged on the closet shelves, and a blue plastic folding chair sits folded at the foot of the bed, ready to provide an alternate seat for Rik to play in or to watch television. A plastic television table doubles as a bedside table. A thin, wheelchair-accessible table is stored in the front entranceway, all but blocking the front door. His parents had the table made when Rik was in preschool, but he does not use it anymore. For more information about the accessibility of Rik's home environment, see Box 8-2.

BOX 8-2   ## Accessibility of Rik's Current Home: Barriers and Benefits

Ben and Jenny were interested in buying a home. They were trying to decide whether to buy the house they were currently renting or to look further. They consulted a physical therapist to assist them in evaluating their home. Together, they identified some barriers and benefits to their current home.

Barriers
1. The house has an inaccessible second bathroom. There is some potential to expand the size or to reconfigure it to make it more accessible.
2. The current bathroom could not accommodate a portable mechanical lift for Rik, but might be able to accommodate a wall- or ceiling-mounted lift.
3. The bedrooms and hallways are small; however, Rik is currently able to negotiate them in his wheelchair. This may change as he grows and needs a larger wheelchair.
4. The standard size doorways have little potential for widening because of the proximity of the bedrooms and bathroom. Rik is able to negotiate the doorways in his current wheelchair, but when he grows out of his pediatric chair, he will have more difficulty.
5. The kitchen appliances are inaccessible for a wheelchair, but there is potential to renovate the kitchen to make it more accessible for Rik.
6. The house has only three bedrooms. With a live-in nanny for Sean and Rik, this prevents each boy from having his own bedroom.

7. Small steps between levels exist to get into the house and to get from the living room area to the family room. These have been made accessible through custom wooden ramps.

Benefits
1. The house is primarily on one level.
2. There is a swimming pool, which can be beneficial for Rik and that the whole family can enjoy.
3. The family living area is continuous and fairly large.
4. There is an enclosed patio area.
5. The house is in proximity to a good elementary school, whose staff are familiar with Rik and are willing to work with the family to include him in regular education classes.
6. The location of the house is close to Ben's job, to a shopping center, and a nice park. It is in a residential neighborhood, which is quiet and peaceful.
7. The house is in an area of the city that is in Ben and Jenny's price range.

Ben and Jenny decided to consult a contractor who specializes in building and renovating homes that are accessible to people with disabilities. They also will explore other houses for sale in the same neighborhood. On the basis of the contractor's estimates for needed renovations, compared with other homes they find for sale in the neighborhood, they will make the decision whether to buy their current home.

Rik's entry into his parent's lives was traumatic and wonderful, as is any child's entry into a family. His subsequent disability and the necessary accommodations challenged his parent's creativity and patience and caused them extreme fatigue, especially during his toddler years. For the first 4 years of Rik's life, his parents took turns getting up an average of eight times per night to change his position in bed. He became uncomfortable after only an hour or so, and cried to be turned. Since he learned to talk and became busier at preschool and kindergarten, he was able to tolerate longer periods without repositioning, and now his parents turn him before they go to bed and get up an average of three times during the night.

Aside from their personal difficulties in reconciling their own needs with Rik's needs and the process they continually go through to come to some understanding of the meaning of his disability in their lives, his parents have been very creative in addressing the practical, everyday needs to allow Rik optimal access to life. They have found commercially available products to allow Rik to participate in family activities, such as his lawn/beach/shower chair, jogging stroller, and lap desk for Rik to eat on when propped in the corner of the couch. They have accessed services in the community to help defray the costs involved in puchasing specialized equipment and services for Rik. They have hired a nanny to take care of Sean during the day and Rik after school until one of them can get home from work. It has not been easy to find someone who is dependable and capable, whom Rik and Sean like, and who gets along with the family.

Each day, his nanny, Melanie, meets Rik at school and waits with Sean while he plays with other children on the playground for about an hour after school. Then they walk home together, companionably wandering down the street, talking about Rik's day or other events of interest. Sean rides in the backpack on Melanie's back. When they get home, Rik is transferred to the corner of the couch where he is propped to eat his snack. He does an aerosol respiratory treatment and plays or watches television. Sean has been home all day and eagerly crawls close to Rik, wanting to be with his older brother. Rik is lifted back into his chair and asks Melanie to call Sara, who lives just down the street, to come over to play. When Sara comes over, they play with Power Rangers or with Sean. Rik has developed a method to teach Sean to walk. He tells Sean to stand up holding onto Rik's footplates and then Rik slowly moves his chair backward, so that Sean has to take steps to keep up. They play at this until Sean tires of it.

When his mother comes home, Rik suggests going to Blimpies for dinner. Sara is included. As soon as his dad walks in the door, they are all outside piling into the van. Rik sits in the front seat, with a toddler seatbelt stabilizer to help him stay upright with the lap and shoulder belts in place (Figure 8-5). Sean sits in the infant safety seat in the back seat. Jenny pulls the ramps out. Two motorcycle ramps have been shortened to fit in disabled parking spaces and are used to put Rik's power chair into the van. Jenny strains a little as she pushes the heavy chair up the steep ramp, but she has learned to use momentum to make the job easier (Figure 8-6). Jenny and Sara sit beside Sean in the back seat, and Ben drives. When they get to Blimpies, the process is reversed. As soon as he is in his chair, Rik is off, trying to push the glass door of the shop open with his metal foot plates until Sara comes and holds it open for him.

After dinner, Sara goes home, and it is bath time for the boys. Sean gets his bath first and comes out all fresh and rosy, while Jenny draws the water for Rik. While the bath water runs, Rik balances on the toilet guarded by his mother (Figure 8-7). His bath chair is put into the tub and bubble bath makes a white carpet of froth. When Rik is lowered into the bubbles, his mother sighs, her back bent over from the waist (Figure 8-8). The layout of the bathroom makes it difficult to use good body mechanics without getting wet, and she has not had time to change from her work clothes yet.

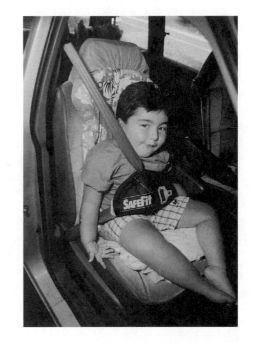

Figure 8-5 Rik sits in a slightly reclined front seat of the car with a toddler seatbelt adapter to help him sit upright.

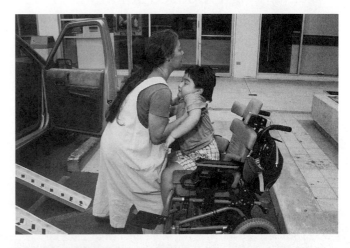

Figure 8-6 Rik's mother transfers him to the van by lifting him under his arms, laying him along her body, and carrying him to the front seat. There is concern about his fragile shoulder girdle, as well as the safety of the caregivers because Rik weighs 70 pounds. The wheelchair is pushed into the van on modified motorcycle ramps.

Rik plays with the bubbles and some small toys, which sit in a basket spanning the width of the tub. Jenny lowers the back of the bath chair to wash his hair and raises it again so that Rik can play. She will not leave him alone in the tub because, if he should slip, he could not recover his balance, and tragedy would result (Figure 8-8). When he is finished playing, he is lifted out of the tub and carried to his bed, where he is thoroughly dried and dressed for bed. There is time before bedtime, so he can play in his wheelchair for awhile.

A few months ago Rik was angry at his parents. He drove himself into his parent's bedroom and backed into the door to slam it shut behind him. He inadvertently fell forward, his arm slipping off the joystick. He could not right himself, nor could he lift his arm to get it back onto the joystick. He was stuck, and his heavy chair was blocking the door so that his parents could not get in to help him.

Jenny and Ben heard a faint voice coming from the bedroom and went to help. They were not sure exactly what had happened and had a hard time understanding Rik's soft voice, which was muffled both by his lap and by the door. They did realize, however, that his chair was blocking the door, and that he could not move. After some frantic moments and futile attempts to push on the door to move the chair, Ben finally went outside and crawled in through the window. Once he got into the room, he easily helped Rik sit up so he could propel himself away from the door. Rik now is much more careful about closing doors.

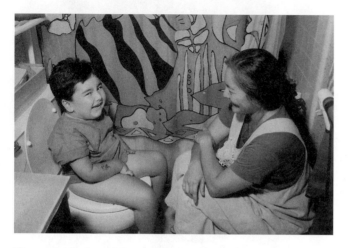

Figure 8-7 Rik can balance on the toilet seat, but he needs a wide base of support, and his mother guards him closely because his balance is precarious.

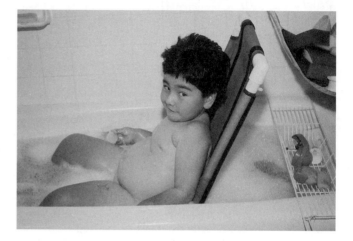

Figure 8-8 Rik enjoys playing in the bathtub in his PVC pipe and nylon mesh bath seat. His bath seat can be reclined to wash his hair.

BOX 8-3   Proposed Solutions to Identified Barriers to Rik's Education

1. The wooden adaptive chair is not providing adequate foot, trunk, or head support for Rik in the classroom.
   - Rik's physical therapist will identify a different adapted chair for Rik's use, which will grow with him over the next few years. It will be adjustable in height and width, will have adjustable trunk supports, adjustable height armrests, adjustable head and foot supports, and will have an adjustable seat to back angle to allow for gravity-assisted positioning, if needed.
2. The television pillow is not providing adequate lateral trunk or head support.
   - A floor sitter on casters will be purchased or found for Rik, which will have head and trunk supports. A Tumble Form floor sitter is one option.
3. The television pillow is not stable enough to allow Rik to be positioned within the larger group of children.
   - Until the floor sitter can be identified, a large piece of Dycem will be used under the television pillow with sandbags to support the pillow from behind so that it can be placed in the middle of the group of children.
4. Rik works alone when sitting in his wheelchair without opportunities to interact with the other children who are working in groups at tables or on the floor.
   - Rik has a small, wheelchair accessible table at home, which his parents had made specifically for his preschool situation. The teacher has identified a place for the table in the classroom and it will be an alternate work center. Other children can stand or sit on stools to participate in an activity alongside Rik.
5. The current method of transferring Rik is difficult for his educational assistant, and is potentially traumatizing his shoulder girdle.
   - An alternate method of transfer was devised and taught to Rik's educational assistant. This entails a seat sling made of heavy fabric that Rik sits on. When being transferred, Rik would be helped to lean forward. His shoulder would rest firmly against the trunk of his caregiver who would then grasp both ends of the sling and lift his bottom and place it on the next positioning device. The sling transfer will not be practical for transferring to the toilet, but in the future, perhaps a modified sling could be made with a hole in it.

BOX 8-3 Proposed Solutions to Identified Barriers to Rik's Education—cont'd

6. Rik has lost range of motion particularly in his knees, elbows, and ankles, which impacts his ability to assume alternate positions. He is developing a scoliosis and his current wheelchair does not adequately support his spine.
   - Range of motion exercises can be provided daily to Rik at school during his naptime by his educational assistant who would be instructed by a physical therapist. Rik's parents will be consulted regarding the implications of his loss of range of motion, so they can decide how vigorous to be in encouraging alternate positioning at home and school to prevent progression of the loss. Alternative seating for his wheelchair will be pursued with Shriners to see whether a more custom back can be obtained for Rik to provide better spinal support.
7. Rik is uncomfortable when positioned on the floor for naptime.
   - A padded sleeping mat will be provided for Rik by his mother. This will be purchased at a camping supply store or a store specializing in exercise equipment.
8. When Rik is in his wheelchair, because of the size of his chair, he cannot be part of the group of children sitting on the floor but needs to stay behind the group.
   - Because his wheelchair is so large, his sitting behind the group may be unavoidable. His educational assistant will take every opportunity to transfer him into a floor sitter, so that he can join the other children, but this will not always be possible.
9. Rik loses class time when using the bathroom.
   - Because of his need for privacy in the bathroom, the timing of his bathroom visits must coincide with the time the other children are in class. If Rik needs to urinate only, a portable urinal can be made available to him so that he does not need to be transferred from his wheelchair. He can use the urinal in the bathroom next to his classroom —the one that all the other children use.

BOX 8-4 Sample Individual Education Program Objectives

By the End of the School Year Rik Will:

1. Use a computer to identify each letter of the alphabet.
2. Use a computer and creative spelling to write at least 10 journal entries about subjects of his choice.
3. Verbally describe for the class a project that he has completed, such as a painting, a Lego construction, or a drawing.
4. Dictate to his educational assistant or teacher at least 10 complete sentences on subjects assigned in class.
5. When given a worksheet scanned into a computer, use the mouse to identify primary colors and color objects appropriately, identify basic shapes (circle, triangle, oval, square, rectangle), and match colors and shapes.
6. Identify each consonant sound and match them to letters or words, either orally or by using a computer.
7. Dictate instructions to a parent, teacher, or educational assistant regarding steps to follow to initiate and complete a project involving scissors and glue.
8. Take turns when speaking in class or participating in group activities.
9. Consistently follow directions regarding rules of classroom behavior, instructions received in class, and rules of playground behavior.
10. Use good judgment to avoid injuring himself or others when operating his power wheelchair in school.
11. Participate in music sessions by singing, dancing in his wheelchair, and using rhythm instruments.
12. Have at least two alternate positions in the classroom so that he can fully participate in a range of activities with the class.

BACKGROUND AND THEORY

Genetics plays a key role in the manifestation of personality, physical characteristics, and abilities that each of us develop. Although we can see that little Emily has Uncle Jim's big nose and Dan has inherited his mother's gentle temperament, genetics plays a more noticeable role in development when things go wrong. Each of 23 pairs of chromosomes in each of our cells has thousands of genes regulating all aspects of our behavior, physiology, and physical characteristics. Possibly all disease processes involve a genetic component through interaction of a genetic predisposition and environmental factors. When genetics plays a direct role in disease processes, however, and if even one gene has a defect, the effects can be profound. Genetic disorders can result in problems as seemingly mild as an extra digit, or as profound as severe mental and physical disability, or death.

It is important for the parents of a child with a genetic disorder to get genetic counseling to assist them in determining the mechanism of transmission of the defect to their child. This knowledge will help alleviate guilt that parents may be feeling for passing on a genetic defect to their child, as well as assist them or their relatives who may share the genetic defect in planning for more children. Physical therapists and physical therapist assistants may see families more often than other health professionals, frequently developing a trusting relationship with them. Although they do not have a direct role in providing genetic counseling, they can refer parents to a geneticist, if needed, and encourage them to follow through with appointments.

This chapter briefly presents the etiology, incidence or prevalence, and underlying neuropathology of a spectrum of genetic disorders. The purpose of surveying an array of disorders is to introduce individual characteristics that will be manifested with specific genetic disorders. Genetic disorders can be differentiated by their specific characteristics.

Subjects discussed in more depth are the clinical symptoms, medical intervention, and the role of physical therapy in treating children with Down syndrome, Prader-Willi syndrome, muscular dystrophy, spinal muscular atrophy, and osteogenesis imperfecta. These disorders were chosen because they represent a range in the classification of genetic disorders, and children with these disorders are frequently seen by a PT for services. We will look at broad and specific treatment strategies for children with these disorders. Many common therapeutic approaches, including working with a team, providing family support, using play in therapy, positioning and handling, and addressing developmental issues, are important for most families and are applied in the context of the specific disease process discussed in the chapter. To get an overview of important therapeutic approaches, the reader is encouraged to read the entire chapter.

An extensive case study of Rik, a boy with spinal muscular atrophy, is presented to stress the importance of understanding the home and school context when working with a child with a genetic disorder.

A special section on handling and positioning (see Applications section, p. 259) presents important concepts for therapy providers that are useful when working with children, or when teaching parents and teachers to handle and position children with disabilities.

Overview of Cellular Reproduction and Its Role in Genetic Disorders of Childhood

The study of genetics is intimidating to many people. It seems complicated and perhaps irrelevant to the day-to-day tasks of working with a child with a disability. It is important, however, to have a grasp of the mechanisms of genetic inheritance to understand differences between types of genetic disorders. This section will provide a basic review, which can be referred to as needed.

As we all learned in high school biology class, deoxyribonucleic acid (DNA) is the genetic material of the cells. All cells have identical genetic material in their molecules of DNA. DNA is composed of two strands of nucleotides (a unit of nucleic acid comprised of sugar, phosphate, and a nitrogenous base). These strands are held together by loose bonds and coiled into a double helix shape. The DNA acts as the structural portion of a chromosome and, along with proteins (which appear to have no effect on the genetic material), forms the chromosomes that are in the nucleus of every cell. Each human cell has 23 pairs of chromosomes.

The function of DNA is to tell the cell how to make certain proteins. It does this through communication with the cell's ribonucleic acid (RNA). Each cell has specific RNA that "reads" various genes in the DNA and then directs the formation of specific proteins, each of which has a particular function within the cell or the body. This difference in specialization explains why some cells in the pancreas make insulin, whereas other cells in the pancreas secrete digestive enzymes. If the genes give erroneous information about how to make the protein, then that protein cannot accomplish the task it was originally intended to do. For instance, in Duchenne's muscular dystrophy, the protein dystrophin is not made. Muscle cells therefore are destroyed, and the result is progressive weakness.

When a cell divides, an exact copy of the DNA is created, so that each "daughter" cell receives a complete copy of the same genetic material. This process is called mitosis. When cell division occurs in the ovum and the sperm, each daughter cell contains only half of the genetic material. This process is called meiosis. When the ovum is fertilized by the sperm, the resultant fertilized ovum has the full complement of genetic material, half provided by each parent.

Problems arise when a disordered gene is duplicated and passed on to offspring, or when a spontaneous mutation occurs to change the function of a specific gene. Problems also occur when a chromosome does not duplicate itself correctly, and a piece or an entire chromosome is either added or deleted from the genetic material in the cell. The following section will give examples of disorders that arise from gene defects or chromosome defects.

Classification of Genetic Abnormalities

Two major types of events can cause genetic defects. These can be classified as chromosomal abnormalities and specific gene defects.

Chromosomal Abnormalities

Chromosomal abnormalities can occur in three ways. The first is a deviation in the number of chromosomes. Monosomies occur when one of the two paired chromosomes in the cells is missing. Children with this type of disorder usually do not live. Autosomal trisomies occur when an extra chromosome is in the pair. Examples of autosomal trisomies include Down syndrome (trisomy 21) (Figure 8-9), Edwards syndrome (trisomy 18), and Patau syndrome (trisomy 13).

A second type of chromosomal abnormality specifically affects the chromosome pair that regulates sexual characteristics. Each child inherits an X chromosome from his or her mother. It is the genetic material inherited from the father that determines the gender of the child. If the child inherits another X chromosome from her father, she will develop as a girl. If the child inherits a Y chromosome, he will develop as a boy. Therefore girls

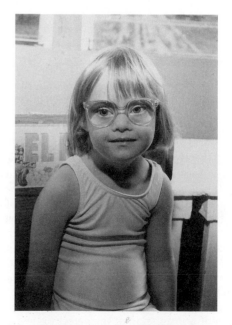

Figure 8-9 Alice is a 5-year-old child with Down syndrome.

have the sex genotype of XX, and boys, XY. Examples of sex chromosome abnormalities include Turner syndrome which is essentially the only viable monosomy. It is also known as gonadal dysgenesis or XO syndrome. In Turner syndrome the paternal sex chromosome is most likely to be missing. Klinefelter syndrome or XXY is the most common sex chromosome abnormality and is due to an extra X chromosome.

The third type of chromosome disorder is a partial deletion syndrome, in which part of one of the chromosomes is missing. Examples of partial deletion syndromes include cri du chat syndrome (5p−), Prader-Willi syndrome (15q−) (see Figure 8-10),

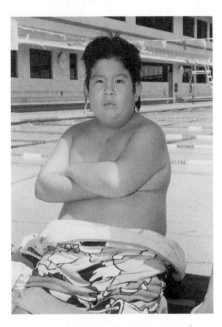

Figure 8-10 Grant is a 12-year-old boy with Prader-Willi syndrome.

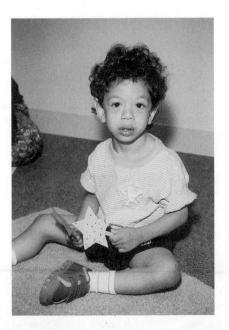

Figure 8-11 Parker is a 3-year-old boy with Williams syndrome.

and Williams syndrome (a deletion near the elastin gene on the seventh chromosome) (Figure 8-11). The notations refer to the number of the specific chromosome pair, the part of the chromosome (p = short arm, q = long arm), and whether a part is missing (−), or added (+).

Each of these syndromes can be detected by prenatal chromosome analysis. Routine screening tests, such as testing the mother's blood for either elevated or decreased levels of maternal serum alpha-fetoprotein (MS-AFP) or ultrasonography of the fetus, can be performed to determine who should get diagnostic tests to rule out chromosomal and other abnormalities. There are several methods of prenatal diagnostic testing for chromosome anomalies, including the testing of amniotic fluid by amniocentesis and chorionic villus sampling. Many mothers do not receive diagnostic chromosome analysis, because they are younger than medical criteria recommends for routine screening by amniocentesis, or parents elect not to do the testing, because they believe the results will not affect their decision of whether to carry the pregnancy to term. Other parents do not have screening or testing available to them, because of lack of prenatal care or lack of financial resources.

Specific Gene Defects

When the disorder is a result of a defect or mutation of a single gene rather than of the chromosome itself, it is called a specific or single-gene disorder. These disorders cannot be detected by chromosome diagnostic tests, and many cannot be detected at all, even by using advanced DNA mapping and linkage procedures. Rapid advances are being made in mapping specific genes, and at least 200 disorders, including Huntington disease, cystic fibrosis, and sickle cell disease, can be detected not only in an affected parent but also in a fetus (Wong, 1995). Direct and indirect genetic tests are run only on persons who are at high risk of having the disorders.

Specific gene defects can occur in one of three ways. The first is an autosomal dominant defect. When a disorder is carried on a dominant gene, only one parent needs to manifest the disorder for it to be present in their offspring. These disorders are sometimes seen as spontaneous mutations in the first generation, but in either case, subsequent generations have a 50% chance of inheriting the disorder. Examples of disorders that have an autosomal dominant inheritance pattern are neurofibromatosis, tuberous sclerosis, and osteogenesis imperfecta.

In disorders with an autosomal recessive pattern of inheritance, the second type of specific gene disorders, each child has a 25% chance of inheriting the disorder from parents who are both unaffected carriers. Each child also has a 50% chance of being a carrier of the disorder and possibly passing it to his or her own children. Disorders that are passed by an autosomal recessive pattern include spinal muscular atrophy (Figure 8-12), sickle cell anemia, Hurler syndrome, and phenylketonuria.

The third type of specific gene disorders are those that are passed through the sex chromosomes and are referred to as sex-linked disorders. The defective gene is usually carried by the mother and passed to her offspring on the X chromosome. If the child is a boy, thereby receiving a Y chromosome from his father, the disorder on the X chromosome is free to manifest itself. If the child is a girl, thereby receiving another X chromosome, the

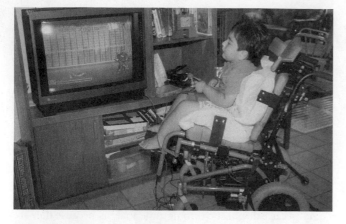

Figure 8-12 Rik, a 5-year-old boy with spinal muscular atrophy, is playing video games. He is sitting in a custom-made foam insert for his wheelchair.

disorder is not expressed because of a second, normal gene on the father's X chromosome. The girl, however, will be a carrier and may pass the disorder to her own children. Examples of specific sex-linked inherited disorders include fragile X syndrome, Duchenne muscular dystrophy, Lowe syndrome, and Lesch-Nyhan syndrome. With few exceptions, all children manifesting sex-linked inherited disorders are boys.

Children with genetic disorders may be seen by a physical therapist in the hospital, outpatient clinic, infant development program, or school for orthopedic and developmental intervention. Services that children might receive from a physical therapist include evaluation, direct therapy, and parent teaching to ameliorate effects of the disability and to optimize functional skills, rehabilitation after surgery, recommendation of equipment to optimize positioning and mobility skills, and coordination with other disciplines who are providing services to the child and family. See Table 8-1 for an overview of the genetic disorders discussed in this section and their typical clinical symptoms.

TABLE 8-1　Overview of Genetic Disorders

Type of disorder	Name of disorder	Clinical features
Chromosome Abnormalities		
Deviation in number of chromosomes	Down syndrome (trisomy 21)	Characteristic facial features including flat occiput, flat face, upward slanting eyes; hypotonicity; broad, short feet and hands; protruding abdomen; mental retardation; possible cardiac anomalies.
	Edwards syndrome (trisomy 18)	Small stature; long, narrow skull; low set ears; hypotonicity; rocker-bottom feet; scoliosis; profound mental retardation.
	Patau syndrome (trisomy 13)	Microcephaly; cleft lip and palate; polydactyly of hands and feet; severe to profound mental retardation.
Deviation in sex chromosomes	Turner syndrome (XO syndrome)	Congenitally webbed neck; growth retardation; ptosis of upper eyelids; lack of sexual development; congenital heart and kidney disease; scoliosis; low normal intelligence.
	Klinefelter syndrome (XXY)	Long limbs; tall and slender build until adulthood when obesity becomes a problem (if no testosterone replacement therapy); small penis and testes; low average to mild mental retardation; tremors, behavior problems.
Partial deletion syndrome	Cri du chat syndrome (5p-)	High-pitched, catlike cry in infancy; microcephaly; low-set ears; hypotonicity; severe mental retardation; scoliosis; clubfeet; dislocated hips.
	Prader-Willi syndrome (15q-)	Low tone with feeding disorder in infancy; insatiable appetite develops in toddlerhood; moderate mental retardation; hyperflexibility; obesity; characteristic facial features including almond-shaped eyes; small stature; small hands and feet; small penis.
	Williams syndrome (deletion near the elastin gene on chromosome 7)	Characteristic facial abnormalities, including prominent lips, medial eyebrow flare, and open mouth; mild microcephaly; mild growth retardation; short nails; mild to moderate mental retardation; cardiovascular anomalies.
Specific Gene Defects		
Autosomal dominant	Neurofibromatosis	Areas of hyperpigmentation or hypopigmentation of skin including "café au lait" spots or axillary "freckling"; tumors along nerves, in connective tissue, eyes or meninges; macrocephaly; short stature. May have skeletal abnormalities including scoliosis, bowing of long bones, and dislocations.
	Tuberous sclerosis	Brain lesions causing seizures and mental retardation; skin lesions on cheeks, around nose; "café au lait" spots; cystlike areas in bones of fingers; kidney and teeth abnormalities.

TABLE 8-1 Overview of Genetic Disorders—cont'd

Type of disorder	Name of disorder	Clinical features
Specific Gene Defects–cont'd		
Autosomal dominant–cont'd	Osteogenesis imperfecta	Type I: Small stature; thin bones; bowing of bones; fractures of long bones; hyperextensible joints; kyphoscoliosis; flat feet; thin skin; deafness in adult life; blue sclerae of eyes; blue or yellow teeth.
		Type II: Prenatal growth deficiency; short limbs; multiple fractures; hypotonia; hydrocephalus; frequent early death.
		Type III: Short stature; bowing and angulation of long bones; multiple fractures; kyphoscoliosis.
		Type IV: Osteoporosis leading to fractures; variable mild deformity of long bones; normal sclerae of eyes; may have poor teeth.
Autosomal recessive	Spinal muscular atrophy	Progressive muscle atrophy and weakness; normal intelligence; normal sensation; weakness may begin before birth, in early childhood, or in later childhood.
	Sickle cell disease	A group of diseases characterized by blood disorders related to hemoglobin defects. Mostly seen in people of African or infrequently of Mediterranean decent. Sickle-shaped red blood cells cause anemia, and crises of blockages in veins, causing a variety of conditions. These include leg ulcers, arthritis, acute pain, and problems in major organ systems, including the spleen, liver, kidney, bones, heart, and central nervous system. Children may exhibit weakness, pain or fever and may have growth retardation.
	Hurler syndrome	Normal or rapid growth during the first year with deterioration during second year; coarse facial features characterized by full lips, flared nostrils, thick eyebrows, low nasal bridge, and prominent forehead; stiff joints; small stature; small teeth, enlarged tongue; kyphosis, short neck; clawhand, hip dislocation and other joint deformities; mental retardation.
	Phenylketonuria	Children cannot metabolize phenylalanine causing mental retardation, growth retardation, hypertonicity, seizures, pigment deficiency of hair and skin if left untreated. Can be successfully treated by limiting amount of phenylalanine in diet.
Sex-Linked Disorders (all affected are boys)	Fragile X syndrome	One of the most common causes of mental retardation in boys. Characteristic facial features include elongated face, large ears and prominent jaw. Other characteristics include enlarged testicles in adulthood, and prolapse of the mitral valve in the heart. Mental retardation is usually in the severe range, sometimes with aggressive behaviors. Some boys will have poor coordination and hypotonia.
	Duchenne muscular dystrophy	Progressive weakness beginning between 2 to 5 years of age; characteristic gait disturbances, including toe walking, abducted gait, lordosis, waddling gait. Progressive weakness leads to wheelchair use, decreased independence in all areas, and finally death by respiratory or cardiac failure.
	Lowe syndrome	Progressive mental deterioration leading to moderate to severe mental retardation, renal dysfunction, cortical cataracts with or without glaucoma leading to blindness later in life, hypotonicity, joint hyperextensibility, growth retardation, large low set ears, pale skin, and blond hair.
	Lesch-Nyhan syndrome	Moderate to severe mental retardation, hypertonicity leading to dislocated hips, club foot, growth retardation, movement disorders including chorea, ballistic movements, and tremor. Self-mutilating behaviors including lip-biting and fingertip-biting characterize this disease.

The Child With Down Syndrome

Incidence and Cause

Down syndrome (DS), also called trisomy 21, is the most common chromosomal abnormality. It occurs in 1:800 live births. Although its cause is unknown, the incidence of DS increases markedly as maternal age increases. Paternal age can also be a factor.

There are three types of DS. Ninety-two to ninety-five percent of all cases are a true trisomy, where an extra chromosome exists on the twenty first pair. The second type (4% to 6% of cases) is a translocation, where the third chromosome is attached to a different pair of chromosomes. This type can be hereditary and is not affected by parental age (Wong, 1995). The third type is a mosaic type, where different cells in the body exhibit either normal or abnormal chromosomes. In this type children's physical and cognitive impairment is related to the percentage of cells that exhibit abnormal chromosomes.

Clinical Features

The physical therapist assistant (PTA) needs to be aware of clinical features of DS. This information impacts how we can assist children to optimize their development, what precautions we need to take when handling them or teaching parents how to handle them, and how we advise family members to encourage their development at home and in the community.

Clinical features are similar among the three types of DS. Common features characterizing infants with DS include low muscle tone; joint laxity; a flat facial profile; upward slanting eyes; a flat nasal bridge; small ears; protruding, large tongue; and broad, short hands with an incurved little finger and a transverse palmar crease. In infants mottled skin, excess skin on the back of the neck, and reduced birth weight are also chara-cteristic.

Children with DS have from severely retarded to low-average intelligence, with most children falling into the mildly to moderately retarded range. Thirty-five percent of children with DS have congenital heart disease. Visual problems, including strabismus, nystagmus, astigmatism, myopia, and cataracts, are common in persons with DS. Hearing impairments are also common, probably as a result of narrow eustachian tubes and frequent ear infections.

Other medical problems include immune deficiency causing frequent respiratory and other infections, an increased incidence of leukemia, thyroid dysfunction, and delayed or incomplete sexual development (Wong, 1995). Orthopedic problems can include atlantoaxial (the first and second cervical vertebrae) instability, causing an increased risk of trauma induced spinal cord injury with resultant paralysis, usually from hyperflexion injuries. According to Blackston (1990), up to 20% of children with DS have cervical instability, so all children should be screened to rule it out before being allowed to play football, gymnastics, or other sports where there is physical contact or potential for trauma. This is a preventable, potentially serious injury that the PTA can take an active role in preventing.

Physical therapy treatment for a child with DS will vary according to the needs and age of the individual child. See Table 8-2 for a sample of long- and short-term goals for a child with DS at different ages. Suggested activities to address the goals are also listed.

TABLE 8-2 Sample Developmental Goals: Child With Down Syndrome

Family or child long-term goal	Physical therapy short-term objectives	Activities to address long-term goals and short-term objectives
Infant		
Family will safely be able to include child on day hiking trip. Problem: Child's head and trunk control is not sufficient to allow riding in child carrier backpack safely.	1. Child will roll independently from prone to and from supine position. 2. Child will hold head up 5 minutes in supported sitting. 3. Child will have independent sitting balance for 5 minutes.	• In therapy, work on rolling activities and reaching for toys. • Teach family how to carry and position child to allow child to practice head control. • Adapt child carrier backpack to provide support for infant. Use Foam-in-Place from Dynamic Systems, carved foam, or towel rolls and duct tape. • Weight shifts in supported sitting on lap while singing. Support initially provided to trunk with guarding for head. As child gets stronger, move hands down trunk, providing lower and lower support. • Facilitated coming to sit on lap or mat. • Have family use gentle swing at home
Toddler		
Child will walk independently. (This is a common goal of families.)	1. Child will creep on hands and knees for 20 feet. 2. Child will stand with support for 2 minutes.	• Create environments in therapy room, classroom, or home that the child wants to move between. • Have child stand in standing frame while playing with parent or siblings at home or in infant program daily for 15 minutes.

TABLE 8-2	Sample Developmental Goals: Child With Down Syndrome—cont'd	
Family or child long-term goal	**Physical therapy short-term objectives**	**Activities to address long-term goals and short-term objectives**
Toddler—cont'd	3. Child will cruise at furniture either direction for 6 feet.	• Child walks from therapist to mom, dad, or sibling, and back. • Ankle foot orthoses to support feet and ankles. • Do dancing or marching activities to music, providing support as needed. • Before asking child to stand, do tone stimulating activities, such as rolling a ball over child when in supine or prone position, marching feet in supine, etc. • Educate family about dangers of child walkers and inappropriateness for children with high or low tone.
Preschooler Child will go up and down five steps to house independently.	1. Child will walk independently. 2. Child will ascend and descend 5 steps with two hands held. 3. Child will ascend and descend 5 steps holding the railing.	• Provide obstacle course for child to go over, through, around, and under objects. • Provide an activity where the child needs to squat repeatedly to pick up toys, color on paper, put stickers on objects, etc. • Work on balance in standing activities, such as walking on a balance beam, a line of tape on the floor, or a string. Make the activity into a game, for instance, the balance beam is a bridge with alligators down below. • Help child go up and down a small slide. • Have parents encourage child to use parent's bodies as an obstacle course. The child would step on parent's feet, bent knees, and stiffly held forearms as they climb over and around adult. • Have child go up and down different steps, stackable steps in therapy room, stairs in house, steps at the mall. Children love to go up and down steps. Give as much help as the child needs.
School-Aged Child Child will play baseball in an after-school program.	1. Child will swing bat and hit ball. 2. Child will run 15 yards. 3. Child will follow the rules.	• Use a plastic bat at home and in therapy with a light ball to practice skill. T-ball with a stationary ball is a good option. • Use dancing at home and in therapy for balance and weight shifts, coordination. • Develop obstacle course outside to develop speed and coordination in fast walking and running. • Coordinate recess baseball games at school. • Consult with baseball coach on strategies to include child. • Advise parents to get cervical spine x-ray examination to rule out atlantoaxial instability. • Work with the family, coach, and IEP team to provide a peer buddy during baseball to help learn the skills, timing of the game, and rules. • Research Challenger baseball in your area. National Little League supports the Challenger division.
Adolescent Child will take the bus to after school job.	1. Child will ascend and descend bus steps independently. 2. Child will learn which bus to take and where to get off.	• Take bus rides with child and to help child figure out how to negotiate steps. • Ask bus driver to remind child when to get off bus. • Practice the route with the child.

The Infant With DS

Although the infant with DS has characteristic facial features and low muscle tone, physical characteristics will also resemble those of parents and siblings. A child's temperament may be fairly placid, but the child will also inherit tendencies for behavior from parents. Motor milestones are delayed, and feeding may be a problem because of a protruding tongue, high palate, and low muscle tone. Physical therapy is usually provided through an infant development program or occasionally as an outpatient in a pediatric clinic. Physical therapy goals should be integrated with other discipline goals in the IFSP and focus on the family's priorities for the child. The IFSP will list goals that are intended to be met in 1 year. For an infant, the first year is full of changes, so a therapist will have to write interim goals and be able to explain to the family how the interim goals relate to the long-term goal.

The medical complications of DS need to be kept in mind when planning activities to meet the goals. A child with cardiac defects will probably have decreased endurance, which, in addition to low muscle tone, will delay motor development. Persons working with the child will have to watch for signs of deoxygenation, such as pallid skin, lethargy, blue lips and nail beds, and sweating.

Physical therapy goals. Physical therapy goals for the child less than 1 year old with DS generally focus on developing motor skills that follow normal developmental patterns and sequences. These can include rolling, coming to sitting position, sitting with and without support, and improving head control. For the very young infant goals may focus on motor expressions of interaction, such as head turning to mother's voice or to the sound of a toy, reaching for a brightly colored toy, or lifting the head when in prone position to see mother or a toy. Other goals may address the family's need to learn how to handle and carry the child. Motor goals can and should be integrated with other discipline goals, such as occupational therapy, speech-language pathology, respiratory therapy, and education.

Family support. The family of a young infant with DS may need time to express their feelings about their child's disability, and may appreciate referral to community resources, such as family support groups, respite opportunities, and special programs. If you are part of a team working with the family, coordinate with the other members of the team to ensure that the family gets all the information they need about their rights as parents of a child with a disability, community resources available to them, including programs and publications as well as specific information about their child's disorder. Do not assume that someone else has given them this information. Even if they have been told once, they may not have heard or grasped all of the information the first time.

Play in therapy. When developing activities to meet therapy goals, it is important to have a repertoire of toys, situations, and skills to draw on. Use the child and family for clues in how to structure your therapy sessions. For example, if the child is tired and cranky, you can teach the mother how to position and carry the infant with a minimum of handling by you. If the infant is eager for interaction, you can model for the mother by playing with the infant on your lap or the mat, stimulating the infant to improve motor skills.

Role of the PTA. The PTA may work in an infant developmental program or acute care hospital and will be responsible for working with infants alongside the PT and other team members to promote developmental skills. The gross motor goals will be set by the physical therapist in collaboration with the team. The PTA will probably treat the child alternating with the PT and should get regular feedback from the PT as the child progresses through developmental changes. It is important to know how gross motor skills develop in infants and direct your treatment strategies toward the goals set by the team. It is also important to know strategies for working with children who have low muscle tone. When working with infants, it is easy to fall back into playing with them without having goals in mind. If you can state a goal-directed reason for everything that you are doing with the child, then you will have a larger picture of the scope of treatment for that child than just the therapy session today. Skills and strategies for working with young infants include teaching parents and others ways to play with the child in a manner that encourages the child's development.

The Toddler and Preschooler With DS

Learning to walk. Almost all children with DS learn to walk by an average of 2 years of age (Pueschel, 1978). Walking comes later than in children with typical development. Physical therapy goals in this age period usually focus on mobility skills, including prewalking skills, such as pulling to tall kneeling and to stand, moving into and out of a half-kneeling position, standing with and without support, and squatting from standing to pick up toys on the floor. Advanced gait skills include walking up and down stairs, walking on uneven terrain, jumping, running, and kicking a ball. See Table 8-3 for a comparison of attainment gross motor and other skills by children with DS, in comparison with children who are typically developing.

Quality of movement. Important integrated skills learned during this age include motor planning, or learning how to plan and coordinate arm, legs, and trunk movement in the right order to achieve a motor goal, such as riding a toy fire engine. A child may need verbal assistance or physical prompts to learn motor planning for particular skills.

Another element of the quality of movement learned during toddler years is the coordination of graded movements. This means that a child learns movement patterns well enough that movements occur in smooth paths rather than jerky movements, which overshoot or miss their aim. An example is a child who can walk in a coordinated fashion with legs closer together versus a child who walks in an immature, uneven gait with legs apart for balance. Practice assists in learning these skills, as does strengthening.

Cocontraction of proximal muscle groups for stability is important for children to be developing throughout infancy and toddlerhood, but particularly for a child with DS who has low muscle tone, weak muscles, and lax joints. Cocontraction refers to appropriate muscle strength on all sides of a joint at the same time to provide stability in that joint. Weight bearing through legs and arms and weight shifts in standing and sitting are good ways to develop better cocontraction. Some activities to promote good cocontraction include standing, one leg standing, cruising, walking, running, jumping, wheelbarrow, and walking with hands and feet on footprints or dots. These activities should be

Comparison of Skills Development: Children With Down Syndrome and Typically Developing Children

TABLE 8-3

Skill	Children with Down syndrome		Typically developing children	
	Average (mo)	Range (mo)	Average (mo)	Range (mo)
Smiling	2	1½-3	1	½-3
Rolling over	6	2-12	5	2-10
Sitting	9	6-18	7	5-9
Crawling	11	7-21	8	6-11
Creeping	13	8-25	10	7-13
Standing	16	10-32	11	8-16
Walking	20	12-45	13	8-18
Talking, words	14	9-30	10	6-14
Talking, sentences	24	18-46	21	14-32

From Pueschel, S. M. (1990). *A parent's guide to Down syndrome: Toward a brighter future.* Baltimore: Paul H. Brookes, p. 97.

performed within the context of an activity, such as standing on one foot to pull on pants, rather than practiced in isolation. For example, rather than asking the child to run from one end of the room to the other, use a game that requires running to play.

Rhythm is another modality for developing skills during the toddler years. Music is a wonderful tool for therapy. Hitting a drum may help develop graded movements, give proprioceptive input for cocontraction, and provide a wonderful avenue to learn rhythm, a necessary element in turn taking, timing, and balance skills. Marching, reciting poetry, and singing are all related activities that combine well with gross motor activity.

 Include other children in your therapy sessions. This could mean "including" the rest of the class during recess to help a child access play equipment or "including" a few peers to play a game that addresses a child's motor skills needs. Including other children not only makes the therapy session more fulfilling; it also allows a child with disabilities to develop friendships.

Role of the PTA. Children may be followed up for PT services in an infant development program or a private or public preschool. The PTA will follow up young children under the direction of a PT and may be responsible for daily or biweekly therapy sessions. In the preschool these sessions can occur during normal classroom routines. Materials and experiences available to all the children can be directed toward gross motor goals. The PTA should also be aware of goals related to language, fine motor skills, and socialization that can be supported in the context of gross motor activities. For example, an activity such as playing "London Bridge" can facilitate social skills and language, as well as walking, bimanual (two-handed) activities, and turn taking. In preschool, it is important to work closely with the teacher to facilitate group activities that will benefit the child with DS (Figure 8-13).

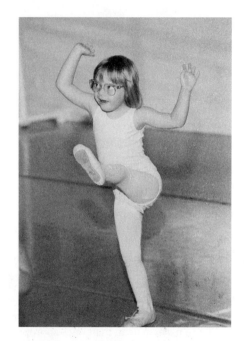

Figure 8-13 Alice, a 5-year-old child with Down syndrome, participates in dance class.

The School-Aged and Adolescent Child With DS

When the child starts attending school, social skills and interactions take on a greater meaning for both the child and family (Figure 8-14). Gross motor goals will focus on developing skills that can help the child healthfully participate in activities that have a social bearing, educational relevance, and later a vocational relevance for the child. For example, a child may want to learn to hold and swing a baseball bat or run between bases.

Exercise. Children with DS have been found to be less active than their siblings, spending more time indoors (Sharav & Bowman, 1992). Twenty-five percent of children with Down syndrome become overweight (Pueschel, 1990). Therefore socially

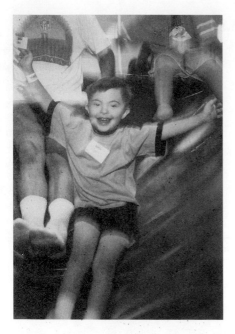

Figure 8-14 Ryan, a 7-year-old child with Down syndrome, plays vigorously.

appropriate gross motor activity should be encouraged. Therapists may find themselves consulting with the after-school dance teacher or athletic coach on how to include the child in team or group activities. Specific exercises may be recommended that would be beneficial for the child with DS and could benefit all of the children who are participating. Individual therapy sessions might be spent in learning rhythm activities to help with dance, or specific skills, such as one-legged balance, hopping, dribbling a ball, or walking on a balance beam, for the specific goal of participating more fully in a group event. All the skills should be reinforced in the group, and therapy sessions should assist the child to meet the goal of participating with the other children.

Consultation. As the child progresses through school, less direct therapy is needed because the child's gross motor skill level allows him or her to participate in many age-appropriate activities, including walking between classes, carrying books, getting on and off the bus, and running on the playground. Child and family energies are directed more toward educational and vocational ends as the child gets older. The therapist might be asked to consult if the child is having trouble with specific skills, such as getting on or off a bus or walking long distances between classes. The therapist might also be consulted if there is regression in gross motor skills. Short-term therapy might be necessary to assist the child to reach a specific goal, such as climbing the steps to a bus without assistance or climbing stairs without railings.

The therapist is a valuable member of the team and can provide insight regarding how to anticipate and avoid obstacles in educational or vocational plans. For example, Johnny has DS. He wants to take a job after school where he will be required to stand up for 3 hours at a time. Johnny has low endurance, and you are afraid that this job may be doomed to failure. You could either suggest alternative job placements, or assist the employer to modify the job requirements so Johnny can work sitting down part of the time as his endurance increases.

Role of the PTA. The PTA is likely to see a child with DS in either special education or regular education classrooms for therapy sessions. Gross motor goals might be addressed in isolated therapy sessions, group activities with children with disabilities, or group activities with the regular peer group. If there is a choice, activities performed in the classroom with the other children promote better peer interactions, better communication among professionals working with the child, and more consistency in providing the experience to the child. A child might be assisted during a group activity for gross motor skills in the classroom or in physical education classes. A daily exercise program might be part of the child's program, which needs to be supervised by the PTA. It is important that the activities be fun for the children. Creativity on the part of the PTA is an essential skill when working with children.

The Child With Spinal Muscular Atrophy

Incidence and Cause

Spinal muscular atrophy (SMA) is a progressive neuromuscular disease that is usually inherited in an autosomal recessive pattern. Both parents need to carry the gene if it is to be manifested in their child. SMA is the cause of the most infant deaths from an inherited disease. Two different genes on chromosome 5 have been pinpointed as the defective gene by two different research groups (Brzustowicz et al., 1990; Melki et al., 1990). Enough information is known that it is now possible to do prenatal diagnosis of SMA in some cases with a family history of SMA. It is thought that both genes play a role in SMA, and researchers are now exploring the different or complementary roles of each site in the disease process. SMA has an incidence of 1 in 10,000.

Clinical Features

SMA is characterized by progressive degeneration of the large anterior horn cells of the spinal cord and resultant muscle atrophy and weakness, which starts proximally and moves distally. Children with SMA are intellectually normal. There are three primary categories of the disease in children, differentiated by age of onset and severity. It is thought that all three types are different mutations of the same gene or of some combination of mutations of the two identified genes on chromosome 5.

SMA type 1. The first type of SMA (type 1), sometimes called infantile SMA, acute SMA, or Werdnig-Hoffman disease, type 1, is the most severe. It is usually detected clinically before 6 months of age and frequently is evident at birth. Children with SMA type 1 have decreased movements, especially against gravity. They lie in a typical "frogged" posture of externally rotated hips and flexed knees and have a weak cry and cough. Their breathing is usually only from the diaphragm because their intercostal and accessory muscles are weak. The infants have alert facial expressions and normal intellect and sensation. Deep tendon reflexes are absent or decreased. Children typically have frequent respiratory infections and may die in infancy or early childhood of respiratory complications.

SMA type 2. Children with SMA type 2 will begin to exhibit symptoms of weakness, delayed or regressed gross motor milestones, and decreased movements between 7 and 18 months of age. As they get older, the symptoms may progress. Most children will not sit up alone or walk, and those who walk will need braces. The progression of the disease process varies between children, and some may die from respiratory infections before they reach adulthood. A pervasive problem for children with SMA type 2 is scoliosis, because of weak trunk muscles. One study involving 37 children with SMA type 2 found that all of them had an early onset and rapid progression of scoliosis before puberty and required spinal fusion (Rodillo, Marini, Heckmatt, & Dubowitz, 1989).

SMA type 3. The third type of SMA, type 3, is the mildest form of the disease and usually manifests itself after 18 months of age. Sometimes this form of SMA does not express itself until late childhood. Children with SMA type 3 usually walk with braces for a time but will eventually need a wheelchair for mobility as they get weaker. They exhibit many signs of low muscle tone and weakness during gait, including lumbar lordosis, genu recurvatum or hyperextended knees, and a waddling gait. Rodillo et al. (1989) found that only 30% of the children with the milder form of SMA had scoliosis. In those children who were able to walk during puberty and beyond, the scoliosis was much milder than those children who lost their ambulation skills earlier.

Physical therapy treatment for a child with SMA will vary according to the needs and age of the individual child. See Table 8-4 for a sample of long- and short-term goals for a child with SMA at different ages. Suggested activities to address the goals are also listed.

The Infant With SMA

Because the infant with SMA is usually very weak with limited voluntary movements, positioning and handling are essential to allow the infant access to the environment. It is important not to fatigue the child but to allow and encourage as much active movement as possible to maintain strength and to encourage normal intellectual development through interacting with the environment. Therapy should be tailored to the individual child, whatever his or her strengths and interests, and should be designed in the context of the family. The strengths and interests of each child will be different depending on the age of onset and progression of weakness and muscle atrophy. Physical therapy goals will typically include normal developmental activities, such as reaching for toys, reaching for and playing with feet, rolling, and sitting with or without support. Goals must be functional, even for a young infant, and can include holding a bottle, bringing a toy to the mouth, and sitting up well enough (with or without support) to be fed with a spoon.

Positioning needs. Traditional infant seats, which cradle the child, work well to position the child in infancy. Rolled towels, cutout foam pads, or commercially purchased car seat infant head supports may be needed to provide extra support. The family should be worked with closely to determine the positioning needs of the child. Positioning needs could include sitting in the kitchen while a parent prepares meals, positioning for meals in a high chair or infant seat, positioning in the car, positioning in the family room during evening television, or outside in the yard while a caregiver gardens or sunbathes. Positioning for sleeping is also important and must be addressed either in a crib, bassinet, family bed, or on a foam mattress on the floor, depending on the habits of the family.

Family support. Families may be wrestling with varied emotions resulting from their child having a significant genetic disorder. If the child has been diagnosed in early infancy, the likelihood is that the prognosis is poor and the child may not live through the first year. Family members may need simply to recount their day-to-day emotions surrounding taking care of their child. They may need to talk about experiences surrounding the birth, diagnosis, and early life of their child. They may need to explore their feelings about death or to gather resources that they can use to plan for their child's future. It is important for the therapist to remember that he or she does not need to have an answer or a solution for every problem. Listening alone can provide immeasurable support.

Family members may be willing or eager to explore resources available in the community, including support groups, books, or medical literature. They also may prefer not to talk about or address more sensitive issues, such as the terminal nature of the disease, for a period. The therapist needs to be sensitive to their needs, while providing information that the family members need to care for their child.

Therapist support. It is also important that the therapist be aware of his/her own feelings about the child and the prognosis. The therapist needs to take care of personal emotional needs through talking with family members, peers, and availing himself or herself of counseling services at the workplace, if necessary.

Role of the PTA. It is important to ensure that there is adequate support from a PT and other staff for the PTA who is treating a child with SMA. Treatments will likely be home based or will occur in an infant development program. Adaptive equipment can be essential for good positioning. Durable medical equipment vendors can be helpful in recommending equipment, but because infants grow quickly, it may be easier to find equipment for the family to borrow, or to be creative in adapting existing equipment. If you recognize a need for positioning, talk with other team members (including parents). Brainstorming how to provide support in a certain position can be more productive with input and ideas from several people. Developing a positive relationship with parents or key caregivers is essential to having an impact with infants because of a sense of trust, shared responsibility, and mutual support which can develop.

The Toddler and Preschooler With SMA

The range of disability can be wide in this age group, depending on the age of onset and the progression of the disease. A particular 2-year-old child with SMA may be too weak to eat independently, while another may still be walking well. The disease may progress and subsequently plateau for a period, perhaps even years. Children with SMA need the same types of intellectual and social stimulation that any child does at this age. Most children with working parents are in daycare or preschool by age 2 or 3 years. At this age, children learn by exploring their environment and manipulating objects. Beginning cognitive skills, such as learning letters, numbers, colors, and shapes, are generally learned in preschool through the use of visual, auditory, and

Sample Developmental Goals: Child With Spinal Muscular Atrophy

TABLE 8-4

Family or child long-term goal	Physical therapy short-term objectives	Activities to address long-term goals and short-term objectives
Infant		
Child will sit up in high chair 30 minutes to eat. Problem: Child's head and trunk control is not sufficient to allow sitting up without support.	1. Child will sit with support for 10 minutes. 2. Child will hold head up without support for 5 minutes. 3. Child will be able to grasp finger foods and bring to the mouth.	• Adapt high chair seat to provide trunk and head support as needed. Use Foam-in-Place from Dynamic Systems, carved foam, or towel rolls and duct tape. • Teach family how to carry and position child to allow child maximum access to environment. • Adapt tray table height to allow child maximum upper extremity function. • Plan other adapted seating to allow the child to sit up in various environments.
Toddler		
Child will have independent mobility.	1. Child will learn to operate joystick. 2. Child will maintain full/functional range of motion in upper and lower extremities.	• Work with occupational therapist on developing switch toys that the child can use in therapy and at home. As child gains proficiency, vary the switch access and use a joystick. • Vary the child's positioning throughout the day at home and school. • Provide equipment for supported standing to promote normal hip development and develop antigravity muscle strength. • Build up to a standing program in a supported position once or twice daily for 30 to 45 minutes. Assess skin, child's fatigue level, and level of alertness to determine standing tolerance. • Have child train on a powered mobile stander to motivate child to stand and develop power mobility skills. • Coordinate obtaining lightweight ankle foot orthoses for the child to support feet and ankles in a neutral position when sitting to prevent drop foot contractures.
Preschooler		
Child will participate in preschool activities.	1. Child will paint independently. 2. Child will accompany class on field trips.	• Modify painting easel to allow child access. Painting on a vertical surface will require too much strength, so place paper on table or lap tray that is at an optimal height to allow child to pivot arms on supported elbows. Provide a lightweight paint brush. • Ensure that positioning is adequate for optimal upper extremity use. This includes trunk and head positioning and upper extremity support. • Provide adapted seating in a preschool height chair, so that child can work at table with other children. • If child cannot manipulate paintbrush, adapt activity so child can use hands, sponges, or other tools to paint. • Ensure child has adequate wheeled mobility with good seating support. • Train child to use power mobility. Advance skills as the child progresses. • Train teacher sand classroom staff to carry and transfer child.

Sample Developmental Goals: Child With Spinal Muscular Atrophy—cont'd

TABLE 8-4

Family or child long-term goal	Physical therapy short-term objectives	Activities to address long-term goals and short-term objectives
Preschooler–cont'd		• Ensure adequate positioning in car or van through 5-point tie down restraint in van for wheelchair, or large car seat with adequate adaptation for positioning. • Train teachers and classroom staff to position child in wheelchair, and to reposition as necessary.
School-Aged Child Child will have independent mobility around the school campus with supervision.	1. Child will drive up and down curb cuts in power wheelchair. 2. Child will drive power wheelchair at a safe speed and not hit other children. 3. Child will drive power wheelchair on uneven ground. 4. Child will negotiate small doorways in power chair. 5. Child will be able to tell someone how to charge wheelchair and perform basic maintenance activities.	• Develop an obstacle course on school campus using architectural features of the school, such as curb cuts, doorways, corners. Develop a chart for the child so progress can be monitored on specific skills. Create a reward system of greater independence as child gains skills. • Develop power wheelchair competitions among local power wheelchair users to provide motivation to develop skills. • Develop a steeplechase event for the class which includes running over uneven ground, going under and over obstacles. Adapt the event for the child using a power chair so full participation can occur. • Modify classroom and regular pathways throughout the school to remove obstacles and allow enough room to maneuver the chair. • Teach the child basic maintenance skills and how to charge the wheelchair.
Adolescent Child will minimize number of school days lost due to respiratory infections.	1. Child will tolerate alternative positions during the school day. 2. Child and family will develop opportunities to provide positioning and percussion for postural drainage each day.	• Provide equipment for alternative positioning including supine stander, wedge for sidelying, or mattress for prone or supine positioning at school. Determine which positions the child can tolerate. Negotiate with child and teachers where and when alternative positioning should occur each day. • Work with family to determine what equipment they need at home for positioning and postural drainage. • Assist the family to schedule daily activities at home for alternative positioning such as sidelying in front of a favorite television show.

kinesthetic tools, such as blocks, pictures, crayons, singing, and recitation. The child with SMA needs access to these tools. Physical therapy goals during the toddler and preschool years can focus on developing functional mobility skills, including walking, walking with assistive devices, or mobility using a wheelchair. Goals may also focus on the child's ability to access the environment through toys, switches, and manipulative tools, such as blocks, or positioning for play at the same level as the preschool classmates.

The child with SMA in a specialized school setting. Frequently, a child will attend a preschool specially designed for children with disabilities who have been determined eligible.

These preschools may be on the grounds of an elementary school or may be freestanding in the community. They are run by the DOE to satisfy legal mandates of providing a free and appropriate education to students with disabilities, per part B of Public Law 99-457, which extended these services from school-aged children to children from ages 3 to 5. Therapy services are also mandated for children who need them.

The child with SMA in a regular school setting. A child with SMA can be included in a regular preschool setting, providing that appropriate supports are provided. These supports can include accessible tables and chairs for the child who uses assistive devices and supports, adapted materials, additional personnel time for physical assistance, and personnel training. The therapist can assist the preschool team to determine what supports are necessary for the child. They may also help adapt existing materials and furniture and rearrange the school layout to accommodate the mobility needs of the child with SMA. The school will have to provide access to a child with assistive devices, such as wheelchair or crutches. Training for school personnel in transfers, lifting techniques, and positioning for the child may also be provided by the therapist.

Upright mobility. A child with SMA may initially walk independently but, as weakness progresses, may need to use knee-ankle-foot orthoses (KAFOs) for support. A lower extremity brace made of molded plastic and aluminum joints can be lightweight and provide specific joint support for children, allowing greater mobility and freedom of movement. Other types of braces include reciprocating gait orthoses and parapodiums, which allow children to ambulate, even with no strength in their legs. Crutches or walkers can help balance when ambulating in braces. The PT or PTA will assist the child to be fitted for braces, teach the child to apply his or her own braces, and teach the child to walk using support, if needed.

Seated mobility. Wheelchair mobility for toddlers and preschoolers with SMA is an option that should be explored. Manual wheelchairs are now being manufactured for children that are light enough for a child to propel. The chairs come in bright colors and child-friendly patterns. Power mobility has been shown to be an important and safe developmental tool for children as young as 2 years old, who do not have the strength to propel a manual chair effectively (Butler, 1990). Children need to move around their environment to explore and to learn to be more independent in their life skills. Independent mobility at a young age is very important to enhance all developmental skills.

Role of the PTA. As children get older, their needs change. The PTA needs to work closely with preschool teachers and classroom staff to ensure that the young child has access to toys and materials in the classroom. Creativity is needed to adapt furniture and equipment to ensure that the child can participate in classroom activities. Raising the height or changing the angle of a lap tray can make a significant difference in a child's ability to use his or her hands. Be aware of slight changes or decreases in strength and communicate well with teachers, families, and the PT to anticipate needs of the child.

The School-Aged and Adolescent Child With SMA

The school-aged child with SMA should be included in a regular education program if possible (Figure 8-15). Children need the social and cognitive stimulation of being with their peers. Social and academic priorities surface during the early years of school. When the question is asked of an early elementary school child, "What is your favorite subject?," many answer, "Recess!" During the early years of school, mobility for gross motor play is very important. Development and support of mobility skills in the preschooler can help a young child better adjust to moving to kindergarten, which can be hard for any child. The therapist should work as part of a team to address how to provide the supports that a child needs during this developmentally crucial time.

Access to academic tasks. Access to academic tasks, such as coloring, writing, and doing worksheets, can be a problem for a child with SMA. A computer can be an important tool to learn and to practice academic skills, at least visually. Some kinesthetic

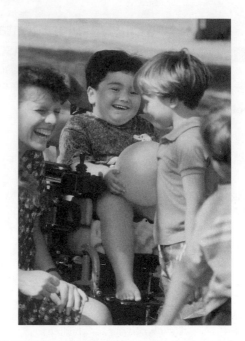

Figure 8-15 Rik, a school-aged boy with spinal muscular atrophy, is included in regular education.

learning should also be provided, if at all possible, through adjusting the height or angle of the work surface, adapting the materials used, and providing hand-over-hand assistance, if needed. It is clear that children learn through all of their senses, and actually moving objects through space provides an important learning clue for young children. Learning by forming letters when moving a crayon across the paper or tracing letters with a finger can be difficult to replace simply by looking at a computer screen.

Positioning and assistive technology. The therapist can provide input to the team regarding positioning the child to access as much as possible. When proximal weakness is a primary problem, support for the trunk and extremities becomes paramount. The height of the arm rests, lap tray, or table can determine whether a child will be able to write or type on a computer keyboard. For those children with less active upper extremity range of motion, a trackball access to an on-screen keyboard may be more functional than a separate keyboard.

Positioning to prevent scoliosis. Another positioning consideration for the therapist working with a school-aged child with SMA is positioning to prevent scoliosis. Adequate trunk supports on a wheelchair are important, and custom molding may be needed to provide maximum support. Most children will develop a scoliosis, but good spinal positioning can minimize the progression of spinal deformity and provide comfort. Respiratory function is also affected by the progression of spinal deformities. A child with good spinal support may maintain adequate respiratory function for longer than a child without.

Surgery. The adolescent with SMA may have medical problems, such as advanced scoliosis that requires surgery. Therapists may be involved in providing care before and after surgery. It is important that the therapist know which surgical procedure was used and understand the precautions well. Information such as this frequently is not communicated to school personnel from the physician or hospital when a child returns after surgery, so it

TABLE 8-5	Types of Muscular Dystrophy Seen in Childhood	
Type	**Age of onset and mechanism of inheritance**	**Typical clinical progression**
Congenital myotonic	Birth (autosomal dominant)	Hypotonia, severe mental retardation, speech disturbances, and spinal deformities, as well as muscle weakness and other problems associated with myotonic dystrophy. Frequent early death. All children are born to mothers with myotonic dystrophy.
Duchenne (pseudohypertrophic)	1-5 years (X-linked)	Progressive weakness from proximal to distal muscles. Child loses walking skills by preteen years, progressively loses other self-care skills. Death by late teens or twenties by respiratory or cardiac causes.
Becker	5-10 years (X-linked)	Similar to Duchenne, but much slower progression. Walks until late teens, death in adult life from respiratory compromise.
Facioscapulohumeral	Variable from infancy to adulthood (autosomal dominant)	Characterized by facial weakness and shoulder girdle weakness. May have hearing or vision problems. There is a wide clinical spectrum of the disease.
Limb-girdle	Adolescence to adulthood (autosomal recessive)	Progressive weakness of proximal muscles of shoulder and hip girdle. Variable age of onset and progression. Lower extremity disability occurs before upper extremity disability.
Myotonic	Adolescence (autosomal dominant)	Muscle weakness, delay in relaxation time of muscle, stiffness. Distal weakness often presents first with proximal weakness occurring later. Cardiac problems, cataracts, and endocrine problems are often seen.

is the therapist's job to inform others how to handle, transfer, and position the child after scoliosis surgery.

Respiratory management. Because of increasing weakness, scoliosis, and poor respiratory hygiene (due to poor cough and lack of movement), the child with SMA will probably have respiratory compromise with frequent respiratory infections. The therapist should fully understand the signs of respiratory distress and maintain communication with the family, the school nurse, and the teacher about the child's respiratory status. Chest physical therapy may be needed in school and could be provided by physical therapy or by the school nurse. Alternate positioning is very important in maintaining respiratory hygiene. The therapist should ensure that the child is placed in different positions several times throughout the day, and that the child is able to tolerate the position without respiratory distress. Positions could include sidelying on a wedge or a cot in the classroom, lying prone over a wedge (although this position is frequently not tolerated well by children with SMA), standing in a standing frame or tilt table, or lying supine on a wedge or cot. Communication with the child and family should be done before deciding on different positions. Cultural values, personal preference, or lack of availability of physical assistance may make lying down in the classroom untenable for a child. The nurse's office or another room where there is supervision may be preferable. Alternatives for positioning may include lying over a therapy ball for postural drainage and positioning, or use of a tilt-in-space or fully reclineable wheelchair for alternate positioning.

Vocational planning. For those children with SMA type 2 or 3 who remain relatively strong during their adolescent years, the therapist can assist in making vocational plans a reality. This may entail assisting the student to learn to drive and to obtain an accessible van or how to use an accessible public city bus system.

Work with a teacher, occupational therapist, speech-language pathologist, or educational assistant as they work with a child on specific skills. You will be able to find ways to integrate the child's gross motor needs into the session, which will benefit not only the child but also yourself and the other professional.

The therapist may help the student think through strengths for a college entrance essay or may help adapt a workplace so that it is accessible.

Role of the PTA. The PTA may not be routinely involved with a child with SMA who is in a regular classroom. Through experience and confidence, the PTA can provide consultative services to the teacher as part of a team, which also includes the PT. The PTA may be asked to adjust braces, teach transfers, or help adapt equipment.

The Child With Duchenne Muscular Dystrophy

Incidence and Cause

Muscular dystrophy is a group of unrelated diseases characterized by four elements: (1) it primarily is a disease of muscle tissue, (2) the course is progressive, (3) it involves degeneration and death of muscle fibers, and (4) there is a genetic basis for the disorder. The diseases included under the category of muscular dystrophies are transmitted by different genetic traits and each differs in its clinical course and expression. See Table 8-5 for a brief description of muscular dystrophies seen in childhood.

Duchenne muscular dystrophy (DMD) is the most common hereditary neuromuscular disease and causes a progressive deterioration of strength and function over time. It is the type of muscular dystrophy most likely to be seen in the clinic, school, or home treatment program. DMD has an incidence of 1 in 3500 live male births (Moser, 1984, Mostacciuolo, Lombardi, Cambilla, Danieli, & Angelini, 1987) and has an X-linked inheritance pattern. Therefore most of the children affected by DMD are boys. About a third of the diagnosed cases of DMD are fresh mutations and a family history cannot be determined (Wong, 1995). The few girls who exhibit symptoms of DMD either have a monosomy of their sex chromosome pairs and so have to manifest the X gene inherited from their mother or have a theorized inactivation of the X chromosome inherited from their father. The defect has been discovered to be a mutation at Xp21 in the gene coding for the protein dystrophin (Koenig, Hoffman, Pertelson, 1987). The absence of the dystrophin protein causes increased permeability of the muscle cell membranes and a resultant build up of calcium level. The calcium activates enzymes that cause a breakdown of muscle cells (Cullen & Fulthorpe, 1975, Mokri & Engel, 1975). Muscle cells are replaced with fat and connective tissue. The breakdown of muscle cells causes weakness, which increases over time.

Clinical Features and Medical Treatment

Clinical features. DMD usually is diagnosed between 3 and 5 years of age; however, clinical signs can be detected as soon as the child begins to walk. Most often parents notice that their children begin to trip, fall, and complain of fatigue while walking or climbing stairs. Children begin to exhibit the Gower sign, walking up their legs with their hands to stand up from the floor. The Gower sign is evidence of weak quadriceps and hip extensor musculature (Figure 8-16).

A child may be hospitalized for necessary diagnostic medical tests, or the tests may be performed as an outpatient. Medical tests to diagnose DMD include blood tests to detect enzymes related to the destruction of muscle tissue, a muscle biopsy, and electromyography (EMG) to test muscle function. Genetic analysis can confirm the diagnosis of DMD.

Clinical evaluation is also very important. A boy with DMD will have enlarged or pseudohypertrophic muscles. Because of this common clinical sign of DMD, the disease is sometimes called pseudohypertrophic muscular dystrophy. Pseudohypertrophy is most evident in the calves, but can also be seen in the deltoid muscles, infraspinatus, quadriceps, tongue, and forearm extensor groups. These muscle groups are firmer than usual to palpation. Other clinical signs include inability to keep up with his peers in play, falling, difficulty climbing stairs or running, Gower's sign, and complaints of fatigue. Toe walking may also be an early sign of DMD.

Other clinical signs, which become evident as the child gets older, include intellectual impairment and cardiac myopathy. Intellectual impairment occurs in all children but is usually in the mild to moderate range. Cardiomyopathy in varying degrees also occurs in all children. The degree of both of these impairments is not related to the degree of skeletal muscle involvement.

As the child loses functional skills due to decrease in strength, a waddling gait or bilateral Trendelenberg and lumbar lordosis will be evident. Scoliosis, joint contractures, muscle atrophy, and obesity occur when a child loses ambulation skills. Respiratory infections occur more readily as a child loses strength in his respiratory muscles. The progression of DMD follows a common pattern and sequence in all children. Variances to the pattern may be related to individual differences between the children, degrees of cardiac or intellectual impairments, or medical interventions. See Table 8-6 for a summary of the clinical signs of

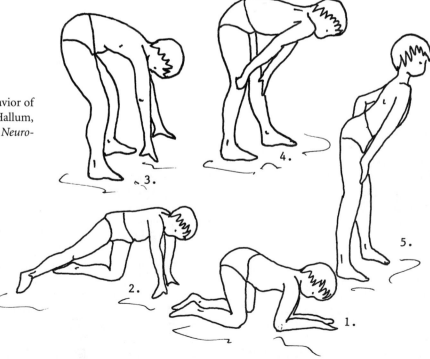

Figure 8-16 The Gower sign is a distinctive behavior of boys with Duchenne muscular dystrophy. (From Hallum, A. (1995). Cerebral palsy. In D.A. Umphred [Ed.], *Neurological rehabilitation* [3rd ed.]. St. Louis: Mosby.)

DMD and physical therapy interventions by general age group of boys with DMD.

Vignos, Spencer, and Archibald (1963) published a functional rating scale for Duchenne muscular dystrophy, which was modified by Brooke et al. (1983) to include the upper extremities (Table 8-7). This scale is useful for denoting functional levels and determining when interventions such as bracing are needed.

Medical treatment. Although there is no cure for DMD, there are several medical treatments that may prolong functional skills, such as ambulation. The prolongation of ambulation can help to delay problems that generally develop once a child begins using a wheelchair full time, including severe scoliosis, severe joint contractures, pathologic fractures due to osteoporosis, and obesity. Surgical tenotomies include lengthening of the

Achilles tendon, tensor facia latae, and hamstring tendons. Transfer of the posterior tibialis tendon to correct for an equinovarus foot has also been successful. In one study, 24 boys with DMD from 8 years to 12 years and 5 months were studied. They were given percutaneous tendo-Achilles lengthening and a transfer of the posterior tibialis tendon when walking became labored because of the foot deformity. After surgery, with bracing, walking was preserved an average of 3.3 years (Hsu & Furumasu, 1993). Some families believe that performing surgery or using braces only prolongs the inevitable decline in function and that the expense and pain to the child are not justifiable. This is a decision that should be made by each family on the basis of their own perspective and values.

Myoblast transfer is a relatively new technique, which is the-

Clinical Features of Duchenne Muscular Dystrophy With Physical Therapy Interventions by Age of Child

TABLE 8-6

Age	Clinical features	Physical therapy interventions
Birth to 2 years	May learn to walk late.	Monitor developmental and functional skills, strength, range of motion (ROM).
3-5 years	Falling, toe walking, clumsiness, reluctance to run, hypertrophy in calves and deltoids, weakness of neck flexors, abdominals, shoulder and hip extensor muscles, Gower's sign.	Teach family ROM of gastrocsoleus and tensor fascia lata groups, positioning, general exercise program, such as swimming, monitor strength and ROM.
6-8 years	Toe walking, lordosis, lack of reciprocal arm swing, cannot climb stairs without support, easily tired, limited ambulation distance, walks with wide-based gait, trendelenberg, cannot rise from floor without help.	General exercise program, such as swimming, monitor strength and ROM, consult with family and school on how to modify activities to avoid fatigue, develop standing/walking program, teach breathing exercises, consult with physical education instructor for ROM program in school, prescribe night splints for ankles, monitor spinal alignment.
9-11 years	Walks with braces, may undergo tenotomy surgeries to prolong ambulation or surgery to stabilize scoliosis, respiratory insufficiency, beginning scoliosis, if no surgery or braces may lose ambulation skills.	Fit and prescribe KAFOs, prescribe and teach to use Rollator walker or parapodium or reciprocating gait orthosis, develop program to integrate walking into school activities, intervention before and after surgery for strengthening/gait training, breathing exercises, manual wheelchair for longer distances with appropriate seating/positioning supports, consider motorized scooter for independent seated mobility, provide ROM, positioning, monitor scoliosis and limb contractures.
12-14 years	Loss of ambulation skills, increasing respiratory difficulty, obesity, increasing contractures at hips, knees, ankles and elbows, progression of scoliosis, osteoporosis, dependent transfers, increasing need for assistance in activities of daily living (ADLs).	Continue with standing program as long as possible; manage obesity and contractures; power wheelchair for independent mobility; instruct family/school on use of mechanical lifting device (Hoyer or other); recommend commode chair, shower chair, other equipment as needed; work with teacher and other team members to develop positioning in classroom and access to computer to facilitate academic work.
15-17 years	Dependent in many ADLs, possible need for assisted ventilation, increased respiratory compromise.	Adapted equipment to assist with ADLs, including a ball-bearing feeder; develop regular schedule and method for pressure relief/monitor skin; adapt power or manual chair for mechanical ventilation, if indicated; teach family assisted coughing, breathing exercises, and postural drainage; monitor respiratory function, consider mechanical or power control bed; comfort mattress, such as air flow or alternating pressure pad; work with child, family and team to assist in planning of vocational goals for child.
18+ years	Need for assisted ventilation, dependence in all ADLs, death comes after a period of declining respiratory function.	May need to adapt controls of power chair to sip and puff or other control that is accessible to individual with DMD, skin care, management of contractures, positioning, consultation regarding access to higher educational or vocational activities, provide support to individual and family, provide family information about accessible transportation for family/child.

TABLE 8-7   Functional Rating Scale for Boys With Duchenne Muscular Dystrophy

Arms	Legs
1. Starting with arms at sides, child can abduct arms in full circle until they touch above head. Can place a weight >0.5 kg on a shelf above eye level.	1. Walks and climbs stairs without assistance.
2. Can raise arms above head as above; cannot place 0.5 kg on a shelf above eye level.	2. Walks and climbs stairs with aid of railing.
3. Can raise arms above head only by flexing elbow/use of accessory muscles.	3. Walks and climbs stairs slowly with aid; >12 seconds for 4 standard steps.
4. Cannot raise hands above head; can raise glass of water to mouth.	4. Walks unassisted and rises from chair; cannot climb stairs.
5. Cannot raise hands to mouth; can use hands to hold pen/pick coins from table.	5. Walks unassisted; cannot rise from chair; cannot climb stairs.
6. Cannot raise hands to mouth and has no useful hand function.	6. Walks with assistance or independently with leg braces.
	7. Walks in leg braces but requires assistance for balance.
	8. Stands in leg braces; unable to walk even with assistance.
	9. Uses a wheelchair.
	10. Confined to bed.

Modified from Vignos, Spencer, & Archibald, 1963; and Brooke et al., 1983.

orized to provide cells with their own method of making dystrophin. Healthy muscle cells have been injected into the muscles of boys with DMD in the hopes that the myoblasts, or precursors to muscle cells, will fuse with the myoblasts in the boys' cells. The results have so far been equivocal. One review of the literature indicated that results of a series of clinical trials have been disappointing (Dubowitz, 1992).

Another controversial treatment is prednisone. Some doctors believe that the side effects of steroid therapy will injure more muscle cells and accelerate the disease process (Khan, 1993). However, DeSilva, Drachman, Mellitis, and Kuncl (1987) found that, in clinical trials, a group treated with prednisone lived 2 years longer than a control group. Clinical trials are continuing with promising results (Reitter, 1995; Sansome, Royston, & Dubowitz, 1993).

Electrical stimulation has been explored as a method of maintaining strength in preserved muscle cells. One trial found that, when a low-frequency chronic electrical stimulation was used on the tibialis anterior muscle in young children, there was an increase in maximum muscle contraction of 47% (Scott, Vrbova, Hyde, & Dubowitz, 1986). There was no effect in older children.

Other conservative medical management includes drugs to maximize cardiac function in those boys with significant cardiomyopathy, diet to control obesity and increase calcium levels to prevent osteoporosis, and aggressive management of respiratory infections.

Physical therapy treatment for a child with DMD will vary according to the needs and age of the individual child. See Table 8-8 for a sample of long- and short-term goals for a child with DMD at different ages. Suggested activities to address the goals are also listed.

The Infant With DMD

Unless an older sibling has been diagnosed with DMD, or there is significant family history, most infants will not be monitored for symptoms of the disease. Some researchers say that motor milestones will be normal (Hsu & Furumasu, 1993), and others say that the infant may be mildly hypotonic, with slight delays in motor milestones (Eckersley, 1993). In those children who are identified early by family history, the Gower sign may be evident as early as 15 months with repeated standing from the floor. In general, however, most children with DMD are not identified until between 3 and 5 years of age.

The Preschooler With DMD

The child who is newly diagnosed with DMD is usually referred to physical therapy for an evaluation and monitoring of his condition. Services may be provided in an outpatient clinic, such as a hospital or a Muscular Dystrophy Association (MDA) clinic. They may also be provided at school if the child is referred and eligible for special education services. Delays in cognitive skills may have been identified in preschool, instigating the referral to special education. The child will have enlarged calf muscles and reluctance to run or attempt advanced gait activities, such as climbing, hopping, or jumping jacks. If the child has existing problems, such as decreased active or passive ankle dorsiflexion, he will be seen intermittently for treatment, otherwise he will be followed on a regular basis to monitor his strength, range of motion (ROM), and developmental skills.

Physical therapy goals. Therapy goals should be functional. Depending on the needs of the child, developmentally appropriate activities may include jumping on two feet, standing and balancing on one foot, walking on heels, squatting to play, or walking up an angled balance beam or ramp. Activities should be incorporated into the normal routines and play at the preschool or at home. Activities should be geared to maintain or improve ankle and hip ROM, as well as balance and motor planning skills. Teaching family members how to do passive ROM, as well as encourage ankle dorsiflexion during daily activities, is important. Family members can be taught to do many of the same activities performed in the therapy session, including playing "Simon Says" to encourage balancing on one foot, jumping in place, or squatting. Other activities can include imaginative play,

Sample Developmental Goals: Child With Duchenne Muscular Dystrophy

TABLE 8-8

Family or child long-term goal	Physical therapy short-term objectives	Activities to address long-term goals and short-term objectives
Preschooler Child will keep up with classmates during preschool activities.	1. Child will maintain ankle range of motion of at least 90 degrees.	• Provide passive range of motion to ankles at least once daily in the context of a regular activity such as putting on shoes. Teach child how to do active stretching with supervision. • Choose class route to recess and lunch that goes up ramps or stairs. • Teach family members and teacher to do passive range of motion when putting on shoes.
	2. Child will play on playground equipment safely.	• Help child go up and down a small slide. • Encourage going up and down steps. • Develop class exercise program to music incorporating activities for strengthening and flexibility, such as jumping, squatting to stand, walking on heels, bear walking, and leap frog.
School-Aged Child Child will participate in after-school swim program.	1. Child will breathe efficiently in the pool.	• Use incentive spirometer to develop and maintain vital capacity. Use a chart to document progress with stickers or stars. • Teach child breathing exercises to do at home to improve strength in respiratory muscles, such as blowing ping-pong balls, using a straw to blow feathers, and deep breathing exercises to do with parents. • Consult with swim coach to encourage child to participate in group pool games, such as adapted water polo to develop respiratory capacity. Modify the rules for the child with DMD if needed, and explain the reasons for the rule modifications to the other children.
	2. Child will swim 25 yards in pool.	• Practice different strokes in individual and group sessions in the pool. • Encourage family outings to pools and other swimming sites to complement activities done in after-school program. • Have child swim using flutter board to optimize upper and lower extremity strength, as well as to ensure safety and success. • Modify activities as needed so child does not get over tired. Stress light general conditioning and aerobic capacity rather than strengthening of individual muscle groups. Instruct the coach to adapt the activities to the child as needed each day.
Adolescent Child will attend junior prom.	1. Child will tolerate an upright seated position for 3 hours.	• Reevaluate seating and positioning. Look at options for seating including tilt-in-space option or recline for pressure relief and intermittent rest. • Gradually build up tolerance to upright position if the child is not currently able to tolerate. • Consider supplementary oxygen on prom night. Work with other team members including family, RN, and MD to determine medical needs and solutions.
	2. Child will dance at the prom.	• Plan dance sequence to music with child who can move power wheelchair to music. • Work with friends and child to design special dance. If child is using a manual wheelchair, a peer can move chair. If power mobility is used, child can propel self. • Ensure that child's driving skills are adequate for power mobility on a crowded dance floor. Design activities to simulate dance floor and practice mobility skills needed. • If needed, work with dance organizers to modify an area for child to dance in wheelchair.

such as making a ramp of a balance beam laid from the floor to a higher stable surface and pretending it is the gangplank of a pirate ship and there are person-eating alligators down below. Play activities, such as being chased by a crocodile or playing the pirate captain demonstrating how to walk the plank, can encourage a reluctant child to walk up a balance beam ramp.

Maintaining range of motion. A 4-year-old has already learned many ways to compensate for tight heel cords and weakness. It is up to an imaginative therapist to encourage him to try activities he knows are hard for him. The family may have a very hard time ranging his ankles and hips every day because he has learned how to manipulate his environment to suit him. The therapist needs to stress the importance of daily range of motion and splinting. Scott, Hyde, Goddard, and Dubowitz (1981) found that children who followed a daily stretching regimen and wore night splints significantly slowed the progression of their heel cord contractures compared with a group of boys who did not comply with the exercises and splint wearing. They were able to prolong their ability to ambulate because they maintained functional range of motion longer.

Passive range of motion for ankles and hips should be planned into the daily routine at home and school. See Figures 8-17 and 8-18 for illustrations of how to stretch these joints for a child with DMD. The therapist can help the family think through the events of the day and decide on the best time to do the exercises. Some appropriate times might be on waking up in the morning, in or after the bath, while watching a particular television show, when putting on shoes, or before the bedtime story. There is no agreement between researchers on how many times passive ROM should be performed during the day or how many repetitions it should encompass (Stuberg, 1994). In general, probably the more often and the more frequent repetitions, the better. Families can be given this information with recommendations to find two times each day and do at least 10 repetitions, holding each for 10 seconds. Range of motion should be done slowly, it should never be forced, and it should not hurt. There is potential to damage muscle fibers and cause more destruction if too much force is used. If a parent is unsure of how hard to push, have the parent try it on you to assess how strong it should be. An important adjunct to passive exercises should be finding op-

portunities for the child to stand or walk with his ankles in dorsiflexion throughout the day, such as standing on a wedge during tabletop activities.

Exercise. A young child is generally interested in keeping up with his peers or siblings. A formal exercise program is not necessary at this age. However, families can be counseled to encourage the child to do age-appropriate activities, such as playing on the playground, running with peers, learning to ride a tricycle, and learning to swim. The child will generally limit his activities to those he can tolerate.

Role of the PTA. The PTA may be responsible for carrying out a regular treatment program with the preschooler who has DMD, under the supervision of a PT. The child may be followed at an outpatient clinic or in preschool. The program will include passive and active range of motion and exercises. The PTA should keep in mind the goals at all times and direct activities toward the specific goals. A child may be unwilling to participate in some of the activities if they are difficult or uncomfortable. Creativity will be needed to encourage the child. Respect for the child's feelings is important to develop a trusting relationship. The primary caregiver will probably feel very vulnerable during these early years as the child develops more obvious signs of DMD. Support and encouragement are important from the therapy provider.

The School-Aged Child With DMD

Gait deviations. Once the child starts school, weakness in his proximal muscles, which progresses symmetrically down his legs, will start to cause gait deviations in a predictable pattern. The child will initially have an increased lateral trunk lean and arm swing to compensate for gluteus medius weakness. The child will then start leaning his trunk backward to compensate for weak hip extensor muscles. Frequently, a child will develop contractures in hip abduction and ankle plantarflexion that will cause him to walk on his toes and keep his hips abducted. He will take smaller steps, increase his lordosis, and move his arms backward to compensate for his more forward center of gravity. An equinovarus deformity may cause him to walk on the lateral border of his foot, and he will fall more frequently because of an inability to keep his knees extended and poor balance (Figure 8-19). At this point, he will need surgery and bracing to continue to ambulate.

Physical therapy goals. Physical therapy goals for the school-aged child will focus on maintenance of ambulation skills, safety,

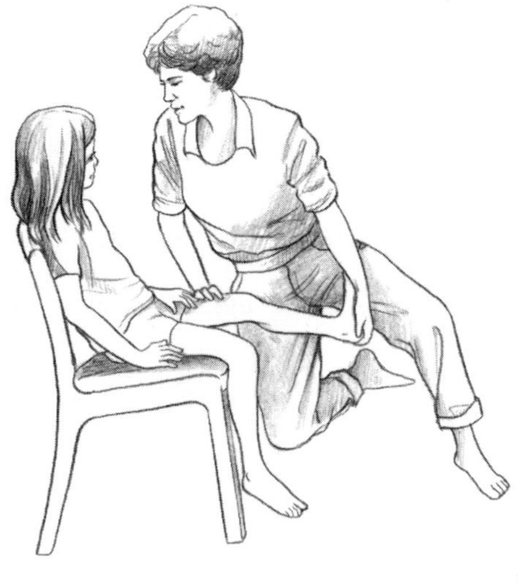

Figure 8-17 Heel cord stretch.

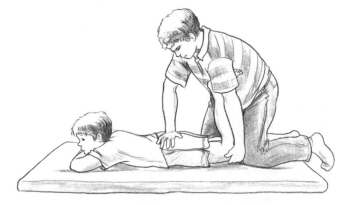

Figure 8-18 Hip flexor stretch.

maintenance of skills of daily living, and conservation of energy during the day. Physical therapy can help a child with DMD remain functional in his daily tasks longer by providing strategies, appropriate equipment, training to use the equipment, appropriate exercises, and intensive intervention before and after surgery. Consulting with other members of the team to assist in making decisions about when or whether to have bracing or surgery and when to transition to a wheelchair are also important roles for the physical therapist.

Surgery and bracing. By the time the child is 8 to 10 years old, he will be having significant difficulty walking, because of weakness of his quadriceps, hip extensors and ankle dorsiflexor muscle groups, and resultant joint contractures. Unless surgery to lengthen his Achilles tendon, iliotibial band, and hamstrings is performed, the child will likely lose his ability to walk because of poor balance from joint contractures. The goal of surgery to release joint contractures is to promote normal joint alignment to allow braced standing and walking. Another common surgery to promote normal foot alignment is a tendon transfer of the posterior tibialis tendon. Immobility from casting or bedrest after surgery can cause the child with DMD to irretrievably lose strength and function. Therefore it is very important that a child be prepared with appropriate splints measured and molded before to surgery, so that he can get up as soon as possible after surgery to stand and walk.

Lightweight braces that provide support at the hip, knee, and ankle are used after tendon releases to maintain joint alignment and to provide stability for movement. Knee-ankle-foot orthoses (KAFOs) may be all that are needed, but sometimes a child will use KAFOs in conjunction with a pelvic belt to provide stability at the hips or thoracic-lumbar-sacral orthosis (TLSO) to provide better trunk stability. Devices for mobility include reciprocating gait orthoses, parapodiums, reciprocating walkers, and front-wheeled walkers. A child will eventually lose his mobility and will subsequently use a stander to maintain standing skills for 1 or more hours each day, until that, too, taxes him too much.

Exercise. Although a specific exercise program can be created for the school-aged child with DMD, a general exercise program, such as swimming or riding a bicycle, may be more socially appropriate and provide many of the same benefits. A child should not exercise to fatigue, as this may damage the intact muscle fibers. If he can exercise with peers, such as in a swimming class or club, additional social benefits can be gained from the activity.

> Make an effort to talk with individuals who interact with the child outside of school to find out what skills the child needs to learn to succeed. This could include the dance teacher, baseball coach, or bus driver. You may learn more than you think!

Specific exercises, if developed, can include strengthening activities for the trunk flexors, hip extensors, hip adductors, knee extensors, and ankle dorsiflexors. A school-aged child will get bored repeating multiple repetitions of quad sets and abdominal curls, so the exercises should be incorporated into a fun routine, if possible. They can be done to music, with a peer group, in a pool, in a park, or with family members. A chart to demonstrate progress would be helpful. A reward system for motivation with the child and family helping to decide on appropriate rewards can help. Examples of rewards could include dinner at a restaurant, a small toy such as an action figure, extra television time, or an extra story read at night.

Standing and walking are very important to maintain upright positioning and mobility, and should be built into everyday routines. Times that might be appropriate for walking are during physical education class, walking with parents or siblings to and from school, walking after school, and walking to a specific class, lunch, or recess. Standing can be incorporated into television time at home, specific academic class time, or physical education class. To maintain ambulation skills, the goal of postoperative physical therapy programs is up to 3 to 5 hours per day of standing and/or walking (Tecklin, 1994). If the child is no longer walking, at least 1 hour per day of standing is necessary for standing with support to be beneficial. Some advocates of standing believe that standing with the spine in extension locks the facet joints, causing a stable spine that will not side bend, thus helping to prevent the development of scoliosis.

Role of the PTA. The PTA will likely be involved with the school-aged child with DMD on a regular basis, providing passive range of motion, helping to put on braces, teaching him to walk with new equipment and devices, monitoring an exercise program, and helping to develop strategies for the child to accomplish needed tasks. It is very important to communicate regularly with the family, teacher, occupational therapist, physical therapist, and other team members about how the child is progressing, so decisions related to changes in equipment or routine can be made.

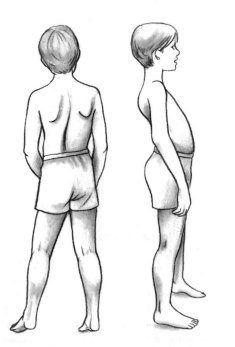

Figure 8-19 This child with Duchenne muscular dystrophy has gait and postural deviations of toe walking, abducted legs with weight on lateral borders of feet, forward center of gravity, arms back, lumbar lordosis. Also note the pseudohypertrophy of calf muscles.

The Adolescent With DMD

Mobility. By the time a child with DMD reaches adolescence, he will likely be using a wheelchair for mobility. Most boys are using a wheelchair by the time they are 12 to 14 years old. Some boys as young as 8 or 9 years old, depending on decisions regarding surgery and bracing, use a wheelchair full time for mobility. For those families who believe that the maintenance of walking and standing skills is important to delay the negative effects of wheelchair use (obesity, joint contractures, scoliosis), it is important to wait as long as possible to begin using a wheelchair full time. A boy with DMD will find that a wheelchair offers him more ease of movement, comfort, convenience, and less fatigue than he has been used to while struggling with his ambulation skills. He may be unwilling to continue struggling with walking once he discovers the convenience of a wheelchair. A phase-in period when a boy can use a wheelchair or scooter for certain social activities, such as playing with friends in the neighborhood, may be advisable.

Power mobility can offer significant independence to boys with upper extremity weakness. Younger boys who have more trunk and upper extremity control can use a powered three-wheeled scooter in school and around the neighborhood. Boys with less upper extremity strength will need the closer joystick that a wheelchair provides. Moving the joystick on a wheelchair from one side of the chair to the other every 6 months may slow down the development of scoliosis. Children often resist changing the joystick position, because they are adept at using their dominant hand.

In any type of wheelchair, positioning is very important, both to allow the child maximum function and to promote optimal body alignment to slow the formation of spinal deformities. Custom-molded seating inserts, modular seating with adjustable lateral trunk supports, or body jackets or corsets can be used for trunk positioning. Each method has its own positive and negative features and should be considered in light of the individual child's needs. At minimum, the pelvis should be securely positioned in neutral, and the trunk should have three points of support. That is, support should be provided at the apex of the scoliotic curve on one side and the pelvis and the ribs on the other side of the trunk. The wheelchair should be very lightweight if it is a manual chair to allow the child independent propulsion. If it is a power chair, it should have a proportional joystick control with the ability to change controls, speed, and power as the child's function changes. The wheelchair should have a manual or power tilt-in-space option to provide for pressure relief, postural relief, and easier repositioning. The back-to-seat angle should be greater than 90 degrees to allow for slight extension of the spine and the resultant locking of spinal facets in a neutral position. A biangular back would be ideal to provide this type of spinal extension. Safety features, including chest straps for stability when riding in a bus or van, should be considered. The chair should be able to accommodate a mechanical ventilator and oxygen canister when the child needs it. A child should be intimately involved in choosing the colors, features, and customization of his wheelchair.

Self-care. Adolescence is a time of significantly less independence in all areas for boys with DMD. Boys will lose functional skills in their upper extremities as well as their lower extremities. Feeding themselves will become a problem, as will independent bladder and bowel care, grooming, and bathing.

Assistive devices, such as a ball-bearing feeder, commode chair, urinal, bath or shower chair, long-handled bath brush, built-up handles on eating and grooming utensils, and transfer boards, may be helpful. Other adaptive equipment that allows longer self-feeding skills include a long straw and elevated lap trays so distance from plate to mouth is shorter. Boys with DMD will eventually need help for transfers and, gradually, will be dependent for all transfers. Parents and caregivers will need training to help them learn how to manually transfer boys to and from their wheelchair, bed, toilet or commode, couch, and car. As boys get older and heavier, mechanical lifting devices will become appropriate, and electrical lifting devices may even be purchased for them. Therapists will need to work closely with the child, his family, occupational therapist, and other team members to determine what equipment and training are needed for safe and efficient care at home.

Sleeping. As boys lose the ability to move themselves in bed, sleeping may become difficult for them. They will need a regular positioning program of turning throughout the night to promote comfort and relieve pressure areas. To relieve the strain on parents and primary caregivers, a hospital bed with an air-flow mattress, alternating pressure mattress, or other pressure relieving mattress will help the child be more comfortable for longer periods. The head of the hospital bed can be elevated to assist with respiratory comfort and care. Frequently, parents do not think to complain about their own lack of sleep from continually repositioning their children at night. The therapist can ask appropriate questions about sleep patterns and can recommend equipment that may help.

Vocational and educational support. Boys may graduate from high school and be interested in taking classes at a community college, four-year college, or vocational school. They also may be interested in working. The therapist will work with the team to decide how to best support the student during the transition from high school to further education or work. This may entail visits to work or school sites, training of aides or other supportive personnel, and problem solving. Issues that need to be resolved could include transportation, accessibility to buildings or equipment, modifying the work/school site and requirements, or funding for supportive personnel or specialized equipment.

Respiratory compromise. Respiratory failure or pulmonary infection is the major cause of death for children with DMD (Bach, Alba, Pilkington, & Lee, 1981). With decreasing pulmonary capacity due to weakening of respiratory muscles, boys with DMD start losing vital capacity at 8 or 9 years old. By the last stages of the disease, they are functioning at only 9% of their total vital capacity (Fukunaga, Okubo, Moritoyo, Kawashima, & Osame, 1993). Boys with DMD and their families need to evaluate the use of mechanical ventilation to help get adequate levels of oxygen. Mechanical ventilation can significantly increase the life expectancy of boys with DMD (Alexander, Johnson, Petty, & Staunch, 1979; Bach, O'Brien, Krotenberg, & Alba, 1987). Families may think that they are only prolonging the inevitable, but studies have shown that the quality of life is perceived as good by children with DMD who elect to use assisted ventilation, and life can be prolonged by 3 to 6 years (Fukunaga, Okubo, Moritoyo, Kawashima, & Osame, 1993; Curran & Colbert, 1989).

Therapists should be able to closely monitor and teach the educational staff how to monitor the respiratory function of boys with advanced DMD. Signs of respiratory insufficiency include decreased alertness, pallor or mottling of the skin, and bluish tinges to the lips and nail beds. If one of these signs is noted, the child should be given oxygen, laid down on his or her side, and help should be obtained.

Pulmonary infection is also a leading cause of death for boys with DMD. Therapists can improve the respiratory hygiene of boys with DMD by teaching them and their families postural drainage techniques, assisted coughing, and breathing exercises.

Boys with DMD on average die by the time they are 18 to 22 years old, although some live through their 20s into their early 30s. If due to respiratory insufficiency, death frequently comes as sleep through a coma induced by hypoxygenation. Therapists need to confront their own attitudes about death and participate as part of a team of people supporting boys with DMD and their families. Listening is very important when people talk about their feelings or fears. The MDA is a valuable resource for families and therapists working with children with DMD. Support groups and literature are available, among other services.

Role of the PTA. The PTA will have less of a direct role to play with the adolescent with DMD than with a younger child. Working as part of a team to provide services and address particular needs, such as refitting splints, repairing adaptive equipment, and problem solving, will be the primary roles of the PTA.

The Child With Prader-Willi Syndrome

Incidence and Cause

Prader-Willi syndrome (PWS) was first named in 1956 by Prader, Labhart, and Willi, and has an estimated prevalence of 1 in 10,000 live births (Donaldson, Chu, Cooke, Wilson, Greene, & Stephenson, 1994). It is caused by a microdeletion, or a small missing section, of the proximal part of the long arm of the paternal chromosome 15 (Donaldson, et al., 1994; Richards, Quaghebeur, Clift, Holland, Dahlitz, & Parkes, 1994). The chromosome in question is the one in the fifteenth pair of chromosomes that was inherited from the child's father. If the same microdeletion occurred on the other chromosome in the pair, the one inherited from the child's mother, a different disorder called Angelman syndrome (also called "happy puppet syndrome") would manifest itself.

A second method of inheriting PWS is that of unimaternal disomy (Chu, Cooke, Stephenson, Tolmie, Clarke, Parry-Jones, Connor, & Donaldson, 1994). With this type of inheritance, both of the fifteenth chromosomes with microdeletions are inherited from the child's mother with no contribution from the father. This method of transmission is more rare than the type manifested on the paternally derived chromosome. Most children with definitive PWS demonstrate one or the other characteristic chromosomal features with genetic testing.

Clinical Features

The infant with PWS is hypotonic at birth and has difficulty with sucking and feeding. Mothers notice decreased fetal movements before birth. Frequently, the infant is in an abnormal position at birth and sometimes has an asymmetric head shape (Cassidy, 1987). During the first several years of life, feeding is very diffi-

cult, requiring tube or gavage feedings. Frequently, an infant with PWS is diagnosed with failure to thrive. Other characteristic features of an infant with PWS are an abnormal or absent cry, genital hypoplasia or small genitals, undescended testicles in boys, delayed motor milestones, delayed speech development, fair hair, blue eyes, and typical facial features. Facial features that are typical of a child with PWS include almond-shaped eyelids, thin upper lip, mouth turns downward, narrow forehead, and light-colored hair and skin (Cassidy, 1987; Donaldson, Chu, Cooke, Wilson, Greene, & Stephenson, 1994). Sticky saliva is another common problem, which contributes to mouth caries in later childhood.

At around 2 to 3 years of age, the child with PWS develops an insatiable appetite, and the family who have been struggling to promote adequate nutrition now has to closely monitor the child for overeating. This insatiable appetite is one of the most difficult aspects of PWS to manage. If not managed aggressively, children will become morbidly obese and die from complications of obesity. If the obesity can be controlled, the child with PWS can live a normal life span.

Other characteristics include speech and motor delays. A child eventually will develop speech, but articulation will be poor and voice quality will be weak. The tone of voice will be high pitched with a nasal quality. Expressive speech skills will be delayed. Gross motor milestones will be delayed because of hypotonia, but fine motor skills usually are age appropriate.

Children with PWS have short stature and typically have small hands and feet with a straight ulnar border to their hands. They bruise easily, are excessively sleepy during the day, and can develop scoliosis during childhood. They are unable to vomit. They frequently have strabismus (eyes do not work together) and myopia (near-sightedness), and may squint to see. Behavior problems that may develop during childhood include skin picking, temper tantrums, stubbornness, manipulative personality, negativism, and depression. These problems generally get worse as adolescence approaches.

Children with PWS will have a delayed or incomplete puberty. Hormone levels are low because of pituitary gland dysfunction. Sixty to eighty percent of girls do not menstruate. Boys have small genitals, and all adults with PWS are infertile. Osteoporosis may be a problem due to decreased hormonal levels (Cassidy, 1987).

Children are usually intellectually impaired with average IQ of 70 and a range from 40 to normal. Twelve percent of children with PWS have IQ within normal ranges (Cassidy, 1987). However, they frequently do not work up to their potential academically, and have more difficulty with mathematics than reading skills. Severe learning disabilities as well as intellectual impairment can affect their academic progress.

As children get older, they may develop a poor self-image that results in poor peer relationships and depression. This poor self-image can be related to obesity, poor performance in school, poor athletic performance, poor communicative skills, and difficulty with self-help skills. Behavior is more difficult for them to manage, and temper tantrums, stubbornness, and manipulation can become more pervasive. Children with PWS generally have a sweet temperament but become easily frustrated. They can be very tedious to their family members and friends through repeating the same information multiple times and can get very concerned if routines change. Obtaining food

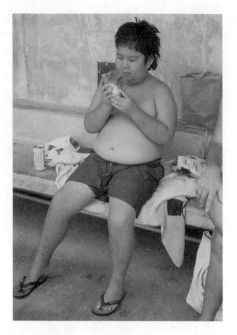

Figure 8-20 Getting food can be all-consuming for children with Prader-Willi syndrome.

can consume their waking hours and can take precedence over all other activities.

Most children with PWS demonstrate creativity and perseverance when it comes to finding food (Figure 8-20). They have been known to unscrew the hinges of locked cabinets, take all the candy from candy dishes in hotels and restaurants, shoplift food and candy from stores, order hundreds of dollars of food-related items from catalogs over the telephone without permission, and forge checks to pay for their food. They also have been known to eat garbage and spoiled food. Because of a lower metabolic rate and less physical activity, persons with PWS need fewer calories than someone without PWS to maintain their weight. They gain weight very fast and do not feel full when eating. Close supervision is essential by everyone around a child or adult with PWS to maintain a healthy level of food consumption.

Medical treatments. There is no cure for PWS, but some medical interventions may provide help in preventing morbid obesity. Growth hormones may help with changing body composition from fat to protein, but results have been equivocal (Donaldson, Chu, Cooke, Wilson, Greene, & Stephenson, 1994). Gastric bypass surgery has been effective in some cases to prevent morbid obesity (Soper, Mason, Printen, & Zellweger, 1975). Drugs to suppress appetite have been tried with mixed results (Donaldson, et. al., 1994). Behavioral control has been most effective to control weight gain.

Physical therapy treatment for a child with PWS will vary according to the needs and age of the individual child. Please see Table 8-9 for a sample of long- and short-term goals for a child with PWS at different ages. Suggested activities to address the goals are also listed.

The Infant With PWS

The physical therapist may become involved with the infant with PWS because of delayed gross motor development and hypotonia. The infant may be seen in an infant development program, outpatient department in a pediatric hospital, or a clinic. Physical therapy goals may include adequate positioning for feeding, positioning while being carried by caregivers, and facilitating early gross motor milestones, such as rolling, sitting without support, and standing with support.

Feeding. A major problem for infants with PWS is poor feeding, and therapists will have to work closely with parents, occupational therapists, and speech-language pathologists to address feeding issues. Because oral feeding is likely to take a long time at each sitting, positioning is very important. It is unlikely that the infant will be able to breast feed because of a poor suck and hypotonia. The mother may express breast milk, or use formula, and feed it to her baby using a nipple with an enlarged opening. The infant's head should be in midline, and the chin should be slightly tucked for easy swallowing. It is important that the infant's head is higher than its stomach. Feeding in the parent's lap is one alternative, or feeding in an infant seat, infant swing, or propped on a couch, are all good positions. It is important that the caregiver understand the importance of face-to-face interaction during feeding in promoting normal social skills. Talking to the infant, smiling, and touching the infant are all important activities to encourage mutual interaction. These aspects of interaction are also important if the parent is tube feeding the child.

Activities to improve oral-motor tone can promote better nippling. These activities can include stroking the lips, gums, and tongue; providing light pressure around the mouth; and facial massage. Discovering the rhythm of the child's eating is also important. How long he or she sucks before taking a break, whether naps are taken during feeding, and how long of a rest is taken in between sucking are all important qualities for parents to recognize. Most parents develop this type of understanding with their child, but it is often more difficult for parents of children with feeding disorders to assess the rhythms of their child's eating patterns.

Positioning. Static positioning and positioning for carrying are important for an infant with low muscle tone, to help him or her access the world visually, as well as to develop strength to interact motorically with the environment. Young infants should be positioned with their heads in midline, their legs in flexion, and their arms close to their sides. This position approximates the physiological flexion of newborns with normal muscle tone. It can be achieved by using blankets for swaddling or by using folded infant blankets under the infant's legs and beside the head, trunk, and arms. A parent or caregiver should hold the infant's limbs close, not allowing them to droop when being carried. An infant will feel more secure when held this way than if the infant were allowed to flop arms and legs out to the side without adequate head support. This position can also be approximated when the infant is on its side or stomach.

Developing gross motor skills. As the infant grows, strength will improve so that the child will be able to reach for toys, roll over, and prop on forearms. By providing facilitation to move between positions and assisting the child to maintain positions for longer periods using assistive devices or an adult body for support, the therapist can help the child develop improved

Sample Developmental Goals: Child With Prader-Willi Syndrome

TABLE 8-9

Family or child long-term goal	Physical therapy short-term objectives	Activities to address long-term goals and short-term objectives
Infant Child will hold bottle independently to eat.	1. Child will play with toys bimanually in supine.	• Place child in a supported sidelying position with toys in front of child. Toys should make noise, be bright colors, and be lightweight, such as plastic keys or other infant toys. Move toys, make noise, and encourage child to reach for them. • Place child in supported sitting with a table at child's chest level to support toys. Encourage active manipulation with both hands. • Provide upper extremity weight bearing activities prior to asking child to reach. Activities could include facilitated propping through hands or elbows while prone over a roll or therapists leg or hand over hand hitting at a large ball or bouncy surface with a flat palm.
	2. Child will hold bottle briefly.	• Use 2- or 4-ounce bottle initially. • Teach parents to do hand over hand holding of bottle with pressure over infant's hands to provide proprioceptive input. This should be done for each feeding.
Toddler Child will run.	1. Child will fast-walk for 10 feet.	• Encourage weight-bearing activities, such as walking, climbing, and squatting. • Hold both hands, and provide upper extremity support while you physically encourage child to walk fast. • While guarding the child, play games that encourage fast walking, such as "I'm chasing you!" games.
Preschooler Child will climb jungle gym.	1. Child will get into and out of a small chair.	• Create an obstacle course with a tunnel, steps to go up and down, and obstacles to climb over. Assist child to complete course as needed. • Model sitting in a chair, or have parent model sitting in a chair next to a small one for the child. Assist the child to climb in and out of chair if needed. • Play adapted musical chairs in a group situation. There should always be enough chairs for everyone.
	2. Child will climb steps to the slide.	• Encourage child to climb stacked stools. Put toys at the top and give upper extremity support if needed. Facilitate upright walking on steps rather than allowing creeping. • Facilitate climbing up steps to slide. Provide support for descending slide as this may be too much for child to do alone. • Facilitate climbing playground equipment with smaller steps than jungle gym. Always be aware of safety for child.
School-Aged Child Child will maintain weight within expected levels for age.	1. Child will tolerate aerobic exercise daily.	• Provide exercise activity for entire class of children. This could include walking around the school grounds, running races, potato sack games, or other activities that children enjoy. Vary the activities to ensure fun. • Encourage family to enroll child in after school sports activity, such as swimming or soccer. For a child with PWS to be successful in after-school activity, the focus should not be competition but learning of skills and fun. Consult with coach of after-school activity on specific needs of the child with PWS. • Talk with family about initiating regular weighing program at home and at school to monitor weight if one is not in place.

Continued

Sample Developmental Goals: Child With Prader-Willi Syndrome—cont'd

TABLE 8-9

Family or child long-term goal	Physical therapy short-term objectives	Activities to address long-term goals and short-term objectives
Adolescent		
Student will be successful in holding part-time job stacking boxes in warehouse.	1. Student will repeatedly lift 20 pound boxes.	• Simulate job site at the school and practice lifting and stacking skills. Use a chart to monitor progress. • Visit the job site with student and consult with supervisor to modify environment for greater likelihood of success. (Examples: Move forklift closer to loading dock so boxes do not have to be carried so far, stack boxes only four high instead of six high.) • With team members, inform work site employees of health needs of student, including closely monitoring food intake. Make sure they understand importance of not eating in front of student or giving food to student.
	2. Child will tolerate working in standing for 2 hours at a time in 4 1/2-hour work shifts.	• Change or add to daily exercise routine to include standing or walking exercises to increase endurance. • Discuss with supervisor the possibility of modifying work requirements until student's endurance levels are improved. For instance, give student a break after an hour instead of 2 hours, or shorten work shift initially.

strength and control to progress in gross motor skills. Depending on the child's developmental level, activities could include:
• Propping prone over a roll to play with toys (facilitates head control, shoulder cocontraction)
• Sitting in a custom chair with trunk support to play with toys (facilitates head control, moving upper extremities on a stable trunk)
• Sitting straddling therapist's or parent's leg to play with toys (facilitates head and trunk control in sitting, moving off the base of support)
• Facilitating propped sitting both forward and to the side (develops cocontraction in the shoulders and head control)
• Facilitated "marching" (moving legs up and down) to music either in supine, sidelying, supported sitting, or supported standing (provides proprioceptive input through lower extremities to promote weight bearing)

Role of the PTA. The PTA will work closely with the PT to develop activities for the infant with PWS. Treatment sessions will usually occur in the home or infant development program, and will focus on parent teaching and positioning of the infant, as well as promoting gross motor skills.

The Toddler and Preschooler With PWS

For the toddler and preschooler, physical therapy goals include gross motor skills, such as pulling to stand, standing with support, squatting to pick up toys from the floor, cruising, walking, jumping, and running. It is during this period that the child with PWS begins to exhibit an insatiable appetite and may gain a significant amount of weight. Most children will not get morbidly obese during this period because their eating is still under their parent's control. It is very important that an accurate diagnosis of PWS be made, however, so that early patterns of healthful eating can be set by the family.

The toddler or preschool-aged child is eager to explore and is motivated to learn to stand and walk. To reach goals of independent ambulation, children need only be presented with situations that will stimulate them to get up and go. Interesting toys can be placed strategically on coffee table height tables to entice children to cruise toward them while holding on. Small play areas can be set up with chairs, so that children want to cruise between them. The hula hoop is an excellent tool for teaching children that they can walk with less support. Have a child hold onto the hula hoop with both hands while you hold it very securely with both of your hands. While singing, the child can be encouraged to walk in a circle holding on. Your support can be decreased until the child is essentially holding the hula hoop alone. Of course, you can always offer immediate support should it be needed. A dish towel or scarf is another way to encourage a child who is close to walking independently. Have the child hold the middle of a dish towel while you hold the ends and pull it very taut. As the child gains more confidence, the tautness can be gradually released so that the towel becomes limp. Eventually, the child is holding the dish towel alone. You must stay close enough to provide support to the child if necessary so that his or her confidence will not be eroded by falling.

Role of the PTA. The PTA may have an active role in the infant development program or preschool with the child with PWS. It is very important that food control needs are understood and communicated to all team members. A regular exercise program may be initiated, and activities to promote gross motor skills can be integrated into the regular preschool routine.

The School-Aged Child With PWS

The early school years are critical for developing routines that encourage normal eating patterns. Three elements must go into any weight control program for a child with PWS. The first is es-

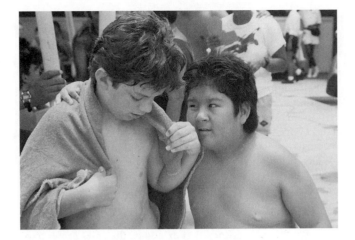

Figure 8-21 Grant *(right)* participates at Special Olympics with his friend Luke. Peer relationships can be difficult, but Grant demonstrates warmth and caring for his friend.

tablishing a good diet and sticking to it. Foods chosen should be low in calories and fat. Foods should be filling. Children with PWS often believe that they have more food if more items, even though lesser amounts, are offered at meals or snacks. Regular snacks that are low in calories should be offered. If a special occasion, such as a birthday party, should occur, the child with PWS should not be excluded. A half portion of treats should be offered and the calories should be subtracted from a meal at another time of the day.

The second component of a weight control program is avoiding temptation. Strict watch over diet is always necessary. For children with PWS, this is not as easy as for other obese children. Because they always want to eat and do not sense when they are full, external controls are needed. Children with PWS cannot develop the self-control needed to control their own diet. It is the responsibility of everyone at home and at school to help them avoid temptation. Therefore no one should eat snacks in front of a child with PWS. Meals should be scheduled and the schedule should not deviate. All food should be kept out of sight and usually behind locked doors. All adults and responsible children should be informed of their responsibility to watch the child with PWS to ensure that extra food is not obtained.

The third component to an effective diet is exercise. Daily exercise is very important. Although a child with PWS has low muscle tone, he or she will be able to carry out a daily walking, running, or swimming program with supervision (Figure 8-21). A child who is very obese may have related health problems, such as diabetes or cardiac insufficiency, which will need to be monitored during exercise.

The Special Olympics is a wonderful arena to develop and implement an exercise program. There are events for swimming, running, and other track and field events. Communities frequently have programs for training before the Olympics in group settings that can help improve the motivation of the athlete. The events themselves are fun, a social opportunity both for children with disabilities, as well as for parents and others who volunteer to help. All participants receive medals or ribbons and hugs and cheers, so the Special Olympics are an opportunity to build self-esteem for the participants, as well as get some good exercise.

Therapists can participate as coaches or volunteers for particular children, agencies, or the community. It is a great opportunity to meet people and benefit the children with disabilities, who we work with every day.

Other community opportunities for exercise include parks and recreation activities run by local government agencies. Activities for children with disabilities are frequently offered. The activities may be limited to children with disabilities or may include them with other children in pool or field games. Even if children with disabilities are not expressly welcomed, a parent can usually approach administrators and arrange to have their child participate. A therapist may provide valuable assistance in adapting the activity for the child with PWS.

Behavior challenges. Behaviors such as lying and stealing, frequently related to food, become common during school-aged years. Strict behavioral supports need to be in place to deal with these issues when they arise. Some of the supports suggested by the Prader-Willi Society include the following:

1. Programs should be intervention-prevention oriented. Plan ahead, lock doors and cabinets, food supplies.
2. Rules should be reasonable, easily enforced, and realistic. Do not nag or argue. Do not ignore bad behavior.
3. A positive reinforcement program should be implemented where there are positive rewards for positive behavior. A token system is an example.
4. There should be opportunity for choice or decision making. No more than two choices should be offered at a time.
5. Routine is important. Plan ahead for changes in routine.

Role of the PTA. Activities for general exercise can be supervised by the PTA. These will be most successful if performed with other children in the class. Specific exercises to strengthen certain muscle groups may also be appropriate. A small group could be gathered to do the exercises, or they could be incorporated into daily routines in school. If a child is unwilling to participate in recommended activities, the family or teacher may be able to suggest motivational strategies that work with the child.

The Adolescent With PWS

As the child with PWS grows older, some of the problems become more difficult to manage. Adolescence is not an easy time for anyone, and children with PWS have more to contend with than most. Self-esteem can be fragile at best; peer relationships can be nonexistent. Behavioral challenges can escalate with temper tantrums becoming more frequent and violent. Time out is a good way to handle behavior crises, because adolescents with PWS cannot reason well, especially when upset.

One role for physical therapy during these years is to continue to support a daily exercise program. Monitoring for scoliosis should be done regularly, as scoliosis can progress rapidly during adolescence. Consulting with the team of people involved with the child, including the family, classroom teachers, physical education teacher, speech-language pathologist, transition coordinator, psychologist, and others, to solve immediate problems and plan for transition to a job or supported employment after high school is essential. The therapist can provide needed information about endurance, strength, and physical capabilities when considering opportunities for the adolescent with PWS after high school. Consideration of alternate residential arrangements may also be addressed, as it may be difficult for the family to support the adult with PWS at home indefinitely. Emotional support for the child and family is very important during these difficult years.

Role of the PTA. A regular exercise program is still important for the adolescent with PWS. Coaching or volunteering with Special Olympics or other after-school athletic activities is a wonderful way to promote exercise for all children with disabilities. Assisting the instructor in school-based physical education classes to include the adolescent with PWS may be effective in maintaining a regular exercise program.

The Child With Osteogenesis Imperfecta

Incidence and Cause

Osteogenesis imperfecta (OI) is a group of diseases, that are characterized by poor collagen synthesis causing fragile bones. It is sometimes called brittle bone disease. Four types of OI were classified by Sillence, Senn, and Danks (1979), based on the mode of inheritance and by how the disease presents itself. Groups II and III are the most severe and have an autosomal recessive inheritance pattern. The defective gene(s) must be carried by both parents, who do not manifest the disorder. Groups I and IV are less severe, but the defective gene may be carried by only one affected parent in an autosomal dominant pattern of inheritance. The disease may also be caused by a spontaneous mutation. Child-ren with type I OI have the mildest course of the disease and are usually ambulatory. Children with type IV have more bone fragility, but are frequently ambulatory with assistive devices. Children with type III have a severe form of the disease and frequently have fractures at birth. Children born with type II OI always have fractures and deformities at birth and usually die at birth or in infancy.

Clinical Features

The clinical features of children with OI vary according to the nature of their genetic inheritance. The most prominent feature is bone fragility, resulting in bowing of the long bones and fractures. Children may be born with fractures, or these may develop later in life. Multiple, early fractures may lead to deformities of the long bones, shortness of stature, and inability to walk. Fractures heal in a normal amount of time, but the callus formation may be large and of poor quality. Fractures tend to decrease as the child ages, especially after puberty. Frequently, children with mild OI are evaluated for child abuse secondary to multiple fractures before OI is diagnosed. This can be traumatic for families. The child with OI usually has normal intelligence and a cheerful personality.

Other features of a child with OI can include blue sclerae of the eye and tympanic membrane. Poor development of the deciduous or secondary teeth is also characteristic, and the teeth that do develop may be brown in color, translucent, and soft. The child may be short in stature, with short limbs, and develop a scoliosis or kyphoscoliosis. The ligaments may be lax, leading to hypermobility and joint dislocations. A triangular face with a wide skull, narrow long bones and osteoporosis on radiographs, and thin skin as a result of poor collagen formation are also char-

acteristic of the child with OI. Metabolic problems can include heat intolerance, increased body temperature, and sweating (Zaleske, Doppelt, & Mankin, 1990). The child may be at risk for developing deafness because of fractures of the small bones in the middle ear.

Medical interventions. Although multiple treatments with vitamins, minerals, and drugs have been tried, none have proved effective in improving bone strength of children with OI (Zaleske, Koppelt, & Mankin, 1990; Albright, 1981). Aggressive treatments of respiratory infections help maintain health.

The surgical intervention of inserting rods into the medulla, or the long axis of the long bones, has proven to be the primary intervention improving the quality of life of children with OI. Intramedullary rods can be used to stabilize fractures, straighten bones with multiple deformities, or to provide stability for bones at risk of fracturing. Rods that extend as the child grows have been used to minimize the numbers of surgeries required. Surgical techniques that allow the rods to be inserted through the skin can allow stabilization of children with severe OI until they are stable enough for the more invasive surgery (McHale, Tenuta, Tosi, & McKay, 1994). Surgery to repair scoliosis can also help a child with severe OI to maintain respiratory function, as well as functional sitting positions.

Physical therapy treatment for a child with OI will vary according to the needs and age of the individual child. See Table 8-10 for a sample of long- and short-term goals for a child with OI at different ages. Suggested activities to address the goals are also listed.

The Infant With OI

Physical therapy goals. Physical therapy goals for a young child with OI will include developmentally appropriate gross motor skills, such as rolling, reaching for toys, and sitting without support. Caretaker ability to handle and carry the child will also be important goals, and home visits may provide the best circumstances for the therapist to work with the family on functional activities. Precautions include prevention and recognition of fractures.

Recognizing fractures. The children most likely to receive early intervention services from physical therapy are those with the more severe forms of OI. The risk of fractures with infants with OI is very high, and sometimes parents are reluctant to handle their infant. Children with OI have normal sensation, and fractures are painful. Even diaper changes and dressing can be traumatic. Fractures can occur through normal handling, weight bearing, bumping an extremity, uneven pressure through the horizontal axis of a long bone, or spontaneously through muscle pull on a bone. It is important not to blame a caregiver or therapist if a fracture occurs. The child and family should be emotionally supported. The fracture should be treated. The reason the fracture occurred should be identified and addressed, although identifying the reason will not be possible much of the time.

Infant cues of crying, vacant stare, hypersensitivity to touch, and decreased interactions can be important clues that something is wrong in the young child. An infant with a fracture will be unwilling to move the extremity that is involved. Classic signs of fracture include redness, swelling, heat, and discoloration at

Sample Developmental Goals: Child With Osteogenesis Imperfecta

TABLE 8-10		
Family or child long-term goal	**Physical therapy short-term objectives**	**Activities to address long-term goals and short-term objectives**
Infant Child will accompany family to grocery store.	1. Child will hold head up 15 minutes in supported sitting.	• Teach family members to provide gentle vestibular input holding child protected on lap while rocking on a rocking chair, positioning child in an adapted infant seat on a gentle porch swing (not an infant swing, which swings too hard), and carrying infant around the house. • Make an adapted positioning device from custom molded foam to position and carry infant in a semi-upright position. • Provide visual and auditory input using mobiles in crib, crib gymnastic toys, and busy boxes for child to look at and reach for. • Encourage parents to alternate which arm in which they carry child, and to change the direction the child lies in the crib every month to encourage head turning to both sides (the child will tend to turn head toward parent or doorway).
	2. Child will sit safely in grocery cart.	• Adapt seating for grocery cart, including providing support and protection for hanging limbs. Straps should be broad and padded. • Encourage sitting balance skills through music games on lap. Sit child on your lap and tip gently by moving your knees while singing a song to child. • Have older infant practice sitting on bolster while reaching for toys. Bolster should be the same height as the infant's knees so both feet can be placed on the floor on either side of the bolster. Songs and gently rocking the bolster while providing safe support are alternative activities on the bolster.
Toddler Child will have independent household mobility.	1. Child will propel a floor cart on casters for 10 feet on a tile or wood surface.	• Provide activities to increase upper extremity strength, including propped sitting, (forward, laterally, and backward) and prone on elbows. Encourage weight shifts through upper extremities in sitting and prone positions, such as leaning through one arm to reach for toys with the other. • Practice propelling floor cart. Assist as needed. Provide incentive such as "Push to Mom!" or "Go get the toy!"
	2. Child will tolerate standing with support for 10 minutes in rolling stander.	• Provide gentle weight-bearing activities through lower extremities, including sitting on your lap or straddling bolster with feet on floor. Gently raise your lap or the end of the bolster, so that more weight goes through the child's legs. This can be done to music or to facilitate reaching for something. • Use air splints to provide lower extremity support in supported standing. • Position the child in a standing frame that has good support and encourage child to play with toys on the tray. • Have child propel rolling stander using hands on large wheels. Include child in mobile game with other children.

Continued

Sample Developmental Goals: Child With Osteogenesis Imperfecta—cont'd

TABLE 8-10

Family or child long-term goal	Physical therapy short-term objectives	Activities to address long-term goals and short-term objectives
Preschooler		
Child will have independent power mobility.	1. Child will start and stop wheelchair on command.	• Practice skills in wheelchair. The activity itself will be intrinsically rewarding to the child. Make sure the seating is adequate for safety in the chair. • Include the child in a game of red light-green light in the power chair. If child's skills are variable, make sure that an adult is close to assist for safety.
	2. Child will have good safety awareness in power chair.	• Create an obstacle course, including driving between two lines, stopping on another line, going through a narrow doorway, and around a corner, driving on a sidewalk with a high curb, negotiating a curb cut, and driving in a crowd of other children. Make the task of succeeding at the obstacle course fun by providing tangible rewards, including stickers or stars. • Have child practice using the power wheelchair in all daily environments, including school, home, the store, getting on and off the bus, and the playground. • Teach parents or caregivers how to operate and care for wheelchair. Child should have a small but important role in taking care of chair, for instance, reminding parents to charge it at night, wiping down the seat every day, or asking to have the water in the battery checked.
School-Aged Child		
Child will participate fully in regular education classes.	1. Child will tolerate being in the classroom all day.	• Ensure that seating position in classroom is comfortable and safe for child. Child should be at the same height as classmates to access tables or desks. • Ensure that child has independent mobility skills to move around the classroom with the other children. • Provide alternative positioning in the classroom, including floor sitting, standing, and a resting position. Teach teacher and classroom aide to transfer and position child. • Encourage awareness of safety among classmates through educating them about child with OI and safety precautions. Have child with OI participate in the presentation to class, and teach other children specifically how they can help (do not bump child with OI, get an adult if help is needed, be aware of their movements around the child with OI).
	2. Child will participate in regular physical education class.	• Consult with physical education teacher to adapt activities for child to be included. • Work with team to provide assistive technology, such as electric pitching device or bowling ramp to assist child in participating.

the site of the fracture. Fever may also occur. These may not be readily apparent in a small child but will eventually appear. The parents and frequent caregivers will come to recognize the signs easily.

Positioning. Positioning to minimize the risk of fractures and maximize social interactions is very important. A crib should be well padded with no openings for limbs to get caught. Crib rails should be padded to minimize damage if legs or arms get bumped. An infant seat with full extremity support is a good positioning device for a small infant who is not mobile. It should be well padded with soft blankets. Side supports made of rolled blankets can provide positioning, so that arms do not flop out

Sample Developmental Goals: Child With Osteogenesis Imperfecta—cont'd

TABLE 8-10

Family or child long-term goal	Physical therapy short-term objectives	Activities to address long-term goals and short-term objectives
Adolescent Student will drive a car.	1. Student will learn skills to drive using adapted hand controls. (Short stature will preclude reaching foot pedals on vehicle.)	• Refer to adaptive driving program in your area. • Make any modifications needed on wheelchair to accommodate needs for driving. • Provide input to vendor, family, and adaptive driving program on seating needs and needs for wheelchair-accessible van, including lift and adapted driving controls. • Assist in finding funding to pay for van, controls, and training.

to the side. Parents may prefer to carry a small infant on an adult-sized bed pillow, which will provide a large base of support. For children with severe OI, sometimes custom-molded foam cushions are made from Foam-in-Place for carrying and positioning. If the child is carried directly in the caregiver's arms, all the extremities and the head should be well supported. Varied carrying positions should be used and the child's position changed throughout the day to allow for varied visual input, vestibular input, and opportunity for movement against gravity. Care should be taken not to support the child across the axis of the long bones, which could cause fracture. This means that the entire length of the long bones should be supported rather than holding in the middle of the thigh or arm. A child with OI should not be lifted by the arms, held by the hand or arm, or carried so that the legs or arms dangle. The infant should be rolled on and off a diaper with legs and hips fully supported rather than lifted by the ankles to change a diaper.

Role of the PTA. The PTA may not have a direct role in treating an infant with OI, because of the medically fragile nature of the child. If a PTA is treating an infant with OI through an outpatient clinic, inpatient facility where the child is hospitalized for a fracture, or through an infant development program, awareness of safety precautions to prevent fractures is important. Support from the PT and other team members is essential. Activities will likely be directed toward positioning and carrying the child and promoting gross motor skills.

The Toddler and Preschooler With OI

Independent mobility. Independent mobility is an important developmental goal for toddlers and preschoolers. It can be achieved through independent creeping, cruising, walking, propelling a scooterboard or cart, scooting on buttocks, or powered mobility. Scooting on buttocks is a common method that children discover to move around the house. Although functional for them, it can be slow and tiring. It is important to encourage weight bearing through arms and legs to promote active bone strengthening and to allow the child to be as functionally independent as possible. Propelling wheeled devices can facilitate upper extremity weight bearing and strengthening. Wheeled de-

vices can be faster than scooting to move around the house, playground, or school. Independent creeping, cruising, and walking are possible for children with mild or moderate disease. They may need bracing to support extremities during these activities. For children with severe OI, power mobility is a good option. Power mobility allows them the opportunity to explore their world and to keep up with peers. Training is important, so the children are safe with the heavy power devices and do not injure themselves or others. The mobility devices that a child needs may change as new skills are learned, strength is achieved, and the child grows.

Bracing. Long leg braces can provide external support to the long bones of the leg that will promote independent ambulation skills, as well as minimize fractures and bowing of the long bones. Frequently, because they are lighter, braces or splints are used instead of casting for fractures. The therapist's role is to assist the orthotist to measure for braces, monitor the fit, teach the child how to put on and take off the braces, and how to walk with them. Air splints are an effective alternative for bracing either legs or arms for weight bearing. Assistive devices, such as rolling walkers or crutches, will probably be necessary for balance and support.

Role of the PTA. Treatment will be directed toward teaching mobility skills, self-help skills, encouraging head and trunk control to facilitate sitting up and moving through space, and facilitating early weight-bearing skills (Figure 8-22). Therapy sessions may occur in the home, the infant development program, or, for preschoolers, in a preschool setting. The child with OI may be afraid to move because of fear of fractures or may reflect parent's fears and be unwilling to move. The PTA will need to develop a positive and respectful relationship with the child and family, be confident, and be very aware of safety for the child. The PT and other team members will be valuable resources for the family.

The School-Aged Child With OI

Frequent hospitalizations. The school-aged child with OI may have frequent hospitalizations to promote healing of fractures. These hospitalizations may interfere with school progress, socialization, and confidence in gross motor skills. Efforts to en-

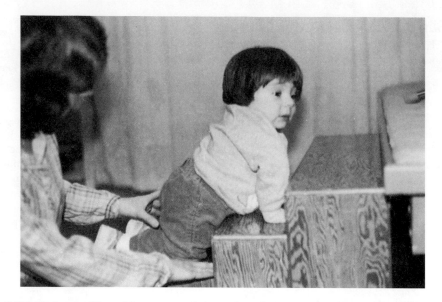

Figure 8-22 Chris, a toddler with osteogenesis imperfecta, learns to ascend steps. (From Harris, S.R., & Tada, W.L. [1990]. Genetic disorders. In D.A. Umphred [Ed.], *Neurological rehabilitation* [2nd ed.]. St. Louis: Mosby.)

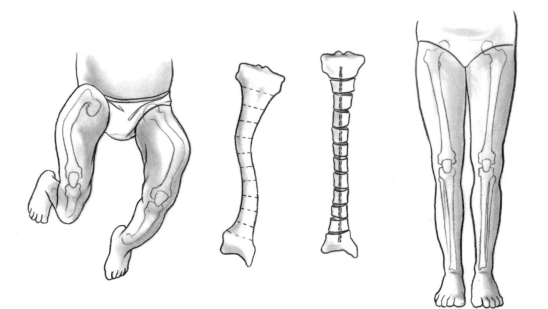

Figure 8-23 Intramedullary rods.

courage movement in a safe environment as early as possible after a fracture will be helpful.

Surgery and bracing. Among almost all children with OI, fractures will occur and require surgical repair. Intramedullary rods (Figure 8-23) may be placed after the child is 4 or 5 years old. Indications for intramedullary rods are frequent, recurring fractures and long bone deformity. The therapist will need to monitor the rod sites for slippage of the rods, as well as teach other team members how to monitor the rods. A change in the orientation of the limb, length of the limb, or a bruise or bump at the end of the long bone, indicating that the rod is

closer to the skin, can be cause for concern. The family should be notified immediately if any changes are noticed, and the physician informed. Slippage of the rods can be life threatening. Bracing with thermoplastic materials is an important adjunct to surgically implanted intramedullary rods to provide external stability.

Gait training. Most children with OI will be able to walk with long leg braces and an assistive device. Initial training begins with standing using splints or braces and a standing orthosis, such as a prone or supine stander, usually when the child is a toddler. When the child is comfortable standing, gait training can begin. The pool is an excellent place to begin gait activities, because the water supports the child in an upright position. Braces or splints and a walking aid, such as a rolled walker with trunk and pelvic support, a two-wheeled rolled walker, or forearm crutches, can help with balance and provide support. The walking aids can be progressed as the child gains skill. Once the child is walking well, walking should be incorporated into the school routine every day to maintain independent mobility, bone strength, and muscle strength. Opportunities to walk during the day may include between classes, to lunch, and during physical education (PE) class.

Physical therapy intervention. Physical therapy may be involved with the child with OI at school or in the clinic. At school, activities may include daily exercise, gait training, and teaching the child to put on and remove braces. Facilitating the child's participation in school activities, such as walking through the lunch line, going on field trips, and participation in PE classes is important to maintain the child as part of the school community. Adaptive equipment may be needed because of the child's short stature, including adapted chairs, floor sitters for young children, and reachers or computers for those children who have difficulty moving. Physical therapy intervention in the clinic is usually related to acute needs, including prescribing braces, wheelchair, or rehabilitation after an injury.

Role of the PTA. The PTA working in the schools will likely take an active role working with a child with OI. Gait training, strengthening activities, teaching the child to use braces and adaptive equipment, assisting with standing activities for weight bearing, and teaching mobility skills in a wheelchair or with powered mobility are some of the activities that a PTA might be involved with.

The Adolescent With OI

Scoliosis. Spinal deformities, including kyphosis and scoliosis, usually progress during adolescence, and surgery may be required. Spinal bracing may not be effective with children who have OI, because the external brace may hold the ribcage, but the ribs may bend and allow the spine to continue its progressive curve. Surgical correction with internal fixation is usually recommended (Gitelis, Whiffen & DeWald, 1983). The therapist may be involved with strengthening before surgery, or rehabilitation after surgery. It is important to get the child with OI up and moving as soon as possible after any surgery or fracture to decrease the length of time in bed. Disuse increases bone demineralization and osteoporosis, leading to more risk of bone fractures.

Transition. The child with OI is likely to be a productive member of society and will need help to explore options for work, further education, social opportunities, and recreation after high school. The therapist, as a member of the interdisciplinary team, can provide valuable assistance to the planning process by providing information about adaptive equipment, community transportation, community programs, local colleges with comprehensive programs for students with disabilities, and strategies for adapting work sites for accessibility.

Role of the PTA. Direct physical therapy may not be necessary for an adolescent, but consultation may be needed for specific problems that arise. The PTA can monitor the needs of a student with OI as they regularly treat other students at the school. Checking in with the teachers and student can help bring problems to light. Attending team meetings, even though direct services are not needed, can provide an important resource to the child, teacher, and family.

APPLICATIONS Handling and Positioning for Fun and Learning

Children play, learn, and live in a variety of environments, including home, school, Grandma's house, the neighborhood playground, and the store. Children with motor disorders that do not allow them the postural control to sit, stand, or maintain a position without assistance need help to function optimally in each environment. Help can occur through appropriate handling and positioning by competent adults or peers, the use of appropriate adaptive equipment, and teaching adaptations and skills to the child. Appropriate positioning is necessary to assist a child to maximize potential learning in the classroom, perform self-help skills, such as eating or grooming, and enjoy recreational and leisure activities, such as watching television or riding a bike. With creativity and a positive sense of possibilities, we can help children access activities and environments previously thought impossible, such as sailing with the family on a small boat, playing in the sandbox with friends, helping Mom garden, or hiking a local trail with dad (Figure 8-24).

Besides the functional benefits of appropriate positioning, there are also physiological benefits (Figure 8-25). A child who is able to access a variety of positions throughout the day, including lying down, sitting, and standing, can improve the function of major organ systems, including respiration, bowel and bladder function, and skin integrity. Changing positions helps respiratory hygiene by allowing gravity to assist in the removal of secretions. Upright positions help improve respiratory function by allowing maximal expansion of the thoracic cavity. Upright positions also help bowel and bladder elimination by using gravity to assist with evacuation. By improving elimination, some medical problems common to children with movement disorders, such as urinary tract infections and constipation, can be minimized. Other physiological benefits include improved blood flow, improved oxygenation to the tissues, decreased potential for contractures, improved muscle tone and function, improved sensory awareness, and decreased bone loss.

The child whose position is varied in different environments benefits by improved self-esteem, better social skills, and a more active personality. He or she is able to initiate physical or social interaction with people, interact with toys and learning materials, or actively move within the classroom and playground. Because the child's visual orientation and ability to interact is changed, there is potential for a changed view of the self, from that of a passive, dependent observer to that of an active, participating peer.

Adaptive equipment is useful for helping children with severe motor deficits maintain positions. Although most people think of adaptive equipment as being commercial, expensive, available

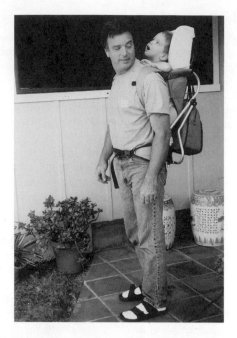

Figure 8-24 Ian uses a custom-made foam head support in his commercially available toddler backpack so he can hike with his parents.

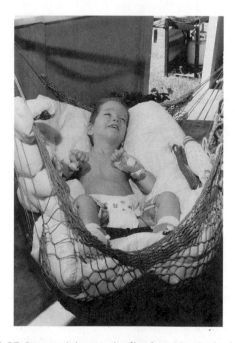

Figure 8-25 Ian can sit in a semireclined position in this hammock his parents adapted for him. His mother thinks his constipation problems are much better since he has been able to be more upright.

only from durable medical equipment dealers, and (sometimes) reimbursable by medical insurance, many other types of equipment can be useful to help a child achieve and maintain a functional position. This section will refer to commercially available equipment but will also challenge the reader to use everyday fur-

niture and objects to help children to be included in everyday life. Adaptive equipment for positioning can include pillows, sandbags, armchairs, wagons, wheelchairs, fences, standers, and power mobility equipment. With creativity and some locally available materials, almost anything can be created to assist a child's positioning to access multiple environments. Many of the case studies in this book illustrate creative adaptations for positioning for specific children.

Therapists, teachers, parents, and others who care for children with severe motor deficits lift, carry, roll, pull, and push children and heavy equipment frequently throughout the day. Using poor body mechanics can cause injury to the caregiver that is caused by repeated misuse of muscles and joints. It is important for caregivers to be aware of proper body mechanics for their own health and safety, as well as that of the child or children they care for. Although much of this material is well known, a brief review will be provided to stress its importance.

Body Mechanics
Back Care

Most of us know the fundamentals of caring for our backs when lifting, as summarized in Table 8-11. Becoming aware of and changing habits of movement and posture that we have held for years is not easy, however. Attention to our own posture and movement can help us become more aware of our predispositions for back injury and can result in positive changes in our own behavior. It may also help us become more aware of the posture and movement of others. As caregivers, we are trying to help to lift or carry children more efficiently, including children with posture and movement disorders. As physical therapy providers, it is posture and movement that are the core of our practice!

Transfers

Lifting should be performed only when necessary, so in the context of moving children with motor disabilities, it will be discussed as part of a transfer from one position or piece of equipment to another. The purposes of transferring a child usually will include teaching the child mobility skills and providing a change of position for comfort or functional activity. Before any transfer, the caregiver should know (1) why the child is being moved; (2) characteristics of the child to be lifted, including general weight, muscle tone, ways in which the child can assist in the transfer; (3) precautions for moving the child, such as osteoporosis or seizure activity; (4) what position the child will be in when lifted; (5) where the child is to be moved; (6) what position the child will assume once moved; and (7) how to use any equipment involved in the transfer, including mechanical lifts, wheelchairs, standers, or other positioning equipment. Before the transfer, the caregiver should arrange the equipment so that it is in close proximity, get others to help if needed, and discuss the move with the child to plan how the child will help.

The following scenarios illustrate different methods of transfer, as well as different types of positioning equipment.

Transfer using a mechanical lift: wheelchair to plinth and plinth to commode. Rik is a 5-year-old boy with spinal muscular atrophy (see p. 219). He independently drives a power wheelchair for mobility but is dependent on others for transfers. He

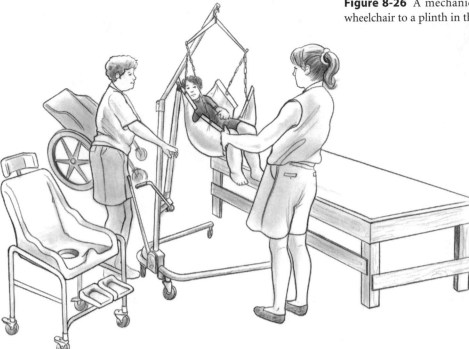

Figure 8-26 A mechanical lift is used to transfer Rik from his wheelchair to a plinth in the bathroom.

Principles of Back Care for Lifting a Child

TABLE 8-11

1. Plan each lift or transfer from beginning to end before starting the lift.
2. Enlist the help of others, if needed. Make sure the child helps as much as he/she is able. Discuss the lift thoroughly with partners.
3. Ensure an obstacle-free environment. The floor should be clear and dry, the equipment (wheelchair, tilt table, prone stander, bed, etc.) close to the child, and the equipment should be locked and safe.
4. Move from a stable base of support. Your feet should be shoulder width apart, shoes should be flat, and obstacles removed.
5. Hold the child close to you as you lift.
6. Keep your back straight and use your legs to lift.
7. Move smoothly, not jerkily during the lift.
8. Never twist your body. If you need to turn, take tiny steps with your feet to turn your body.
9. Ensure the child and equipment are safe before moving away. Pelvic belts should be fastened, equipment locked, and child comfortable.

asks to be transferred to the toilet. Rik is overweight at 70 pounds, has extreme weakness and flaccidity, moderate flexion contractures especially at his elbows and knees, and poor head control. He can assist verbally in the transfer. He is being moved from an upright sitting position in his power wheelchair to a supine position on a plinth, so that his pants can be removed be-

fore subsequently being transferred to the rolling commode chair in the bathroom at school (Figure 8-26). The chair will then be rolled over the toilet. Rik's wheelchair locks automatically when the power is turned off. The plinth is stabilized against the wall, and the commode chair has manual locks on the two rear wheels for safety. Rik's classroom aide, Mrs. Young, is using a mechanical lift to help with the transfers.

Mrs. Young first ensures that Rik has moved his wheelchair alongside the plinth and has turned the power off. Then she attaches four hooks from the lift to the four grommets in the sling that Rik sits on in his wheelchair, with the hooks facing away from Rik for safety. She ensures that the sling is positioned correctly to support his head and legs. Because the school policy requires two people to assist with this type of transfer, she then uses the intercom in the bathroom to call an aide from another classroom to assist. When the aide arrives, Mrs. Young asks Rik to tell her when he is ready. At his prompt, she undoes Rik's pelvic belt and pumps the hydraulic lift so that Rik is lifted in a reclined sitting position into the air over his wheelchair. With the other aide stabilizing his legs, they swing him over the plinth and gently let him down into a supine position. Without undoing the sling from the lift, Mrs. Young slides his pants off. The other aide, meanwhile, has positioned the commode chair where Rik's wheelchair used to be. At Rik's signal again, Mrs. Young pumps the lift and gently sits him down on the commode chair. The other aide slips out back to her classroom, and Mrs. Young buckles the pelvic strap, pulls the sling away from his legs, and rolls Rik over the toilet. When he is finished, she will call the other aide to come back to assist in transferring him back to his wheelchair.

One person–dependent transfer: stroller to mat. Matthew is a 2-year-old boy with cerebral palsy and deafness (see Case Study, Chapter 11). He is being transferred by his PTA, Kelly, from sitting

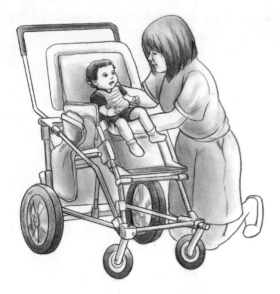

Figure 8-27 Matthew is transferred from his stroller to the mat during a therapy session.

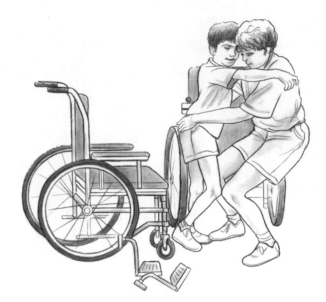

Figure 8-28 Cyril can assist with a standing pivot transfer to the power wheelchair.

in his adapted stroller to lying down on a mat on the floor for physical therapy (Figure 8-27). Matthew weighs about 30 pounds, has underlying low muscle tone, has high tone with effort or excitement, and likes to wildly move his arms when he is excited. He can stiffen his body somewhat to help with transfers. His stroller has a locking feature on the back casters.

Kelly signs to Matthew that he is going to go onto the mat, using a sign he is familiar with. She then locks the casters of his stroller and lifts the stroller bar over Matthew's head. She undoes his pelvic belt and moves to the side of the stroller. She gets down on one knee next to the stroller and puts one arm behind Matthew's shoulders with his head resting on her forearm. The other arm goes under his legs. She makes sure Matthew is looking at her face while she counts to three, and then scoops him close to her body as she stands up. She turns toward the mat and goes down on one knee with Matthew resting on the knee that is up. Then she sits down, pulling him into her lap. Once she is stable, she shifts him off her lap onto the mat and helps him reach for toys that she has ready.

Standing pivot transfer: chair to chair. Cyril is a 14-year-old boy with cerebral palsy (see Case Study, Chapter 7). He is being transferred from his manual wheelchair into a power wheelchair for training (Figure 8-28). Cyril weighs about 75 pounds. He has increased tone in all of his extremities with effort but is able to bear weight on his left leg and hold his trunk and head up in standing. He is unable to balance in this position, however, and his right hip is painful when bearing weight. Cyril's educational assistant, Mrs. Moore, pulls his manual wheelchair to a 90 degree angle next to the power chair. She talks to Cyril about what she is doing, and moves the chair a little closer, based on his suggestion. She asks Cyril to undo his pelvic belt, and she flips down the abductor wedge on his wheelchair so he can slide out more easily. She makes sure the power chair is locked, and clears the pelvic belt off the seat. Standing in front of Cyril, she reaches forward and puts her hands behind his hips. Then she moves her

whole body in a shuffling motion, her arms alternately pulling one side, then the other, of his hips as she guides them forward on the seat. When Cyril's bottom is at the front of his seat, she helps him sit upright, places his left foot on the floor, and anchors it in place with her foot. His right leg is shorter than his left, and does not reach all the way to the floor. Cyril holds on to Mrs. Moore around her shoulders, and she asks him to count. On the count of three, Mrs. Moore shifts her weight backward with her hands on Cyril's waist. As Cyril stands up, Mrs. Moore's body moves back and down. She keeps her knees bent and close to Cyril's knees to block them from buckling. Cyril enjoys standing, and they smile at each other for a fraction of a second as they balance in this standing position. Each is holding the other up, although Mrs. Moore is in control of their movement. She helps Cyril pivot to the left, and moves her body backward as she guides his hips into the power wheelchair seat. Cyril is able to push his hips back when Mrs. Moore places his foot on the footrest. He struggles to buckle his own pelvic belt, as Mrs. Moore moves his manual chair out of the way.

Two person–dependent transfer: tilt table to mat. Mattie is a 15-year-old girl with severe developmental disabilities. She has been diagnosed as profoundly mentally retarded with spastic quadriplegia. Her muscle tone is generally low, although she is active when she is excited and can be strong when she hits someone by mistake when she flings her arms. She has fair head control and is able to hold her head up for 3 to 5 minutes at a time. She cannot maintain a sitting position by herself, and needs support for trunk control, as well as balance. She does not take any weight through her legs and tends to sink immediately to the floor if put on her feet. She has severe osteoporosis and has recently recovered from a fractured right radius. No one could remember an incident to explain how the bone was fractured. Mattie is short and is overweight at 90 pounds. The PTA is helping the special education teacher transfer Mattie from the tilt table to the mat after she participated in a cooking activity while stand-

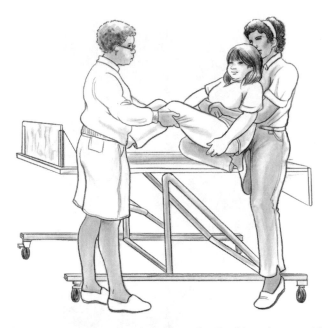

Figure 8-29 Mattie is transferred from the tilt table to the mat with a two person–dependent transfer.

ing (Figure 8-29). Mattie will lie in a prone position over a wedge to join other students who are on the floor watching a movie.

The electric-powered tilt table is brought gently to the lowest horizontal position, moved against the wall for stability, and the casters locked. While talking to Mattie, telling her what they are doing, and where they are going, the teacher undoes the tilt table straps, making sure to stand close to the open side of the table for safety. The PTA drags the mat close to the table and places the large wedge in the center of the mat, facing the television. The PTA then moves to Mattie's head, and the teacher to her legs. The PTA again tells Mattie what they are going to do, then looks at the teacher and obtains eye contact. The two women discuss the transfer, where they will go, and how they will do it. They slide Mattie further toward the wall and help her roll to her side facing out into the room. With Mattie's feet off the table, the PTA rolls Mattie's shoulders forward and pivots Mattie up into a sitting position.

The teacher grasps Mattie's thighs, while the PTA reaches her hands around Mattie's trunk, sliding through her arms, and grasping Mattie's wrists. Mattie is shifted somewhat to the side so that the PTA can reach under both arms and grasp her forearms. The PTA has one knee up on the tilt table, so that she does not have to twist her body. Once they feel secure, the teacher and the PTA catch each other's eye, and the PTA counts to three. On three, they smoothly move Mattie off the table and bend their knees to sit her at the base of the wedge. Mattie is sitting partially on the PTA, who slides out from under her and helps Mattie roll over onto her stomach. The two women make sure that both of Mattie's arms are off the wedge and are positioned so that she is weight bearing through her elbows. They place saddle-type sandbags across Mattie's hips, with the sand supporting Mattie's hips laterally. These are for safety, so she will not roll off the wedge. A padded bench is moved in front of Mattie, so that she can put her head down to rest when she is tired.

Handling Children With Neuromuscular Disorders

To position a child with a neuromuscular disorder, handling may be necessary to obtain optimal posture and range of motion. Handling or touching a child in a therapeutic or educational context can be for the purposes of positioning, facilitating movement, facilitating improved posture, helping the child learn a skill, controlling behavior, or communicating with a child. Handling is a form of sensory input. It provides tactile and proprioceptive input to a child and can provide physical guidance for subtle movements or weight shifts. The tactile and proprioceptive input provided during handling can augment other means of communication, such as auditory or visual.

Each child is an individual, as is each child's particular manifestation of muscle tone, strength, deformities, medical condition, and personality. It is these individual traits that dictate how to interact with and handle a child. There are some considerations, however, that can help a person working with a child with a neuromuscular disorder, such as cerebral palsy, traumatic brain injury, spinal cord injury, or Guillain-Barré syndrome, plan their physical interactions.

Effects of Environment, Health, and Emotions on Muscle Tone

A calming environment, including quiet or soothing music, lack of extraneous activity, slow rhythmic movements, dim lights, and gentle handling, will calm most people. On the other hand, an exciting environment with vigorous movements, rough textures, loud music, bright lights, and many people moving about will tend to cause most of us to increase our energy level significantly. These environmental influences will affect the muscle tone and emotions of children with neuromuscular disorders in the same ways, sometimes markedly. A child seen for therapy in the lunchroom at school will respond much differently than when seen alone in a dimmed therapy room. The choice of therapy environment is important and can affect the outcome of therapy. The environment must be appropriate to the activity, however. For example, many children with high muscle tone can and should learn to eat lunch in a crowded cafeteria rather than being secluded alone in a separate room. A child should usually learn to function in the natural environment, but it is important that the therapy provider understand the effects of environmental stimuli.

Emotion can also affect the child's responses to handling. A child will tend to be more relaxed if the therapist is trusted and the child feels safe, listened to, and accepted. A child who feels angry, irritated, embarrassed, or excited may respond with increased muscle tone and decreased motor control than in other circumstances. Emotions generated from environments other than the therapy session can also influence the child's responses. A fight at home, teasing on the playground, or an earlier accident in the classroom may need to be identified and addressed to help the child benefit maximally from the therapy session.

Health issues, including acute illness, pain, or change in medications, can also affect the child's responses to handling. In a nonverbal child, changes in muscle tone or responses to handling can be indications of illness or pain from injury. Sensitivity to environmental, emotional, and health issues can assist the PTA in providing appropriate interventions to children with neuromuscular disorders.

Handling to Increase Motor Output

A child with low muscle tone may need vigorous tactile input to elicit more energetic movement. Techniques, such as tapping, brushing, vibrating, rubbing, or providing deep pressure to a muscle or skin, have been found to increase motor response. Vigorous vestibular input, including spinning, swinging, and bouncing, are also useful in stimulating postural muscles. These techniques can be even more effective when combined with other sensory input, such as providing instruction in a loud and insistent voice, varying the voice tone, demonstrating visually, and physically guiding a child through a movement pattern from the shoulders or hips. A child with low muscle tone may have hypermobility at key joints, including shoulders, hips, knees, elbows, and wrists. To stimulate improved contraction of muscles on both sides of a joint (cocontraction), and therefore improved stability of the joint, facilitated weight bearing and moving over a stabilized joint can be helpful. Examples include having a child lean onto an extended arm while reaching for toys or school materials, or weight shift over a stable foot to play a game. A more vigorous activity is having the child walk on hands while you support the trunk and legs, sometimes called a "wheelbarrow game." Activities such as these can be integrated into physical education or classroom and recess games. Pressure through proximal joints, called approximation, can stimulate postural reactions, such as sitting up straighter or weight bearing through the legs. This pressure can be given manually by pressing down through the shoulders or hips while the child is sitting or standing or can be given through a weighted belt or vest.

Handling to Reduce Excessive Motor Output

The child who has increased muscle tone will benefit from relaxation techniques and handling to facilitate more functional movement. Gentle rhythmic movements, such as rocking a child, moving a body part slowly and consistently, singing, or providing relaxing music can be helpful when assisting a child to relax (Figure 8-30). Touching the child firmly and avoiding loud noises or bright lights can also help to relax a child with increased muscle tone. It is important not to provide stimulating tactile input directly over spastic muscles. Therefore attention to hand placement and pressure is vital when handling a child. Hand placement should be over muscles that are not spastic, usually those on the outside of limbs. Pressure should be firm, but not heavy. Touch should be through the palm or flat surface of the hand rather than fingertips, which can cause discomfort. Other sensory input that can help a child relax includes warm water, warm colors, such as pink, and for some children, wrapping in a soft blanket or sheet.

Handling to Facilitate Functional Positions

Children with brain injuries, such as cerebral palsy and traumatic brain injury, frequently have nonfunctional movements and postures dictated by abnormal reflex patterns. These are dis-

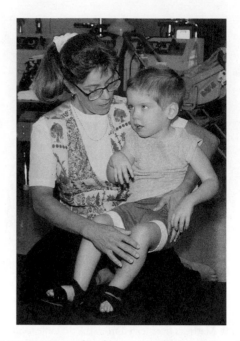

Figure 8-30 Singing and rocking are methods to help a child with high muscle tone to relax.

cussed more fully in Chapters 3 and 7. Avoiding positions that stimulate abnormal reflex activity is essential in helping children attain and maintain functional positions. Encouraging midline orientation of the head by helping the child look forward rather than to the side can help avoid asymmetry from an asymmetrical tonic neck response. Encouraging a neutral anterior/posterior position of the head can help avoid abnormal postures from an symmetrical tonic neck response. Maintaining an upright position can help avoid postures and muscle tone related to the tonic labyrinthine response.

Rotation is a key. Children with spasticity may tend to move in characteristic patterns of flexion or extension, depending on where the injury occurred in their brain. To preserve joint motion and to allow maximum postural adaptability, movements in all planes need to be encouraged. It may be difficult for a child to move out of a typically occurring pattern without assistance. Rotation is frequently a key in helping a child move out of a locked position, either in flexion or extension. If the arms are rotated outward, the muscles generally relax so that the joints can be moved throughout their range. If the legs are rotated outward, the muscles in the legs relax, allowing much more movement. To help a limb outwardly rotate, stand to the side of the child who is either lying down or sitting up, place the flat part of your hands firmly on the inside of the upper part of the limb nearest to you, and roll gently but firmly toward you, allowing the limb to rotate and move toward you. You may have to give a consistent firm pressure for a few seconds before you feel the tone relaxing and the limb begin to move. It should be clear to you when the pattern of tone has relaxed. At this point, you will be able to move the limb throughout its maximal range, and help the child to move or attain a more functional position.

Key points of control. Children with neuromuscular disorders, particularly those with cerebral palsy, have poor control of their trunk muscles, which leads to poor skills in balance, pos-

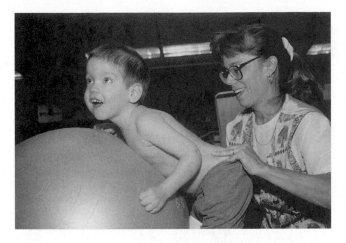

Figure 8-31 Using key points of control at the shoulders and the pelvis is more effective than holding a child's hands to help him or her achieve movement transitions.

ture, head control, and functional hand use. Berta Bobath and others found that by facilitating movements and posture of a child proximally, rather than through the extremities, they could best encourage more normal movements. For example, when helping a child come to sitting from lying supine on the floor, place your hands on the child's pelvis and shoulders to encourage rolling, pushing up through the hands, and movement into an upright position (Figure 8-31). This is more effective than grasping the child's hands and attempting to cue them how to move appropriately. The pelvis, hips, shoulders, and head are sometimes called "key points of control" and are seen as places where, through handling, a therapist can most effectively break up abnormal movements and facilitate normal postural reflexes and active movements.

Positioning and Carrying Children and Infants With Neuromuscular Disorders

Appropriate positioning depends on the specific needs of the individual child, the activity, and the environment, but there are general considerations for positioning that should be kept in mind.

Positioning for Function

Positioning should always be done in a specific environment for a specific activity. In other words, the position is not an end in itself; it is a means for a child to be somewhere and to do something. An inappropriate positioning goal for a child at school would be the following: Cody tolerates 30 minutes in the prone stander. A more appropriate goal would be the following: Cody stands in the prone stander for 30 minutes without complaints while actively participating in music class (tapping a tambourine, shaking a gourd, or vocalizing with the class to music he is familiar with). The prone stander is a means for Cody to participate with his peers in music class. The position should also match the activity. For instance, lying on the floor is appropriate

for watching a movie on television or resting but inappropriate for playing ping-pong or attending mathematics class. Table 8-12 lists some functional positions, common postural problems, and adaptations for children with low or high muscle tone.

Goals of Positioning

Positioning is not static. For a typically developing child, achieving one position is simply a stepping off place for getting into another position. Children do not sit still for long but move frequently, subtly shifting their position even while sitting in one place. Many children with severe disabilities are not able to move, except in gross patterns, which may not be functional for achieving a stable new position. They are not able to subtly shift their position for comfort, weight shift, or attending to a different task. We can, however, provide the child with a positioning device or manual support that can help in attaining and maintaining a stable position, yet allow for some degree of active movement. These children may need to stay in one position for a length of time. If they cannot change positions without help, it is important that their position be changed for them when an activity changes. In this way negative effects of staying in one position for too long, such as skin breakdown, joint contractures, negative behaviors because of discomfort or boredom, and learned helplessness from being solely a passive observer in school or at home, can be minimized.

Midline orientation. The head, trunk, and extremities should be kept in midline as much as possible (Figure 8-32). This means the trunk should be centered, not curved to the side, rotated, flexed forward, or allowed to hyperextend backward. In the midline position, the trunk has the most stability. The head should be facing forward, not tilted to the right or left, and not in flexion or hyperextension. In this position a child can best visually access the environment. The extremities should be supported, if necessary, in a neutral orientation near the midline of the body. In this position there is the most potential for using the extremities functionally. Table 8-13 outlines ideal positions for sitting, standing, supine, and sidelying. Keep in mind that each ideal position will have to be modified to accommodate the specific needs of individual children.

Symmetrical positioning. In general, children should be positioned symmetrically, with both arms and legs supported in a similar manner, and the head and trunk in midline. There are some exceptions to this, for instance, in a sidelying position where the upper leg or arm may be more bent or posterior to the lower leg or arm.

Positioning the child with low muscle tone. A child with low muscle tone has difficulty holding head, trunk, and extremities up against gravity. Therefore this child will tend to sink toward the supporting surface, whether that be a parent's lap, the floor, or a positioning device. If position is not attended to carefully, deformities of the spine, including scoliosis or kyphosis, of the extremities, including elbow, knee, and hip flexion or ankle plantarflexion contractures, and asymmetries or flattening in skeletal features, such as the face, skull, and rib cage, may result.

A useful strategy in positioning a child with low muscle tone is to use gravity to assist, rather than fighting gravity, to maintain a position. For example, tilting a seat with posterior head support, yet supporting the head in some flexion so the child can see straight ahead, may allow upright sitting for longer periods.

TABLE 8-12 Ideal Positioning

	Supine	Prone	Sidelying	Sitting
Pelvis and hips	Pelvis in line with trunk. Hips in 30 to 90 degrees of flexion. Neutral rotation of pelvis. Hips symmetrically abducted 10 to 20 degrees.	Pelvis in line with trunk. Hips in extension. Neutral rotation of pelvis. Hips symmetrically abducted 10-20 degrees.	Pelvis in line with trunk. Hips in flexion. Neutral rotation. Hips in 10 to 20 degrees abduction.	Pelvis in line with trunk. Hips at 90 degrees flexion. Neutral rotation of pelvis. Hips symmetrically abducted 10 to 20 degrees.
Trunk	Straight. Shoulders in line with hips. Neutral rotation of trunk.	Straight. Shoulders in line with hips. Neutral rotation.	Straight. Shoulders in line with hips. Slight sidebending okay.	Straight. Shoulders over hips. Not rotated.
Head and neck	Head in neutral position. Facing forward. Slight cervical flexion.	Head in neutral position. Facing to one side. Slight cervical flexion.	Head in neutral position. Facing forward. Slight cervical flexion.	Head in neutral position. Facing forward. Head evenly on shoulders.
Shoulders and arms	Arms fully supported. Arms forward of trunk. Forearms rest on trunk or pillow.	Arms fully supported. Arms forward of trunk. Flexion at shoulders. Flexion at elbows.	Both arms supported. Lower arm forward. Not lying on point of shoulder. Lower arm neutral rotation. Upper arm may have 0 to 40 degrees internal rotation.	Arms fully supported. Elbows in flexion. Zero to 45 degrees internally rotated shoulders.
Legs and feet	Knees supported in flexion. Feet held at 90 degrees.	Knees extended. Feet supported at 90 degrees.	Knees in flexion. Feet positioned at 90 degrees. Pillow between knees.	Knees at 90 degrees. Ankles at 90 degrees. Feet fully supported. Thighs fully supported.

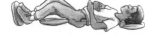 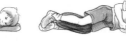

Using a supine stander with posterior head support at about 70 degrees, rather than a prone stander that requires a child to hold up the head, may allow a more functional standing position. The degree of tilt tolerated in sitting or standing will depend on the child's strength, sensory skills, and size.

The extremities of a child with low tone should always be supported, rather than allowed to hang over the side of a positioning device. This is important for safety, aesthetics, and function, as well as to avoid potential pain and discomfort associated with poorly supported, lax joints. Therefore good foot and leg rests, arm rests, or tray tables are essential.

Positioning the child with high muscle tone. The child with high muscle tone will not usually accommodate to a supporting surface, such as a chair, the floor, or a positioning device. This means that the child's body will generally not contact the supporting surface well and will move stiffly according to stereotypical or gross patterns. The trunk and limbs will be stiff, and the child's muscles will be excessively firm and tight. Good posi-

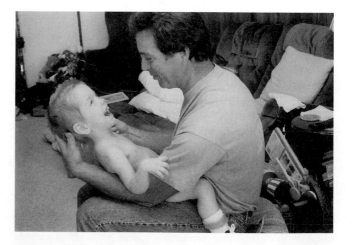

Figure 8-32 Ian's father supports his trunk and head in midline and supports his legs and arms as he plays with Ian in his lap.

Functional Positions and Possible Adaptations for Children With Severe Disabilities

TABLE 8-13

Activity/positioning devices	Functional goal	Possible postural problems	Possible adaptations
Activity: Child sleeps in supine position. *Devices:* Crib Bassinet Blanket Adult arms or lap Bed Mat	The infant or child will maintain a neutral alignment of the head and trunk with age appropriate flexion of the extremities while sleeping in supine position.	Infant or child with low postural tone: • Unable to keep head in midline. • Excessive passive extension in arms and legs. Infant or child with high postural tone: • Strong influence of ATNR causing head to turn to side and trunk to arch. • Asymmetry in posture caused by ATNR.	• Purchase or make a U-shaped towel roll to put around child's head. (Works better for infants and small children.) • If the towel roll gets pushed out of position, attach a flat surface for the child to lie on to anchor the device. • Make a double wedged pillow that will guide the child's head to midline. • Use towel rolls to encircle an infant's body, or sandbags/bolsters/stuffed animals supporting the arms and legs of a child in a symmetrical flexed position.
Activity: Child plays with toy truck in prone position. *Devices:* Crib Blanket Adult lap Adult body Mat Carpeted floor Scooter board Wedge Bolster	Child will move toy truck at least 3 inches across floor using arm to propel.	Infant or child with low postural tone: • Unable to lift head and upper trunk. • Unable to lift arms to reach. • Arms and legs in excessive passive extension. Infant or child with high postural tone: • Strong influence of STNR causing difficulty extending arm when head is extended. • Unable to maintain head in midline to look at toy. • Movements are jerky and poorly graded. • Unable to extend arm when head is in midline.	• The child may need a small roll, pillow, or wedge under the chest so the head is not forced into hyperextension when prone, and to allow the arms to fall into flexion. • Both arms can be supported at the elbow to prevent asymmetries of trunk and head position. • Lateral trunk pads can give extra stability to allow arm movement.
Activity: Child goes to the beach with family. *Devices:* Car seat Infant seat Beach chair Lawn chair Bath seat or ring Jog stroller	Child will play with sand toys while sitting on the sand at the beach.	Infant or child with low postural tone: • Sits with rounded trunk, unable to lift head to see or interact. • Unable to lift arms to reach. • Arms and legs in excessive passive extension. • Unable to grasp or lift toy. Infant or child with high postural tone: • Tends to arch and move out of the sitting position. • Unable to maintain head in midline to look at toys or friends. • Movements are jerky and poorly graded. • Unable to extend arm when head is in midline.	• Use gravity to help with head control. Recline the device if it has posterior head support. A base can be created to allow variations of recline. • Create posterior head support by building a padded solid seat insert, or a custom foam insert. • Use a plastic-molded lawn chair with a high back. Either bury the legs so the chair seat is on or below the level of the sand, or cut off the legs. • Use a pelvic belt/strap in the lawn chair to hold the pelvis in place. • Make a wedge to hold the head in slight flexion to decrease effects of extension pattern of movement.

Continued

TABLE 8-13   Functional Positions and Possible Adaptations for Children With Severe Disabilities—cont'd

Activity/positioning devices	Functional goal	Possible postural Problems	Possible adaptations
			• Cut out a cardboard box to use as a table for toys. • Dig out the sand so legs, knees, hips, and ankles can be supported at 90 degrees or appropriate angles by the sand. • Build up lateral trunk supports that can be placed in lawn or beach chair. Towel rolls or foam blocks work well. • Use a wide strap that can be pulled through cut out slots in the back of the seating device for trunk support.
Activity: Child plays with toys standing at a coffee table. *Devices:* Infant walker Low table Playpen Stander Ring walker Pick up walker Rolling walker	Child will play with toys while standing at the coffee table for 5 minutes.	Infant or child with low postural tone: • Unable to bear full weight through legs. • Unable to free arms to play with toys. • Poor foot and leg position in standing. • Difficulty holding head upright for extended periods of play. Infant or child with high postural tone: • Stands on toes with poor lower extremity alignment. • Poor balance in standing. • Movements are jerky and poorly graded. • Difficulty using arms in standing.	• Manually support the infant or child's head. • Use a soft, thick, foam collar supporting occiput and chin, which is resting on the chest to allow free breathing while supporting the head upright. • Provide graded posterior support either using an adult's body, or a sturdy chair. • Use orthotics to facilitate lower extremity alignment in standing. • Place furniture next to child to help with balance. • Use a stander with support at feet, knees, hips, and trunk as needed for stability.

tioning can prevent deformities from repetitive posturing because of the influence of primitive reflexes, contractures from limited ranges of movement, and injury because of poor motor control, as well as maximize the child's participation in different environments and activities.

The key to helping a child with high muscle tone maintain a specific posture is to eliminate or mediate the effects of primitive reflexes by avoiding positions that stimulate them. A midline posture, as described above, can avoid stimulating most reflexes, and will provide the most stable base from which to move. Positioning the hips at a greater than 90 degree angle can prevent a strong extensor thrust of the legs and trunk (Figure 8-33). This can be helpful in sitting, supine, or sidelying. It is important to be aware of the position of the pelvis when bending the hips and be attentive to causing posterior pelvic tilt through too much hip flexion. Posterior pelvic tilt may be difficult to avoid, but strategies such as using a snug pelvic belt at a 45 degree angle to the pelvis, using a strap behind the pelvis in a sling type of seat, or customizing foam cushions to support the pelvis adequately may

help. A posterior pelvic tilt can decrease the stability of a sitting position. Attention to head position can also be important to maintaining a good posture. Positioning the head in slight flexion with a pillow or wedge can help minimize extensor postures in sitting, supine, and sidelying.

For a child with strong extensor posturing, maintaining a neutral pelvic position is very important. In sitting, the pelvic belt is essential to maintain an upright pelvis. Many caregivers believe that a snug belt may be uncomfortable for a child, so they loosen it, causing significant postural problems. Actually, a snug belt at a 45 degree angle around an upright pelvis, which crosses just below the anterior superior iliac spines (ASIS), is more comfortable for a child than a looser belt, which a child has leverage to push against and which crosses the pelvis at a more vulnerable place. It is very important for children to maintain the pelvis in an upright position by using an appropriately positioned belt. In other positions, such as prone or supine, supports—including saddle sandbags, tubular sandbags, wedges, and cushions—can help maintain pelvic position.

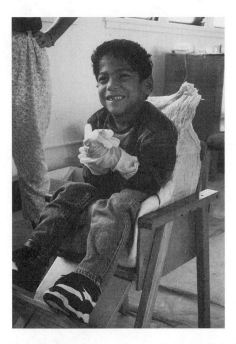

Figure 8-33 Paul sits with more than 90 degrees of hip flexion to control his extensor thrust. He is sitting in a custom-molded Foam-in-Place seat.

Providing adequate postural support is also essential to help a child maintain a functional position. Provision of lateral trunk supports, hip guides, and head supports in supine, prone, sidelying, and sitting can help a child stay comfortable. Because the child with high tone does not conform well to a support surface, to provide adequate postural support, the support surface may need to conform to the child. See the Applications section in Chapter 9 for ways this can be accomplished for wheelchair seating. The same concepts can be applied to other forms of positioning, such as bed, mat, and standing positions. A commercially available postural support system can be adapted to contour more fully to a child by adding materials such as soft foam and duct tape, or a device can be constructed by carving foam, building a plywood and foam system, or pouring liquid foam to conform fully to the child. More information on liquid foam for positioning (Foam-in-Place) can be obtained from Dynamic Systems (Rt. 2, Box 1828, Leicester, NC 28748).

Positioning the child with deformities or medical conditions.
Besides accommodating for individual variances in skills, muscle tone, age, and size; postural supports also have to accommodate musculoskeletal deformities. Common problems may include hydrocephalus, joint contracture, scoliosis, myelomeningocele, or hip dislocations. Medical conditions, such as skin breakdown, respiratory problems, or seizures, and medical appliances, such as ventriculoperitoneal shunts or feeding tubes, may also need to be accommodated in a positioning device or program.

Most of these conditions necessitate adapting positioning equipment to accommodate them. The provision of lateral trunk supports can provide enough support to allow even a child with severe scoliosis to sit upright. In the past, many children with scoliosis who could not tolerate stabilization surgery were always positioned lying down, to reduce the effects of gravity. Muscle pull, however, is a stronger influence on the development of spinal deformities than gravity, and individuals are now positioned as up-

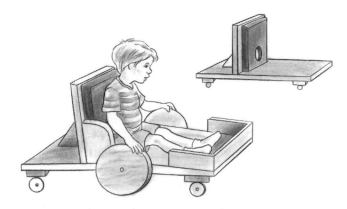

Figure 8-34 Cutting out the back support around the site of injury can allow a child with a myelomeningocele to sit upright or lie supine.

right as possible to minimize abnormal reflexes and maximize functional benefits. Children with advanced hydrocephalus who had not been able to be shunted were also positioned lying down to prevent injury to their neck or head. With adequate head support, however, most children with uncontrolled hydrocephalus can sit up to go to school, participate with their peers, and enjoy a variety of activities. A myelomeningocele can be accommodated by cutting out the back support around the site of injury, and padding to support the myelomeningocele (Figure 8-34). Most children who have a pressure sensitive area surrounding or over a myelomeningocele, can lie on their back and sit up in a chair using adapted positioning devices, to allow them greater access to their environment.

Lower extremity joint contractures and hip dislocations can be accommodated by changing the seat to back angle, angling half of the seat to allow for a unilateral hip extension contracture, building in asymmetries in abduction using custom molding or placement of hip guides, or incorporating extra padding where needed. Upper extremity deformities can be accommodated with asymmetrical arm supports, such as arm rests or lap trays, attention to the placement of trunk supports, or the use of custom adaptations, such as shoulder protractors, neoprene cuffs, or lap tray arm guides.

Medical conditions or appliances can be accommodated in positioning devices as well. Placement of a pelvic belt can be varied for a child with a gastrostomy (abdominal feeding tube). Head supports can be custom fitted to accommodate for an unusual shunt placement. Children with respiratory difficulties can use seats, which tilt-in-space or recline, to allow easy position changes, and special foams and other cushioning surfaces are available for children with pressure sensitive skin. Belts, helmets, and other supports, such as a lap tray, can be useful to protect the child with uncontrolled seizures.

Carrying the child with disabilities. Principles of carrying the child with a disability follow the same pattern as those of positioning the child. For a child with low postural tone, the head, trunk, and limbs should be fully supported. A child with a tendency for higher muscle tone should be carried, keeping in mind some of the reflex inhibiting postures, such as keeping the hips and knees abducted and in more than 90 degrees of flexion for the child with extensor thrusting, keeping the hips and knees

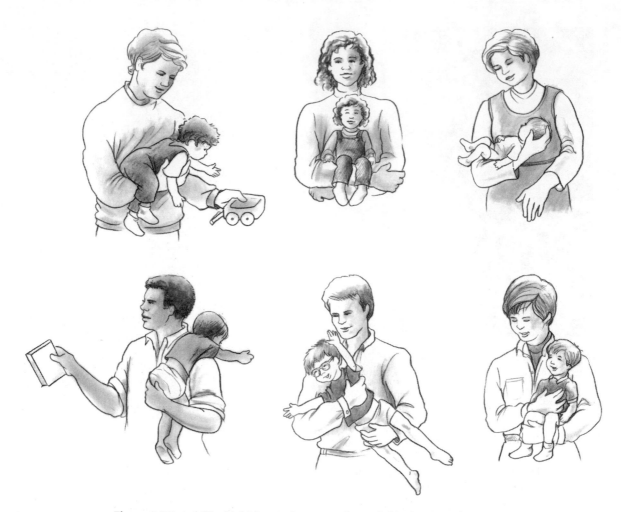

Figure 8-35 A child with high muscle tone can be carried in a variety of positions.

flexed, while encouraging trunk rotation for the child with strong extension patterns of movement, keeping the neck in some flexion for the child who tends to arch backward, and maintaining a face forward position to eliminate the effects of the ATNR (Figure 8-35).

Some accidental fractures in children with osteoporosis occur when an unsupported limb hits the edge of a chair or bed, or is subjected to unusual pressures when a child is moved. Careful attention should be paid to the extremities when moving or carrying a child.

The Infant With Positioning Needs

Infants have not yet developed the postural control needed to achieve and to maintain upright positions. Yet, to grow and develop, children need to be a part of their environment. They need to interact with people and objects around them. Commercial infant positioning devices and toys have been developed to encourage and allow infants to participate fully in the world around them, and many available devices can be used or adapted for infants and young children with postural and movement disorders. Particular considerations need to be kept in mind for infants and children with specific needs, however.

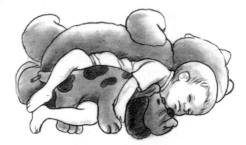

Figure 8-36 The child born prematurely with low muscle tone needs to be supported to maintain physiological flexion.

The premature infant. Although PTAs will not work in the neonatal intensive care unit (NICU), they may work alongside a PT with medically fragile or very young children after they have "graduated" from the NICU and are being followed in an infant development program. Teaching parents appropriate ways of handling and positioning their infant or child is an essential part of providing services to them.

Supporting physiological flexion is very important for a young child born prematurely. When the child is positioned in prone, the limbs should be flexed under the child's trunk. A pil-

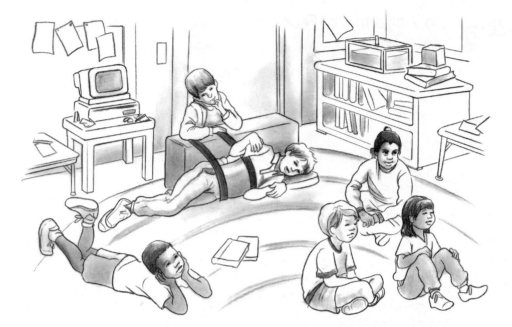

Figure 8-37 Andrew can lie on the floor with his classmates while listening during story hour at school.

low or sling may be necessary to allow the child to support the limbs in flexion. In sidelying, the limbs should be supported around a stuffed animal or pillow to give the child a sense of security and allow the arms and legs to maintain a flexed position. Small sandbags or stuffed animals can be used to keep the child's head in midline or slight flexion (Figure 8-36). In supine or a semireclined position, pillows or stuffed animals can be used under the knees to keep the hips and knees in flexion, and pillows beside the head and trunk help the child maintain a neutral position of the head and trunk, as well as the arms in flexion. Early experiences in weight bearing, such as an infant in utero experiences through kicking, can help the normal development of active movement and can be provided through toys placed at the feet, or with the child placed at the end of a bassinet or solid crib side so the feet can push against a solid surface.

As the premature infant matures and gains more skills, less postural supports will be needed, unless the infant develops postural or movement problems.

Adaptive Equipment for Positioning

Identifying Appropriate Equipment

The key to identifying appropriate and functional adaptive equipment for an infant or child with postural disabilities is to look at where the equipment will be used, and its purpose. Rather than deciding that you need a piece of equipment to position a child in sidelying because you think the child needs an alternative position in the classroom, think about what it is that you want the child to do. For instance, the kindergarten class has a story time when children can lie down in a carpeted area and listen to the teacher read. You want 5-year-old Andrew (see Case Study, Chapter 7), who has cerebral palsy, to be able to lie on the

carpet with his classmates and see the teacher as the book is read. A cumbersome padded wooden sidelyer, which you might have chosen before thinking of the context of the activity, would separate Andrew from his classmates who touch each other, wiggle, and giggle as the story is being read. A covered foam block or wedge with a wide strap on one side can effectively help Andrew maintain sidelying so he can see the teacher, and will allow him to lie amidst his classmates, wiggling, giggling, and touching (Figure 8-37). His classmates can sit on the block, push against it, lean against it, or roll over it to interact with Andrew during this activity. These interactions may not be possible with a heavy commercial sidelyer, which has sharp corners and metal hardware. A few other foam blocks or wedges in the area can help other children be comfortable and prevent Andrew from being singled out.

Catalogs, venders, teachers, therapists, and parents can all be resources for figuring out what sort of adaptive equipment might work in various situations. The vender can be a valuable resource in describing the features of commercially available equipment, matching the needs of the child with what is available, and quoting prices. Even if there is no budget to purchase equipment, a team of people can usually figure out resources to either purchase or make a piece of adaptive equipment, if they are committed to the child and the idea.

Making or Buying Adaptive Equipment

Each piece of equipment for a child at home, in a classroom, or in a community setting needs to be purchased, created, or adapted for the specific circumstances. The question of how to obtain the equipment can best be made by the team of people who have decided that it is necessary. For instance, the foam block with a wide belt that the team decided would be most ap-

TABLE 8-14   Buying, Adapting, or Fabricating Positioning Equipment: How to Decide

	Benefits	Difficulties	Use this method if you:
Commercially available equipment	• Durable. • Vender support for defects or problems. • Has been thought about carefully by many design professionals. • May be purchased by medical insurance or other third-party funding.	• Expensive. • Heavy. • Imposing. • May be more complicated than needed. • Usually takes a long time to obtain if waiting for funding.	• Can get medical insurance coverage. • Need the special features built into the device. • Do not have time to adapt or fabricate device. • Do not have skills to adapt or fabricate device.
Adapted equipment	• May be able to complete sooner than getting commercially made equipment. • Can customize to specific needs and desires. • Able to use equipment and materials on hand. • Designing and adapting device promotes team building.	• Takes time. • Takes creativity to design. • Materials may be difficult to obtain. • May be less durable than commercially made equipment.	• Have equipment that can be adapted. • Have skills to do the adaptation. • Have materials and time to do the adaptation. • Need the device quickly.
Fabricated equipment	• Can customize to specific needs and desires. • May be able to get it completed in a timely manner. • May be less expensive than commercially available equipment. • Team building when designing and doing adaptation.	• Takes time to make. • Takes creativity to design. • May need specific skills like sewing, carpentry, or metal work. • May have difficulty finding materials or resources to fabricate. • May be less durable.	• Have skills and resources to fabricate equipment. • Do not have money to buy equipment. • Need the device quickly. • Need equipment not available commercially.

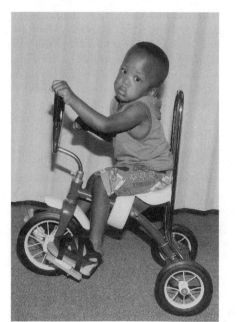

Figure 8-38 Chris rides an adapted tricycle. The wooden pedal blocks were purchased but could easily be made from wood and screws.

propriate for Andrew is not available commercially. The team then has to decide whether to make it themselves, adapt something else, such as a foam wedge or a bolster, for Andrew's use, or whether a commercial product, such as a Sidelyer Adaptive Positioner from Skillbuilders, would meet Andrew's needs. Table 8-14 outlines some benefits and difficulties of each approach.

Paying for Equipment

The issue of cost and who will foot the bill is very important when deciding on a piece of adaptive equipment. The most common funding sources for children's equipment are medical insurance, the DOE, and the child's family. Alternative funding sources are fundraisers, local grants, local service agencies, such as Lions Club or Rotary Club, or a loan bank or recycling center for used equipment. The team should decide how they will approach the funding issue, make a list of priorities of who to approach for funding, and decide who will write the letters or make the necessary phone calls. Each funding method has particularities that need to be addressed, and it is helpful to have someone on the team who has experience with that method of funding and can assist the process. Some durable medical equipment companies have materials and sample letters that describe strategies for approaching insurance companies (Prentke Romich, Co., 1022 Heyl Rd., Wooster, OH 44691).

Summary

Children with postural abnormalities can benefit from handling and positioning to allow them greater access to their environments. Handling can decrease abnormal postures and movements related to atypical muscle tone, as well as facilitate maximum postural response and functional skills for a child. Proper handling may assist a child to attain and maintain a more functional position to participate in school, sports, or family activities. Positioning devices also help a child maintain functional positions for self-care, recreational, or learning activities. These devices can be purchased commercially, adapted from mainstream furniture or positioning aids, or fabricated from scratch (Figure 8-38).

It is important for a therapy provider to be aware of handling techniques that can be useful for children with a variety of postural problems, as well as the range of positioning devices that are available commercially or can be constructed. Being aware of these techniques and devices is only the first step, however. A PTA, teacher, or educational assistant must be willing to work with others to decide the specific needs of a child in different environments and how these can best be met. Working as a team to plan the incorporation of handling techniques and positioning in adaptive equipment throughout a child's day, as well as using creativity and being open-minded, can expand options for children and allow them to be fully included at home, school, and in the community.

EXERCISES

1. Research the addresses and services provided by local branches of agencies and organizations that support families who have children with genetic disorders.
2. Attend a family support group for children who have a genetic disorder.
3. Make a simple adaptive device (for a specific child, if possible). This could include a sandbag, a pillow, or a seatbelt for a chair. What problems did you have making it? What might have made your job easier?

QUESTIONS TO PONDER

1. You find out during a prenatal test that you are (or your wife is) carrying a child with a significant genetic abnormality.
   a. What factors will you and your spouse consider to make a decision about whether or not to carry this infant to term?
   b. How will your decision affect the way you interact with families who have a child with a significant genetic abnormality?
   c. Should personal views (religious, medical, etc.) affect professional relationships with children and families?
2. You notice that a teacher you work with is lifting improperly. She has been defensive in the past when you tried to give her some pointers on lifting technique. You are concerned that she is going to injure herself. What are some ways you could approach this situation?

Annotated Bibliography

Stray-Gundersen, Karen (Ed.) (1986). *Babies With Down Syndrome: A New Parent's Guide.* U. S. A.: Woodbine House.

This easy-to-read book is targeted at new parents of infants with Down syndrome. It was recommended to me by a parent who loaned me a well-worn copy with underlined sections and bookmarks to designate often used pages. The book covers basic information ranging from medical etiology to daily care, family life, growth and development of the infant, and legal rights. It gives a good idea of what family concerns may be regarding the child with Down syndrome and includes important community resources and support agencies for families. The book provides a healthy departure from medical-based texts and allows therapists to become familiar with family concerns regarding children who have disabilities.

Diamont, R. B. (1992). *Positioning for Play: Home Activities for Parents of Young Children.* Tucson, AZ: Therapy Skill Builders.

This accessible book with simple illustrations gives many ideas for positioning young children. Easily available materials, including pillows, swim rings, laundry baskets, towels, and your own body, are used to help children attain functional positions from which they can play. Activities are suggested for play, and rationale for each position is explained simply. The pages can be copied to give to parents and make a great teaching tool.

References

Albright, J. A. (1981). Management overview of osteogenesis imperfecta. *Clinical Orthopedics, 159,* 80-87.

Alexander, M. A., Johnson, E. W., Petty, J., & Staunch, D. (1979). Mechanical ventilation of patients with late stage Duchenne muscular dystrophy: Management in the home. *Archives of Physical Medicine and Rehabilitation, 60,* 289-292.

Bach, J. R., Alba, A. S., Pilkington, L. A., & Lee, M. (1981). Long-term rehabilitation in advanced stage of childhood onset, rapidly progressive muscular dystrophy. *Archives of Physical Medicine and Rehabilitation, 62,* 328-331.

Bach, J. R., O'Brien, J., Krotenberg, R., & Alba, A. S. (1987). Management of end stage respiratory failure in Duchenne muscular dystrophy. *Muscle and Nerve; 10,* 177-182.

Blackston, R. D. (1990). Medical genetics for the orthopaedist. In R. T. Morrissy (Ed.), *Lovell and Winter's pediatric orthopaedics* (3rd ed., pp. 143-174). Philadelphia: J.B. Lippincott.

Brooke, M. H., Fenichel, G. M., Griggs, R. C., Mendell, J. R., Moxley, R., Miller, J. P., Province, M. A., & the CIDD Group. (1983). Clinical investigation in Duchenne dystrophy: Determination of the "power" of therapeutic trials based on the natural history. *Muscle and Nerve, 6,* 91-103.

Brzustowicz, L. M., Lehner, T., Castilla, L. H., et al. (1990). Genetic mapping of chronic childhood-onset spinal muscular atrophy to chromosome 5q11.2-12.3. *Nature, 344,* 540-41.

Butler, C. (1986). Effects of powered mobility on self-initiated behaviors of very young children with locomotor disorders. *Developmental Medicine and Child Neurology, 28*(3), 325-332.

Cassidy, S. (1987, June). *Characteristic clinical features of Prader-Willi syndrome.* Paper presented at the 9th Annual Prader-Willi Syndrome Association (PWSA) Conference, Houston, TX.

Chu, C. E., Cooke, A., Stephenson, J. P. B., Tolmie, J. L., Clarke, B., Parry-Jones, W. L., Connor, J. M., & Donaldson, M. D. C. (1994). Diagnosis in Prader-Willi syndrome. *Archives of Disease in Childhood, 71* (5), 441-442.

Cullen, M. J., & Fulthorpe, J. H. (1975). Stages in fibre breakdown in Duchenne muscular dystrophy: An electron-microscope study. *Journal of Neurologic Science, 24,* 179-200.

Curran, F. J., & Colbert, A. P. (1989). Ventilator management in Duchenne muscular dystrophy and postpoliomyelitis syndrome: Twelve years' experience. *Archives of Physical Medicine and Rehabilitation, 70,* 180-185.

Cumming, W. J. K. (1993). Neuromuscular disorders. In P. M. Eckersley (Ed.) *Elements of paediatric physiotherapy.* Edinburgh: J.B. Lippincott.

DeSilva, S., Drachman, D. B, Mellitis, D., & Kuncl, R. W. (1987). Prednisone treatment in Duchenne muscular dystrophy. *Archives of Neurology, 44,* 818-822.

Donaldson, M. D. C., Chu, C. E., Cooke, A., Wilson, A., Greene, S. A., & Stephenson, J. B. P. (1994). The Prader-Willi syndrome. *Archives of Disease in Childhood, 70,* 58-63.

Dubowitz, V. (1992). Transferring myoblasts in Duchenne dystrophy. *British Medical Journal, 305,* 844-845.

Fukunaga, H., Okubo, R., Moritoyo, T., Kawashima, N., & Osame, M. (1993). Long-term follow-up of patients with Duchenne muscular dystrophy receiving ventilatory support. *Muscle and Nerve, 16,* 554-558.

Gitelis, S., Whiffen, J., & DeWald, R. L. (1983). Treatment of severe scoliosis in osteogenesis imperfecta. *Clinical Orthopedics, 175,* 56.

Hsu, J. D., & Furumasu, J. (1993). Gait and posture changes in the Duchenne muscular dystrophy child. *Clinical Orthopedics and Related Research, 288,* 122-125.

Khan, M.A. (1993). Corticosteroid therapy in Duchenne muscular dystrophy. *Journal of Neurological Science, 120*(1), 8-14.

Koenig, M., Hoffman, E. P., & Pertelson, C. K. (1987). Complete cloning of the Duchenne muscular dystrophy (DMD) cDNA and preliminary genomic organization of the DMD gene in mouse and affected individuals. *Cell, 50,* 509-517.

McHale, K. A., Tenuta, J. J., Tosi, L. L., & McKay, D. W. (1994). Percutaneous intramedullary fixation of long bone deformity in severe osteogenesis imperfecta. *Clinical Orthopaedics and Related Research, 305,* 242-248.

Melki, J., Sheth, P., Abdelhak, S., Burlet, P., Bachelot, M-F., Lathrop, M. G., Frezai, J, Munnich, A., & The French Spinal Muscular Atrophy Investigators. (1990). Mapping of acute (type 1) spinal muscular atrophy to chromosome 5q12-q14. *Lancet, 336,* 271-273.

Mokri, B., & Engel, A. W. (1975). Duchenne dystrophy: Electron microscopic findings pointing to a basic or early abnormality in the plasma membrane of the muscle fiber. *Neurology, 25,* 1111-1120.

Moser, H. (1984). Duchenne muscular dystrophy: Pathogenetic aspects and genetic prevention. *Human Genetics, 66,* 17-40.

Mostacciuolo, M. L., Lombardi, A., Cambilla, V., Danieli, G. A., & Angelini, C. (1987). Population data on benign and severe forms for X-linked muscular dystrophy. *Human Genetics, 75,* 217-220.

Naganuma, G. M., Harris, S. R., & Tada, W. L. (1995). Genetic disorders. In D. Umphred (Ed.). *Neurologic rehabilitation* (3rd ed.). St Louis: Mosby.

Pueschel, S. M. (1978). *Down syndrome: Growing and learning.* Kansas City: Andrews & McMeel.

Pueschel, S. M. (1990). *A parent's guide to Down syndrome: Toward a brighter future.* Baltimore: Brookes.

Reitter, B. (1995). Deflagacort vs. Prednisone in Duchenne muscular dystrophy: Trends of an ongoing study. *Brain Development, 17* Suppl, 39-43.

Richards, A., Quaghebeur, G., Clift, C., Holland, A., Dahlitz, M., & Parkes, D. (1994). The upper airway and sleep apnea in the Prader-Willi syndrome. *Clinical Otolaryngology, 19,* 193-197.

Rodillo, E., Marini, M. L., Heckmatt, J. Z., & Dubowitz, V. (1989). Scoliosis in spinal muscular atrophy: Review of 63 cases. *Journal of Child Neurology, 4,* 118-123.

Sansome, A., Royston, P., Dubowitz, V. (1993). Steroids in Duchenne muscular dystrophy: Pilot study of a new low-dosage schedule. *Neuromuscular Disorders, 3*(5-6), 567-569.

Scott, O. M., Hyde, S. A., Goddard, C., & Dubowitz, V. (1981). Prevention of deformity in Duchenne muscular dystrophy: A prospective study of passive stretching and splintage. *Physiotherapy, 67,* 177-180.

Scott, O. M., Vrbova, G., Hyde, S. A., & Dubowitz, V. (1986). Responses of muscles of patients with Duchenne muscular dystrophy to chronic electrical stimulation. *Journal of Neurology, Neurosurgery and Psychiatry, 49,* 1427-1434.

Sharav, T., & Bowman, T. (1992). Dietary practices, physical activity and body-mass index in a selected population of Down syndrome children and their siblings. *Clinical Pediatrics, 31*(6), 341-344.

Sillence, D. O., Senn, A., & Danks, D. M. (1979). Genetic heterogeneity in osteogenesis imperfecta. *Journal of Medical Genetics, 16,* 101.

Soper, R., Mason, E., Printen, K., & Zellweger, H. (1975). Gastric bypass for morbid obesity in children and adolescents. *Journal Pediatric Surgery, 10,* 51-58.

Stuberg, W. A. (1994). Muscular dystrophy and spinal muscular atrophy. In S. K. Campbell (Ed.). *Physical therapy for children* (pp. 295-324). Philadelphia: WB Saunders.

Tecklin, J. S. (1994). *Pediatric physical therapy* (2nd ed.). Philadelphia: J.B. Lippincott.

Vignos, P. J., Spencer, G. E., & Archibald, K. C. (1963). Management of progressive muscular dystrophy. *Journal of the American Medical Association, 184,* 103-112.

Wong, D. L. (1995). *Whaley and Wong's nursing care of infants and children* (5th ed.). St Louis: Mosby.

Zaleske, K. J., Doppelt, S. H., & Mankin, H. J. (1990). Metabolic and endocrine abnormalities of the immature skeleton. In R. T. Morrissey (Ed.). *Lovell and Winter's pediatric orthopaedics* (3rd ed.) Philadelphia: J.B. Lippincott.

Traumatic Disorders

traumatic brain injury
open head injury
closed head injury
shaken baby syndrome
concussion
near-drowning
pediatric spinal cord injury
spinal shock
hydrotherapy
transfers
ambulation
burn injury
dressings
contractures
scar formation
school reentry
pediatric seating
pediatric wheelchair
stroller
seating principles
simple contour
generic contour
intimate contour
wheelchair accessories
tilt-in-space

Noelle, A Young Child With Severe Burns

The toddler wandered out of the bedroom, looking for Grandma Grace. She walked into the kitchen where she had heard someone rummaging around. Standing quietly inside the doorway, she watched her grandmother make a cup of tea. Grandma carefully poured the hot water from a saucepan into her mug on the counter. Then she put the pan back on the stove. She found a tea bag in the cupboard and plunked it into the cup, moving it up and down a few times, then draping the tag over the edge of the cup as it steeped. She left the cup steaming on the countertop while she moved over to the cupboard and looked for a cookie.

Noelle watched the pan on the stove and the cup on the counter. She watched the steam rise into the air. The pan beckoned her, its handle stuck out over the edge of the stove. She edged nearer to it. Reaching up toward the pan, she glanced over at her grandmother who was busily looking in the cupboard, unaware of Noelle's presence. Noelle grasped the handle and pulled it closer to her so that she could see inside. She screamed as the pan tipped over, spilling near boiling water over her head, face, arm, and chest.

Noelle had an uneventful birth, although her conception and gestation were far from uneventful because of the young age of her mother. Leila was 13 years old when she came home with hickeys on her neck and was beaten by her father. Angry and rebellious, she called the police and turned her father in for child abuse. It was not the first time he had hit her. Leila was placed in a foster home, from where she repeatedly ran away. When her grandmother, Grace, realized that Leila was pregnant, she offered to take her in as a foster child. Grace had four grown sons and felt that she might be able to help her granddaughter. Leila agreed to try the arrangement; she had been living with Grace most of the time since just before the birth of her daughter. Others who lived in the house included Grace's husband, their son and his wife (Leila's uncle and aunt), and Leila's two brothers. Leila was 13 when Noelle was born. After her birth, there were four generations of women living in the house: Grace, Leila's aunt, Leila, and Noelle.

Even after moving in with her grandmother, Leila had a hard time. Child Protective Services monitored both Leila and Noelle, although the only active case was Leila's. Social Services wanted Leila to be an effective parent and helped her learn to care for her daughter. However, Leila was not consistent about her school attendance and repeatedly ran away to spend time with her friends, who were older and out of high school. She was bored staying at home taking care of her daughter. Grace became the primary caretaker for Noelle, as well as the legal guardian for Leila. Because no neglect or abuse had been documented for Noelle, Leila was legally her daughter's guardian.

At 15 years of age, Leila was still in the ninth grade. She had a steady boyfriend; he was a 20-year-old unemployed man who was not Noelle's father. Leila took care of Noelle sometimes and liked to take her out for rides with her boyfriend in his car. Grace was reluctant to allow Leila to take Noelle out of the house too much, but she wanted Noelle to develop a relationship with her mother. When Leila was angry at her grandmother, she threatened to take Noelle away from her.

Noelle was 15 months old at the time of her accident (Figure 9-1). She stayed home with her great-grandmother Grace during the day and sometimes saw her mother in the evenings when Leila came home early enough. Noelle had a regular schedule of two naps per day and went to bed at 8:00 PM. It was getting close to her bedtime, and she was playing with her uncles in the bedroom on that evening when she wandered out to find her grandmother.

Noelle was only wearing a disposable diaper when she spilled the boiling water over herself. When Grace heard the screams, she turned around and saw immediately what had happened. She ran to put cold water on the burns. She called to other family members for help, hoping that the burns would not be as bad as she feared. Noelle's aunt tried to help by putting aloe on Noelle's face and arm. When Grace saw Noelle's eyelids start to blister, she immediately rushed her to the emergency department.

Noelle was transferred to the children's hospital in the city and stayed there for 2 weeks. Her face, scalp, neck, chest, upper arm, axilla, and anterior thigh had partial thickness burns, with some deep areas on her chest and face. Her diaper had saved her perineal area from injury.

Grace sat with Noelle all day, every day. She felt responsible for the accident because her lack of awareness had allowed Noelle to be near the stove and reach the pot of water. Visiting Noelle was hard for other family members because the hospital was over an hour's drive from home. Leila came sometimes on the bus.

The first few days were filled with pain and drugs for the toddler. She had a Foley catheter so that her fluid output could be carefully monitored. She had an intravenous (IV) line in her foot to replace fluids, balance electrolytes, and provide nutrition. She also had a nasogastric tube for the first few days for feeding. Dressing changes occurred twice daily; her nurse, physical therapist (PT), and occupational therapist (OT) provided exercises to maintain her range of motion at her right shoulder, elbow, and hip, the joints most badly burned (Figure 9-2). Noelle was heavily medicated before the dressing changes to help her tolerate the pain, but she cried anyway. The therapists worked with the nurses to encourage Noelle to move her arm herself, and to move it passively as far as she would allow them. Doing the exercises effectively without traumatizing the toddler too much was a challenge.

Noelle could not move too far from her bed because of the length of her IV tubing. When her foot became swollen and tender, the IV site was changed to her hand. When her hand became tender, it was changed to her other foot. It was changed every 3 to 5 days. When the IV was in her foot, she could not stand or walk. When it was in her hand, she could not use both hands to play. Noelle stayed in her bed most of the time for the first week. Grace read to her or talked to her. Grace was not comfortable with too much talking, so there were hours of si-

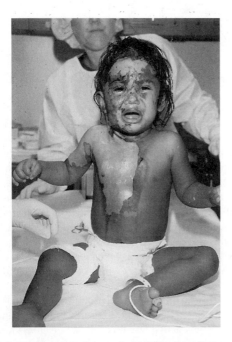

Figure 9-1 Noelle was unhappy during dressing changes. She was premedicated, but the procedure was painful anyway.

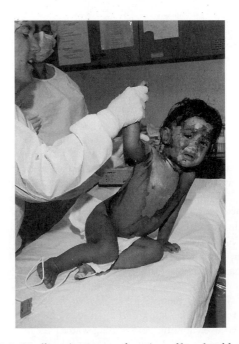

Figure 9-2 Noelle resists range of motion of her shoulder because of pain.

lence when the older woman just sat beside the toddler's crib. Noelle did not feel too well those first days and slept most of the time.

A social worker from Child Protective Services visited Grace to determine if the burns had occurred through abuse, neglect, or an accident. The social worker made sure that Grace's story matched the one that had been told when Noelle was brought to the emergency department. Grace understood very well how the accident could have been prevented and chastised herself for not being more careful. The social worker knew the family and could determine fairly easily that Noelle was not at risk in the house. Her burns were an accident, an avoidable accident, but an accident nonetheless.

During the second week of her hospitalization, when Noelle felt well enough to get up, her grandmother took her to the playroom. Sometimes the PT, Elise, met them there; she encouraged the toddler to use her arm actively to reach, throw, and point at toys. Although Noelle clung to her grandmother, the therapist invited her to walk between play areas. She was encouraged to push a shopping cart and fill it with toys that she could take off the shelves herself. Some toys were so big that she needed to use two hands. Grace watched these interactions and began to imitate some of the games with Noelle, even when Elise was not there.

Dressing changes continued to be painful and scary for Noelle, but she was a social child and enjoyed interacting with the nurses and therapists. Her burns were healing well; by the last few days of her hospital stay, she did not need dressings on her face, arm, or leg. Some of the more deeply burned areas on her chest continued to be at risk of infection, so those were dressed. Because Noelle was healing so well and because she had recovered nearly full active and passive range of motion of her

arm, she did not require regular outpatient physical or occupational therapy once she was discharged from the hospital. Although her scars were lighter than the rest of her skin, they were flexible and congruent. They were not raised or keloid. Pressure garments were not warranted (Figure 9-3).

Before discharge Elise assessed Noelle's gross motor skills, which were appropriate for her age. She was walking independently, climbing the equipment in the playroom, and playing actively with both hands. She used her right arm less than her left while playing, but she could be coaxed to reach almost to full range actively. Because of the asymmetrical functional use of her arms, the therapist performed one follow-up home visit for reassessment and family teaching.

A follow-up visit to the home to assess Noelle's recovery 1 week after discharge found her driving her toy electric car through the house, smiling and laughing (Figure 9-4). She was using both arms for bilateral activities in reaching and playing. She had full active and passive range of motion in her shoulder and elbow. She demonstrated full spontaneous active range of motion of both arms during play. Her scars were fading. The deeper areas on her chest were healing well. Noelle was happy and demonstrated good attachment to and comfort with both her grandmother and mother, who came home during the afternoon.

Although Noelle looked happy and healthy, Elise noticed that only a few toys were out. She was concerned about safety with some of the toys she saw. Grace had probably cleaned in preparation for the therapist's visit, but Elise decided to use the time for general teaching, using modeling and play with Noelle, about Noelle's development.

Noelle warmed to Elise quickly and was easy to engage in play. The therapist pointed out Noelle's wonderful skills and capabilities by exclaiming about them as they exhibited themselves. Noelle's use of words, her ability to climb in and out of the car, ability to use gestures and facial expressions to communicate and receive what she wanted, and her ability to point and to steer the car were all mentioned. In addition, Elise taught Grace and Leila what to expect next in Noelle's development and how to en-

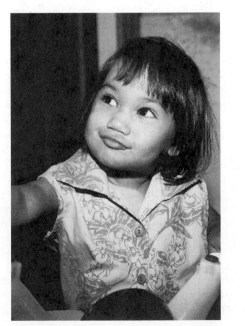

Figure 9-3 A few weeks after returning home, Noelle's face shows only light patches where her skin was burned.

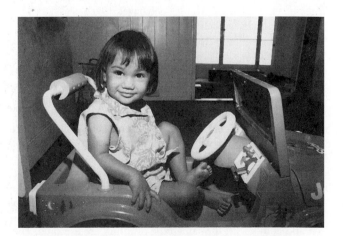

Figure 9-4 Noelle demonstrates how she can drive her electric car. Her burn scars are evident on her face and arm, but the scar tissue is soft and pliable.

courage her gross motor, fine motor, language, and social skills while playing with her (Figure 9-5). She modeled talking to Noelle about her toys and activities to encourage language skills. She played gross motor games that encouraged running, stopping, and balance skills. She encouraged Grace to let Noelle feed herself independently and provided her with hints on how to set up the area around the table to minimize the clean up after a meal. She discussed safety with the toy car and helped Grace to create a barrier around the step that led from the family room into the living room. Grace mentioned her attention to turning the handles of pots so they did not protrude over the edge of the stove.

Elise determined that further home visits were not necessary, but she discussed with Grace the possibility of enrolling Noelle in a play group where Grace could receive some peer support from other parents and caregivers. Grace could also learn appropriate games and activities for toddlers that she could use at home. Grace expressed interest in the idea. As she walked to her car, Elise heard Leila laughing and exclaiming to Grace about Noelle's skill at balancing standing on top of the toy car. Elise hoped she would not see Noelle in the hospital again!

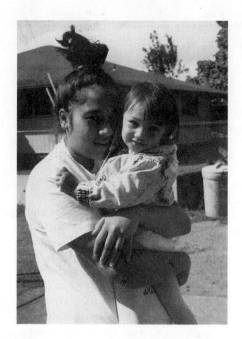

Figure 9-5 Noelle enjoys spending time with her mother.

BACKGROUND AND THEORY

Childhood accidents cause more death and disability than all childhood illnesses combined. After congenital anomalies and disorders related to the birth process and sudden infant death syndrome (SIDS), accidents are the leading cause of death in infants under 1 year. After 1 year of age accidents are the leading cause of death for all children. Of all children who die between the ages of 5 and 19, injuries account for 70% of the deaths (Centers for Disease Control and Prevention, 1990). Many more children are left to cope with lifelong disability from accidents than die in those accidents. Motor vehicle accidents, drowning, and burns from fires are in the top five types of accidents leading to death in every age group of children. Firearms are the second leading cause of death in children from 10 to 19 years of all ethnicities (Svenson, Spurlock, & Nypaver, 1996).

Motor vehicle accidents are the leading cause of traumatic death of all accidental means for children older than 1 year (Centers for Disease Control and Prevention, 1990). Included in this category are children who are occupants in cars, pedestrians hit by motor vehicles, and riders on motorcycles/bicycles. Seat belts and bicycle helmets are unable to prevent trauma to those who do not use them. Some parents do not realize the benefits of these safety precautions until it is too late. Trauma can be intentionally or accidentally inflicted on a child, but either way the results can be very serious.

In this chapter childhood disabilities related to traumatic brain injury, near-drowning, spinal cord injury, and burns are discussed. The acute phase of each disability, the rehabilitation phase, and specific information about the difference between children and adults with the same type of injury are explored. The previous case study of a young child who suffered severe burns over her face, scalp, arm and chest highlights the importance of safety for children to prevent burns, as well as the role of physical

therapy with a young child who has an acute burn. An Applications section on seating, positioning, and wheeled mobility provides an overview of seating and mobility principles for the child with mobility impairment and neuromuscular disability.

Child Abuse

Reports of a parent being led away in handcuffs while a severely injured child recovers in the hospital are commonly seen in today's news. Frustrated parents shake their infants when they will not stop crying. Children are hit, dunked into scalding water, held under water, or locked in rooms with no toilet or food. Child abuse is a common cause of traumatic injury to children. All service providers should be aware of signs of abuse and the role of each person in reporting suspected abuse. Service providers may work with families who have abused their children to the extent of causing permanent damage. The way in which these circumstances are handled may affect the child's recovery.

Child abuse is actually more prevalent than is seen on the news. The National Coalition for the Prevention of Child Abuse (NCPCA) reported in 1993 that a child was abused every 13 seconds in the United States, and more than three children died each day as a result of maltreatment (ChildHelp USA, 1996). In 1992 over 2.9 million reports of child abuse were made. As reported by the U.S. Department of Health and Human Resources in 1993; 44% of the substantiated cases of abuse constituted neglect, 24%, physical abuse; 15%, sexual abuse; 6%, emotional maltreatment; 2%, medical neglect; and the remaining 9%, other or unknown forms of maltreatment (ChildHelp USA, 1996). One child in every hundred is abused in the United States, with physical abuse occurring in almost half of the cases (Pecora, Wittaker, Maluccio, Barth, & Plotnick, 1992). The other types of abuse are emotional and sexual. It is thought that only half of the cases of severe abuse are reported (Lister, 1996). Statistics show that child abuse is rising, perhaps due to an increased occurrence or to improved reporting.

Before 1962 no states had laws to protect children from abuse and neglect. In a seminal paper Kempe, Silverman, Steele, Broegemueller, & Silver (1962) defined the "battered child syndrome" and brought medical and legal attention to this common occurrence. The Federal Child Abuse Prevention and Treatment Act of 1974 defined abuse and neglect and set guidelines for reporting these acts to authorities. It also set into place intervention procedures. The 1980 Adoption Assistance and Child Welfare Act (PL 96-272) expanded interventions to protect children, including support of the natural family to keep their children and financial support for foster and adoptive placement when the natural family is unable to care for the child. Every state now has laws mandating reporting of suspected abuse and neglect of children. Medical professionals should be familiar with reporting procedures in their own state.

Child abuse is especially important to those in medical service professions. Children with disabilities are four to ten times more likely to be sexually abused than their typically developing peers. Physical therapy providers are often in positions to identify abuse and are under legal obligation to report any suspected abuse, with legal ramifications if it is not reported. PTs and physical therapist assistants (PTAs) are likely to handle children and to remove clothing for evaluation or treatment. Assessing a child's emotional response to these activities, relationships to parents and other adults, and observations of the signs of physical abuse can occur during the therapy session. Some signs and symptoms of physical abuse include fractures, welts, bruises, burns, soft tissue injuries, and internal injuries. Sexual abuse is more difficult to see, but children have typical behaviors that can range from fear, extreme shyness, extroversion, or hostility. A change in the child's behaviors may be the clearest sign of sexual abuse, but it is important to have other team members corroborate because such behaviors can have multiple causes.

Suspecting child abuse can be difficult for a therapy provider. A strong relationship with the family has frequently been established. To suspect wrongdoing toward their child can feel like breaking a trust. However, the first allegiance must be to the safety of the child. When abuse is suspected, confronting the adult whom you suspect is not the appropriate step. Each state has specific protocols for reporting suspected abuse that should be followed. Many states have anonymous hotlines; however, following the protocol of your own employer may provide the most support for you. You may find that others have also suspected the abuse but have not been confident enough to come forward.

Besides the physical therapy provider's role in identification of abuse, the PT and PTA also treat children who have suffered physical harm at the hands of adults. Common methods of physical abuse include shaking; hitting with a fist, open hand, or object; pushing or shoving; burning with a cigarette; holding under water; or scalding in hot water. A pattern of abuse may involve several methods of inflicting harm. Abuse can be verified by a series of broken bones over time, frequently untreated; a brain injury consistent with shaking an infant with little head control; certain patterns of scalds; or injuries that do not fit the adult's

description of the event in which they occurred. If a parent is the suspected abuser, the child is usually placed in foster care during any investigation. Child Protective Services usually encourages a maintenance of relationship between the parents and child, and therapy providers may find themselves teaching handling and other skills to the very person who caused the injury in the first place.

It is important to recognize that a child abuser is wrestling with issues of his or her own, such as an inability to control anger, poor control over outside circumstances in life, a history of abuse as a child, an abusive spousal relationship, and other stresses. Most people who cause injuries to children are not thinking of the possible outcomes of their actions, and suffer significant remorse for injuring their child. Abusing a child is never acceptable, but compassion for the abuser can help a therapy provider continue to work with the family in a productive manner. Trying to work with family members in the present and putting aside what has occurred in the past can also be an effective strategy.

The Child With a Traumatic Brain Injury

A 5-year-old boy falls out of a tree onto a concrete sidewalk. A 7-year-old boy is hit by a car while he is riding his bicycle. He was not wearing a helmet. A 12-year-old girl is thrown from the back of a pickup truck during a minor traffic accident. A 17-year-old boy is involved in a major traffic collision on the evening of his senior prom. He was not wearing his seat belt. All of these children suffer traumatic brain injuries. All of these injuries could have been prevented by using proper safety procedures. However, children explore and take risks by nature, and underestimating the importance of safety procedures by adults can have severe consequences.

Traumatic brain injury (TBI) has been defined as trauma sufficient to result in a change in level of consciousness and/or an anatomical abnormality of the brain (Michaud & Duhaime, 1992). The federal government has defined traumatic brain injury for the purposes of defining eligibility for special education as the following:

. . . an acquired injury to the brain caused by an external force, resulting in total or partial functional disability or psychosocial impairment, or both, that adversely affects a child's educational performance. The term applies to open- or closed-head injuries resulting in impairments in one or more areas, such as cognition; language; memory; attention; reasoning; abstract thinking; judgment; problem solving; sensory, perceptual, and motor abilities; psychosocial behavior; physical functions; information processing; and speech (Federal Register, 1992).

Although most mild brain injuries appear to heal completely, the 5% of children with more severe injuries have deficits that last the rest of their lives. It is this 5% that the federal definition addresses.

Incidence and Cause

Estimates range from 78,000 to 600,000 to 2 million occurrences of new traumatic brain injuries in children per year in the United States (Greenspan, 1996; Massagli, et al., 1996; Jaffe, Polissar, Fay, & Liao, 1995). The figure is dependent on how the traumatic brain injury is defined. Most of these injuries are mild, but approximately 5% lead to death or permanent disability. The incidence of head injury is approximately 219 per 100,000 per year for children under 19 years old (Rouse, Eichelberger, & Martin, 1992). It is the most common cause of acquired disability in childhood (Krause, Rock, & Hemyari, 1990).

The most common cause of head injury in children less than 1 year is violence related to the shaken baby syndrome, described later. Children older than 1 year generally sustain head injuries related to a motor vehicle accident, either as an unrestrained passenger, pedestrian, or bicycle rider involved in an altercation with a car. Other causes include falls, sports- or recreation-related accidents, physical abuse, or trauma related to gunshot injuries.

Boys sustain TBI at least twice as often as girls. One study found that over half of children with TBI had previously existing learning disabilities, attention-deficit hyperactivity disorder (ADHD), or other personality/characterological disorders (Mahalik, Yalamanchi, Ruzicka, & Bowen, 1990). The incidence of head injuries among children with these preexisting disorders could relate to more risk-taking behavior, impaired judgment, or poor impulse control related to their preexisting diagnoses.

Clinical Features

TBI entails the injury to the scalp, skull, meninges, or brain as a result of mechanical injury (Figure 9-6). The age at which a child sustains a TBI is a factor in the outcome. Younger children do worse than older children. Toddlers and preschoolers have more disability related to TBI than adolescents, possibly because of the impairment of their ability to learn. Depending on the mechanism of injury, children with TBI can have several different patterns of brain injury.

Open head injury. Depressed skull fractures, gunshot wounds, severe trauma, or other injury resulting in an open wound exposing brain tissue to the environment can result in severe brain injury, infection, and other complications in chil-

Figure 9-6 The head comprises the bony structure of the skull, as well as the softer tissues contained therein, including the brain, meninges, and blood vessels. A mechanical trauma can result in several types of injury to the brain caused by coup, contrecoup, and shear forces on the brain tissue.

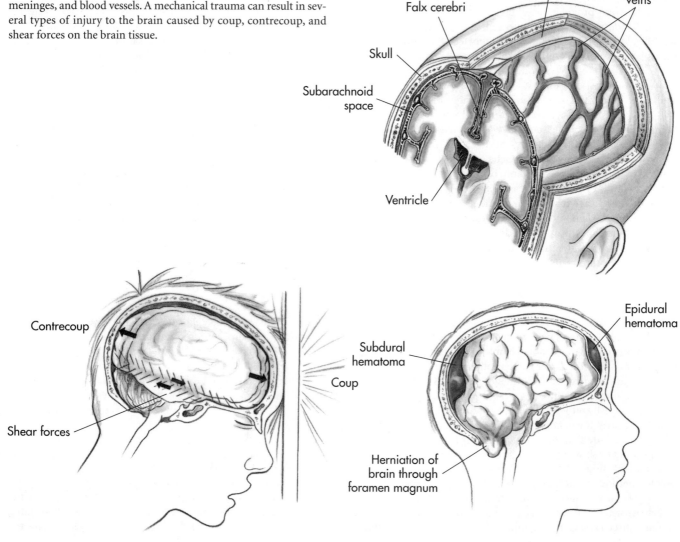

dren. These injuries are less common but cause similar deficits to the closed head injuries, which are discussed next.

Closed head injury. The function of the skull is to protect the vulnerable brain tissue that rests inside. The skull is a solid bony case with limited space. Directional forces on the skull can cause a variety of injuries to the brain itself, even if the integrity of the skull is not breached. Acceleration and deceleration forces on the head can cause the brain to move slower or faster than the bony skull, thus causing injury to the delicate tissues. Shear forces inside the brain tissue itself can cause disruption as well.

A direct injury to the brain is called a *coup injury.* If the head suddenly decelerates in force, such as when a child's head hits the windshield in a moving car or the pavement when falling from a tree, the soft brain tissue hits the skull and bounces back, causing an injury to the opposite side of the brain as it hits the other side of the skull. This secondary injury is called a *contrecoup injury.* Acceleration of the head, such as when a standing car is hit from behind at a high speed, can cause similar injuries. *Shear stresses* occur when different brain tissues move in different directions or in the same direction at different rates of speed. Shear forces usually occur at the intersection of different types of tissues, such as the gray matter (brain cells) and the white matter (axons). They can cause stretching and trauma to nerves and blood vessels, causing the most serious injuries at the surface of the brain and at the brain stem where vital functions such as breathing are regulated.

Related problems with TBI

Skull fractures. Skull fractures occur in 25% of TBIs. The occurrence of a fracture does not indicate the severity of the accompanying brain injury. The most common type of skull fracture is the *linear fracture,* which occurs at the site of injury and is dictated by the site and velocity of the impact. In children with more mature bones these fractures often heal without accompanying brain injury. However, if they occur over an important cerebral artery, damage from bleeding or anoxia to the brain tissue can be extensive. *Depressed fractures* occur when the skull is deformed and depressed into the brain tissue. These are serious injuries and usually cause substantial damage to brain tissue. Children with immature bone may present with a dent or bending of the skull, which does not result in a fracture, but may cause tissue damage.

Hematomas. Hematomas, or bleeding, can occur with a TBI. *Epidural hematomas* occur with a direct injury to the brain, such as a depressed skull fracture. Bleeding occurs into the spaces between the skull and the dura. Rapidly accumulating hematomas can be very serious, causing damage to the neural structures. Surgery to stop the bleeding and remove accumulated blood is imperative. Acute *subdural hematomas* form under the dura of the brain and over the brain tissue itself. They are caused by shear forces to the blood vessels supplying the brain and usually accompany a major injury. Relief of the pressure from the blood clot does not often significantly affect the recovery of the child. This factor reflects the extensive brain damage that is caused by forces strong enough to cause rupture of the blood vessels on the surface of the brain.

Increased intracranial pressure. *Cerebral edema* often accompanies a TBI. Trauma to the brain causes increased capillary permeability, which allows fluid to build up slowly in the brain. Excessive fluid that cannot escape the brain cavity can cause increased intracranial pressure and lead to herniation of the brain. If the brain tissue is forced through an available opening such as the foramen magnum, the child will sustain severe brain damage and probably death. Cerebral edema can peak up to 72 hours after a brain injury. A child who is at risk for increased intracranial pressure is usually observed in intensive care with a pressure gauge inserted through the skull to monitor pressures until the danger period has passed.

Shaken baby syndrome. Many adults do not realize the fragile nature of the infant's head. A child's head is much bigger in relation to his or her body than that of an adult. Because of poor strength and muscle control, the young child cannot compensate for accelerations or decelerations in movements of the head (Figure 9-7). Shaking is most dangerous in infants under 6 months. Even if the child's head were supported, the forces on the immature brain can cause damage. Most shaken babies incur injuries from parents or caretakers who have difficulty controlling anger or frustration. Infants who are colicky may cry a lot, frustrating caregivers who do not know how to console them. They pick up the infant and shake vigorously to stop the child from crying. Shaking does not have to be overly vigorous to cause harm. Other injuries are caused by more aggressive abuse: shaking accompanied by other trauma such as violently throwing the child on the bed or against the wall or floor.

Parents may bring the child to the emergency department because the child is throwing up or is unresponsive. They may not even realize that they caused the injury. The abuse may occur in one episode of shaking or a series of episodes taking place over time. Obvious injury may not be apparent, but x-ray examinations can demonstrate the classic pattern of injuries accompanying this type of abuse. Shaking injuries will include acceleration injuries to the brain. Coup and contrecoup injuries will be apparent, as well as injuries related to shear forces in the brain. A common related injury is detached retinas, causing visual impairments in these children.

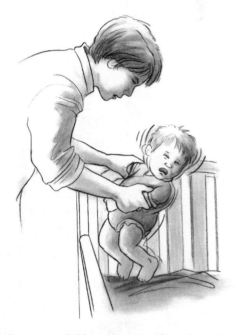

Figure 9-7 A young child can incur significant brain damage when shaken.

Concussion. Concussion is a common brain injury that usually resolves without long-term neurological damage. An external force to the head causes loss of awareness and responsiveness, which could last for minutes or hours. Amnesia related to the traumatic event itself and to events preceding the trauma is characteristic; although some memory of events can return, some amnesia will always remain. Concussion can occur during sports that involve physical contact, such as football, or during a fall. Most children have no long-term sequelae from concussion.

Assessing severity of TBI. The Glasgow Coma Scale (GCS) is a common instrument for assessing the severity of head injuries in adults. Its adaptation for children, the Pediatric Coma Scale (PCS), is reproduced in Table 9-1. The PCS assesses eye opening, motor response, and verbal response. Scores on all three areas range from 3 to 15; a score of 3 indicates a child who is completely unresponsive, and a score of 15 indicates a child who is alert and oriented and follows verbal commands. The severity of TBI in children, unlike adults, is not closely related to their scores on the GCS. Children with low scores on the GCS may die; however, if they recover from the brain injury, they will recover more fully than adults with similar scores. Some researchers think that prognosis is better predicted by the duration of posttraumatic amnesia, the period of time around and after the trauma that the child cannot remember. Posttraumatic amnesia of less than 24 hours is considered a mild TBI; between 24 hours and 7 days is considered a moderate TBI; longer than 7 days is considered a severe TBI. Outcome of brain injury is influenced by the part of the brain that was damaged.

Table 9-2 outlines the major structures of the brain, their functions, and dysfunction that may ensue with damage.

Recovery patterns. Children with more serious brain injuries have a characteristic pattern of recovery. The Rancho Los Amigos Scale (1989) designates eight levels of recovery and is often used in acute care and rehabilitation centers to describe a child's behavior. Behavior often initially presents as completely *unresponsive.* The child will eventually develop *generalized responses,* particularly to pain. As the child becomes more alert, he or she may develop a *localized response* to stimulation. At this point the child may smile or squeeze a parent's hand in response to a command. This state changes to *confused and agitated* as the child becomes more alert. At this stage verbalizations and behaviors may be disinhibited; a child may swear or become violent, even when these behaviors were not part of his or her repertoire before the injury. A gradual return of cognitive and functional skills occurs as this agitated state fades; however, confusion may still be present, and the child's actions may be inappropriate. This is called the *confused, inappropriate, nonagitated* level of recovery. As the child gains alertness, actions may be more appropriate, but the child may still be confused. This is the *confused appropriate* stage. He or she has some awareness of self and others but has difficulty with memory and may need verbal cueing to relearn self-care skills. As the confusion resolves, the child may appear to move in a robotlike manner doing what is asked but may have difficulty with problem solving, judgment, and planning skills. He or she is in the *automatic ap-*

| TABLE 9-1 | Pediatric Coma Scale |

Category of assessment	Score			
		Over 1 year	**Less than 1 year**	
Eyes opening	4	Spontaneously	Spontaneously	
	3	To verbal command	To shout	
	2	To pain	To pain	
	1	No response	No response	
		Over 1 year	**Less than 1 year**	
Best motor response	6	Obeys		
	5	Localizes pain	Localizes pain	
	4	Flexion withdrawal	Flexion withdrawal	
	3	Flexion—abnormal (decorticate rigidity)	Flexion—abnormal (decorticate rigidity)	
	2	Extension (decerebrate rigidity)	Extension (decerebrate rigidity)	
	1	No response	No response	
		Over 5 years	**2-5 years**	**0-23 months**
Best verbal response	5	Oriented and converses	Appropriate words and phrases	Smiles, coos, cries appropriately
	4	Disoriented and converses	Inappropriate words	Cries
	3	Inappropriate words	Cries and/or screams	Inappropriate crying and/or screaming
	2	Incomprehensible sounds	Grunts	Grunts
	1	No response	No response	No response
Total	3-15			

Modified from the Glasgow Coma Scale. From Wong, D. L., Whaley, L. F., & Kasprisin, C. A. (1990). *Clinical manual of pediatric nursing.* St. Louis: Mosby, p. 393.

propriate level of recovery. The final stage of recovery sees the return of *appropriate and purposeful* activity. The child's personality may be permanently altered, however, with persisting deficits in problem solving, tolerating stress, and abstract reasoning. Any preexisting behavior problems may be greatly exacerbated in the child with a TBI.

Motor functions may be impaired in children with TBI. Depending on the area or areas of brain injury, the child may have spasticity, ataxia, or tremor. Patterns of motor deficits may include hemiplegia, double hemiplegia, or more global motor impairment. As with adults with acquired brain injury, motor impairment may manifest itself as hypotonia initially, with spasticity emerging throughout the recovery period. As a result of the crossing over of motor pathways, injuries to one side of the brain will cause motor and sensory impairment on the opposite side of the body.

Because of the plasticity of pediatric brains, children can recover functions of language better than adults and do not usually have long-term problems with unilateral hemineglect, agnosia (inability to recognize objects), or dyspraxias (inability to carry out a specified motor behavior), although these may occur in the short term. These problems are common to adults who suffer brain injuries including stroke or TBI. Feeding disorders related to motor deficits are common with more severe injuries. Deficits

TABLE 9-2 Brain Structures and Implications for Injury

Brain structure	Function	If injured
Frontal lobes of the cerebrum	Abstract thinking, recognition of cause-and-effect relationships, expressive language, basis for social interaction; posterior portion contains cells that control motor activity throughout body	Personality changes, altered intellectual functioning, memory deficits, language deficits, impaired motor skills
Parietal lobes of the cerebrum	Appreciation of sensation, somatic (sensory) interpretation and integration	Language dysfunction, aphasia (inability to formulate and use symbols such as words), apraxia (inability to carry out on request a complex or skilled movement); motor and sensory loss to lower extremities; atopognosia (inability to localize tactile stimuli)
Occipital lobe of the cerebrum	Visual cortex, spatial orientation, visual recognition	Impaired vision, functional blindness
Temporal lobes of the cerebrum	Receives and interprets stimuli for taste, vision, sound, smell; converts crude visual impressions into recognizable images, interprets images; primary speech, hearing, receptive language areas	Inability to interpret sensory stimuli; difficulty understanding higher levels of meaning of body sensory experiences; aphasia (ability to formulate and use symbols such as words); hearing dysfunction
Cerebellum	Refinement and coordination of all muscle movements including walking, talking, control of muscle tone, and balance	Dysmetria, ataxia, dysarthria (inability to form words), hypotonia, nystagmus, dystonia; tremor at rest
Basal ganglia	Unconscious or automatic control of lower motor centers; excitation causes inhibition of muscle tone throughout body	Movement disorders including chorea, athetosis, dystonia, tremor at rest
Diencephalon (thalamus and hypothalamus)	Major relay station for sensory impulses to cerebral cortex, activates cerebral cortex. Vital control centers for involuntary functions (e.g., blood pressure, satiety, hunger, rage, feeding, water conservation, temperature, sleep regulation, libido); secretion of tropic hormones	Impaired consciousness. Alterations in vegetative functions; somnolence, coma; anorexia, loss of weight, fever, diabetes insipidus, loss of libido; endocrine disorders
Brainstem (mesencephalon, pons, and medulla)	All cranial nerves except I, eye movement, vital centers for respiration and vasomotor control	Impaired eye movement; deep, rapid, or periodic breathing; impaired function of facial muscles, flaccid muscle tone, absent deep tendon reflexes, no response to stimuli; impaired vital functions (e.g., respiration, vasomotor control)

Modified from Wong, D. L. (1995). *Whaley and Wong's nursing care of infants and children* (5th ed.). St. Louis: Mosby, pp. 1672-1673.

in vision or hearing may impede rehabilitation. Psychosocial problems can be related to a changed self-image in a child and occur even more so in an adolescent who is already struggling with issues of self and peer relationships. Family dynamics will probably be affected strongly by this significant change in one family member. Family stress may come to a peak several years after the injury when the extent of disability is clear.

Cognitive and academic problems may be immediately apparent. Children with milder injuries may grow into cognitive problems that are not apparent when they are younger; these may cause problems with self-esteem and academic performance in adolescence. Special education may be involved to help the child succeed in school.

Intervention for Acute TBI

Medical intervention for the child with an acute traumatic brain injury focuses on preserving life while minimizing secondary injury from cerebral edema and increased intracranial pressure. Supportive measures may be necessary in the acute phase of an injury to support respiration, blood pressure, nutrition, and other physiologic functions. Surgery may be necessary to stop hemorrhaging, repair fractures, and address concurrent injuries. Most children with a moderate or severe injury are monitored in intensive care for at least 24 hours and may need mechanical ventilation, intravenous fluids and nutrition, and medications to decrease edema or control seizures.

It is important for hospital personnel to know who the child was before the injury. Photographs of the child participating in school, sports, and home activities can be placed near the child's bed for the encouragement of the family, staff, and child. Family members should be encouraged to talk about the child's likes, activities, and dislikes. Some of this information can be used to plan therapy sessions or to build conversations between the therapy provider and the child, which can sometimes seem very one-sided.

Physical therapy intervention. Initial intervention efforts support the child to avoid secondary injuries or disabilities from the acute TBI. Physical therapy may make splints to prevent plantarflexion contractures as the child lies in a coma. During this acute phase of the injury, the child should be allowed deep rest so the healing process can begin without increasing intracranial pressure. Gentle range of motion to preserve joint mobility may be indicated. It is important to watch the intracranial pressure monitor when interacting physically with a child, to ensure pressure in the brain does not exceed safe levels. Range of motion can become more vigorous after the first few days of recovery. Helping the nurses position the child in partial sidelying as well as supine positions can help avoid pressure areas to the skin, as well as provide comfort to the child. It is unlikely that a PTA will be asked to see the child with a TBI during the first few days after injury. However, if you find yourself in this situation, rely heavily on the nurses to tell you what is safe and what is not.

Teaching family members ways to touch and interact with the child can help them feel useful and productive as they wait for the child to recover. Providing auditory input may help the child become more alert. This can include family members and friends talking on tape or in person; favorite music or stories; and taped sounds of familiar environments such as a classroom cacophony, foghorns, traffic noises, or ocean sounds. Tactile input may also help the child become more alert. Encouraging family members

to massage gently, rub with a towel, stroke, or otherwise touch a child can be comforting.

Intervention in the Rehabilitation Phase

Medical intervention continues to be directed toward preserving physiological functions and repairing related musculoskeletal and visceral injuries.

Physical therapy intervention. Once a child is moved out of intensive care and is medically stable, more vigorous rehabilitation can begin. Varied sensory input can be provided to help the child increase alertness. Getting the small child into the lap of a family member to rock in a rocking chair can provide vestibular input. A larger child can be briefly sat up on the side of the bed to change the child's orientation to the world. Sitting up with support, even for a comatose child, can help increase alertness. Because these activities may initially fatigue children, resting after a short time should be allowed.

As soon as a child is medically stable, he or she should be encouraged to get up and move around. Even a child who appears to be in a coma can be sat up at the side of the bed with support or sat in a wheelchair to be pushed around. Standing on a tilt table can provide yet another orientation to the world to help a child relearn head control, trunk control, and beginning postural extension and equilibrium responses. Because the child's blood pressure may drop when getting upright for the first few times, it should be monitored throughout a sitting or standing session until it stabilizes.

Communication skills should be encouraged. If a child's verbal language skills do not return soon, assistive devices to help communication can be as basic as using a switch to make a toy fireman climb up a ladder. Simple messages can be placed along the ladder to indicate "I'm tired," "I'm hungry," "I want Mom," or "I have to use the bathroom." Simple signs, facial expressions, or hand squeezes can be worked out for communication strategies. Everyone working with the child should know the communication strategies that are being used.

Skills will return quickly once the healing process has begun. Goals to encourage functional skills to help the child be more independent at home are very appropriate. Mobility skills using a wheelchair, crutches, or a cane can precede independent gait. Splints to prevent genu recurvatum or foot drop may be needed only temporarily or may be needed for an extended period of time, depending on the child's individual pattern of recovery.

Once the child is discharged from the rehabilitation center, outpatient therapy may be allowed by third-party coverage. Goals should always be measurable and functional. Significant return of neuromuscular and cognitive function generally occurs within the first year after the injury and lessens after that. As the child becomes more independent with walking, advanced gait skills should be tackled to help with balance, timing, and muscle control. The child's judgment and the family's ability to follow through at home should help determine home programs. The child will learn to cope with residual deficits in gross motor skills and should be encouraged to participate in an exercise program to promote strength and endurance, as well as preventing joint contractures in spastic muscles and soft tissue. Participating as part of a group doing individual types of exercise, such as swimming or weight training, may particularly help an adolescent receive peer support and socialization while continuing to work on rehabilitation goals.

Outcome for a child with TBI can be variable. Some children recover almost complete motor skills. Others have subtle deficiencies in balance and coordination. Still other children may have overt physical disabilities, such as hemiplegia or ataxia. The most severely involved children have quadriplegia and are not able to regain ambulation skills. For these severely involved children, physical therapy emphasizes positioning; assistive technology, especially a well-fitting wheelchair; and prevention of secondary disabilities including contractures. Working with teachers can help integrate gross motor activities into a classroom environment.

Role of the PTA. The PTA is unlikely to work directly with a child with a TBI immediately postinjury during the medically unstable phase of recovery. If working in the hospital, however, the PTA could accompany the therapist to the child's bedside and observe interventions from the beginning of his or her recovery. If a referral for PT is not initiated early, visits to the child's bedside to meet the family can encourage them to look forward to future rehabilitation, as well as build early relationships. The PTA can learn information about the child, which may help during later therapy sessions.

When working with a child in the agitated and confused stage of recovery, ignoring irrational and even violent outbursts, adhering to planned activities to give a structure to the child's day and interactions, yet listening and responding compassionately to the core messages of confusion and distress from a child can reassure a child and family members. Although interventions should be planned before the therapy session, it is important to remain flexible to new skills that may emerge during a session. The child in this stage of recovery is almost always in the hospital.

Your body is one of the most adaptable supporting surfaces that you can find. Using your own body, support a young child coming to stand. Have the child straddle your knee when you are kneeling, while the child faces mom or dad, then slowly raise yourself into a tall kneel position. The child will gradually come to a standing position and may not even realize that he or she is supporting most of his or her own weight! You can easily adjust the amount of support you are providing.

A child may be seen for active rehabilitation by a PTA in an acute hospital setting or in an inpatient rehabilitation setting, depending on the age of the child and the settings available in that location. During the first year postinjury, recovery is rapid with new skills or refinements emerging almost daily, especially during the first weeks and months of recovery. The PTA needs to work closely with the PT to adapt goals and objectives as new skills become evident.

The PTA may also see a child with a TBI in school, after the initial stage of recovery and rehabilitation. The child may not be recovering skills at the same pace as initially but will continue to improve and learn. Depending on the age of the child, therapy may be direct or may be provided as consultation to the classroom teacher, physical education teacher, or special education teacher. Specific behavior challenges may need to be addressed during therapy sessions. Talking with parents, teachers, and other team members who know the child well can help the PTA use strategies that are consistent across domains at school and home to address these behaviors. The team may identify specific skills for the child to learn, such as climbing the stairs to the bus, descending a set of stairs to the cafeteria, walking a prescribed distance between a classroom and the library, or throwing a ball to participate in recess games. Integrating training for these activities into the child's day can be a successful way of providing therapy, depending on the child's age and the willingness of teachers to incorporate gross motor skills into their activities.

Adaptation of wheelchairs and other assistive devices is a regular part of service provision. Adaptations include maintaining or fixing equipment as well as adapting seating supports, wheelchairs, walkers, and other devices as a child's postural control changes or the child grows. The PTA needs to work closely with the PT and school maintenance staff or vendors who may provide support for these functions.

Adolescents are concerned about transition between high school and the world of work or higher education. Most high schools will develop a transition plan for the child in special education, usually by the time the child is 14 years old or in the ninth grade. The interdisciplinary team should formulate the plan, which outlines classes the child should take, skills the child needs to be successful after high school, and any learning opportunities that will help the child develop these skills. Learning opportunities can include community-based instruction where the child and teacher, by themselves or in a group with others, travel to community sites to work on skills. Skills can vary between practical life skills, such as shopping or using the bus, to vocational skills, including working at a fast-food restaurant or office. The physical therapy provider can help the team support the child by participating in the plan formulation, identifying gross motor skills the child needs to be successful, and working with the child to develop those skills. The PTA may provide direct services on the school campus or at community sites. Instructing job trainers, teachers, or educational aides in methods to help the child develop certain skills can ensure greater integration of skills into daily tasks, and therefore, greater success.

The Child With a Near-Drowning Injury

Drowning is the second most common form of traumatic injury for a child younger than 5 years. It is a devastating injury to families partly because it is an inherently preventable occurrence. Most drownings occur in swimming pools under unsupervised situations. Others occur in bathtubs; large bodies of water, such as ponds, lakes, or oceans; or in very small bodies of water, including toilets or buckets. Most deaths and injuries from near-drowning are accidental, but some are inflicted by adults as child abuse. Near-drowning is defined as survival at least 24 hours after submersion in a fluid medium. Children who survive near-drowning have specific problems that differentiate their recovery from children with TBI and other brain injuries.

Incidence and Cause

Incidence of near-drowning varies according to the state but can be estimated at 2.8 per 100,000 (Ellis & Trent, 1995). Children less than 5 years and adolescents between 15 and 18 years account for the highest risk for this type of injury (Nieves, Buttacavoli, Fuller, Clarke, & Schimpf, 1996). Swimming pools are the site of submersion in over 60% of the cases. The site of submersion varies according to the age of the child, with bathtubs being the most common for infants younger than 1 year, swimming pools the most common for toddlers and preschoolers, and large bodies of water the most common for older children and adolescents. From 26% to 67% of children injured in bathtubs may be a result of child abuse (Gillenwater, Quan, & Feldman, 1996; Lavelle, Shaw, Seidl, & Ludwig, 1995).

Clinical Features

The most common outcome of a near-drowning incident is hypoxia, or too little oxygen to the brain and other organs. This can result in death of brain cells, as well as significant damage to other organ systems, especially the lungs and heart. The brain suffers irreversible damage after 4 to 6 minutes of anoxia, and the heart and lungs can survive almost 30 minutes. The *diving reflex* can be stimulated in some young children who are submerged in very cold water. The stimulation of cold water on the face causes blood to be shunted away from the periphery of the body and concentrated in the brain and heart. The heart rate decreases, but available oxygen is supplied to these essential organs. Some young children submerged in very cold water can survive longer periods of submersion because of this reflex.

Other medical concerns include aspiration of fluid into the lungs and hypothermia for those children who are submerged in water with a temperature lower than the body's. Children who are injured in bathtubs and hot tubs generally do not have hypothermia. The degree of hypothermia can be indicative of the length of time submerged. Management of the lowered body temperature is important because increasing body temperature too quickly can cause a decrease in core blood pressure, causing further hypoxia. Aspiration of fluid can cause pulmonary edema, inflammation, and a further decrease in the oxygen supplied to the tissues.

Infections from the fluid a child aspirates is dependent on the environment of the accident. Toilets and hot tubs harbor microorganisms, which can cause infections. Submersion in salt versus fresh water has not been shown to affect a child's prognosis.

Outcome from a near-drowning incident is dependent primarily on the length of time submerged. Children submerged less than 5 minutes have a good chance at recovery. After 10 minutes there is likely to be severe neurological impairment or death. Children with a mild submersion injury can be awake and fully conscious with mild abnormalities in blood gases. These children may sustain no appreciable brain damage. Children with moderate submersion can be obtunded with decreased alertness and respiratory distress. Children who survive more severe submersion injuries will be comatose and may have seizures, dysrhythmias, and severe anoxia causing abnormal posturing.

Anoxia tends to affect the brain globally, so motor problems after a near-drowning injury will be global rather than specific. A child may have rigidity, spasticity, and abnormal posturing, which will affect the entire musculoskeletal system. A child is likely to have cognitive impairments if the motor system is damaged.

Intervention

Initial medical intervention is focused on maximizing oxygenation to the brain and other tissues. Intubation and mechanical ventilation in the intensive care unit for children with severe injuries allows them to rest and reduce energy expenditure to allow maximum recovery. Some children remain comatose and may need support for respiration for extended periods. Support for nutrition through intravenous lines or nasogastric tube and medications to control seizures, adjust blood gases, and treat infections are other common medical interventions.

A child may have cerebral edema, causing increased intracranial pressure. Children with this complication have a worse prognosis for recovery than those without it.

Physical therapy intervention. Physical therapy provides support to prevent contractures and pressure sores for those children who are comatose for extended periods or for those with abnormal posturing. Splinting, positioning, and range of motion can all be initiated while the child is in intensive care (Figure 9-8). After the initial recovery period parents or caregivers should be taught how to provide some of these interventions so they feel more involved in the child's recovery process.

Physical therapy intervention is similar to that for a child with TBI. As a child becomes more alert, working toward improved postural control, equilibrium responses, and functional use of extremities can be achieved through play activities and movement transitions. Weight bearing through arms and legs and weight shifting in prone, supine, and sitting positions can be incorporated into play activities such as reaching for toys. Early sitting, standing, and mobility can help improve a child's level of alertness. Development of functional goals for the child is important at each stage of recovery. For those children who do not regain ambulation skills, positioning, seating, and mobility with the use of appropriate assistive devices is essential.

Role of the PTA. The PTA may see a child in an acute stage of recovery in the hospital or may work with a child as an inpatient or outpatient during rehabilitation. When the child starts school or returns to school after the accident, physical therapy may be a related service to help the child benefit from the educational environment. Becoming aware of the differences between a child with a TBI and a child who is the victim of a near-drowning injury can help the PTA be more effective at helping a child reach therapeutic goals.

The Child With a Spinal Cord Injury

Only 5% of spinal cord injuries occur in children under 16 years of age (Chao & Mayo, 1994). The overall incidence is approximately 5 individuals per 100,000, which translates to 0.25 children under 16 years with a spinal cord injury (SCI) per 100,000 population. This is a very low incidence. However, the challenges of working with a child with a spinal cord injury are considerable. The differences between a child presenting with a spinal cord injury and an adult can be substantial. Although the child has the same result from a partial or complete injury to the

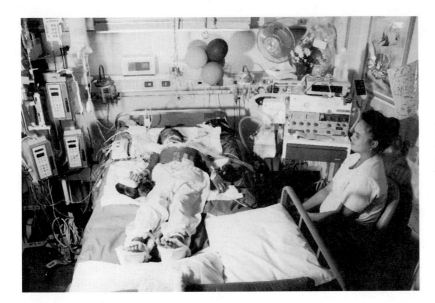

Figure 9-8 This child with a traumatic brain injury has decorticate posturing and is using prefabricated splints to hold his ankles in a neutral position to prevent contracture at the ankle.

spinal cord, the mechanism of injury, the effects of development on functional skills, and the effects of the spinal cord injury on development are very different in a child and an adult. The types of injuries sustained by children tend to vary by age and type of accident. Understanding these differences will help a therapy provider be more effective at working with children who may need extensive physical therapy to maximize independence in the face of changing size, skills, and developmental needs throughout childhood.

Causes

Most children with injuries to their spinal cord sustain congenital neural cord injuries such as myelomeningocele. These conditions are considered in Chapter 5. In this chapter the effect on children of injuries that occur after birth is discussed. Most, but not all, are related to trauma. As with TBI, the most common mechanism for SCI in a child is a motor vehicle accident. Young children can sustain cervical cord injuries when involved in an accident even when restrained in a car seat, if facing forward. Older children who are restrained by lap and shoulder belts may sustain a cervical cord injury as a result of poor placement of an adult-sized shoulder belt or because of a securely restrained torso, weak neck muscles, and a large head causing hyperflexion. This event has been termed the *pediatric cervical seat belt syndrome* (Hoy, & Cole, 1993). Traumatic brain injury and injury to anterior structures of the neck are likely to accompany a cervical spinal cord injury in these children.

Other mechanisms of traumatic injury include falls, diving into shallow water, sports injuries such as football or surfing, trauma from shaking in young infants, birth trauma, gunshots, and stabbing with a knife. Mechanisms of SCI that are not traumatic include tumors of the spinal cord and transverse myelitis. Children with other developmental disabilities, including Down syndrome and juvenile rheumatoid arthritis, are at risk for atlantoaxial or atlantooccipital dislocations, which can cause SCI either slowly and progressively or through a specific incident or trauma. Children under 5 years or over 10

years are more likely to sustain spinal cord injuries than children in the middle years.

Clinical Features

Children are more likely to sustain cervical cord injuries than thoracic or lower cord injuries. Most lower cord injuries in children occur through trauma such as stabbing or gunshot wounds. Very young children are more likely to sustain high cervical cord injuries. Preteenagers are likely to sustain middle cervical cord injuries, and adults, lower cervical cord injuries (Apple, Anson, Hunter, & Bell, 1995). Injuries at different levels produce very different patterns of disability. These are outlined in Figure 9-9. Table 9-3 outlines the functional effects of different levels of injury to the spinal cord.

> To remember the key autonomic functions of the spinal cord, which helps when working with children who have SCI-related problems with respiration and elimination, remember:
> "C3, 4, 5 keeps the diaphragm alive."
> "S2, 3, 4 keeps the urine off the floor."

Levels and types of SCI. Five different types of spinal cord injuries can occur, indicating different amounts of damage to the cord, as indicated by the ASIA Impairment Scale from the American Spinal Injury Association (1992). ASIA level A is a *complete injury,* meaning that no sensory or motor function is present below sacral levels 4 and 5. Most children sustain this type of injury. An *incomplete injury* with sensory but no motor function present below the sacral levels 4 and 5 is ASIA level B. ASIA level C indicates an incomplete injury with both motor and sensory preservation below the level of injury, but motor strength is less than grade 3, or good strength, in a manual muscle examination. If a child has motor and sensory preservation

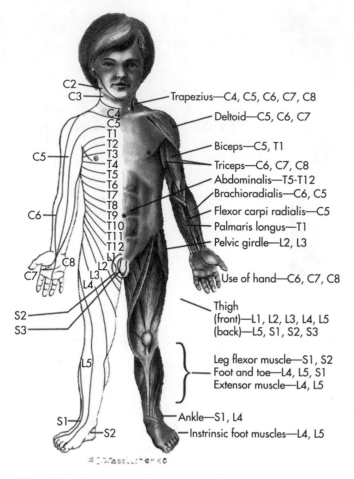

with strength greater than grade 3 below the level of injury, he or she has an ASIA level D injury. Children with complete recovery of sensory and motor tracts have an ASIA level E injury.

Children may sustain incomplete injuries, which result in patterns of motor and sensory recovery that are similar to those of adults. *Brown-Séquard* is an injury to half of the spinal cord. It is more common with stabbing injuries than other types of trauma. The child with a Brown-Séquard syndrome generally has a hemiplegia with motor and some sensory pathways interrupted on the same side of the body as the injury. Pain and temperature pathways are damaged on the opposite side of the body but intact on the same side, as a result of crossover of these tracts in the spinal cord. The child with Brown-Séquard syndrome will probably learn to walk with assistive devices and will usually preserve function of bowel and bladder. Children with an *anterior cord injury* have impairment of motor functions as well as sensations of pain and temperature at and below the level of the injury, but sparing of proprioception, kinesthesia, and vibration senses. This pattern of injury is usually caused by a partial dislocation or fracture in the cervical spine. The child with an anterior cord syndrome is probably not able to walk or preserve bowel and bladder control. A *central cord syndrome* is also usually located in the cervical spine and is characterized by increasing disability in sensory functions, especially pain and temperature, as well as motor dysfunction that is more severe in the arms than the legs. Children with *cauda equina* injuries have a flaccid paralysis of muscles in the lower extremities.

Stages of recovery from traumatic SCI. Immediately after injury the child experiences the effects of edema and trauma to the spinal cord, leading to the appearance of a complete transection of the cord. This is called *spinal shock syndrome.* Manifestations of spinal shock include absence of reflexes below the level of the injury; flaccidity of deinnervated muscles; loss of complete sensation; and autonomic dysfunction including hypotension, abnormal body temperatures, loss of bladder and bowel function, and autonomic dysreflexia. This stage is shorter in children than adults and lasts anywhere from 1 to 6 weeks

Figure 9-9 Dermatomes are sensory distributions at discrete spinal levels. Different levels also innervate muscles used for specific functional tasks. (From Wong, D.L. [1995]. *Whaley and Wong's nursing care of infants and children* [5th ed.]. St. Louis: Mosby.)

TABLE 9-3   Functional Effects of Spinal Cord Lesions at Different Levels

Highest intact cord segment	Functional limitations/capabilities	Physical therapy/functional goals
C1-3	• No voluntary musculoskeletal control below the chin • Complete respiratory paralysis • May have bradycardia, tachycardia, or vomiting	• Comfortable midline seating position, with ventilator tray • Pressure relief mechanism in seating such as tilt-in-space or power recline with low shear for older children
C4	• Neck movements intact • No voluntary function of upper extremities, trunk, or lower extremities • Dependent on ventilator support for breathing	• Sip'n puff control mechanism for power mobility (chin control possible for C4 injury), environmental control • Mouthstick for functional tasks • Respiratory hygiene • Provide alternative positioning and cushions to prevent pressure sores, range of motion to prevent contractures • Switch access for computers

Highest intact cord segment	Functional limitations/capabilities	Physical therapy/functional goals
C5 Muscles innervated include partial deltoid, biceps, most rotator cuff muscles, diaphragm	• Can abduct, extend, and flex shoulder • Some flexion of elbow • Abdominal respiration as a result of no accessory respiratory muscles; poor respiratory reserve • Cannot roll over or get into sitting position without help • Abdominal breathing	• Adapted joystick mechanism on power wheelchair and environmental control devices • Standing pivot transfers with assistance • Use adapted devices (universal cuff, mouthstick, switch interface) for grooming, self-feeding, and accessing computer • Respiratory hygiene • Pressure relief cushions • Older child may be able to do independent pressure relief through hooking arm and leaning if biceps strong enough
C6 Muscles innervated include pectoralis major, serratus anterior, latissimus dorsi. Complete deltoid and brachioradialis; partial triceps	• Good elbow flexion • Adduction and internal rotation of shoulder • Wrist extension • Abdominal breathing	• Propels wheelchair using hand rim extensions • Independent pressure relief • Can use sliding board for transfers with assistance • Assists in dressing and standing pivot transfers • Uses universal cuff to write, eat, use computer keyboard • Pressure relief cushion • Respiratory hygiene
C7 Muscles innervated include triceps, finger flexor and extensor muscles, shoulder depressor muscles	• Can lift body weight using shoulder depressors • Has weak grasp and release, poor coordination	• Independent manual wheelchair propulsion • Needs minimal assistance with transfers • Needs minimal assistance with lower extremity dressing • Can scoot on mat long distances • Can roll over, sit up independently
T1-10 Muscles innervated include all upper extremity muscles, trunk muscles above level of injury	• Full use of upper extremities • Poor trunk balance • May use braces for standing	• Independent manual wheelchair mobility • Adolescents can use hand controls to drive car or van • Trunk balance and upper extremity strength can improve • Independent pressure relief
T10-L2 Muscles innervated include abdominal and upper trunk muscles	• Good trunk balance • Good respiratory reserve • Can accomplish moderate hiphiking using external oblique and latissimus dorsi muscles	• Ambulation with bilateral long leg braces and crutches is possible but energy consuming • Can stand or walk functionally in school within small areas • Independent scooting, rolling on mat or floor • Uses a wheelchair for most mobility • Trunk strength and balance skills can improve
L3 or below Muscles innervated include quadriceps muscle, partial gluteus and hamstring muscles, partial lower extremity muscles depending on level of injury	• Poor control of ankles • May have lumbar lordosis	• Ambulates well, may use short leg braces, walker, crutches or cane • Will need ankle foot orthoses for ankle stability • Creeps on all fours, can roll, come to sitting, push up to stand • May not use wheelchair • May have difficulty getting up from sitting • Be aware of skin integrity in feet—possibility of sores if unseen cuts fester

(Yoshimura, Murakami, Kawamura, & Takayanigi, 1995). The shorter the duration of spinal shock, the more neurological the return can be anticipated.

The second stage of recovery heralds the end of flaccidity in affected muscles, and the beginning of spasticity and/or neurological return. Autonomic changes include the potential for reflex emptying of bladder and bowels and increased potential for *autonomic dysreflexia*. Autonomic dysreflexia is a disinhibition of the sympathetic nervous system and can occur in people with injuries above T6. A full bladder or bowel causes sensory input to the spinal cord where it is blocked because of the spinal cord lesion. Sympathetic nervous system inputs travel to the heart via the vagus nerve and cause bradycardia (slow heart rate). The body is not able to inhibit the sympathetic stimulation because it cannot obtain sensory input through the spinal cord. Autonomic dysreflexia can be life-threatening; it is an emergency situation. Causes and symptoms of autonomic dysreflexia as well as appropriate responses are outlined in Box 9-1. Fewer children than adults have autonomic dysreflexia; approximately 25% of children with lesions higher than T6 will have it within 1 year after the injury (Kewalramani et al., 1980). This condition will be a potential danger for the rest of the child's life, but he or she will begin to recognize the early symptoms and will learn to take precautions to avoid antecedents.

The third stage of recovery involves a stabilization of loss and recovery of spinal functions. The emphasis is on rehabilitation and return to typical life activities.

Effect of age and level of injury.   A child's age at the time of injury, as well as the level of injury sustained, can have a significant impact on recovery and on the learning of functional skills. Many children sustain additional injuries to the SCI, including head trauma, musculoskeletal trauma, and internal injuries. If involved in a motor vehicle accident, some children may lose family members to death or significant disability as well. This loss can affect the child's recovery.

Very young children commonly sustain high cervical cord injuries, resulting in the need for mechanical ventilation, and affecting communication as well as motor abilities. The child who has significant skeletal growth yet to occur is at higher risk for developing deformities in the spine or extremities. A problem common to children with SCI is the development of spinal deformity as the child grows. Scoliosis and kyphosis are common, and lordosis may occur if contractures are allowed to develop in the hip flexor muscles. Children may have spinal stabilization with rods, may wear external spinal supports such as body jackets, and may use supportive seating such as a custom-molded seat in the wheelchair to minimize possible deformity.

Children with such a severe injury undoubtedly undergo a change in body image and self-image as a result. The onset of SCI during adolescence when a child is engaged in developing an independent self-image can certainly create problems with depression and lack of self-esteem. The isolation an adolescent is likely to undergo as a result of long-term hospitalization, rehabilitation, and absence from school and friends can exacerbate the difficulty of rebuilding a self-image that is compatible with the disabilities acquired and the life a child envisions for him or herself. With support, most children are able to continue with their lives. Research has demonstrated that children with SCI are no more at risk for long-term psychosocial problems, such as depression, decreased self-esteem, or altered self-perception, than adults with similar injuries (Kennedy, Gorsuch, & Marsh, 1995). Age and level of injury are not correlated with psychosocial problems later in life. Two factors that are correlated with an individual's recovery and psychosocial adjustment after a severe injury are the personality before the injury and the influence of significant others (Bracken, & Shepard, 1980).

Intervention for Children With Spinal Cord Injuries

The three stages of recovery have very different interventions from both the acute medical and rehabilitation professionals. A team of nurses, physicians, therapists, social service personnel, teachers, and family members forms quickly to support a child who has been hospitalized for an acute spinal cord injury. Intervention is addressed in terms of stages of recovery.

Initial stage of recovery.   Medical intervention includes stabilization of the unstable spine; support of physiologic processes such as respiration, nutrition, and elimination; and prevention of secondary problems such as pressure sores, contractures, and further injury to the spinal cord through edema or inflammation. Any other injuries incurred during the accident also will be treated.

BOX 9-1   ## Symptoms of Autonomic Dysreflexia

Causes	Symptoms	Responses
Full bladder	Pounding headache	Alert medical personnel
Bladder infection	Nausea	Monitor blood pressure
Full bowel	Dangerous hypertension	Remove irritating stimuli
Other visceral irritation	Shivering and goosebumps	Empty bladder or unkink bladder drainage device
Pressure sores	Initial fast pulse	Evacuate bowel
Other skin irritation	Subsequent bradycardia	Loosen clothing
Prolonged muscle spasm	Pallor below level of injury	Sit person upright to try to decrease blood pressure
Constricting clothing or appliances	Flushing face and trunk above the level of injury	Identify and correct other visceral irritation
Sudden change in room temperature	Sweating above the level of injury	If corrective measures are not successful, vasodilator given
Congested lungs	Nasal congestion	Continue to monitor blood pressure

Surgery may be performed immediately to decompress the spinal cord after injury and to correct any vertebral bony injuries to prevent further damage to the cord. Surgery may also be postponed until the initial trauma has resolved. The child with a cervical injury may receive initial spinal stabilization through a halo-ring cervical traction device before or after surgery. A circular "halo" of metal is anchored directly to the child's skull using pins. Because the child's skull is thinner than that of an adult, a greater number of pins are used for stabilization, perhaps as many as eight or nine. The halo is attached to a rigid, molded trunk orthosis made of plastic or plaster using metal bars and metal distraction bolts and can be adjusted as needed. This mobile traction device allows children to get up and move sooner than immobilizing traction in bed and is appropriate for the adolescent, but it may be difficult to handle for the young child because of weight and balance. The halo or the body jacket should never be grasped to move or transfer the child. The child should always be lifted through the trunk, while the head and neck are stabilized. The young child with a cervical cord injury may receive traction in bed using tongs that are pinned to the skull.

If the injury is lower in the spine, the child may be stabilized using a body jacket or orthosis. The body jacket provides less stability than a halo, so precautions to avoid excessive spinal movement should be taken when moving a child who is using one.

The child with a high cervical injury needs support for respiration and is intubated with mechanical ventilation. The child will be unable to talk, even when awake, because the endotracheal tube passes directly through the vocal cords, not allowing air to cause vibrations and sound. Even the child who receives a tracheostomy is unable to talk because the air exits the larynx before passing over the vocal cords. Although some tracheos-tomy devices allow speech, they are usually not fitted during the acute phase of recovery and require training to be used effectively.

The child usually receives supplementary nutrition intravenously or through a nasogastric tube until he or she is able to eat orally. Other medical supports may include special mattresses of water, gel, air, or pressure-relief foam, or special bed frames that rotate to provide pressure relief. Temperature regulation is important because the child may be unable to regulate skin or body temperature. Medications to control electrolyte balance and infection or to treat other medical conditions that may be present are administered intravenously.

Physical therapy intervention. Physical therapy for the child with a spinal cord injury should be initiated right away. Resting ankle splints prevents contractures in the calf muscles during the initial period of flaccidity. Regular range of motion at least once or twice per day helps avoid contractures from immobility. Care should be taken not to stress the spine when doing exercises. Some children have shoulder pain and stiffness during this period of immobility. Positioning to allow scapular freedom when doing full passive and active range of motion may help, and positioning the upper extremity in abduction and external rotation in supine, with the lower arm resting on pillows may also help (Schneider, 1990). Opportunities for variation in positioning may be limited as a result of restrictions from poor spinal stability. If the child is stabilized in a halo or body splint, more vigorous rehabilitation can be started after the first few days.

Chest physical therapy to encourage deep breathing and mobilization of secretions is important to avoid pulmonary infections.

Every child with a spinal cord injury above T12 will have decreased respiratory function. Assisted coughing, quick stretches to assist expiration and inspiration, intercostal mobilization to maintain rib mobility, and incentive spirometry can help maintain pulmonary hygiene. Games to encourage the young child to use breath or voice can be helpful. Blowing a ping pong ball across a table, singing loudly, and even spitting contests can help a child develop increased respiratory capacity. The Applications section in Chapter 11 more fully addresses ways to assist pulmonary hygiene.

Early mobilization can occur once the spine is stabilized through surgery or proper application of an orthosis. Getting the child upright should be done gradually because of potential problems accommodating to changes in position. Blood pressure should be monitored so that excessively low pressures from orthostatic hypotension and excessively high pressures from autonomic dysreflexia can be detected and treated. If a child feels nauseous, lightheaded, disoriented, or starts breathing faster, low blood pressure should be suspected, and the child should immediately be repositioned in supine. The tilt table is the most logical appliance to help with gradual increase in upright orientation. Sitting a child on the side of the bed can also be done, as well as gradual propping higher and higher sitting up in bed. When using the bed to increase upright tolerance, the foot of the bed should be dropped to simulate a dependent position of the legs. Any child should be monitored continuously when changing upright orientation.

Involving the child and family members in rehabilitation from the very beginning is important. In the emotional upheaval of recent injury, they may not be able to articulate goals beyond wanting their child to walk and go to school again; however, their awareness of the process of rehabilitation and their feelings of inclusion are important. The family is a key element in ensuring the best outcome for the child.

Second stage of recovery. Medical intervention during the second stage continues to emphasize support of physiological functions. A child with a high cervical injury may still require ventilatory support, supplementary nutrition, and medications to decrease secondary effects of the injury. Surgery may be undertaken during this phase if the child was not stable enough to tolerate a surgical procedure earlier or if the medical team decided to wait until the recovery pattern was clearer. Usually a child will be moved to a rehabilitation facility during this phase of recovery. Most adolescents are comfortable in a facility for adult rehabilitation where many of the people receiving help for SCI are young adults. Children, however, have different needs and may be followed in a pediatric acute care facility if a pediatric rehabilitation facility is not available.

Role of physical therapy. Rehabilitation during this stage is exciting, because neurological return may be occurring. Monitoring the child's sensory function, muscle tone, muscle strength, and range of motion; avoiding secondary problems such as contractures and pulmonary deficiencies; and working toward functional goals are the primary tasks of therapy. Functional goals depend on the age of the child and the level of injury, but they can include bed mobility skills, which can be expanded to include the floor and mat. Transfers and wheelchair mobility issues are also addressed, such as using a manual or power wheelchair. If the lesion is low enough, ambulation might be considered using assistive devices. Each of these goals and activities is considered in light of the role of the PTA.

Monitoring muscle tone, strength, range of motion, and sensation. Although the PTA is not directly involved in assessment of a child with SCI, monitoring of muscle strength, range of motion, muscle tone, and sensory function are part of the repertoire of the PTA and can occur within the context of a therapy session. The PTA, working closely with the PT, should be aware of the sensate dermatomes of the child. Through daily monitoring any changes in the pattern of sensory awareness can become clear. Light touch, deep pressure, and pain and temperature are some of the sensory tracts that can be tested.

An effect of decreased or absent sensation is the potential for pressure sores, sometimes called *decubitus ulcers*. When a child cannot move independently nor feel pressure, he or she is at risk for developing pressure sores. Teaching children ways to relieve pressure on their ischium can be challenging. Children with a low SCI can simply push down with their hands to lift their hips off the support surface for a few seconds. This can be done every hour or two throughout the day to avoid ischemia to the tissues. Children with high thoracic and cervical injuries are not able to perform this task; if strong enough biceps function is present, they can lean forward after hooking an arm through a strap to relieve pressure through the sitting surface. Children with higher injuries need a mechanical means to relieve pressure. This can include a reclining back to the wheelchair or a tilt-in-space seating system. These mechanisms may have manual control, where a caregiver can operate them, or may have power control, where a child can access a switch to change alignment of the seating system. If a reclining back is used, attention should be paid to obtaining a system with low shear so the skin will not be stretched each time the back is reclined. The child needs to relieve pressure through changing positions every few hours throughout the day.

Muscle testing can occur within the context of activities or can be tested formally. Children under 5 years are difficult to test formally, but muscle strength can be seen and muscles palpated within the context of therapy activities. For instance, testing ankle dorsiflexors for trace, poor, or fair strength in a young child with an incomplete cervical spinal lesion can be done by placing the child in a supported sitting position, then displacing the child gently backwards. Dorsiflexion, if available, can be recruited as part of a balance reaction.

Range of motion can likewise be tested formally using goniometry or through activities. Rather than asking a young child to raise his or her arm as far as possible and hold it there while you measure, a child could be asked to reach for a toy that is held up in the air. The PTA or PT can palpate the scapula, humerus, shoulder, and trunk muscles to assess for scapular winging, muscle contraction, and excursion of movement during the activity. Eyeballing the range is not as accurate as goniometry but can be adequate.

Changes in muscle tone should be obvious through handling of the child. Flaccidity usually changes to spasticity during this stage of recovery. Problems related to spasticity could arise including potential for contractures, difficulty maintaining or changing positions, and hyperreflex activities. Clonus, a spinal reflex causing repeated stretch reflex reactions when disinhibited after a spinal cord or brain injury, can impair a child's ability to maintain a good seated position and can be very distracting. Teaching the child or family member techniques for inhibiting clonus is part of a rehabilitation program (Figure 9-10).

Managing hypertonicity and contractures. Managing hypertonicity is another skill that should be taught to the family and the child. Placing the limbs in reflex-inhibiting postures of flexion and abduction can avoid spasms into extension. Warm baths, relaxation techniques, range of motion, and massage can all reduce spasticity, at least temporarily. Individuals with SCI have expressed that range of motion before going to bed can help them sleep better by reducing spasms. Range of motion upon arising can help them meet the day in a more controlled manner through reducing spasms.

Contractures may begin to occur as the spastic muscles hold the limbs in particular positions for long periods of time. Although spasms tend to be in the direction of extension, sitting in a wheelchair can cause tightness in flexor muscle groups leading to contractures. A child with an SCI is at risk for developing joint contractures in ankle plantarflexion and flexion in the hip, knee, elbow, and fingers. Range of motion can address this risk, but it is not enough to avoid contractures by itself. Orthoses can help avoid contractures as a result of the pull of gravity and may also help control spasticity. Assuming a variety of positions throughout the day can counter long hours in a wheelchair. Some alternative positions include standing with support and lying prone to stretch out hip and knee flexor muscles (Figure 9-11). Care should be taken, however, if a hip flexion contracture is present because lying prone may cause an increased lumbar lordosis to

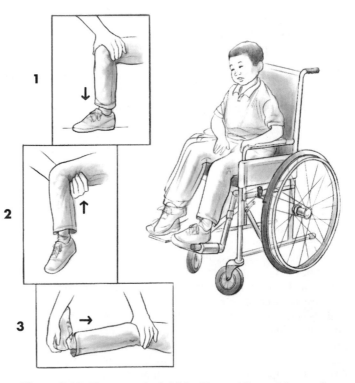

Figure 9-10 Clonus can be inhibited by avoiding quick stretch to the muscle. This can be done by (1) pressing down firmly through the joint so the muscle has no excursion when it contracts, (2) taking the foot off the supporting surface so gravity cannot provide a stretch when the muscle relaxes, and (3) stretching the muscle to its full range.

compensate. If this is the case, using a pillow to support the hips in slight flexion can decrease stress on the lumbar spine.

An older child with sufficient strength and function can be taught to range his or her own limbs. A strap with a loop can be useful to grasp and move the lower extremity if the child cannot reach independently. If the child is responsible for at least some daily range, it should be a regular part of the daily routine. An example might be for the child to range both legs before donning pants each morning. Teaching range of motion can occur alongside teaching self-help skills like dressing. Some children may not have either the strength needed to work through strong tone or the control over muscles needed to do the range. The child may be too young to understand the exercises and to be able to follow through on them. In these cases help will be required from a parent or caregiver.

Pulmonary hygiene. Focus on pulmonary hygiene is not as crucial in this phase of recovery when the child is more often upright and is moving more. However, depending on the level of injury, pulmonary hygiene is still very important. If the child should become sick, the risk of serious illness and death is high. Children with high lesions continue to need help to clear secretions and to improve inspiratory volume and expiratory pressure. This help may include full chest PT with percussion and drainage or simply assistance with coughing.

Home evaluation. A home evaluation should be done not only to ensure optimal access in a wheelchair at home but also to help the family plan where the child should sleep, how to access the bathroom for bathing, and how to plan for other activities of daily living. The home evaluation should be performed by a team and include the occupational therapist and the physical therapist. The PTA may be asked to participate in the home evaluation as well, particularly if therapy will be continued in the home after discharge from the rehabilitation facility.

Mat mobility. Functional skills during this stage of recovery begin with mobility issues on the mat or in bed and can include rolling, sitting up with or without assistance, and scooting. The skills learned depend on the level of injury, the strength of the child, and the functional needs of the child. Learning these functional skills often includes strength training, balance training, and stretching, as well as learning specific ways to move to accomplish movement and balance tasks.

Strength and balance training. Most spinal cord rehabilitation clinics for adults have group classes with weight training; group or individual mat mobility training; and therapy activities to improve balance and strength, such as tossing a medicine ball, using pulleys with weights, or exercising individually with Theraband, an elastic material with variable resistance. A child will quickly become bored with repetitive activities such as these. Incorporating strengthening activities into play can be done numerous ways depending on the age of the child. To strengthen deltoid muscles in shoulder abduction and flexion, for instance, activities such as writing or drawing on a blackboard, dancing to favorite music with wrist weights, finger painting in shaving or whipped cream sprayed on a vertical board or wall, or painting on an easel may accomplish the same tasks. Although these activities may require more time to set up and clean up than those for adults, they will be more effective for children.

Learning independent transfers. Independence in transfers can help to develop some control and self-determination for children. Very young children and children with cervical lesions above C7 are not usually able to transfer independently, but children with lesions at C7 and below are eventually able to transfer between two flat surfaces at similar heights. A transfer or sliding board may be useful. Some more intricate plastic transfer boards have "lazy susan" devices that allow a person to pivot easily, then slide the length of the board without the added resistance of friction between the child's skin or clothing and the board (Beasy-Trans from Beatrice Brantman, Inc., 207 E. Westminster, Lake Forest, IL 60045). Transfer training involves the practice of particular skills, which can be incorporated into games or contests if the child becomes bored. A chart documenting progress can be a useful motivation device for an older child or adolescent who is flagging in enthusiasm. Transfer training should be incorporated into other activities throughout the child's daily routine, such as transferring in and out of bed or on and off the mat.

For children with higher lesions transfers are accomplished using a standing pivot with assistance or a mechanical lift. Skills to assist with either of these types of transfers can be taught to children. They may help by verbally initiating the transfer through counting or holding on to the caregiver. The prescription of a mechanical lift should be a team decision. Many lifts are quite large and can be cumbersome in a private home. Mechanical lifts are frequently purchased and left unused when the family discovers that their size is inconvenient. Exploring all other options for transfers in the home before purchasing a large mechanical lift is prudent.

Transfers to and from a car are an issue as soon as the child begins to have day or weekend trips home from the rehabilita-

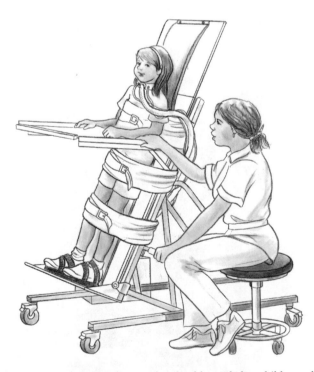

Figure 9-11 Daily standing on the tilt table can help a child stretch hip and knee flexors to avoid contractures. Other benefits include upright positioning to facilitate bowel and bladder evacuation, increased respiratory function, and upright orientation at the same level as peers.

tion facility. Depending on the child's level of injury and the type of family car, most children need assistance with these transfers. Some families of children with high level injuries opt to purchase a van with ramps or an electric lift, which can accommodate a wheelchair.

Learning wheelchair mobility. Wheelchair mobility is another key to independence. Depending on a child's age, level of injury, and cognitive status, a manual or power wheelchair may be considered. Power wheelchairs can be important developmental tools for even a very young child, and children as young as 18 months with normal cognitive status and good parental supervision can be successful drivers. It is important to remember that all toddlers require constant attention for safety, whether they are using the power mobility of a wheelchair or their own two legs to explore their surroundings. Children with injuries as low as midthoracic levels may need a power wheelchair because of low strength and endurance, even if they have full use of their arms. Most children require a manual wheelchair or stroller as a backup if the power chair breaks down and to allow parents to easily transport them to medical appointments, shopping, or other family outings. For children whose homes are not accessible, school may be the only place they are able to use power mobility functionally. If possible, they should be supported to use a power chair at school, rather than foregoing this mode of independence because the home is not accessible.

Proper positioning is essential to minimize postural deformity. The pelvis should be level in the seat and the trunk well supported laterally to avoid slumping to the side. Even strollers used in the home should be evaluated for postural control. Many strollers are available with built-in postural supports. A creative therapy provider can use foam blocks, plywood, and vinyl or cloth covering to create satisfactory inserts in commercially made products. The Applications section in this chapter addresses positioning for seating.

Third stage of recovery. During the third stage of recovery most neurological return has already occurred. The child and family are learning to cope with the daily issues of living with a significant disability. Medical intervention is focused on ongoing issues of medical care including management of spasticity through drugs, optimizing nutrition and weight, and ensuring prompt recovery from respiratory illness or skin breakdown. Methods and behaviors to control potentially dangerous health issues such as pressure sores, urinary tract infections, and respiratory infections should be taught to the child and family. Medical problems that could persist for the child with a midthoracic level SCI or above include orthostatic hypotension, impaired temperature regulation, autonomic dysreflexia, deep vein thrombosis, neurogenic pain, and spasticity.

Physical therapy intervention. Physical therapy intervention continues to focus on the learning of functional skills and the refining of these skills as the child matures. Continuing with daily activities including range of motion and strengthening to maximize function is important as the child grows. New needs will present themselves as the child matures. These can include the need for greater independence, such as graduation from a manual to a power chair; or incorporation of ecological control devices to turn on and off lights, television, or radio; or figuring out computer access for a child with minimal gross and fine motor skills. Being able to access a computer may be essential to success in school. The therapy provider should work closely with the teacher and other team members to ensure proper positioning for access to switches, keyboards, and other devices to help the child learn academic skills.

Helping the child and family cope with the disability as new challenges arise can be an ongoing process. Working out accessibility at summer camp, helping adjust a new van and lift, adapting seating as the child grows, and helping to adapt a wheelchair for a ventilator and/or oxygen tank are only some of the challenges that may present themselves.

Ambulation. The child with a low injury may be able to ambulate with assistive devices. Young children with higher lesions are able to ambulate while they remain small but may need to use wheelchairs full time as they grow and walking requires more energy. Assistive devices to help a child stand or walk are varied. The parapodium supports the lower trunk and supports the child's legs in an extended position (Figure 9-12). The child can swing the upper body from side to side, rocking from balancing on one side of the device to the other. This motion will propel the device forward. Children with congenital spinal cord injuries, as well as those with traumatic injuries, may use the parapodium. Children may need crutches for balance and control. Another mobility device that requires less energy than the parapodium is the Orlau walker (Figure 9-13). A sensitive mechanism allows a small lateral weight shift to move "feet" alternately forward to propel the device. These devices can be used only on flat surfaces. If a child has hip control, knee-ankle-foot orthoses (KAFOs) or braces that support the hip can be used with crutches for ambulation (Figure 9-14). These are extremely energy consuming, taking two to four times the energy of normal walking. All these devices require assistance for the young child to put on or take off. Both the energy required for this plus that for ambulation with the device may be workable when a child is

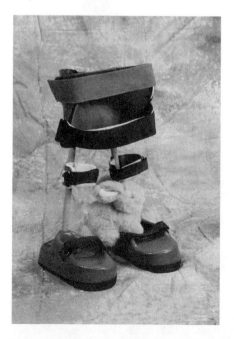

Figure 9-12 The parapodium can give mobility to a young child with a low spinal cord injury.

small, but as a child grows he or she may prefer to spend energy in more efficient ways and use a wheelchair for mobility.

Some research centers are having positive results with using surface or implanted electrodes to exercise denervated muscles and even to produce coordinated muscle contractions to allow controlled walking in individuals with SCIs. The research in this field continues to emerge but most involves young or middle-aged adults.

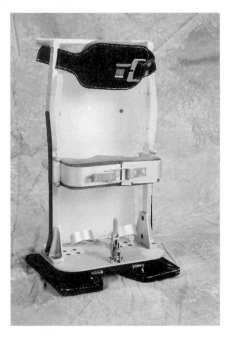

Figure 9-13 The Orlau walker requires a minimum of energy in lateral weight shifts to move forward.

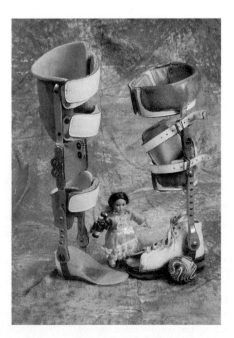

Figure 9-14 The knee-ankle-foot orthosis can support a child's lower extremity to allow ambulation.

Growing older with an SCI. Children who sustain SCIs usually reach adolescence and adulthood. Issues such as intimacy and sexuality, having children, higher education, and vocation may take on different importance as a child matures. It is important to address these issues as they become developmentally appropriate. The PTA may, by virtue of spending long hours with the child, become a trusted confidante. Level of comfort in discussing sensitive topics, as well as awareness of how they affect an individual with a SCI, determines the effectiveness of the PTA in this role. If a PTA should find himself or herself in this position, consulting other team members for support and information may be warranted. The PTA may refer or accompany the child to other team members for information on specific topics. The school psychologist may be able to help with issues regarding self-esteem, sexuality, and intimacy, and the guidance counselor can explain options for higher education or work.

As children become adolescents, driving independently becomes an option. Many rehabilitation facilities have driver training programs with adapted vans. Adapted controls are available and can be used by individuals having voluntary control of shoulder flexion, extension, adduction, and abduction. An adolescent or young adult should be medically stable before learning to drive. An episode of autonomic dysreflexia when in the driver's seat could be disastrous. The cost of an adapted van can be very high, but the benefits of independence in community mobility are even higher. Independent community mobility can allow a young person to hold a job more easily, go to school, and sustain a social life.

The Child With a Burn Injury

Children exploring their environment may play with matches, flammable liquids, hot water, and chemicals. They are also at risk from accidents or abuse. A burn injury can be devastating to a child and family. Besides the extended illness, pain, medical costs, and functional limitations from scarring and contractures, a child can receive disfiguration that will remain his or her entire life.

Working with a child who has had a significant burn injury can be very difficult for a physical therapy provider. A child will have significant pain, anxiety, and psychological trauma from the process of injury and recovery. Part of the intervention includes causing pain to a child through debridement of the wound, maintenance of range of motion, and dressing changes. These functions are essential for optimal recovery but can be difficult to perform because of reluctance to cause pain. Involvement of family members and other team members in the procedures can help relieve the stress for everyone involved.

Incidence and Cause

Burns are caused by thermal (heat or cold), electrical, chemical, or radioactive agents. Most children receive burn injuries from thermal agents including fire, hot liquids, and hot solid objects. Electrical and chemical burns are far less common in children, and radioactive burns are rarely seen in the pediatric population. Almost twice as many boys as girls sustain burns (Morrow, Smith, Howell, Nakayama, & Peterson, 1996). From 70% to 90% of all children under 5 years who receive burn injuries are 2 years or younger, and most receive scald injuries from spilling hot liquids in the kitchen or immersion in hot water in the bathtub (Ray, 1995; Simon & Baron, 1994). Children older than 5 years have more flame injuries than scald injuries. Fireworks, hot grease, radiators or hot stoves, and fires also cause burns in children. The incidence of burn injuries needing hospitalization in children is 40.5 per 100,000 children in the Denver, Colorado, area, which may or may not be representative of the rest of the country (Simon & Baron, 1994).

Most burns are accidental, but about 9% may be a result of abuse (Silverstein & Wilson, 1988). The most common patterns of inflicted burns on children are multiple burns from objects such as cigarettes, and certain patterns of scald injuries such as the buttocks, feet, and backs of the thighs and calves from forcible immersion in a scalding bath.

Clinical Features

Depending on the mechanism of injury, the causative agent, and the circumstances surrounding the injury, burns may be distributed over any part or parts of the body. The severity of burns is indicated by the depth of the burn, part of the body injured, extent of the injury, and any other medical issues accompanying the injury such as trauma or illness. Children are almost always admitted to the hospital if the burn is on the scalp, face, or genitals, or if it occurs in an infant or toddler under 2 years. These young children have a far greater mortality for the same type of burns as older children and adults because of thinner and more immature skin and immature organ systems, particularly the renal system, which is important in balancing the body's fluids and electrolytes.

Extent of injury. Determining the extent of injury is essential in a child because it is an important measure of the severity of injury. This task is more difficult in a child than an adult. The "rule of nines" for adults, where the body can be easily divided into nine areas with the same relative area, does not hold true for children. Children's body proportions change as they grow and are very different at 2 years old, 5 years old, and 15 years old. Figure 9-15 provides a drawing of how the body proportions change with age.

Depth of injury. Burns can be categorized according to their depth. Burns used to be characterized in terms of degrees but now are listed as partial or full thickness to reflect their effect on the skin (Figure 9-16). Table 9-4 lists the various classifications for the spectrum of depth of burns, as well as the characteristics and common mechanisms of injury for each.

Severity of injury. The severity of injury is usually classified by the American Burn Association Classification system. Major burn centers generally treat severe injuries, including partial thickness burns over 20% of the total body surface area (TBSA); full thickness burns over 10% of the body; inhalation injuries; burns involving hands, face, eyes, ears, feet, or perineum; and complicated injuries involving a very young child or additional trauma. Those with moderate injuries, generally 10% to 20% of the TBSA for partial thickness burns or full thickness burns of less than 10% of TBSA, are treated at a hospital familiar with burn care. Children with mild injuries, less than 10% TBSA of partial thickness burns, or less than 2% TBSA of full thickness burns can be treated as outpatients. Noelle, the child in this chapter's case study, has partial thickness burns over about 20% of her TBSA, which are complicated by involving her face and

eyes. Therefore, she would be classified as having a severe burn injury. She was treated at a local children's hospital because of the absence of a burn center in the vicinity.

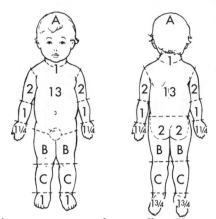

Relative percentages of areas affected by growth

AREA	BIRTH	AGE 1 YR	AGE 5 YR
A = ½ of head	9½	8½	6½
B = ½ of one thigh	2¾	3¼	4
C = ½ of one leg	2½	2½	2¾

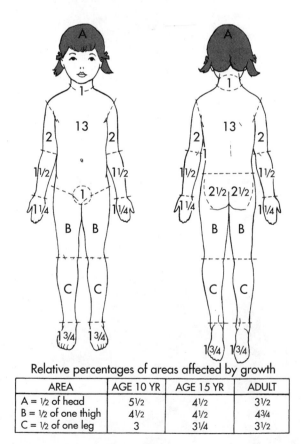

Relative percentages of areas affected by growth

AREA	AGE 10 YR	AGE 15 YR	ADULT
A = ½ of head	5½	4½	3½
B = ½ of one thigh	4½	4½	4¾
C = ½ of one leg	3	3¼	3½

Figure 9-15 Because children's body proportions are changing as they grow, the estimation of total body surface area changes according to the age of the child. (From Wong, D.L. [1995]. *Whaley and Wong's nursing care of infants and children* [5th ed.]. St. Louis: Mosby.)

Burn centers may be hundreds of miles from the family's home. Children with severe burns treated at these centers generally require extended time to heal and rehabilitate. The distance from home, as well as the severity of the injuries, can cause significant stress on the child and family. Some regions have hospitals that are designated to treat people with burn injuries. If these hospitals do not have pediatric expertise, young children with moderate burns may be kept at the regional pediatric hospital for treatment.

Stages of recovery. Three major stages of recovery for a severe burn can be identified. The emergent phase includes maintenance of physiological functions during the body's initial re-

TABLE 9-4 Classifications of Burns

| Classification | Partial thickness | | | Full thickness | Full thickness plus underlying tissue |
| | Superficial | Deep | | | Char |
	1st Degree	2nd Degree		3rd Degree	4th Degree
Depth of burn	Superficial skin only	Epidermis and a small part of the dermis	Epidermis and a deeper portion of the dermis	All of the epidermis and dermis	Epidermis, dermis, and underlying structures of fat, muscle, bone
Appearance	Red, dry, blanches with pressure	Red, blisters, moist, blanches with pressure	Marbled white, red, mottled, blisters	White, brown-black, dry, tough, does not blanch with pressure	White, brown-black, dry, tough, does not blanch with pressure
Sensation	Painful	Very painful	Very painful	No pain or temperature sensation	No pain or temperature sensation
Type of burn	Sunburn, brief scald	Scalds, flash flame	Scalds, flash flame	Flame, contact with hot objects	Flame, contact with hot objects

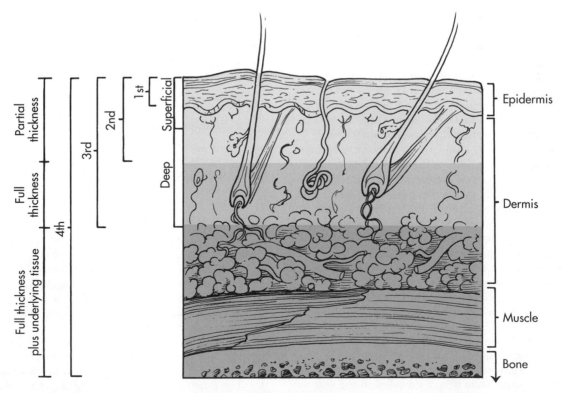

Figure 9-16 The extent of burns can be measured by how deep into the skin and underlying structures damage occurs.

sponse to the trauma. The acute phase begins when the child is medically stable. Efforts are focused on prevention of infection, closure of the wound, and prevention of secondary impairments. The rehabilitative phase begins when the wound is closed and medical issues take a back seat to functional issues. Of course, rehabilitation begins when the child is initially injured, but it takes more of a prominent role after medical concerns have been stabilized.

Intervention for the Child With a Burn Injury

A team approach for a child with a severe burn injury is essential. Nursing, medical staff, physical therapy, occupational therapy, social services, nutrition, psychology, and the family all need to work together from the beginning of a child's course of recovery to ensure the best possible outcome. Other team members may include child life specialists, teachers, orthotists or prosthetists, and recreational therapists. Most burn centers have strong interdisciplinary teams to support the child and family through the trauma of the initial injury, the pain and uncertainty of the acute phase, and the planning and hard work of the rehabilitation phase. The specific role of each team member varies slightly from center to center, but core duties will remain similar.

Emergent phase. Medical emphasis in the emergent phase is in supporting physiological functions of breathing, nutrition, and adequate fluid and electrolyte balance. Pain control is also initiated during this period. Establishing and maintaining an airway with endotrachial intubation if necessary, covering wounds with sterile dressings to decrease fluid loss, monitoring electrolyte balance through constant measuring of fluid input and output, establishing an intravenous line for fluid replacement and electrolyte balance, and maintaining body temperature are some of the most important medical interventions.

Children with an injury of over 12% of the body surface or infants under 1 year with less injury may have burn shock. The fluid lost through the injured skin contains a high amount of protein. Loss of this protein causes osmotic fluid drawing from capillaries into surrounding cells throughout the body. Unless the fluid in the bloodstream can be restored, the child faces the risk of circulatory collapse. Massive amounts of fluid replacement in the first 24 to 48 hours after injury usually controls this complication.

Dressing changes. Dressing changes usually occur two to three times per day and involve removal of the old dressing, debridement, and replacement with new dressings. Dressings encourage healing by providing a moist environment, protecting the wound from infection, absorbing blood and exudate, reducing pain and exposure to environmental irritants, and applying medication to the wound. Sterile technique must be maintained to avoid introducing infectious agents. The dressing change is a good opportunity to range each affected joint, because bulky dressings are removed. The child may feel significant pain during dressing changes and will usually require sedation or treatment with pain medications before the procedure.

Role of physical therapy. During the emergent phase of injury when the child is medically unstable, physical therapy can assist with range of motion during dressing changes. Splinting may be needed if the injury crosses joint spaces. Resting splints may be made for the ankle to maintain neutral dorsiflexion, the knee to maintain extension, or upper extremity joints to support in a neutral position so healing may occur. An occupational thera-

pist usually fabricates splints for the wrists, hands, and fingers; but may collaborate with the physical therapist on making the splints. Table 9-5 delineates common splints for burns. The PTA may assist with range of motion during dressing changes or in the fabrication of splints.

Establishing a relationship with parents or caregivers during this unsettling period of time is important. Some studies have indicated the major role of parents in helping their children reduce their experience of pain during invasive procedures (George & Hancock, 1993). Some parents may find it difficult to participate in procedures that cause their children pain, but others recognize the benefits of parental support. PTs need supportive relationships with parents and caregivers during the later phases of hospitalization and rehabilitation. The early hospitalization is a good time to initiate these relationships so that parents do not have to meet new service providers each step of the way.

A relationship with the child may be difficult to establish during this emergent phase because the child may be sedated during dressing changes or may connect the therapist with the pain related to dressing changes and range of motion. Visiting the child during nondressing change times, providing positive interactions, and developing a collaborative relationship with trusted family members can all help. The therapy provider must be sensitive to the emotional issues the child may be having. Very young children may have separation anxiety when hospitalized and parents cannot be with them all the time. Fantasies about the accident being a punishment or guilt about the role the child played in the accident may be causing acute anxiety to the preschool or school-aged child. Psychological support for the hospitalized child can help the rest of the team become aware of issues the child is struggling with, as well as appropriate methods to support the child and family during the child's recovery.

After an aversive procedure, spend time with the child in a positive manner. This will help maintain trust between you and the child. For example, after a dressing change for a child with burns, you may take the child to the playroom in the hospital. Another example is if a child cried while on the tilt table, allow the child to operate the controls (with supervision) while you lie on the table.

Acute phase. After the emergent period of medical fragility has passed, healing of the wounds must be facilitated while encouraging normal developmental skills. Medical intervention is aimed toward preventing infection, closing the wound as quickly as possible, ensuring proper nutrition to allow healing, and managing the complications that can occur during this phase such as pressure sores, contractures, infection and pain. Eschar is thick, necrotic tissue that inhibits wound healing and is found in deep partial thickness and full thickness wounds. Early excision of eschar is necessary to allow healing and reduce the threat of infection. This excision is usually done surgically. The child will continue to have discomfort during daily dressing changes and will need medication to manage the pain (Figure 9-17).

TABLE 9-5	Common Splints for Burns That Cross Joints		
Joint or body area	**Optimal position**	**Potential contracture**	**Splint/position**
Anterior neck	Neutral flexion and extension	Cervical flexion	• Neck conformer—maintains chin to chest distance • No pillow in bed
Posterior neck	Neutral flexion and extension	Cervical extension	• Neck conformer—maintains length in posterior neck • Pillow in supine • Pillow under chest in prone
Anterior chest	Shoulder retraction	Shoulder protraction	• Body jacket with neck conformer • In supine no pillow, shoulders abducted and externally rotated
Axilla	Shoulder abduction	Shoulder adduction	• Airplane splint—maintains shoulder in abduction
Anterior elbow	Extension	Elbow flexion	• Posterior splint
Anterior wrist and hand	Neutral flexion and extension of wrist, extension and abduction of fingers	Wrist and hand/finger flexion	• 15-degree wrist extension splint, finger troughs for finger abduction
Posterior wrist	Neutral flexion and extension of wrist	Wrist extension	• 15-degree wrist flexion splint
Anterior hip	Extension	Hip flexion	• Prone positioning • Supine with hip and knee extended, externally rotated, and abducted, pillow under hips for increased extension
Posterior knee	Extension	Knee flexion	• Posterior knee splint • No pillow under knees in supine
Posterior or anterior ankle	Neutral flexion and extension	Ankle plantar flexion or dorsiflexion	• Ankle foot orthosis at 90 degrees • Anterior ankle conformer

Temporary skin coverings. Temporary skin coverings may be used during the initial phases of recovery to encourage epithelialization (regrowth of skin tissue), decrease infection, decrease fluid and protein loss, and encourage more pain free range of motion. Skin coverings can be used over any depth of injury and range from human skin available from skin banks, to porcine skin from pigs, to synthetic skin coverings. All of these skin coverings are temporary and encourage wound healing; they must be used early over a clean wound to be effective.

Antimicrobial dressings. If skin coverings are not used, an antimicrobial dressing over the wound discourages infection. The choice of agent depends on the properties of the wound and the child (Figure 9-18).

Permanent skin coverings. Skin grafts are permanent skin coverings used for some deep partial thickness burns and all full thickness burns. Skin grafts may be taken from intact skin of the child (autologous) or a compatible donor (isologous). A split-thickness graft preserves the donor site and consists of epithe-

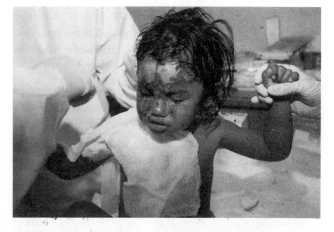

Figure 9-17 Noelle has been medicated for pain but still feels the pain and anxiety during dressing changes. The team of nurses and therapists reassures her while working as quickly as possible.

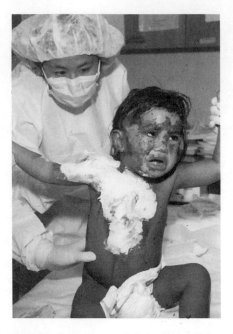

Figure 9-18 Topical agents retard the growth of bacteria on denuded skin.

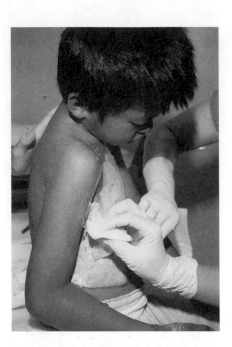

Figure 9-19 Physical therapists often debride burn wounds.

lium and a portion of the dermis. After the donor site has healed, it can be used again, but the quality of the graft is not as good. The split thickness graft is either a sheet graft, which is used over areas where cosmesis is important, or a mesh graft, in which the skin is passed through a mesher and small slits are inserted to allow it to spread and cover from 1½ to 9 times the area of a sheet graft. These grafts are done early to facilitate wound closure but must be done over clean skin. Immediately after a skin graft has been done, care must be taken to avoid any infectious agents and excessive trauma to the wound including range of motion and dressing changes. Early vascularization of the grafted tissue occurs after 3 days, and healing is complete with connective tissue in place by 10 to 14 days. Physical therapy intervention may be limited for 1 to 2 weeks after a graft has been placed to avoid trauma to the healing tissues. Range of motion of joints immediately distal and proximal to a graft site must be avoided during the first 5 to 7 days.

Role of physical therapy. Physical therapy is directed toward preventing functional loss and optimizing developmental skills. Methods to reach these goals involve range of motion, stretching of healing skin, and activities to work toward coordination, strength, endurance, and functional independence.

Working with children. Children should be told in advance what to expect during physical therapy and should be encouraged to assist with all aspects of their care. This assistance can be as simple as holding the roll of gauze during a dressing change, helping to peel off old dressings, turning on the agitator in the whirlpool, or stating when they are ready to start an exercise. Helping gives them some control over the painful and difficult process of healing and develops a sense of trust.

Positioning. Children with severe burn injuries or concurrent injuries, such as fractures or TBI, may be lying in bed and at risk for decubitus and contracture. Positioning is an important element in the healing of these children. The physical therapy provider should work closely with nursing staff to ensure frequent changes of position and adequate support in different positions.

Wound management. The physical therapy provider is usually involved in the daily wound management. This includes daily or twice daily dressing changes, with active and passive range of motion exercises during the dressing changes. Children should be adequately medicated at least 20 minutes before any dressing change. *Debridement* is the removal of dead or necrotic tissue from a wound. This can be done through manual means, rubbing or cutting the damaged tissue out of the wound, or through the more gentle action of water movement. Removal of the dead tissue is necessary to speed healing and avoid infection. Using gauze pads to remove dead tissue from open wounds is a common method of debridement and can be painful for the child (Figure 9-19).

Hydrotherapy. Hydrotherapy has been used as a modality to assist the child to be more comfortable during dressing changes, allowing water to help soak off adhered bandages and water action to help debride sensitive skin. This method of debridement is usually more acceptable to a young child, although sometimes manual means are needed to supplement the water action.

Range of motion in the warm water can be accomplished more easily because the water itself is a distracter and the warmth promotes comfort. Most children enjoy the whirlpool action. Some younger children, however, may be traumatized by the whirlpool and should be introduced to it slowly. Introducing the child to the tub with the agitator off may be a necessary first step, then increasing the agitator action slowly as the child gets used to it. A young child may need this process each time the whirlpool is used. Safety in the whirlpool is important, and children should never be left unattended. For very young children and children who are heavily sedated, extra precautions should be taken such as maintaining constant hands-on contact with the child.

Different facilities have different policies and procedures not only for use of the whirlpool but also regarding the chemicals and medications put in the water to retard infectious agents and methods for cleaning the bath to prevent growth of bacteria. Procedures should be followed carefully to avoid contamination and cross-contamination.

Managing contractures. Splints and passive range of motion may continue to be used throughout the acute phase of recovery to minimize contractures from healing tissue or disuse, especially as wounds cross joints. Serial casting has been shown to be effective with reducing contractures that splinting and exercise cannot reduce (Johnson & Silverberg, 1995). As the child becomes more active, however, more active means of range of motion should be encouraged. Early ambulation helps promote extension in the hips and knees and maintain functional range of the ankles. Children may need assistance initially from an adult's hand, a pediatric walker, or a children's toy such as a toy shopping cart until confidence is regained. For younger children, creeping, rolling, or scooting can promote range of motion, as well as stimulate cognitive development, social development, strength, and endurance. Motivating strategies may vary for children of different ages.

Developmental activities. Children should be encouraged to get up and move around as soon as possible. Encouraging movement through play and developmental activities can sometimes distract the child from pain and fear of movement and encourage early mobilization. Developing a trusting relationship with the child; incorporating family members, toys, and other motivators into the play; and being able to recognize the child's nonverbal cues of pain or discomfort can all help to encourage early mobility. If the child has sustained burns on the feet or lower legs, ambulation may be difficult, but research has shown that ambulation in the first 7 days after grafting leads to decreased hospital stays (Schmitt, French, & Kalil, 1991). Soft foam shoes or slippers, padded bandages, and spiral wrapping may help children be more comfortable on injured feet.

Rehabilitation phase. Rehabilitation, of course, begins on admission to an acute care hospital and continues until the child has attained optimal function in the community. Intervention after the acute care process has been completed and when a child is ready to reenter the family home, school, and community changes perspective. The team may change to include community members such as teachers, school administrators, and employers. Team members including the physical therapist may change from hospital-based professionals to school-based professionals. The emphasis changes from a medical recovery and prevention of secondary disability to that of relearning overall and specific functions in daily life and reintegrating into daily routines.

Reconstructive surgery. Children with severe burns leading to tissue destruction and contractures may have surgery for reconstruction of damaged or contracted tissue during this phase of recovery. They need specific rehabilitation to support surgical goals including increased range of motion. Orthopedic problems occurring from burns that may need treatment include osteoporosis, stunted growth of phalanges and limbs, osteomyelitis, ankylosis or fusion of joints, and resorption of terminal phalanges (Pandit, Malla, Zarger, Kaul, & Dev, 1993). The child with severe burns may continue to have problems with adequate nutrition. Most young children who suffer severe burns have

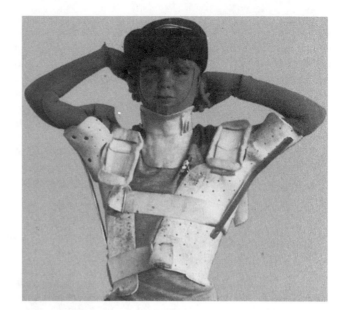

Figure 9-20 William wears bilateral airplane splints and an anterior neck conformer to control contractures, and pressure garments to control hypertrophic scar formation. (From Wong D.L. [1995]. *Whaley and Wong's nursing care of infants and children* [5th ed.]. St. Louis: Mosby.)

growth retardation after the injury (Mittendorfer, Hildreth, Desai, & Herndon, 1995).

Controlling scar formation. Controlling the formation of scarring to prevent keloid or overgrowth of scars may be an important consideration in some children. Some children are more at risk for hypertrophic scar formation than others by virtue of genetics, the agent of injury, and the depth and type of injury. People with dark skin are more at risk than people with light skin. As a precaution, all burns deeper than superficial levels should be treated to prevent or manage this occurrence. Hypertrophic scarring reaches a peak at 4 to 6 months into the healing process, and most scars become inactive 1 to 2 years after injury.

The best method of prevention is uniform pressure over the healing site. Pressure decreases the blood supply and helps the collagen in the developing scar tissue to align itself. Pressure should be maintained over the developing scar at all times to avoid allowing the blood supply to increase even briefly.

Several methods of applying pressure can be used including wrapping with elastic materials such as Ace wrap or Coban, use of splints, or application of pressure garments. For children with extensive burns, pressure garments are the most effective. Materials for the garments vary and should be chosen on the basis of the type and area of the burn. Garments can be purchased premade or can be custom made. Pre-made garments are not usually as effective as those that are custom made. The therapist and the orthotist who is ordering the garments need to make careful measurements to ensure the proper size. Measurements are usually done before discharge from the hospital so that the garments are ready before the scar formation is excessive. Once the pressure garments are received, the therapist may be responsible for fitting and monitoring the fit as the child grows. The child may wear the garments for several months up to 2 years, until the scar is mature and supple (Figure 9-20).

Reentry into school. A child with significant change in appearance because of a severe burn may have a difficult time returning to school. Children can be very cruel to each other, and school personnel may not be comfortable with helping a child with severe disfigurement or disability. Reentry programs where concrete factual information is given to the child's peers and school personnel can help to address concerns and expectations to facilitate the adjustment of both the child and the school community (Bishop & Gilinsky, 1995).

Parental and child adjustment after a severe burn injury. Most children with severe burns are perceived as having a difficult time adjusting psychologically to their injuries. Parents' perceptions of children's adjustment difficulties may be more sensitive than perceptions of either the children themselves or their teachers (Blakeney et al., 1993; Meyer et al., 1995; Meyer, Blakeney, LeDoux, & Herndon, 1995). Parents may be very sensitive to the difficulties their children are experiencing during the reintegration into daily life after a severe burn injury. These difficulties may include behavior problems, poor self-esteem, and academic problems. Therapy providers should be sensitive to parental perceptions about their children and work closely with parents and teachers to ensure the best outcome for the child.

● **APPLICATIONS** # Functional Seating and Wheeled Mobility for Children
LORRAINE SYLVESTER

Seating systems and mobility bases for children differ from those for adults because of the unique nature of children. Not only are children smaller than adults, but also their needs differ because of developmental factors. Children's skills develop as they grow and mature, and even children with significant disabilities change as they grow. Functional tasks for children are different from those of adults and may include learning in a classroom, accessing playground equipment, or socializing at floor level. A final consideration is that children are growing physically as well as developmentally. A pediatric seating system and mobility base should be able to accommodate growth changes for at least several years.

A PTA may not be independently evaluating or prescribing equipment but will likely be part of a team giving recommendations and troubleshooting problems with seating and mobility. Therefore a PTA needs to be familiar with pediatric seating and mobility systems and their features. This section describes the benefits of positioning and use of postural supports for the child, a standard child's wheelchair or stroller, and special adaptations that can provide additional postural support for a child with special needs. It also presents guiding principles to use when providing or modifying a seating and mobility system for a child.

Anatomy of the Wheelchair or Stroller

Each part of the wheelchair is specifically ordered and fitted to the individual child. A wheelchair consists of two basic elements that must be addressed for each child: the mobility base and the postural support system. Most of the time, special seating supports are incorporated on a mobility base that moves with the child throughout the day, such as a wheelchair or stroller. The child may be dependent in mobility and rely on others to push the chair, or mobility can be independent through manual or power propulsion.

The most recognizable aspect of the wheelchair is the mobility base, consisting of the tubular frame and push handles, the large rear wheels, smaller front casters, armrests, legrests, and wheel locks. A general use wheelchair also includes a standard seat and a backrest (Figure 9-21). Many standard child stroller bases have similar components, but the wheels are smaller and a stroller base cannot be propelled by the user. There are three different kinds of mobility bases: caregiver propelled (dependent); user propelled by hand or foot (manual independent); and user propelled electronically (power independent). Children may need to use a variety of mobility options to move through different environments, and they will always require a good postural support system on the mobility base.

The child or caregiver will not be able to move the wheelchair if the child's postural control is not stable. A very large or complicated postural support system may also make it difficult for a child to move the chair independently. The family may have difficulty transporting a large or heavy system. For example, Cyril (Case Study, Chapter 7) uses a stroller for quick trips because it is easier for his mother and father to put in and out of their small car. He uses a more sophisticated positioning system in a heavier manual wheelchair base for school, but he relies on the school bus with a lift to transport him. The stroller provides mobility for Cyril and his family but sacrifices postural support and independence. The use of a stroller for an adolescent can be socially inappropriate. Although Cyril expresses his embarrassment at using a stroller, his parents feel they have no option.

Assessing Features of the Standard Mobility Base

Size and fit of the mobility system are important to optimize the child's function in the wheelchair and cost effectiveness of the equipment. The system also needs to adjust to accommodate growth of the child. Features that provide good postural support and provide for growth can prevent potential postural damage from systems that are too big (Figure 9-22). Aesthetics are important for social acceptance and to maintain self-esteem. Therefore, color and "look" of the wheelchair are not minor factors. Many pediatric wheelchair manufacturers have a wide variety of colors to choose from and have incorporated child-friendly names and aesthetics into the design.

The seat surface may be vinyl or fabric, or it may have a firm (planar) surface. Sling seats usually allow the chair to fold up and be more portable, such as in an umbrella stroller. Solid seats may be inserted (plywood base under foam), or may be attached to the chair, and still allow the chair to fold by using hinges or other hardware.

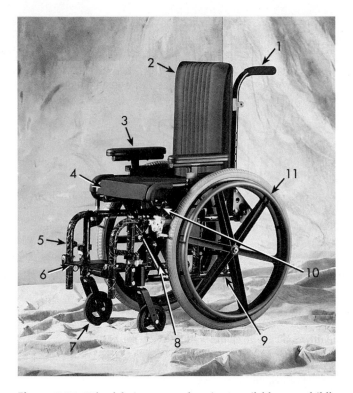

Figure 9-21 Wheelchair parts and options available on a child's chair (Kid's Quickie 2). (Courtesy Quickie Designs, Inc.) *1,* Handgrips/push handles; *2,* back upholstery/cushion; *3,* armrests; *4,* seat upholstery/cushion; *5,* front rigging/legrest; *6,* footplate; *7,* front casters; *8,* crossbraces; *9,* tipping lever/anti-tippers attach; *10,* wheel locks; *11,* mag style wheel and handrim.

Seat length. The seat of the stroller or wheelchair must provide support along the length of the child's legs (femurs) from buttocks almost to the back of the knee. Allow about 1 to 2 inches gap behind the knee to prevent pressure on the popliteal space. If the seat is too short for the child, excessive skin pressure or postural instability will result. When possible, allowance should be provided for growth. For example, Ian's Snug Seat (Box 9-2) has been able to grow with him as he has gotten taller because the foam pieces from behind his back can be removed. This makes his sitting depth longer (he can sit further back into the seat). Other systems allow the seat base to be moved forward or the backrest to be moved backward, all allowing for growth in seat length. Generally speaking, children grow more quickly in length (get taller), compared to their width or girth measurements.

Seat width. The wheelchair or stroller width must allow adequate room for the child and potential growth, as well as allow the child to reach the wheels to self-propel if needed. Most important, it must provide adequate postural support. If a chair is too narrow, it will cause pressure or skin problems along the sides of the hips and sometimes at the shoulders. If is it is too wide, the child may be unable to reach the wheels to propel or may develop a functional scoliosis from leaning to one side or the other.

Most pediatric wheelchairs and strollers are made with built-in adjustment for width to accommodate growth and to extend

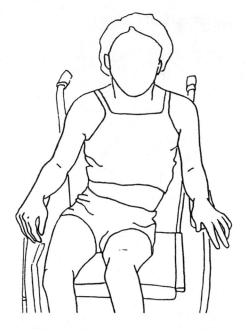

Figure 9-22 If the wheelchair is too wide, pelvic obliquity and secondary spinal scoliosis could result. (Courtesy Jay Medical, Ltd.)

the life of the chair. A chair can be made wider by expanding an adjustable solid seat or by getting a larger cross frame, a more expensive option.

Back surface. Like the seat surface, the back rest is often made of flexible vinyl or fabric. It may have a solid insert or a removable solid back cushion with foam. Sling fabric allows the chair to fold easily. Some solid back inserts may be removable to allow the chair to fold.

Height and position of the backrest. If the child will propel the chair independently, then it is important not to have the back height higher than the scapulae. Blocking the shoulder blades prevents efficient use of the arms in propelling the wheels. If the child is dependent in mobility, does not have adequate trunk control, requires more postural stability, or will be using powered mobility, then the back should support all the way up to the top of the shoulders.

Seat height. This measurement describes the distance from the floor to the sitting surface of the wheelchair or stroller (Figure 9-23). For adult chairs standard floor-to-seat distance is 19 to 20 inches. Hemi-height or low-riding chairs are available for shorter people and are usually about 17 to 17 ½ inches from the seat to the floor. Pediatric chairs have wheels and casters that are smaller in diameter than adult chairs, allowing children to be lower to the floor and closer to the level of their peers.

Seat-to-back angle. The position or angle of the backrest is usually set near 90 to 100 degrees, relative to the seat. There are times when the child may have hip extension contractures that prohibit full upright sitting at the 90-degree seat to back angle. This would require the backrest to angle backward, or recline, in relation to the seat, thus opening up the hip angle beyond 90 degrees. Children with severe kyphotic deformity of the spine may

BOX 9-2   Case Study: Ian—Benefits of Proper Positioning

1. Neutralize abnormal muscle tone

Ian is a 2-year-old child with hydrocephalus and cerebral palsy. Like many children with cerebral palsy, his muscles are "stiff" or "floppy" at different times. When he is unsupported, he tends to use his muscles inefficiently causing stiff, awkward, poorly graded, and poorly controlled movements. Ian's seating system provides external stability through total contact support for his body, giving him the postural control that he needs to sit up, eat, and play. He is able to look around, use his hands, and express himself with less interference from his muscle tone.

2. Enhance body functions

In his stroller Ian is upright with midline stability and can interact with his family and environment. A secure and stable upright sitting posture with good head control helps Ian be alert, facilitating his learning. Respiration and elimination are enhanced, and aspiration or choking are minimized with good head, neck, and trunk position.

3. Increase function

Children with cerebral palsy and other neuromotor disabilities often expend a lot of energy just to remain stable in their seat. When Ian's pelvis is firmly and securely rooted to the sitting surface, then he has less difficulty maintaining trunk control and is able to use his hands more easily because he does not need them for stability. Other supports, such as a lap tray and head support, provide additional support so that he can attend to activities for a longer time. While sitting in his stroller, he has learned to operate a switch to play with toys and use his computer.

Using a custom-contoured seat in an electric car, Ian is able to access a switch to move himself, and enjoy independent movement for the first time in his life. With a stable seated position, he has a greater opportunity to learn and interact with his peers as he grows older.

4. Prevent musculoskeletal abnormalities

Because of his lack of neuromotor control, Ian has learned ways of moving using asymmetrical motor patterns, putting him at risk for muscle shortening and contractures as he grows. He is at risk for developing asymmetries in his oral and facial muscles, as well as his trunk. Facial asymmetries could make eating and speaking difficult. Asymmetry in the trunk could contribute to scoliosis of the spine, which in turn may cause difficulty with breathing and digestion. Early intervention with a stable base of support and external support for postural control will limit development of these deformities.

Ian recently had surgery to release tight muscles and reposition his left hip to prevent dislocation. His seated position is now even more critical to maintain his hip range of motion and stability. Because of his surgery and asymmetrical muscle tone, Ian's pelvis tends to be positioned asymmetrically, causing his spine to curve. Special foam blocks help position his pelvis in a neutral alignment, and firm foam along his back and sides helps to keep his spine straight.

Ian has difficulty keeping his head in a neutral position; it often falls backward causing difficulty with swallowing, breathing, and vocalizing. It is very difficult for him to see things around him when his eyes gaze toward the ceiling. In his stroller special foam pieces placed around his head help Ian to keep his head more stable in midline so he can look forward and minimize the development of spinal deformities.

5. Prevent pressure sores

Ian is at risk for the development of pressure sores. When he sits for long periods, he cannot shift his position, to redistribute pressure. Changing his position frequently from sitting to lying down to standing prevents excessive pressure to any one part of his body. The development of pressure sores can also be minimized by using cushions or supports that help to equalize pressure distribution in his seating system. Custom contouring Ian's seat helps to decrease pressure in any one area by spreading out the contact of his body with the seating system.

6. Promote comfort

Ian uses chest and shoulder straps to help maintain his shoulder position, so that he can more easily control his head. While he tolerates these during meals and during transportation in the family van, he complains if they are on for long periods of time. The stability of his head is compromised at times by relieving the straps, although they are not necessary for the short times when Ian can maintain postural control on his own. To maintain his comfort, compromises are made that may sacrifice postural control at times. If Ian is not comfortable in his seating system, it cannot be helpful to him. His comfort is a primary objective.

7. Decrease fatigue

By using an appropriately fitted seating system in his stroller, Ian has more energy to expend on daily activities and play instead of spending his limited energy staying upright and balancing in his chair. His parents can interact with him and introduce him to toys, switches, and motorized cars rather than constantly repositioning him in his stroller.

8. Facilitate normal development

Ian is now almost 3 years old and is about to enter preschool. Typically developing children his age walk, talk, and play actively. Appropriate use of positioning equipment can facilitate normal developmental skills for Ian. When he uses his customized seat in his motorized car, he is able to drive the car independently using a switch. Although he is not yet using words for communication, when he is properly supported in his stroller, his vocalizations become more understandable. He is also beginning to use an augmentative communication device to help others understand his needs. To operate the device he needs the use of his hands and a steady gaze, both of which are afforded him through proper positioning.

9. Facilitate maximum function with minimal pathology

By supporting Ian in a stable upright posture, his positioning equipment allows him to access his environment as he grows using the most normal types of movement, communication strategies, and visual orientation possible. Ian can learn to function to his maximum capacity without developing as many contractures, abnormal movement patterns, or a skewed view of his environment that an unsupported position would facilitate. Ian's underlying disability may not change; however, optimal postural control may help him to gain functional use of his body to accomplish desired tasks and to learn additional ways to communicate and move within his environment.

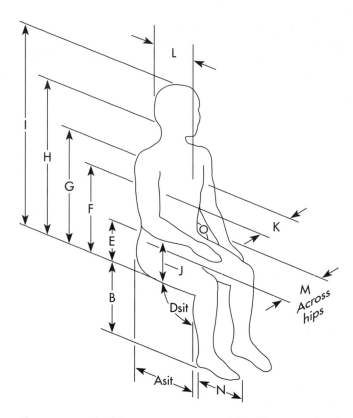

Figure 9-23 Wheelchair measurements: *A,* Behind hips to popliteal fossa (R & L); *B,* popliteal fossa to heel (R & L); *D,* knee flexion angle (R & L); *E,* sitting surface to pelvic crest; *F,* sitting surface to axilla; *G,* sitting surface to shoulder; *H,* sitting surface to occiput; *I,* sitting surface to top of head; *J,* sitting surface to hanging elbow; *K,* trunk width; *L,* trunk depth; *M,* hip width; *N,* heel-to-toe length; *O,* Hip flexion angle. (From Bergen, A.F., Presperin, J., & Tallman, T. [1990]. *Positioning for function: Wheelchair and other assistive technologies.* Valhalla, NY: Valhalla Rehabilitation Publications, Ltd.)

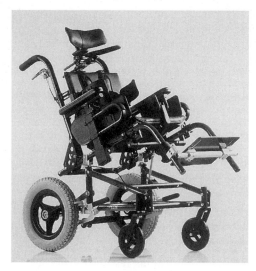

Figure 9-24 Tilt-in-space wheelchair frame with a fixed backrest angle. (Courtesy Quickie Designs, Inc.)

also need a reclined backrest to accommodate their deformity. Otherwise, the kyphosis may push their head forward, making it difficult to see. Finally, lack of trunk control against gravity as seen in a child with low postural tone may require a slightly reclined back to maintain an upright position. When ordering a seating system, the angle of recline can either be fixed or adjustable (Figure 9-24).

Wheels and tires. A wheelchair usually has two large rear wheels with two smaller front rolling casters. The rear tires may be pneumatic (air filled), hard rubber, or pneumatic with a solid core. Pneumatic tires usually are fatter, more comfortable to roll on, and may decrease pressure over the buttocks when going over bumps. They are easier to propel over loose surfaces, such as dirt or firm sand. However, they lose air and need to be filled like a bicycle tire. Hard rubber tires are more sturdy and durable; however, they are not as comfortable when rolling over rougher terrain. Wheels may have spokes (more lightweight), or mags (heavier, but more sturdy). Spokes tend to get bent and fall out and may cause damage to the wheel. Mags are good for children who can propel independently but have less strength (see Figure 9-21).

Handrims. Handrims may be plastic-coated which helps increase friction for easier manual propulsion for children who have limited use of their hands. Quad knobs placed on the handrim provide projections that allow children with less strength or hand function to propel the chair. Quad knob projections placed vertically to the axis of the wheel may make the chair effectively wider and more difficult to push through narrow doorways.

Sometimes there are two handrims on one wheel, allowing both wheels to be operated from one side. This is called a one-arm-drive propulsion system. A child with functional use of only one arm can propel this system, although it requires more strength and cognitive skills than a basic mobility base.

Wheel locks. Wheel locks stop movement of the wheels (see Figure 9-21). They will not slow down the wheelchair and so are not called *brakes*. They may be mounted low or high on the rear wheels, depending on the needs of the user. Low-mounted wheel locks do not interfere with independent propulsion, but high-mounted locks are easier for a caregiver to access. Wheel lock levers may be pulled or pushed to engage. Wheel lock extensions allow a person with decreased strength or range of motion to access the wheel locks effectively, or allow easier use by caregivers.

Tip bars. Tip bars are located on the back lower ends of the wheelchair frame (see Figure 9-21). They can be used to assist the caregiver to tip the chair back slightly when ascending a curb or step. Anti-tip bars prevent unwanted tipping back of the chair while the child is in it.

Armrests. Armrests provide positioning and support for the arms. They also provide a surface to support a tray or work table on the wheelchair (see Figure 9-21). Armrests may be completely removable, fixed to the frame, or hinged to flip up or swing out of the way. Flip-up or removable armrests allow more freedom for transfers. Removable armrests allow a child to roll up to and under a table or desk. Full-length armrests provide a stable surface for a tray table as well as lateral support for the user. Desk length armrests are shorter and allow the chair to roll up closer to a desk. Elevating armrests support the arms allowing better trunk control. Elevating armrests are important for growing children and those who need a change of arm position for different activities.

Chair weight. Pediatric wheelchairs vary significantly in weight depending on size, type, and seating components. Lighter weight chairs help maintain independent mobility for children with limited strength or endurance. A lighter weight chair should be also considered for parents who frequently need to lift the chair into a car. Power wheelchairs are always significantly heavier than manually propelled chairs. The increase in weight and size may decrease independent mobility because of home and car access concerns. For example, although Cyril (Case Study, Chapter 7) demonstrated independent use of a power wheelchair, it was inappropriate for home use because of his family's small apartment and car.

Designing the Seating System

Children with disabilities use the seated position for most of their daily activities including resting, eating meals, toileting, riding in the car, attending classes, going to the movies, or watching TV, to name only a few. In the classroom the seated position is important for children to be able to function and participate effectively. This position may be difficult for a child with postural disabilities to attain or maintain. Just as the standing child needs to use all body parts in synergy to have smooth, balanced, functional movement, so the seated child must have balance in the trunk and extremities to give postural stability and allow functional movement. If a child does not have the internal muscle control to support or balance independently, adaptive equipment is available to provide these supports externally. A variety of adaptations such as structured chairs, padding, straps, or other supports can be used to hold a child's body stable and secure in an upright and forward-facing position. A functional sitting posture should be comfortable, stable, and should afford access to desired activities. In a forward-facing seated position a child can access other forms of assistive technology, such as computers and augmentative communication devices to support educational and social goals.

The postural support, or seating system, fits onto the mobility base. For children with neuromotor impairment, proper body alignment is critical to prevent deformities and optimize functional skills. For a postural support system to be effective in allowing the child to participate in activities across environments, it should provide at least nine basic benefits to the child as described in Box 9-2.

Principles for Achieving Postural Support and Stability in Sitting

The following principles for achieving postural support in sitting should be considered when designing or prescribing a custom seating system for a child with a disability. While these features are generally applied to special pediatric strollers or wheelchairs, they may also be used to modify a classroom or alternative chair for a child.

Build support from the back, then sides, then front. When choosing, adapting, or fabricating a seating system for a child with a movement deficit, it is most important to look for the point where the child has the *most* control with the *least* amount of restriction. Stability and support should be considered and provided in the following order: posterior, lateral, then anterior.

Posterior support. Whatever contacts the back and underside of the sitting child is posterior support. The seat and back surface may provide very little support as with sling or fabric surfaces. A planar or flat surface provides greater support. A child may need maximum posterior support such as a custom contoured seat or back. Other types of posterior support include lumbar pads, neck and head rests, and leg or foot support.

Lateral support. Features that help to control the child's movements or asymmetries in the frontal plane are lateral supports. These supports include hip guides, lateral trunk supports, and hip adductor or abductor pads.

Anterior support. Features that keep the child's body from moving out of the seating system in a forward direction in the sagittal plane are anterior supports. These usually include pelvic belts, chest belts and panels, shoulder straps, forehead straps, and lap trays. Anterior supports are usually provided as a last resort; their use should be minimal if proper posterior and lateral support has been addressed. One exception is the pelvic positioning belt. This anterior support assists in maintaining posterior and lateral support and stability of the pelvis. The pelvic belt helps keep the child's pelvis in contact with the seat, in an upright, neutral alignment.

Provision of postural support is often attempted in the opposite order, for example, when an anterior chest panel or belt is inappropriately used to help a child stop leaning to the side. The chest panel used in this way may cause bruising on a child's neck and does not solve the underlying problem of inadequate posterior and lateral support. When an anterior support is applied in this way before giving attention to posterior and lateral support, the result is ineffective at best and dangerous at worst (Figure 9-25).

Build support upward from the foundation. A child needs a solid base of support to be posturally stable and allow for functional movements.

The pelvis is the foundation for control and stability. If the pelvis is allowed to remain asymmetrically positioned, the trunk will be out of alignment as well. The pelvis can be compared with the foundation of a house. If the foundation of a house is unstable, structural deficits in the walls and possibly even a shifting of the supporting structures occur. Doors do not fit properly and windows may not function. Likewise, the pelvis as a foundation for postural support can be responsible for shifts or asymmetries in the trunk, head, and neck, as well as dysfunctional use of extremities.

Appropriate fit to the body and extremities must be achieved. Proper seat depth, width, and angle at the hips and knees is needed to facilitate neutral tilt of the pelvis, erect spine, and functional position of the arms and legs. The size of the postural support system also affects a child's ability to propel the chair independently.

A firm seat and back surface is essential. Think of how you sit in a hammock or sling swing. Now picture sitting on a church bench. The first seat would promote rest and a curved position of your pelvis and back, with your hips turning inward and moving together. The second position promotes more alertness and an upright posture. A firm seat support allows your thighs to be evenly supported and your pelvis to maintain a neutral orienta-

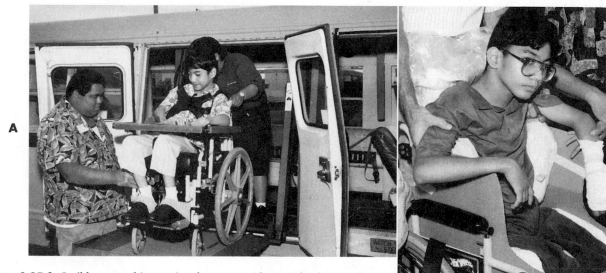

Figure 9-25 A, Cyril hangs on his anterior chest support because he does not have good posterior support. **B,** Cyril sits better in his wheelchair after posterior support is provided. A Foam-in-Place seat and back are being made for him to improve his wheelchair positioning.

tion, not tilted. The firm back support provides input to your nervous system and muscles to sit taller and gives your spine more support. Firm back and seat surfaces provide control at the pelvis and trunk to maintain postural stability.

Variations in types of seat and back surfaces. The range of contoured seat and back cushions available goes from simple or generic, to more aggressive and intimate contours. While the solid seat and back supports previously described provide firm support for the body, it is important to consider that human beings are not flat on our posterior surfaces. While we typically have many natural curves, children with postural deformities may have even more curves because of muscular weakness or postural deformity, such as kyphosis or scoliosis. A contoured surface provides better input to a child's nervous system for stability, as well as sensory feedback to find and maintain a neutral position. It also provides a home base to which the pelvis and trunk return each time the child sits. Compare the sling (hammock) and planar (church bench) seats to the driver's seat of a sports car. The sports car seat is very contoured, and you can probably adjust the backrest to match the natural curves of your lumbar spine. When you take turns sharply, this contouring helps you to remain stable in the seat. If you were to sit on a bench seat rather than a contoured seat, you might need to grip the steering wheel more tightly as you complete the turn. Likewise, contoured seat and back cushions provide stability for the child who has difficulty achieving postural control. Merely providing the natural body curves will greatly enhance overall stability so that a child's hands can be free to do something functional.

Simple or generic contouring. This "off-the-shelf" type of contour is comparable to the contours in your car, your "lazy boy" chair, and some ergonomic desk chairs. In a wheelchair seating system the seat and back can be purchased with basic body curves already built in. For example, Jay Medical, Ltd., provides special generic or simple contoured seat and back cushions to use with children (Figure 9-26). These seats and backs can be

made more aggressively contoured through use of add-on positioning pads and pieces. The pieces of foam can add effective contouring, while being adjustable for growth and change in posture. In another example, the Snug Seat uses a similar modular system where pieces of foam can be added or removed depending on the child's size and postural changes. These are just a few of the possible examples.

Intimate contouring. Custom-fitted contouring is possible for children with such severe deformities or postural needs that an "off-the-shelf" seating system for stable posture is not sufficient. Some examples of intimate contour include a custom-molded liquid foam, which is formed around a child held in an optimal position (Figure 9-25, *B*). Another type of intimate molding is made from a negative cast mold taken from a seating simulator (Figure 9-27). Intimate molding or contouring is necessary for children who have extremely low muscle tone and require total support for postural alignment to be upright against gravity. Conversely, children with extremely high muscle tone and resulting stiffness may benefit from intimate molding to help maintain a more relaxed position while sitting upright. The child with high tone may use less energy for postural stability with a contoured seating system, allowing more functional activities while sitting. Intimate contouring will also provide more support for children who have severe contractures and postural deformities.

Children who have difficulty with temperature regulation may have problems with intimate contours because there is less air circulation in the seat than with more open systems. Children with athetosis or excessive movement may find a contoured seating system to be confining and restricting. A compromise may need to be made to provide enough support for the child to be stable, without restricting movements or causing discomfort.

Additional considerations for seating support

Hip supports. Hip guides or lateral thigh supports can be used to maintain pelvic alignment in neutral. These lateral sup-

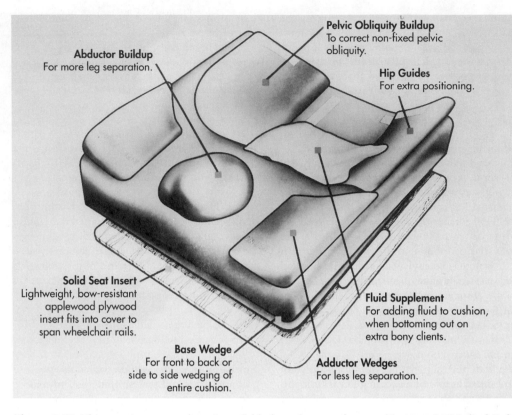

Abductor Buildup
For more leg separation.

Pelvic Obliquity Buildup
To correct non-fixed pelvic obliquity.

Hip Guides
For extra positioning.

Solid Seat Insert
Lightweight, bow-resistant applewood plywood insert fits into cover to span wheelchair rails.

Fluid Supplement
For adding fluid to cushion, when bottoming out on extra bony clients.

Base Wedge
For front to back or side to side wedging of entire cushion.

Adductor Wedges
For less leg separation.

Figure 9-26 This generic contoured seat is available from the manufacturer. (Courtesy Jay Medical, Ltd.)

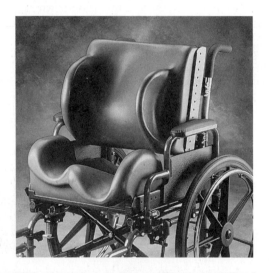

Figure 9-27 This intimate contoured foam seat was made to the exact shape of a child's body. (Courtesy Pin Dot Products.)

ports can be placed beside the buttocks to guide the hips into a stable position or more distally on the lateral aspect of the thighs as adductor supports, preventing excessive hip abduction or "frogged" hips.

Abductor supports. Also called medial thigh supports, this padded piece helps to keep the legs in a neutral position. It is often mistakenly used to help keep the child's pelvis back in the chair. A child without sufficient posterior support may slide for-

ward in the seat resting the genitals against the abductor. This can cause discomfort and injury. The abductor support should not be a weight-bearing surface for the perineum or genitals; it should be used only to maintain neutral alignment of the legs and must be used with caution (Figure 9-28).

Trunk supports. These lateral supports are used to maintain neutral alignment of the spine. They may be attached to the wheelchair frame or molded into a contoured cushion. If used to control a scoliosis in a traditional "three-point control," the pads are placed at the apex of the curve on one side and at the top and bottom of the rib cage on the other side. Care must be taken to monitor skin integrity when pads are used in this way.

Leg and foot supports. Posterior supports for the leg and foot must be measured accurately to accommodate for any foot or knee deformities such as a knee flexion or plantarflexion contracture. Legrests support the child's leg from the knee to the foot. The foot plate supports the child's foot. When measuring, it is important to be aware of the type of shoes the child may be wearing in the wheelchair, because this may affect the length of the lower leg segment. Legrests may be fixed or detachable, and swing away. Proper length allows for optimal foot placement to propel the chair, as well as for ease of transfer into and out of the chair. Elevating legrests are frequently used to position the legs to prevent swelling or circulatory problems that occur when the feet hang down in a dependent position. If children have tight hamstring muscles, elevating legrests will cause the pelvis to tilt posteriorly and result in the child sliding forward out of the seat. Elevating the legrests is an ineffective way to stretch tight hamstring muscles, causing discomfort and poor positioning in the wheelchair.

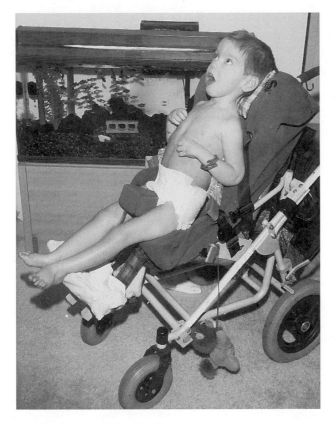

Figure 9-28 This abductor support is being misused to keep Ian's pelvis back in the chair. Damage to the genitals can result from such misuse.

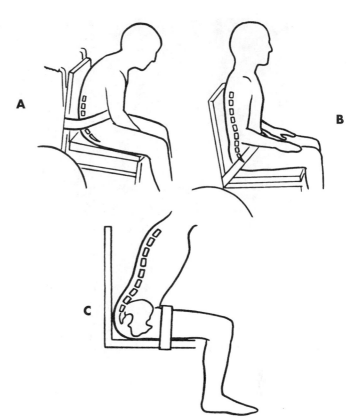

Figure 9-29 The placement of the pelvic belt can affect the overall positioning of the child in the seating system. **A,** A belt below the pelvis encourages posterior pelvic tilt. **B,** A belt placed at the femoral/pelvic junction allows neutral position of the pelvis, with some forward weight shift of the trunk. **C,** A belt placed over the upper thigh will allow the pelvis to tilt forward naturally during weight shift. (From Bergen, A.F., Presperin, J., & Tallman, T. [1990]. *Positioning for function: Wheelchair and other assistive technologies.* Valhalla, NY: Valhalla Rehabilitation Publication, Ltd.)

If a child exhibits very tight plantar flexors, angle-adjustable foot plates may be the only way to get total contact of the foot on the footplate. Heel loops are often added to keep the child's feet from sliding off the footplate into the front casters. Ankle straps may be added to maintain foot position, prevent forward sliding, or prevent spasms of the legs off the footplates. Care must be taken with use of ankle straps, because they may hold shoes in place better than feet.

Head and neck supports. Before adding a posterior head rest, a neck collar, or an anterior forehead strap, the team working with a child should try adjusting the angle of the wheelchair and providing adequate posterior and lateral supports for the seat and back. When the pelvis, trunk, and extremities are positioned well, the head may not need extra support. Posterior or lateral head support may be needed for safety, however, when being transported in a vehicle, or if the chair is tilted back in space. In this case the head should be supported at the occiput so that the neck is in neutral flexion and extension relative to the trunk. If the support is too high, the child's neck will tend to hyperextend as the head slides down on the support.

In a few cases tilting the chair, providing adequate seat and back support, and using a posterior head support is not enough to control the head position. In this case a cervical collar, which rests on the chest to support the chin, can keep the head upright and prevent the head from falling forward. This should be used as a last resort, because collars tend to be hot, cumbersome, and socially inappropriate. An anterior head strap is not usually useful because it tends to encourage neck hyperextension. There are

a few anterior supports available now that prevent hyperextension, but they are more cumbersome to use and quite expensive.

Positioning belts and straps. The most important belt is the pelvic positioning belt. This belt prevents the child from inadvertently falling out of the chair and keeps the pelvis in a neutral, upright alignment. The pelvic belt acts somewhat like the laces of a shoe holding our foot securely inside. It is important to have the pelvic belt placed correctly so as not to impede pelvic mobility and weight shifts. Having a pelvic belt placed too high can block the pelvis, causing it to tilt more posteriorly so the child will slide down and out of the chair. A belt placed below the anterior superior iliac spines (ASIS) allows beneficial forward weight shifts and movement of the pelvis (Figure 9-29).

Chest and shoulder straps or panels, such as a butterfly or X-shaped panel, may be used to help keep the child's trunk contacting the back rest. Shoulder straps may be used in combination with chest straps to improve head and neck position by keeping the shoulders down and preventing them from rolling forward. When chest or shoulder straps are used, they should never be connected to the pelvic positioning belt because this connection decreases the effectiveness of both strapping systems. Belts and straps can be valuable assets to the overall postural

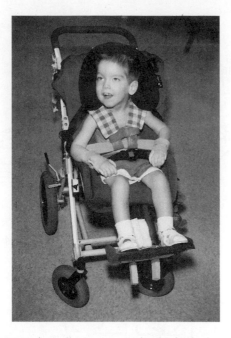

Figure 9-30 Ian's stroller is contoured to his body shape using removable foam pads. His stroller base allows variable tilt-in-space positioning that helps him keep his head and trunk upright.

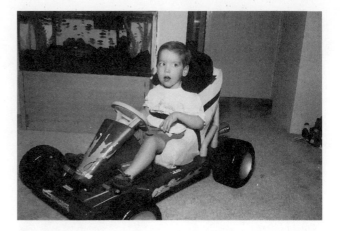

Figure 9-31 Ian uses a custom molded seat to sit in an electrically powered car. With his increased stability, he can operate a switch to drive the car.

control system; however, their use must be judicious and well planned. These are anterior supports and should be used as a last resort, after all other postural supports have been addressed.

Tray tables or lap boards. These anterior supports allow proper positioning of the arms, as well as providing a surface on which the child can eat, play, or work. The tray table may provide anterior trunk support as well.

Tilt-in-space. Variable orientation of the chair or stroller in space (Figure 9-30) is a commonly used feature to relieve pressure or to help the child sit more upright. Tilting the entire base back in space a few degrees, while keeping the back to hip angle constant, may provide enough stability to allow the child relative upright positioning. *Tilt-in-space* is different than *recline,* which allows variable hip to back angle by changing the back angle relative to the seat. The tilt-in-space feature allows maintenance of optimal hip to back angles to control inefficient movement patterns (extensor thrust) or to allow gravity-assisted positioning, yet prevents sliding down in the chair that a reclined angle of seat to back may encourage. Sometimes tilting the frame forward slightly can help a child access postural control to sit more upright. Some pediatric wheelchairs may offer both a tilt-in-space feature and a recline feature. These features may be adjustable by the caregiver as needed or may be locked in at the initial fitting of the chair.

Summary

Children with severe disabilities who cannot walk or sit by themselves may spend their life lying on the floor or being carried. Without proper seating they cannot move, socialize, play, and learn like other children. They may develop stiffness, contractures, or deformities that further restrict movement. With proper

seating most children can improve their social skills, functional skills, and physiological functions. Talking, writing, playing, eating, and even breathing can be easier.

Many children need more support than a typical wheelchair can provide. Special seating inserts can be placed on typical mobility bases that are propelled either by caregivers or independently by the child. Most strollers and wheelchairs have standard seating features that can be customized; other additions can be made to ensure optimal postural support and alignment. It is important that the stroller or wheelchair fit appropriately and allow the child to grow. Postural supports can also be placed in alternative sitting situations, such as a classroom chair, high chair, or alternative mobility base (Figure 9-31).

Postural support systems must be comfortable, safe, and attractive yet provide support and stability. They should not cause undue pressure on sensitive skin. Providing total contact in a seat or back cushion may help prevent excessive pressure from developing. Use of the postural support system should improve body functions for the child such as breathing, alertness, digestion, and elimination. It should also help to improve the child's own ability to function, allowing the child to look around, speak, or use hands for activities. Finally, the postural support system should be capable of change to allow for growth and changing function of the child. Even though a child may need almost total support initially to stay upright, less support may be needed with maturation. Support should be reduced or removed as the child gains skills. Consideration should be given to the function of the equipment in a given environment, such as fitting through doorways or folding and fitting into a car or truck. When determining the best features for a child's positioning and mobility system, it is critical to work as a team with the child, family, caregivers, teacher, vendor, and others to ensure that the best match of features to function occurs.

EXERCISES

1. Look up support agencies in your community. Are support groups available for families of children with severe traumatic injuries such as TBI or SCI? Visit a group for one or more sessions to get a sense of what the issues are for families.

2. Find out the reporting procedures for suspected child abuse in your state, community, and local institutions (e.g., schools, hospitals).
3. From the Internet find out what information is available to families of children with traumatic injuries. Read families' stories on their own home pages. Print these out and share them with your classmates.

QUESTIONS TO PONDER

1. How should government be involved in the prevention of injury to children? Laws have been passed in various states disallowing anyone riding in the back of a pickup truck, enforcing the wearing of seat belts, enforcing the use of child safety seats in automobiles, mandating fences around swimming pools, and enforcing the wearing of helmets on motorcycles and bicycles. Should more laws be enacted enforcing the wearing of protective devices when rollerblading, lifejackets when boating, etc.? What other means are there to reduce the number of injuries and death resulting from accidents?
2. Should children be rehabilitated in the same facilities as adults? What are the unique needs of children that may or may not be met in adult facilities?
3. You are treating a young child with a severe TBI in the hospital. The parent asks you about recovery and prognosis for the child. How should you respond? Should other team members be involved in answering this question with you? What kind of response would you want if you were the parent?

Annotated Bibliography

Bergen, A. F., Presperin, J., & Tallman, T. (1990). *Positioning for function: Wheelchairs and other assistive technologies.* Valhalla, NY: Valhalla Rehabilitation Publications, Ltd.

When this book came out in 1990, therapists who were involved in providing seating and mobility to individuals with severe disabilities were thrilled. This book not only discusses principles of seating and positioning but also reviews equipment that is available commercially. The information supplied is technical and complete; however, some is significantly out of date. The manufacturing companies reviewed still comprise a major segment of the rehabilitation community, however, and their equipment continues to be widely used and prescribed. Reviewing this book, even though some of the equipment and companies reviewed may have been updated or significantly changed, gives the reader a sense of the scope of equipment available. The case studies, photographs, and problem-solving strategies continue to be appropriate and helpful. This book continues to be a mainstay in the field of seating and positioning. We only hope that a more current edition is being planned.

References

American Spinal Injury Association. (1992). *International standards for neurological and functional classification of spinal cord injury.* Chicago: Author.

Apple, D. F. Jr., Anson, C. A., Hunter, J. D., & Bell, R. B. (1995). Spinal cord injury in youth. *Clinical Pediatrics, 34,* 90-95.

Bishop, B., & Gilinsky, V. (1995). School reentry for the patient with burn injuries: video and/or on-site intervention. *Journal of Burn Care and Rehabilitation, 16,* 455-457.

Blakeney, P.E., Meyer, W., Moore, P., Murphy, L., Broemeling, L., Robson, M., & Herndon, D. (1993). Psychosocial sequelae of pediatric burns involving 80% or greater total body surface area. *Journal of Burn Care and Rehabilitation, 6(14),* 684-689.

Bracken, M. B., & Shepard, M. J. (1980). Coping and adaptation following acute spinal cord injury: a theoretical analysis. *Paraplegia, 18,* 74.

Centers for Disease Control and Prevention. (1990). Childhood injuries in the United States. *American Journal of Disabilities in Childhood, 144,* 627-646.

Chao, R. & Mayo, M. E. (1994). Long-term urodynamic follow up in pediatric spinal cord injury. *Paraplegia, 12(32),* 806-809.

ChildHelp USA. (1996). ChildHelp USA National Statistics. *Voices for children* [on-line]. Venture Publications. Available: www.serve.com/vfc/facts.html.

Ellis, A. A., & Trent, R. B. (1995). Hospitalizations for near drowning in California: Incidence and costs. *American Journal of Public Health, 85,* 1115-1118.

Federal Register (September 29, 1992). Part II, Department of Education, 34 CRF Parts 300 and 301, Assistance to States for the Education of Children with Disabilities Program and Preschool Grants for Children with Disabilities, Final Rule, *57(189),* 44801-44802.

George, A., & Hancock, J. (1993). Reducing pediatric burn pain with parent participation. *Journal of Burn Care and Rehabilitation, 14,* 104-107.

Gillenwater, J. M., Quan, L., & Feldman, K. W. (1996). Inflicted submersion in childhood. *Archives in Pediatric and Adolescent Medicine, 150,* 298-303.

Greenspan, A. I. (1996). Functional recovery following head injury among children. *Current Problems in Pediatrics, 26,* 170-177.

Hoy, G. A., & Cole, W. G. (1993). The paediatric cervical seat belt syndrome. *Injury, 5(24),* 297-299.

Jaffe, K. M., Polissar, N. L., Fay, G. C., & Liao, S. (1995). Recovery trends over three years following pediatric traumatic brain injury. *Archives of Physical Medicine and Rehabilitation, 76,* 17-26.

Johnson, J. & Silverberg, R. (1995). Serial casting of the lower extremity to correct contractures during the acute phase of burn care. *Physical Therapy, 75,* 262-266.

Kempe, C. H., Silverman, F. N., Steele, B. F., Broegemueller, W., & Silver, K. H. (1962). The battered child syndrome. *Journal of the American Medical Association, 181,* 508-518.

Kennedy, P., Gorsuch, N., Marsh, N. (1995). Childhood onset of spinal cord injury: Self-esteem and self-perception. *British Journal of Clinical Psychology, 34,* 581-588.

Kewalramani, L. S., Krause, J.S., & Sterling, J.M. (1980). Acute spinal cord lesions in a pediatric population-epidemiological and clinical features. *Paraplegia, 18(3),* 206-219.

Krause, J. F., Rock, A., & Hemyari, P. (1990). Brain injuries among infants, children, adolescents, and young adults. *Archives in Pediatric and Adolescent Medicine, 144,* 684-691.

Lavelle, J. M., Shaw, K. N., Seidl, T., Ludwig, S. (1995). Ten-year review of pediatric bathtub near drownings: Evaluation for child abuse and neglect. *Annals of Emergency Medicine, 25,* 344-348.

Lister, L. (1996). *Child abuse and neglect.* Unpublished manuscript, University of Hawaii at Manoa.

Mahalik, D. M., Yalamanchi, K., Ruzicka, P. O., & Bowen, M. (November, 1990). Spontaneous recovery following pediatric traumatic brain injury. Presented at the National Head Injury Foundation's Annual Conference, New Orleans, LA.

Massagli, T. L., Jaffe, K. M., Fay, G. C., Polissar, N. L., Liao, S. & Rivara, J. B. (1996). Neurobehavioral sequelae of severe pediatric traumatic brain injury: A cohort study. *Archives of Physical Medicine and Rehabilitation, 77,* 223-231.

Meyer III, W.J., Blakeney, P.E., Holzer, C.E., Moore, P., Murphy, L., Robson, M.C., & Herndon, D.N. (1995). Inconsistencies in psychosocial assessment of children after severe burns. *Journal of Burn Care and Rehabilitation, 5,* 16.

Meyer III, W.J., Blakeney, P.E., LeDoux, J., & Herndon, D.N. (1995). Diminished adaptive behaviors among pediatric survivors of burns. *Journal of Burn Care and Rehabilitation, 5(16),* 511-518.

Michaud, L. J. & Duhaime, A. C. (1992). Traumatic brain injury. In M. L. Batshaw & Y. M. Perret, *Children with disabilities: A medical primer.* Baltimore, MD: Brookes.

Mittendorfer, B. , Hildreth, M. A., Desai, M. H., & Herndon, D. N. (1995). Younger pediatric patients with burns are at risk for continuing postdischarge weight loss. *Journal of Burn Care and Rehabilitation, 16,* 589-595.

Morrow, S. E., Smith, D. L., Howell, P. D., Nakayama, K. K., & Peterson, H. D. (1996). Etiology and outcome of pediatric burns. *Journal of Pediatric Surgery, 31,* 329-333.

Nieves, J. A., Buttacavoli, M., Fuller, L., Clarke, T. & Schimpf, P. C. (1996). Childhood drowning: Review of the literature and clinical implications. *Pediatric Nursing, 22,* 206-210.

Pandit, S. K., Malla, C. N., Zarger, H. U., Kaul, A. & Dev. G. (1993). A study of bone and joint changes secondary to burns. *Burns, 19,* 227-228.

Pecora, P., Wittaker, J., Maluccio, A., Barth, R., & Plotnick, R. (1992). *The child welfare challenge.* New York: Aldine De Gruyter.

Ray, J. G. (1995). Burns in young children: A study of the mechanism of burns in children aged 5 years and under in the Hamilton, Ontario burn unit. *Burns, 21,* 463-466.

Rouse, T.M., & Eichelberger, M.R. (1992). Trends in pediatric trauma management. *Surgery Clinics of North America, 72(6),* 1347-1364.

Schmitt, M.A., French, L., & Kalil, E.T. (1991). How soon is safe: Ambulation of the patient with burns after lower extremity skin grafting. *Journal of Burn Care and Rehabilitation, 12(1),* 33-37.

Schneider, F. J. (1990). Traumatic spinal cord injury. In D. A. Umphred (Ed.), *Neurological rehabilitation.* St. Louis: Mosby.

Silverstein, P. & Wilson, R. (1988). Prevention of pediatric burn injuries. In H. F. Carvajal & D. H. Parks (Eds.), *Burns in children: Pediatric burn management.* St. Louis: Mosby.

Simon, P. A., & Baron, R. C. (1994). Age as a risk factor for burn injury requiring hospitalization during early childhood. *Archives in Pediatric and Adolescent Medicine, 148,* 394-397.

Svenson, J. E., Spurlock, C., & Nypaver, M. (1996). Pediatric firearm-related fatalities: Not just an urban problem. *Archives in Pediatric and Adolescent Medicine, 150,* 583-587.

Yoshimura, O., Murakami, T., Kawamura, M., & Takayanigi, K. (1995). Spinal cord injury in a child: A long term follow-up study—Case report. *Paraplegia, 33,* 362-363.

Sensory, Processing, and Cognitive Disorders

10

CASE STUDY — Luke, A Boy With Autism

Luke sat quietly, watching the other participants get ready for their heats. The pool was a cool shade of blue. Luke was sitting in the full sun on a plastic chair on the cement apron of the pool. He blinked his eyes frequently as sunscreen and sweat from his forehead dripped into them. He rubbed his eyes with his fist and allowed his mother to gently wipe his eyes with a damp towel.

The overhead announcer called for the next heat. Luke's mother took his hand and said, "It's your turn Luke. It's time to get in the water. Let's go swimming." She tugged on his arm to help him get up from the chair. Luke shook his head. He pulled back strongly.

"No swimming! No swimming! No, no, no," Luke shouted in his breathy voice as his mother struggled with him over to the pool. People nearby were watching them, not sure whether to help or not.

When Luke reached the side of the pool, he calmed down. His mother helped him sit on the side of the pool. Then she helped him shift his weight to the spill guard and then down into the water. Luke hung on tightly to the side of the pool, kicking his feet in a pedaling motion and lifting his face so it would not get wet.

The starter checked to make sure all the athletes were ready and then fired his gun. "Go Luke! Swim!" his mother encouraged him. Luke slowly left the security of the pool side and struck off into his lane using a modified side stroke. His mother ran to the other end of the pool and called to him, cheering, as he made his way across the blue water.

When Luke arrived at the far end, his parents and friends greeted him (Figure 10-1). His mother pulled him out of the water, wrapped him in a towel, and gave him a hug. Luke stood, dripping, the towel draped over one shoulder and falling off the

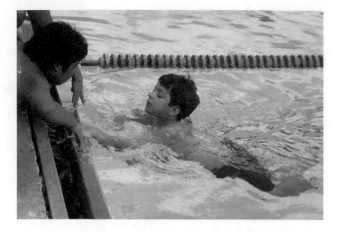

Figure 10-1 Luke finishes his heat of freestyle swimming in the Special Olympics. His friend Grant greets him.

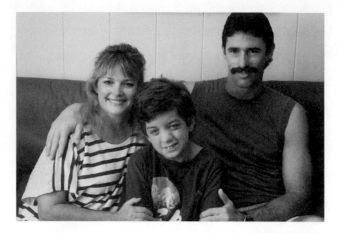

Figure 10-2 Family portrait. Note Luke's quality of eye contact.

other. Athletes milled around with family members and supporters, cheering and hugging. Luke stared into the distance, smiling and shifting from foot to foot, until his mother took his hand and guided him to a plastic chair to wait for his next event.

Developmental History

Luke is the only child of Sam and Camilla Tate (Figure 10-2). He was born after an uneventful pregnancy through spontaneous vaginal delivery and weighed 8 pounds, 2 ounces. When he was 2 days old, he began to have seizures and the long process of adjusting various seizure medications began. Camilla and Sam were very concerned about their son's seizures but never dreamed that he would end up with a permanent disability. They worked closely with pediatric neurologists to adjust his seizure medications and blamed his developmental delays on the medications.

Luke sat up alone at 9 months. He crawled at 1 year, and was cruising along furniture by 1½ years. He walked at 2 years but needed to be carried for longer distances even when he was 3 and 4 years. His mother took him to a baby gymnastics class when he was a toddler and remembers painfully that he was the slowest toddler there. Luke had a permanent bump on his forehead from frequent falls.

Luke began to talk at a little over 1 year old but lost words after he had learned them. "Down," "mama," and "dog" were some of his early words. He learned words in a different order than other children, learning "mama" before "dada," and then losing both of them.

Luke was always finicky about foods. He liked bland foods but did not like spicy or acidic foods, such as those with tomato sauce. At 8 months old, he refused to take the bottle, and his mother hand-fed him with a cup. He did not seem interested in finger foods, and even at 9 months old, he would not take any finger foods, such as toast, crackers, or cookies. His mother fed him with a spoon, and he did not indicate interest in using the spoon himself until much older.

Camilla was very proud of his intelligence. She noted that Luke would spend hours with a shape sorter toy and could put the correct shapes in the holes of an 18-sided shape sorter be-

fore he was 1 year old. He was also very good at puzzles that did not have interlocking pieces.

Luke's doctor noticed the delays in his development, but attributed them to seizures and the medications he had been on since birth. "Boys are slow" was a comment he made to explain Luke's lack of progress. Camilla had no other children to compare Luke's development with, but she spent a lot of time with a friend who had a child the same age as Luke. It was difficult to ignore the differences between the two children. Once, when they were having a picnic, her friend remarked that "Luke's development seems fractured." Camilla took deep offense at the remark and stopped seeing her friend.

When Luke was 2 years old, the family moved and changed physicians. The new physician diagnosed developmental delays and started Luke in an infant development program. Camilla and Sam had to work through many of the feelings they had been putting aside for 2 years. One refrain that Camilla found running through her head was, "There is no one with disabilities in my family, how could I have a disabled child? This isn't happening to me."

Once they accepted that Luke needed special help, the problem of defining or diagnosing Luke's problems seemed very complicated. At 3 years old, he went through a developmental assessment at a major university. Mental retardation, emotional disorder, and autism were all considered as potential diagnoses. Finally, he was diagnosed with pervasive developmental disorder (PDD), not otherwise specified (NOS). This diagnosis did not have much meaning for his parents. In the meantime, Luke started in a special school for children from ages 3 to 22 years and received services to help him improve his communication, gross motor, fine motor, social, cognitive, and self-help skills.

When he was 5 years old, the family moved again, and Luke began kindergarten in the public school system. He was placed in a fully self-contained classroom with other children who had emotional disorders or mild to moderate mental retardation. His diagnosis was changed to mental retardation with autistic tendencies. He received services from physical therapy, occupational therapy, speech-language pathology, and psychology to help him improve his balance, strength, self-help skills, communication skills, and coping behaviors.

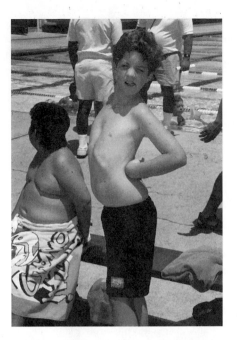

Figure 10-3 This is a characteristic posture for Luke. Note the lumbar lordosis, anterior pelvis, and arms back. His weight is on the balls of his feet with his hips flexed. Note the lack of eye contact.

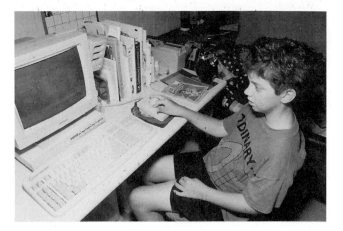

Figure 10-4 Luke is working on his computer at home. He is fully engrossed in the task.

His physical therapist worked with Luke on strengthening activities to help him with advanced gait skills. Luke had a daily exercise routine of pelvic bridges, curl ups, and creeping on hands and knees. He did his exercises alone or with several other children in a group. He was also encouraged to climb the slide and slide down, climb up and down stairs, and walk over uneven surfaces (Figure 10-3).

Luke was generally cooperative, but when he did not want to participate, he would sit down on the ground and stay there until he was ready to get up. His mother and father developed strategies for getting his cooperation, which incorporated many of the routines Luke felt compelled to include in his life. For instance, to get his attention, they asked him to turn off the television set. Also, they waited while he leaned over to turn off the surge protector under the bed. Unless this was done, he did not feel that the task was complete.

Luke's language developed to the extent that he was able to repeat what others said to him, but only rarely was he able to initiate his own verbalizations. When his mother asked him, "Luke do you want a cookie?" Luke would answer, "Want a cookie?" He communicated well with facial expressions that his peers, teachers, and family understood. He also used gestures, such as shaking his head for "no," pointing, and vocalizing to get someone's attention. His parents became used to his communication style and consulted with speech language pathologists at school to help him increase his options for communication. They tried teaching him simple signs and used a communication board with pictures for pointing to things he wanted. Sign language was not effective for Luke as it seemed to add another layer to his communication efforts, but the family continued to work with the communication board, gestures, and verbal language.

Camilla and Sam worked with Luke at home on academic skills, using flash cards and books every night beginning when he was in kindergarten. Luke was able to answer simple questions and recognize important written words, such as danger, exit, and stop.

Camilla and Sam became involved in the Autism Society when Luke was in the third grade. They discovered that many of the symptoms Luke exhibited, such as poor verbal skills, lack of eye contact, and the need for predictability of routines to cope with life, fit into the diagnosis of autism. They enjoyed going to conferences and talking with professionals and other parents. They were able to learn about new treatments and behavior strategies, that seemed to work well with many children with autism. Camilla changed Luke's diagnosis to autism in her own mind, even though the medical diagnosis did not officially change until Luke was in fifth grade.

During this year, his aunt gave the family a computer. Luke used it at home with his parents, and it changed his life. The computer allowed him to repeat things over and over, which his parents did not have the patience for. He was able to start learning rudimentary academic concepts and also enjoyed the games and activities that the software offered (Figure 10-4).

The summer before fourth grade, Luke had been involved in an auditory integration training program that helped him learn to differentiate between sounds. Camilla learned about the training through the autism society. Even though Luke had a bad seizure that made him miss the end of the program, his mother believed that he had benefited from the program by understanding spoken words better. In fourth grade, Luke's teacher changed teaching strategies from sight learning to a phonics approach for teaching reading.

That year Luke also started taking megadoses of some vitamins including B6, magnesium, and dimethylglycine (DMG), all recommended and available through the autism society. The theory is that the drugs would counter some of the negative effects of the seizure medications, such as sleepiness, decreased alertness, and poor attention. Luke's parents noticed that he was more alert, had better eye contact, stuttered less, and was not as sleepy when he took the vitamins.

Luke learned to read in the fourth grade. His mother attributes his learning of this important skill primarily to the repetitive teaching of the computer, and secondarily to the hours that she and his father had spent with Luke on flash cards and books. She believed that the phonics, the auditory integration course, and the vitamins may also have helped.

In the fifth grade, the school finally provided a computer in the classroom for Luke to use, and Luke's father taught the teacher how to use the software that Luke used at home. His reading skills improved, probably as a result of having the computer in the classroom.

Luke at School

Luke is now in sixth grade. He has been fully integrated into a regular sixth grade class along with his friend Grant, a boy with Prader-Willi syndrome. One educational aide in the classroom is designated to assist both Luke and Grant, but strategies have been devised to include the boys into the regular routines of the day through the use of peer support. He has had a recent physical therapy evaluation, which is summarized in Box 10-1.

BOX 10-1   Physical Therapy Evaluation Summary: Luke

Social and Medical History
Addressed in the Case Study.

Range of Motion
All within normal limits except for the following:
Hip straight leg raise: Approximately 40 degrees bilaterally
Ankle dorsiflexion: -5 degrees bilaterally
Luke has an increased carrying angle of his elbows bilaterally.
Spine: Luke has a hyperlordosis with an anteriorly tilted pelvis.

Muscle Strength, Tone, and Bulk
Although strength was not tested formally, his upper extremities were grossly within good/normal ranges with trunk and lower extremities in fair/good ranges. Luke is able to do at least 10 bridges and 10 sit ups without assistance but demonstrates decreased functional pelvic girdle strength by his waddling gait. His muscle tone is on the low side of normal, and bulk is within normal limits.

Reflexes and Functional Skills
Primitive reflexes appear to be appropriately integrated and do not interfere with Luke's motor patterns. He has functional balance reactions in sitting with protective extension to all directions. In standing he has fair/good balance reactions. He has functional protective extension in all directions, but it is delayed and he is not secure with his balance when challenged. He attempts to stand on one foot on either leg and is able to do so briefly bilaterally. He rises from the floor by turning onto all fours and standing up using a modified bear position. Luke is very mobile and walks using a waddling gait with his hips externally rotated and abducted, his knees held fairly straight, and his trunk has a lateral sway to both sides. His arms are held back, behind his center of gravity, perhaps to compensate for his hyperlordosis, and he walks on the balls of his feet using short steps. He is able to run short distances. Luke does not like high places, edges, such as curbs, or climbing. He ascends and descends steps by putting both feet on each step. Luke swims independently using a modified dog paddle/side stroke for at least 25 yards. He enjoys swinging but does not pump to propel himself. He used to like slides but no longer likes them. He has difficulty walking on uneven surfaces, climbing over obstacles, and negotiating ladders and steps.

Posture
Luke stands with his lower back in a hyperlordosis and his pelvis in an anterior tilt. His upper trunk is extended with his arms held behind his center of gravity. He stands on the balls of his feet and his head is forward. In sitting he tends to cross his legs (tailor sit), sitting with an upright posture (brief) or sits with his pelvis upright and his trunk leaning backward or rounded. He can also assume a short sitting position with his legs over the side of the bed or chair.

Adaptive Equipment
Luke has the following games and adaptive equipment for learning, leisure and communication:
- Computer with various types of software for spelling and math activities.
- Handheld video game electronic toy.
- Television with VCR.
- Poster-sized cardboard communication board in his room. Pictures of food, objects, and activities are pasted on the board. Luke is encouraged to point to things he wants. He usually points to what he wants after he is encouraged to do so by his mother.
- Loose, comfortable clothing that he can put on himself. Pants have elastic waistbands.
- Grab bar in the tub. This is not effective because Luke will not touch it when it is wet.

Activities of Daily Living
Luke can assist with most skills of daily living:
- Bathing: Addressed in Case Study.
- Eating: Addressed in Case Study.
- Toileting: Luke is independent in toileting skills, except needs help with wiping after a bowel movement.
- Dressing: Luke can dress himself with minimal help but is inconsistent and frequently puts his shirt on inside out or backward. He can put his shoes on but is inconsistent with getting them on the correct foot. He refuses to wear certain clothes, such as shirts with appliqués that feel different against his skin. He prefers soft fabrics. He does not like buttons.
- Oral care: Luke needs close supervision and hand-over-hand assistance to ensure adequate toothbrushing.

Recreation and Leisure
Luke has been involved with challenger baseball, therapeutic horseback riding, and swimming in Special Olympics over the past year. His parents or another adult accompany Luke to all of his activities. Luke enjoys hiking on relatively even terrain with his family, going out to movies, shopping, and going to his friend's house. When he gets restless in the movies, his mother gives him a napkin to shred.

Luke is driven to school on a special education bus that picks him up outside his house. He has trouble with the bus's high step, and his mother moves a low stool under the step to help him. He has difficulty climbing stairs and ladders in a variety of environments (Figure 10-5). Luke is careful to always sit on the same seat on the bus. If that seat is taken already, he has a very hard day. At school, Luke has his own desk and puts his books away neatly. During the Pledge of Allegiance and the America song, Luke stands with the rest of the class with his head cocked to the side appearing to listen closely, with his eyes unfocused.

When everyone sits down to begin the mathematics lesson, Luke goes to a group of four children who have specifically asked to work with him. Henry and Maya write math problems for Luke and help him work through them. Luke does not write his answers down or show his work on the paper. He punches the numbers into a calculator and is able to speak the answer that shows on the display. He also can choose between answers his classmates write for him on paper. He chooses by pointing to the correct answer or smiling if someone else points to it. When a classmate says something, such as "That's right, Luke!," Luke echoes it, saying, "That's right, Luke!"

While the rest of the class moves on to more advanced math, Luke works on the computer with the aide, Mr. Tino, to refine his skills at adding and subtracting double digit numbers. The computer program provides the questions, as well as appropriate praise when Luke is correct. Luke moves the mouse as if it is part of his hand. He skips quickly and expertly through the dancing rabbit reward to get back to the problems.

At lunch time, Luke gets into line with his class and walks to the cafeteria. He carries his tray by himself without spilling. Luke sits down at the cafeteria table next to Mr. Tino. He is able to eat by himself using a fork, but he pokes at the meat, which is covered with tomato sauce. Mr. Tino cuts it up for him, but Luke is not interested in eating it. He eats all of the mashed potatoes and

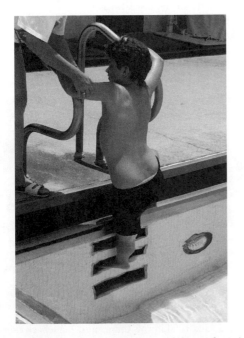

Figure 10-5 Luke needs help getting out of the pool. He is unable to climb the ladder without assistance.

the vanilla pudding but needs prompting from Mr. Tino to eat some of the green beans. Luke's father had taught him to drink his milk right out of the carton, but he needs help opening the carton and will not use a straw. When he finishes eating, Mr. Tino helps him bring his tray to the lunch counter and separate his dishes for washing.

In English class after lunch, Luke again is in a small group. Classmates have written short stories about themselves that they read to Luke and the rest of the group. They then formulate simple questions about the stories and pose them to Luke. The other children in the group do the exercise as both a written and oral exercise, but Luke only participates orally. He pays attention to the stories as they are read, even though he appears to be looking off into space. He is able to answer simple "who" or "what" questions either by speaking one word answers or by gesture and facial expression. He smiles when his classmates laugh.

After the group exercise, Luke goes to the computer to write his own essay. He types with his two index fingers and writes very simple sentences. Mr. Tino sits with him to prompt him on how to do the task. When he is finished writing, he reads his essay out loud to Mr. Tino and then hits the key to print it. When his essay comes out of the printer, Mr. Tino uses a hand-over-hand technique to help Luke write his name on the top. Luke has been tested as being able to read very advanced text, but his comprehension of what he reads is very low, perhaps only at a preschool level. After his essay is finished, Luke can play on any of the computer games or educational software that he chooses. He chooses a spelling program with a complicated maze. It is clear that he is very proficient at negotiating the maze, as well as spelling individual words. When the other students finish their tasks, some of them gather around Luke to watch him play on the computer. His classmates talk to each other and to Luke about the words he is spelling on the screen.

At recess, Luke goes out to the playground with the other students. He and Grant are encouraged by Mr. Tino to run around the playing field. Some of the other students run twice around the playground with them. Grant eagerly joins the others, but Luke hangs back until Mr. Tino takes his hand and encourages him to run with them.

During music class, Luke sits quietly with a tambourine in his hands. He attempts to shake it when the music teacher encourages him and allows a classmate to show him how to do it. When the song starts, however, Luke sits quietly with the tambourine in his lap. When a song comes up that he knows, Luke sings.

Luke's parents have been very happy with his experience in an included setting. They are worried about next year when not only does Luke transition into junior high school, but the family will be moving to another state. They have made contact with the neighborhood school in the town where they will be moving, and Sam has met with the special education staff there to plan Luke's placement for seventh grade. He will be placed in a fully self-contained classroom for the first year. Camilla has already researched the closest therapeutic horseback riding center and Special Olympics activities in their new town. She has asked his current interdisciplinary team to formulate some needs and recommendations for Luke that she can take with them to the new school.

On the basis of the team's evaluations, the following needs have been identified for Luke:

1. Luke needs support to enhance his receptive and expressive language skills at school and at home.

2. Luke needs to improve the strength of his trunk and hip muscles so that he can climb and run better.
3. Luke needs to prevent further loss of range of motion in his ankles to preserve his mobility skills (walking, running, etc.).
4. Luke needs to maintain and improve his aerobic fitness level to continue to participate in family hikes, Special Olympics, and other activities.
5. Luke needs more independent bathing skills.
6. Luke needs more independent toothbrushing skills.
7. Luke needs to participate with regular peers in school to develop better social and academic skills.
8. Luke needs to continue his academic progress in both verbal and quantitative skills.
9. Luke needs regular routines during the day to maintain his coping skills.

After you have considered these needs, turn to Box 10-2 at the end of the Case Study (p. 319) to see what Luke's team recommended to address them. Then refer to Box 10-3 (p. 320) to see some sample integrated IEP objectives that were developed for Luke at his new school.

Luke at Home

Luke's mother greets him when he arrives home after school. She hugs him, and Luke squeezes her back. She taught him to squeeze when hugged and prompts him by saying "squeeze!" Only when he is sick does he encourage or seek out physical contact.

He avoids the family dogs who are locked in the backyard and goes straight to his room. When he is asked to pet the dogs, he reaches out one arm as far as he can from his body and briefly touches a dog with one finger. The dogs move in unpredictable patterns, and Luke is very uncomfortable with them. Once in his room, he takes off his shoes and picks up his handheld video game, sitting cross-legged on his waterbed to play. All of his attention is on the game. He usually plays with his video game, watches videotapes, or plays computer programs when he gets home from school.

Luke's room is small and packed with many of the things that one would expect to see in a 12-year-old boy's room. On his desk sits a computer, a monitor, and a keyboard. Stacked next to the computer are a children's dictionary and other reference books. On his dresser is a photograph of Luke with his challenger baseball teammates, all holding trophies. In the picture, Luke is sitting on the ground in front of a boy in a wheelchair, holding his trophy close to his chest. The bookcase at the head of his bed is filled with books, many of which are spilling out onto the bed. At the foot of the bed is a television and a VCR on a stand. Shoes and a few clothes are strewn on the floor. His school backpack hangs on his closet door, next to a poster-size cardboard communication board onto which his mother has glued magazine pictures of different foods and activities.

Camilla comes into Luke's room, and asks him, "Do you want something to eat?"

He replies, "Want something to eat."

"What do you want?"

Luke looks at her.

Camilla prompts him, "I want . . ."

"I want a peanut butter sandwich, please." He speaks very softly, and she encourages him to show her what he wants on his communication board. Luke leans over to point to the picture of the peanut butter sandwich. This is what he wants every day. Camilla is glad to see him make the effort to communicate with her. She brings him his snack and puts it on the floor next to his bed. Luke looks up and blinks at her.

She smiles at him. "Say, 'Thank you, Mommy.'"

"Say thank you Mommy," he repeats.

"You're welcome."

After an hour, Camilla comes into Luke's room again. He does not look up from the small video screen but acknowledges her presence by hunching his shoulders. "Luke, it is time to go to therapeutic riding. Get up." Luke looks up at her. While helping him find his shoes and put them on, she discusses with him what he might do at his riding lesson today. The instructor had been on vacation for a few weeks, so Luke has not been riding in a while.

When they walk into the living room, Luke's dad comes in the door. He grasps Luke on both cheeks and leans his face close. "Hi, beautiful." "Hi, beautiful," Luke tells his dad, and smiles. Luke's dad tells him that he just went hiking up on the mountain to hunt for crickets to feed their Jackson chameleons. "Next time you can come with me." Camilla helps Luke into the car and buckles his seat belt. It is a 20-minute drive to the riding stable.

Luke wears a bicycle helmet and riding boots when he rides. Grant is there too, and Camilla and Grant's mom talk while the boys have their lesson. The teacher yells, "Sit tall, Luke. I'm . . ." Luke finishes the statement, "I'm sitting tall," and straightens his back a little. The instructor smiles. Luke is able to direct the horse to turn either direction, to trot, and to walk on command. The instructor stays close by Luke and his horse while Luke is riding, and a volunteer walks with Grant. Soon they leave the ring to go for a short trail ride. Luke tends to lean back when riding but will sit up straight when reminded. He bounces around a good deal when the horse trots, but he is able to stay on. Some of the benefits that his mother sees from the therapeutic horsemanship include better balance, posture, and strength. Luke also tolerates the touch of the horse under him and will even pat the horse when asked to do so (Figure 10-6).

When they arrive home, it is time for Luke's bath. His mother helps Luke take off his clothes and climb into the tub. He hangs

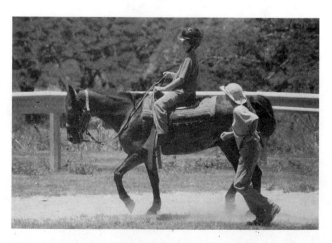

Figure 10-6 Luke is taking his therapeutic horseback riding lesson. Note the lack of ankle dorsiflexion and the leaning back of his trunk.

onto the grab bar that his dad installed on the inside wall of the bathtub. Luke sits on the floor of the tub and looks down while his mother pours water over him from a plastic pitcher. She has learned that, although it is uncomfortable for Luke, pouring water directly over him takes less time and trauma than trying to use the shower. She gets him to help soap his body, but he stops when she is not directing him. Finally, she pours water directly over his head to get his hair wet. Luke squirms and moans as the water rolls over his face, and his mother hands him a towel and helps him dry his eyes. She soaps his hair and again pours water over his head to rinse it. Luke complains and reaches for the towel again. By the end of the bath, they are both very wet. Luke refuses to hold onto the grab bar to get up because it is wet, so his mother waits for him to climb out by himself. He is getting too

---

BOX 10-2 ## Proposed Recommendations Addressing Identified Needs for Luke

1. Luke needs support to enhance his receptive and expressive language skills at school and at home.
   - Continue supporting Luke's communication skills using whatever media is helpful, including spoken language, communication board, facial expressions, and gestures. Luke's parents and the new school should continue to teach him ritualized speech for use in certain circumstances to promote better safety and social skills. These words and phrases can include "please," "thank you," "no thank you," "my name is Luke Tate," "my address is . . . ," "my telephone number is . . . ," and other phrases that are appropriate for his life.
2. Luke needs to improve the strength of his trunk and hip muscles so that he can climb and run better.
   - Rather than being pulled out of class to do individualized physical therapy for strengthening, Luke's exercises should be incorporated into his normal routine. Specific exercises, such as sit ups and bridges, are difficult to get Luke to do and can get boring for anyone. More general exercises, such as walking, climbing stairs, swimming, and horseback riding, can be helpful in improving the strength of specific muscle groups, as well as promote aerobic fitness. Encouraging Luke to learn to swim using a different stroke (breaststroke, butterfly, backstroke, or dolphin kick) than his usual modified side stroke can help develop strength in his abdominal muscles, hips and shoulders. Strokes may have to be modified because he will not tolerate putting his face in the water yet. Temporary use of a flotation device, if tolerated, may encourage Luke to learn a different stroke.
3. Luke needs to prevent further loss of range of motion in his ankles to preserve his mobility skills (walking, running, etc.).
   - Teaching Luke supervised active stretching exercises can be more effective than applying passive stretching. He can lean into a wall or lunge to stretch his heel cords. If the stretching exercises are built into his routine, such as whenever he puts on his shoes or changes his clothes, they can be done more regularly and be more effective. Other activities to help stretch his heel cords can include having him walk up a small grade (on a weekly family hike and between classes at school), active stretching in regular physical education classes in which Luke is included, walking up and down stairs on his way to classes at school, squatting activities on the floor during regular activities at home and school, and a trial of high-topped shoes to encourage more normal ankle alignment.
4. Luke needs to maintain and improve his aerobic fitness level.
   - Luke should continue to participate in family hiking activities, as well as Special Olympics, challenger baseball, and therapeutic horseback riding. These types of aerobic activity can allow him access to varied social situations, as well as help him maintain and improve his strength and cardiovascular conditioning. Individual exercise, including swimming, stationary bicycle, walking or running, would be appropriate for Luke. Team sports are more unpredictable and would be difficult for him.
5. Luke needs more independent bathing skills.
   - His parents intend to get a temperature-regulated faucet after they move, so that Luke can have more independence in drawing his bath. A long-handled, soft bath brush may help Luke to be more independent washing himself. Because he has difficulty in touching the grab bar in the tub when it is wet, perhaps drying both the bar and Luke's hand at the end of the bath, or placing a dry washcloth on the bar will make using it more acceptable to him.
6. Luke needs more independent toothbrushing skills.
   - A mechanical toothbrush may help Luke be more independent in brushing his teeth, although he may not tolerate the vibrations. Trials of various types may be necessary to find one he will use.
7. Luke needs to participate with regular peers in school to develop better social and academic skills.
   - Luke should be included in regular education activities whenever appropriate with a goal of full-time inclusion. This may be more difficult as Luke progresses into high school. He responds to peers and is aware of and enjoys his interactions with others. He is capable of academic work and is able to participate with others in a small group. Luke's physical therapy goals should be integrated into his overall educational plan. Rather than being pulled out of class for individual therapy, his exercise needs should be included into the routines of the day to be done with peer support and participation.
8. Luke needs to continue his academic progress in both verbal and quantitative skills.
   - Luke's educational goals should include academic progress in both verbal and quantitative skills. He needs to use a computer in the classroom and at home for repetition of skills and to maintain his interest.
9. Luke needs regular routines during the day to maintain his coping skills.
   - Change is difficult for Luke. Each day should have the same routine if possible. If the routine is changed, he needs to be given adequate preparation. Extra supervision and support from family or familiar school staff should be given if a major change in routine is expected.

BOX 10-3   Sample Individual Education Program Objectives

By the end of the school year Luke will:

1. Respond using three to four word responses to questions from classmates or teachers during an academic activity.
2. With verbal prompts, such as "my name is . . . ," state his name, address, and telephone number.
3. Read a 4-page book and correctly answer five questions out loud requiring two- to three-word answers regarding the content.
4. Write a complete sentence on the computer with verbal prompts.
5. Add and subtract three-digit numbers using the computer or a handheld calculator, and speak the answer when asked. Number places need to be included (e.g., one hundred twenty-five, rather than one-two-five).
6. Greet three new classmates by name when prompted.
7. Actively stretch his heel cords three times per day at home and at school with verbal and physical prompts.
8. Learn a new swimming stroke and be able to swim half the length of a standard pool using the new stroke in 5 minutes with verbal prompts.
9. With one-on-one assistance of a peer, aide, or instructor, follow along and approximate the exercises during a standard 5-minute stretching routine in physical education class.
10. Run around the entire athletic field with his class without stopping. Verbal and physical prompts are acceptable.
11. Climb out of the swimming pool using the ladder with stand-by assistance during three consecutive swimming sessions.

---

heavy for her to lift. Sometimes it takes him 10 minutes to get out of the tub.

Luke sits with his mother and father at the table to eat dinner. Fish sticks are one of his favorite dishes, and he stabs the fish cakes onto his fork carefully. The television is on, and a show has just ended. Luke watches the credits roll by, his favorite part. He waits to take another bite until they have finished.

After dinner his mother helps him brush his teeth. He needs hand-over-hand help to do a good job. He swallows the toothpaste and makes a spitting sound when his mother asks him to spit it out. After brushing, he goes into his room to watch videos until bedtime. His favorite videotape uses cartoon characters to teach small children how to brush their teeth. Luke loves it and laughs out loud at his favorite parts. His mother comes in to turn off the light and give him a kiss goodnight. Luke smiles at her and turns over to go to sleep. His eyes close right away.

● BACKGROUND AND THEORY

Most of us have been educated to believe that intelligence is a linear trait that can be measured, and that persons with different amounts of it are worth more or less in society. How simple it would be if all people could be categorized in terms of their intelligence. Students who are alike could be grouped together to give them the exact intervention that would help them succeed. Students could be guided to the occupations that were suited to their particular intelligence.

This view of intelligence as an innate linear property that can be measured is being challenged by new theories of multiple intelligences, which are changing the face of many classrooms. The decreased emphasis on the linear concept of intelligence as measured by linguistic and logical skills, with a greater emphasis on diverse skills and behaviors has also changed the definition and treatment of mental retardation. Rather than grouping children with cognitive and other "differences" together, and either accepting or looking to remedy their weaknesses, service providers are now searching for the strengths and skills that each child possesses and building on these to help children be functional members of society.

In this chapter, developmental disorders, including mental retardation, autism, pervasive developmental disability (PDD), learning disorders (LD), and attention-deficit hyperactivity disorder (ADHD), will be discussed from the perspective of a provider of physical therapy services. Developmental problems related to exposure to environmental threats, such as maternal alcohol and drug use, and maternal exposure to cytomegalovirus, will also be discussed. Finally, sensory disorders, including blindness, deafness, and multiple sensory impairments, will be explored.

A case study of Luke, a boy with autism, will help the reader understand the extended effects of this disorder on a child and his family. A special section on positive behavioral supports provides an overview of current theory addressing severe behavioral challenges. This perspective focuses on providing positive supports for persons and views challenging behaviors as having important communicative functions. The section also gives ideas to prevent or address behavior problems of a milder nature.

Developmental Disability

According to the Comprehensive Services and Developmental Disabilities Amendment of 1978 and Public Law 95-602, a *developmental disability* is a severe, chronic disability that:

- Is a mental and/or physical impairment;
- Is manifested before the age of 22;
- Is likely to continue throughout life;
- Substantially limits functioning in three or more of the following areas: self-care, receptive and expressive language, learning, mobility, self-direction, capacity for independent living, economic self sufficiency; and
- Results in a need for individualized, interdisciplinary services of extended duration.

Many severe disorders of childhood fall into this category, and many, but not all, disorders described in this chapter are de-

TABLE 10-1 Categorization of Mental Skills by IQ and Functional Skills

Intelligence quotient score	Older educational designations	DSM-IV definition of mental retardation	Description of typical functional skills
70-75 to 125-130	Average intelligence	Average intelligence	Average functional skills.
50-55 to 70-75	Educable retarded	Mildly retarded	Development in language and other skills is slower than normal. Can learn academic skills to a third to sixth grade level. Can be self-supporting with appropriate social skills and some support.
35-40 to 50-55	Trainable retarded	Moderately retarded	Development noticeably delayed in all areas. Needs support for life skills including self-care. Can work in a sheltered environment. Does not learn reading and arithmetic to a functional level.
20-25 to 35-40	Dependent retarded	Severely retarded	Marked delay in developmental skills. May not develop speech. Can be taught to do some self-care skills, such as self-feeding. Can conform to daily routines but needs a protected environment for continuous support and supervision.
Below 20-25	Life support	Profoundly retarded	May develop physical skills, such as walking, but needs total care in all areas. Will not develop speech. Responds emotionally to situations by smiling or becoming angry. Profound retardation may accompany other disabilities, which are severe in nature.

velopmental disabilities. Children with mental retardation, autism, and multiple sensory impairments may fall under this definition. Other disorders covered in this chapter, including some cases of blindness, deafness, learning disorders, developmental coordination disorders, and attention deficit hyperactivity disorder, fall more loosely under the umbrella of developmental disorders and are included in this chapter because they share many related issues.

Developmental Delay

Young children with differences in developmental skills are usually diagnosed with developmental delay. Developmental delays in young children frequently involve language skills but may also include social skills, gross motor, or fine motor skills. These delays may develop into a developmental disability or, with maturation, may fade as the child catches up with peers. Children whose early diagnosed delays in development fade may experience learning disabilities or other differences when they reach school age, or the children may develop typically as they grow older. For this reason, physicians are reluctant to diagnose mental retardation, autism, or mild cerebral palsy when children are young.

Children With Mental Retardation

The definition of mental retardation that is widely accepted today was developed by the American Association of Mental Retardation (AAMR) in 1992.

Mental retardation refers to substantial limitations in present functioning. It is characterized by significantly subaverage intellectual functioning existing concurrently with related limitations in two or more of the following applicable adaptive skills areas: communication, self-care, home living, social skills, community use, self-direction, health and safety, functional academics, leisure, and work. Mental retardation manifests before age 18 (American Association on Mental Retardation, 1992, p. 1).

Although the 1992 definition is in current use, reviewing parts of the 1983 AAMR definition of mental retardation is prudent, as many service providers are still using some terminology defined there. In the 1983 definition, a person with mental retardation was classified as mildly, moderately, severely, or profoundly retarded, based on his or her score on an IQ test. Although limitations in adaptive skills were included as part of the definition, emphasis was on the quantification of intellectual skills to categorize people with mental retardation and reflect a prognosis for future functioning.

This quantification is not a part of the 1992 definition of mental retardation. In 1992 the AAMR revised the definition to emphasize a person's functional or adaptive skills rather than the IQ score. Both definitions rely on the same factors of (1) a low IQ score, and (2) deficits in adaptive skills. The newer definition, however, does not quantify the level of mental retardation according to the IQ test results but relies on a description of a child's strengths, weaknesses, and needs that details the child's present function and a prognosis for function in the future.

Both the low IQ score and the described adaptive skill deficits must be manifested before the child's eighteenth birthday. If these signs occur later, the deficits are classified as dementia or adult onset cognitive deficit rather than mental retardation.

Some controversy exists today around the new definition (Palmer & Capute, 1994). Detractors believe that a description of the child's skills is not adequate to predict future functioning. Their opponents believe that the greater emphasis on adaptive functioning is more reflective of the child's skills and prognosis than IQ scoring. Regardless of your position, it is important to be familiar with categorization based on IQ scoring. Many of the "old" terms used to describe mental retardation related to the IQ score continue to be used and, in fact, are incorporated into other commonly used current definitions. The most recent *Diagnostic and Statistical Manual of Mental Disorders,* fourth edition *(DSM-IV),* of the Americal Psychological Association (1995) categorizes mental retardation according to scores on IQ tests. Table 10-1 outlines different categorizations of persons with mental retardation throughout recent history.

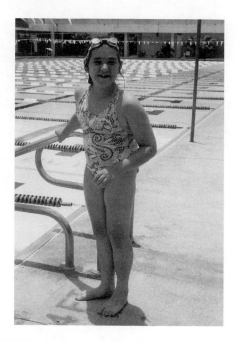

Figure 10-7 Dawn, a 17-year-old girl with mental retardation, enjoys swimming in the Special Olympics. She is smaller than other girls her age.

Incidence and Cause

The incidence of mental retardation is approximately 1% of the general population (Figure 10-7). Causes are varied but can be divided into biological, organic, and sociocultural reasons. Common biological causes of mental retardation include genetic defects, such as Down syndrome and fragile X syndrome; organic causes, including maternal drug abuse, alcohol abuse, and viral infections; or perinatal causes, including asphyxia and birth trauma. Sociocultural causes can include neglect and abuse; environmental deprivation arising from poverty, lack of education, lack of opportunity; and cultural differences, which may not be accounted for using a standardized test.

The most common understood cause of mental retardation in the United States is Down syndrome, comprising approximately 8% to 10% of persons with mental retardation (Aman, Hammer, & Rojahn, 1993). Down syndrome is discussed at length in Chapter 8. The second most common chromosomal abnormality causing mental retardation is fragile X syndrome, which is described further in this chapter. Although some causes of mental retardation are known, 50% to 65% of all cases arise from poorly understood factors that occurred before birth (Kolb & Brodie, 1982).

Most mental retardation is caused not by one factor alone but by a constellation of factors. An example might be a child born with mild fetal alcohol syndrome who lives in an abusive home and is not sent to school. Although this child will have intrinsic difficulties caused by the alcohol exposure in utero, the potential he or she is capable of may not be reached because of the limited environmental resources.

Fifty percent of the children identified with mental retardation will have only mild deficits, 30% will have moderate retardation, 15% will have severe retardation, and 5% will have pro-

found retardation (Baroff, 1986). The majority of children with moderate to profound retardation will generally need supportive services throughout their lives, whereas the majority of those with mild levels will be more independent.

Clinical Description

Because the causes of mental retardation are varied and multifactorial, children with mental retardation can look very different from each other. A spectrum of clinical pictures of children with mental retardation are described in other sections of this chapter and in other chapters of this book. In some of the disorders described, all the children affected may have some degree of mental retardation, and in other disorders only some will have mental retardation. Chapter 7 describes cerebral palsy. Chapter 8 discusses disorders related to genetic causes, including Down syndrome and Prader-Willi syndrome. Chapter 9 describes children with traumatic injuries that may lead to mental retardation, including traumatic brain injury and near drowning accidents. Children with each of these disorders may look very different from each other.

Language deficits are usually the first to surface in a child with mental retardation. Also common are mild motor delays in those with mental retardation as a primary diagnosis. Of the children with mental retardation, 10% to 20% will have significant auditory or visual deficits, 20% to 30% will have motor deficits, 10% to 20% will have a seizure disorder, and 30% to 40% will have neurobehavioral or psychiatric disorders (Palmer & Capute, 1994). Short stature and facial dysmorphia are seen in children with mental retardation more commonly than in typically developing children. Behavior problems, such as stereotypical or purposeless behavior, self-abusive or aggressive behavior, and hyperactivity, are also seen more frequently in children with mental retardation. Many children are not identified as having mental retardation until school age, when problems with academics become apparent. Children from lower socioeconomic groups are more likely to have mental retardation than children from higher socioeconomic groups. This reflects, in part, the effects of environment on the development of cognitive functioning.

Fragile X syndrome. Fragile X is a sex-linked chromosomal abnormality of the X chromosome that is most frequently and most severely manifested by male offspring of female carriers of the disorder. Although only identified in 1969, it is today recognized as one of the most common genetic causes of mental retardation, second only to Down syndrome (Dykens, Hodapp, & Leckman, 1994; Hagerman, 1987). It occurs in 1 in 1000 males, and 1 in 750 females. Although females are usually carriers, they may also manifest some characteristics of the disorder.

Classic characteristics of males with fragile X syndrome include mental retardation, a long narrow face, large protruding ears, a prominent forehead, a prominent chin, a high palate, flattened nasal bridge, large hands and feet, and large testes after puberty (Figure 10-8). Boys may have temper tantrums, learning problems, and speech difficulties, which may include rapid speech, stuttering, and repetition of words (Levine, Carey, Crocker, & Gross, 1992). Some boys will exhibit autism. Some children with fragile X syndrome may have hypotonia, poor coordination and motor planning, seizures, and scoliosis. Most will have a prolapse of the mitral valve in the heart. About 20% of

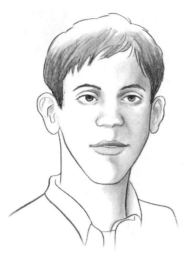

Figure 10-8 Classic features of a boy with fragile X syndrome include a long face and large ears.

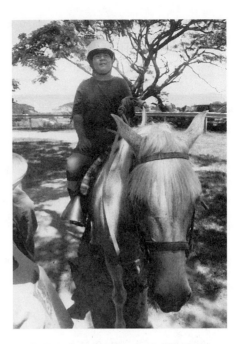

Figure 10-9 Grant, a boy with Prader-Willi syndrome, was given physical therapy as a young child for hypotonia and delay of gross motor skills.

boys with the genetic defect will not have the classic characteristics, but they will transmit the gene to their offspring. The degree of mental retardation is variable from severe to borderline, with most children falling into the severe to moderate range. The degree of mental retardation may increase as the child gets older and increasingly complex activities are required.

Up to 50% of girls who have the gene will have some cognitive or neuropsychiatric symptoms, such as a learning disorder, including 30% to 35% with mild mental retardation (Palmer & Capute, 1994).

Rett syndrome. Although much less common than fragile X syndrome, Rett syndrome is increasingly recognized by clinical symptoms. It is thought to be genetically passed because it only affects girls, although a genetic marker has not yet been identified. It affects about 1 in 15,000 female births. Girls with Rett syndrome have progressive loss of hand function, changes in muscle tone, and severe to profound mental retardation. Symptoms are not evident until about 6 to 18 months of age, when progressive microcephaly, hypotonia that develops into hypertonia, ataxia, and seizures develop. Scoliosis is not uncommon, and stereotypic behaviors of hand wringing, clapping, tapping, and rubbing, as well as episodes of hyperventilation, are common. Lack of communication skills and social isolation also characterize girls with Rett syndrome. Because this disorder is diagnosed by progressive symptoms in a classic pattern, diagnosis cannot usually be definite until about 2 to 5 years of age.

Treatment

Some forms of mental retardation can be prevented. Preventable causes include traumatic brain injury; mental retardation related to untreated phenylketonuria, a genetic inability to metabolize certain proteins; and abuse and neglect. Efforts are being made throughout the country to minimize trauma to children related to motor vehicle accidents, bicycle accidents, and other recreational and sporting accidents. Bicycle helmets, seatbelts, infant and toddler car seats, and other safety devices are reducing deaths and injuries related to these events. Child protective ser-

vices, although overwhelmed in many parts of the country, is addressing issues of abuse and neglect in individual cases. Head Start and other early childhood programs to reach families at risk are very successful in providing support to families to reduce the incidence of environmental deprivation. Public education about the negative effects on a fetus of maternal drinking and ingestion of drugs is addressing these problems. Medical advances in recognizing and early treatment of phenylketonuria and other metabolic diseases that can be treated to minimize negative effects on children continue to be made. Although efforts are being made to prevent mental retardation, there is still much progress to be made to combat all the negative social and medical circumstances that can lead to this disorder.

Children with mental retardation can receive help to optimize their development and to manage related disorders, such as cerebral palsy, blindness, deafness, language delays, deficits in adaptive skills, and behavior disorders. With appropriate intervention, children will develop more skills and become more functional in society than without intervention.

Physical therapy intervention. A child with mental retardation may be seen by physical therapy for related motor problems, such as cerebral palsy, hypotonia, or ataxia (Figure 10-9). Children may also be seen for orthopedic problems related to congenital disorders, such as clubfoot, or related to injury, such as a lower extremity fracture. Each of these disorders is considered in detail in other chapters, yet there are some issues about working with a child with mental retardation that are important to note.

Each child is unique, with his or her own personality, behaviors, physical characteristics, coping mechanisms, and support system. It is important to have a general picture of the child and to be aware of specific needs and interventions that may affect the delivery of physical therapy services, such as a behavior plan; likes and dislikes; family structure, involvement and concerns;

Supportive Practices for Child With Mental Retardation

1. Keep concepts clear and simple.
2. Break down activities into small steps.
3. Ask a child to do only one or two steps at a time.
4. Talk to child. Do not turn to parent or caregiver assuming child cannot respond.
5. Use same tone of voice you would use with other children of similar age.
6. Use visual, auditory, and tactile cues. Demonstrate activity, point to object, repeat concepts in several different ways so child can understand.
7. Ask if the child wants help before stepping in.
8. Allow the child extra time to respond. He or she may take more time to organize thoughts or become aware of you.

Ask family members, teachers, peers, and classroom aides for clues to the meaning behind the behavior of a child who is not verbal. Siblings frequently have unique insights. This understanding can make the difference between feeling a connection to the child or not.

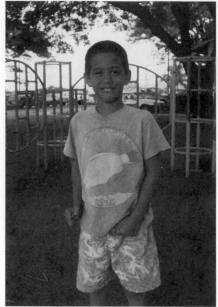

Figure 10-10 Daniel, a boy with probable Asperger syndrome, was willing to smile for a photograph and wanted to look closely into the lens to see how it worked.

and medical history. Related disorders, including blindness, deafness, severe behavioral challenges, or sensory defensiveness, need to be considered when planning interventions for a child with mental retardation.

Children with mental retardation need help and encouragement to succeed at activities other children can do by themselves. Box 10-4 outlines supportive behaviors that can be helpful when working with a child with mental retardation.

The Child With a Pervasive Developmental Disorder

The term *pervasive developmental disorder (PPD)*, as defined by the *Diagnostic and Statistical Manual of Mental Disorders,* fourth edition *(DSM-IV)* (American Psychological Association, 1995), indicates a class of developmental disorders with five subcategories: autistic disorder, Rett's disorder, childhood disintegrative disorder, Asperger disorder, and pervasive developmental disorder not otherwise specified (PDDNOS). Children with PDD have impairment in social interactions; have deficiencies in verbal and nonverbal communication; and have restrictive, repetitive, and stereotyped patterns of behavior (American Psychological Association, 1995). These three qualities are called the triad of symptoms characteristic of PDD.

Asperger Syndrome

Asperger syndrome, described by Hans Asperger in 1944, shares many of the core problems of autism, but differs from it signifi-

cantly, as well. Deficits in social interaction, differences in speech and language, poor nonverbal communication, rigid routines and interests, and clumsiness characterize a child with Asperger syndrome (Figure 10-10). The child will be more functional than a child with autism, but will have many similar features, including decreased facial expression, peculiar voice characteristics, and difficulties with communication. The child with Asperger syndrome will usually have verbal skills and will be able to attend to information in an educational environment. Scores on IQ tests are usually normal (Szatmari, 1991). A main differentiating feature of Asperger syndrome from autism is that with appropriate accommodations and educational methodology, persons with Asperger syndrome may achieve "near-normal behavior" (Frith, 1991).

Autism

Autism is a spectrum of disorders, all of which have similar features, but in different degrees. Autism is a neurobiological disorder related to specific abnormalities in brain function. It manifests itself in social and communication differences that are related to the deficits in brain functioning. Although each child is unique, several features of autism are common and can be useful to describe the disorder. Children with autism (1) fail to develop normal socialization; (2) have disturbances in speech, language, and communication; (3) have abnormal relationships to objects and events; (4) have abnormal responses to sensory stimulation; (5) have developmental delays and differences; and (6) develop these disorders during infancy or early childhood (Powers, 1989).

Incidence and cause. Autism occurs in 1 or 2 in every 1000 births. This is about as common as Down syndrome. Boys are two to four times more likely to be diagnosed with autism as girls (Frith, 1993).

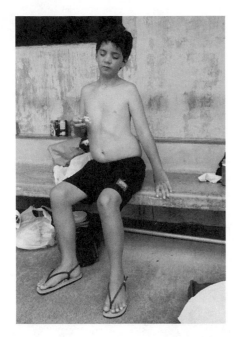

Figure 10-11 Luke perches on the bench to eat his sandwich. He attempts to have the least physical contact possible with the bench.

Autism was first described simultaneously in 1943 in the United States by Kanner and in Germany by Asperger (Frith, 1993). For decades, it was thought to be a psychological disorder caused by a traumatic event, rejection, or poor bonding with a child's mother. Parents were frequently blamed for the disorder, the theory being that rigid, emotionally unreachable parents caused children to withdraw socially. Children often looked physically normal and may have had average intellectual ability, but they withdrew socially and lived in what appeared to be a separate fantasy world. The image of a child in a glass bubble was used to describe the child with autism, with the concurrent belief that if the glass could be shattered, an intact child could be freed to live a normal life.

These theories have now been discounted. Autism is a neurobiological disorder, not a psychological one. Parents are now viewed as valuable resources in helping children learn to live in society and develop to their full potential. It is recognized that there is no glass bubble, and that children with autism have significant disability that is lifelong. The scars from the early attitudes, which blamed parents for their children's disabilities, still hurt, but the positive approaches to helping children develop functional skills are building new ways to reach and help children with autism live in the world today.

Recent studies have demonstrated a genetic factor in at least some cases (Bolton & Rutter, 1990; Smalley, 1991). Structural abnormalities in the brains of persons with autism have been identified, although a specific abnormality is not yet associated directly with the disorder (Frith, 1993). Specific medical conditions frequently associated with autism include fragile X syndrome and tuberous sclerosis, among many others (Gillberg & Coleman, 1996). Autism has been associated with mental retardation, especially in children with low IQ scores (Frith, 1993; Nordin & Gillberg, 1996). All this information leads to the conclusion that autism is a spectrum of disorders related to a specific brain abnormality that can be more or less extensive, leading to a range

Typical Behaviors of Child With Autism

BOX 10-5

A. Stereotypical Movements
   1. Hand flicking
   2. Head banging
   3. Spinning
   4. Rocking
   5. Complex whole-body movements
B. Preoccupation with parts of objects or specific actions of objects
   1. Spinning wheels of toy cars
   2. Lining up toys precisely
   3. Sniffing or smelling objects
   4. Feeling texture of objects repetitively
   5. Carrying around an unusual object (piece of string, dust bunny, cigarette butt)
C. Distress (tantrum) over minute changes in environment (mother sewed a new button on shirt, picture moved a few inches)
D. Distress (tantrum) over small changes in routine (starting in a different isle when shopping, parking in a different spot, taking a bath before supper instead of after)
E. Narrow range of interests (lining up objects, telephone numbers)
F. Speech and language differences
   1. Echolalic speech
   2. Appears to be deaf
G. Poor social skills
   1. Does not mix with other children, stands apart
   2. Poor eye contact
   3. Inappropriate laughing or giggling

of concurrent disorders, such as mental retardation or seizures (Frith, 1993).

Clinical features. The triad of clinical features found in all cases of autism includes impairments in communication, imagination, and socialization. Other features common to children with autism include abnormal relationships to objects and events, abnormal responses to sensory stimulation, and developmental delays and differences (Figure 10-11). Box 10-5 lists some behaviors that may be seen in a child with autism.

Impairments in communication. Communication includes both expressive and receptive language skills, as well as nonverbal communication. Children with autism may not understand or use gestural communication, including waving, beckoning, shrugging, or head shaking. They may develop early vocabulary and sentence patterns that are lost after a few years, but 40% never develop speech at all (Powers, 1989). Those that do develop speech may only repeat what they hear, called *echolalic* speech. For example, Luke (Case Study, this chapter) repeats "Want a cookie?" when his mother asks him, "Do you want a cookie?" Some children are able to repeat entire television commercials. Luke watches videos repetitively, and speaks and sings along with the characters in the videos. A child with autism usually speaks in a voice that is flat and monotonous, or high pitched and loud, but is not expressive of emotion.

Impairments in socialization. Children with autism are not likely to give eye contact or, if they do, it may be vacant or staring. For instance, Luke will smile in response to a social smile but cannot maintain eye contact longer than a second or two. Children with autism do not recognize or respond to social greetings or other social cues and prefer to be alone much of the time. Luke likes to sit alone in his room looking at books, videos, or playing on his computer. Physical contact is often distasteful to children with autism, and they will pull away or resist hugging or kissing. Luke's mother taught him how to hug her when he came home from school, and he tolerates it woodenly. The hugs help his mother feel better.

Impairments in imagination. What used to be thought of as a child's withdrawal into a fantasy world is now seen as a lack of imagination. A child with autism may play with an object in the same way repetitively, such as spinning a plate over and over again, rather than finding new ways to interact with the object. A child with autism is interested in objects and activities that are predictable, such as computer games and video games, rather than objects and activities that require imagination, such as costumes or abstract coloring.

Abnormal relationships to objects and events. Structure and sameness are very important to a child with autism. He or she is much more comfortable when the routine is predictable and has difficulty adapting to changes. An example is Luke's increased anxiety and escalation of abnormal behaviors when his family routines changed during and after their move to a new house. Even seemingly minor changes in routine can wreak havoc in a household. For instance, getting new pajamas, putting a toothbrush away in a different place, a snow day from school, or brushing teeth before a bath rather than afterward could all cause major disruptions. Children with autism tend to interact with objects in stereotypical ways. For instance, rather than building castles or forts, a child with autism may organize the blocks by color or shape or size. Dropping blocks onto the floor to hear the sound may be more engaging than stacking them to create something. Objects, such as ashtrays or plates, may have more attraction than toys because they can be spun, dropped, or categorized.

Abnormal responses to sensory stimulation. Children with autism may have a heightened awareness of some sensory input. Other sensory input may be completely ignored or tuned out. Because of this abnormal response, autism is sometimes seen as being at least partially a sensory processing disorder (Figure 10-12).

Parents sometimes test their children for deafness because loud noises do not startle them, or they do not seem to hear the voices of people speaking. Children frequently cannot tolerate physical contact, including cuddling, hugging, hand shaking, or physical direction. Certain sounds, textures, and sights may be distressing. For instance, Luke refuses to wear T-shirts with an appliquéd design because he does not like the feeling against his skin. Some T-shirts he will only wear inside out. Children may refuse certain foods because of their texture or refuse to go certain places, such as a ferry boat or a department store, because of the sounds (horns, overhead loudspeakers). On the other hand, certain forms of sensory stimulation are sought out. Stereotypical behaviors, such as hand flapping, are thought to provide visual stimulation. Other behaviors, such as spinning, provide vestibular stimulation. Some children with autism are attracted to lights, especially lights that blink or flicker.

Developmental delays and differences. Children with autism may exhibit delays in some areas of development and signifi-

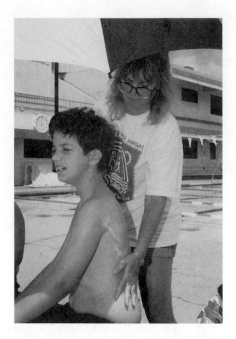

Figure 10-12 Luke hates when his mother puts on sunblock lotion. He squirms and wriggles, and she has to stop frequently to reassure him.

cant differences from other children in other areas. For instance, Luke's mother thought that he was superior to other children in his age group when he was a toddler because he could figure out complex shape-matching toys. Yet he preferred to play by himself and did not develop social skills of interacting with other children. Even in one skill area there may be significant variation in skills. For example, a child with autism may develop an extensive vocabulary but not be able to use the words functionally.

Behavior. Because of difficulty in verbal communication, nonverbal communication, such as screaming, temper tantrums, or social withdrawal, may be common. These behaviors may be related to adverse environmental stimuli, such as physical contact, noises, or changes in routine. Often the cause of the behavior is not immediately clear. These behaviors are often difficult to tolerate by peers, parents, teachers, and other caregivers, because they are either passively or violently antisocial. Until the communicative intent of the behaviors is recognized and the environment can be structured to accommodate the child's needs, the behaviors may not decrease.

Repetitive and apparently purposeless behaviors are characteristic of many persons with autism. These behaviors are commonly known as *stereotypical behaviors*. A classic example is hand flapping near the eyes. Stereotypical behaviors may interfere with education or socialization.

Behaviors that are injurious to the child with autism or to others may occur and are more likely when the child has severe mental retardation, as well as autism. Self-injurious behaviors can be challenging to change because the cause is often not clear. Head banging, skin picking or scratching, face slapping, or hand biting are some self-injurious behaviors that may be encountered. Aggressive behaviors, such as hitting or biting others, also may be difficult to change. Medical treatments to address these behaviors are described in the following section.

Treatment. Autism as a medical condition has not shown significant change from any particular treatment regimen. However, some medical and behavioral interventions are helpful in treating the behaviors that are often associated with autism.

Neuroleptic drugs are tranquilizers that reduce dopamine activity in the brain. Some neuroleptic drugs include thioridazine (Mellaril), chlorpromazine (Thorazine), and haloperidol (Haldol). These drugs have been shown to be helpful in decreasing self-injurious and stereotypical behaviors for children with autism, as well as to increase their attention span, which allows them to learn in school. Side effects of these drugs can be significant, so the team needs to monitor their effects carefully. *Tardive dyskinesia* is a serious side effect that typically occurs after long periods (years) of treatment and includes facial grimaces and unusual movements of the body and hands. It is thought that these abnormal movements come from a changed sensitivity to neurotransmitters that develops after extended periods of using the drugs. Tardive dyskinesia can occur even after the drugs have been stopped and is irreversible.

Structuring the environment can allow the child with autism to improve functional skills within that environment. Attention to maintaining routine and preparing for changes in routine can help a child accommodate minor changes more easily. Giving positive feedback, including praise, may be effective; and using rewards for desired behavior, such as allowing a child extra time on the computer, can also be helpful. Training teachers, peers, and staff at school can help support a child in the school environment. The Applications section in this chapter discusses positive behavior supports, including looking for the communicative function of behavior. These activities can support the child with autism to succeed in school.

Facilitated communication. Facilitated communication was developed in the 1980s as a technique to "unlock" the voice of children with autism and other nonverbal disabilities. A "facilitator" helps the child type his or her message on a typewriter, communication board, or augmentative communication device, simply by holding the child's hand, arm, or sleeve.

After several incidences of children reportedly complaining about sexual abuse through facilitated communication and being removed from their families, many people raised serious questions about the validity of the facilitated communications. When valid research studies were performed on the technique, it was shown that the facilitator controlled the communication in most or all cases, and the child was not actually communicating at all. Most facilitators sincerely believed that they were only "facilitating," and were appalled at the results of studies. This is an example of the "glass jar" myth, misleading people into thinking that they could "unlock" the person inside. Facilitated communication is still being used with some persons with autism and still has proponents, but much of the scientific world has essentially abandoned the technique.

Alternative treatments. Although vitamin therapy has not been approved for autism, many parents are convinced that large doses of some vitamins and minerals, especially vitamin B6 and magnesium, have helped their children with autism to improve behavior, tolerance, and functional skills. Special diets have also been advocated for children with autism, but there has not yet been adequate research to prove the effectiveness of these interventions.

> **BOX 10-6**
> ## Supportive Practices for Child With Autism
>
> 1. Speak clearly.
> 2. Keep instructions simple.
> 3. Try to make sure the child is facing you before talking. This way the child gets visual as well as auditory cues that you are talking.
> 4. Structure your activities the same from day to day.
> 5. Prepare the child for changes in routine.
> 6. Be aware of the child's behaviors and responses to changes in routine, and how to handle adverse behaviors.
> 7. Be patient.
> 8. Encourage verbal and other appropriate responses from the child.
> 9. Involve the child in social situations, even if he or she is reluctant to be included.

Physical therapy intervention. A PT may see the child with autism who has deficits in gross motor skills. Some children are clumsy, have poor balance, decreased strength, or delays in gross motor skills, including climbing stairs, jumping, or running. A child with autism may be seen individually for therapy or may be included in a gross motor group or class that a therapist or physical therapist assistant (PTA) is leading. It is important for the therapy provider to be familiar with the child's behavioral protocol and be comfortable in implementing it. The protocol might include setting limits on certain behaviors or giving particular consequences for certain behaviors. The protocol may also spell out which behaviors are to be encouraged and how this might be done. For instance, a child with autism might be encouraged to work with another child on a particular skill to improve social skills along with the gross motor skills. Box 10-6 lists supportive behaviors that can help when working with a child with autism.

Other Types of PDD

Children with Rett's disorder, also known as Rett syndrome, have been described in this chapter in the section on mental retardation. Children with the triad of symptoms characteristic of PDD who do not display features of autism are categorized as having PDD not otherwise specified (PDDNOS). Other terms that have been applied to these children include atypical autism, autistic-like condition, and autistic "traits" (Nordin & Gillberg, 1996).

Disorders Without Identifiable Neurological Pathology

The diagnosis and treatment of children with clumsiness, incoordination, academic difficulties, attention difficulties, or hyperactivity has been difficult and somewhat inconsistent over the past few decades as efforts have been made to understand these disorders. The term used to describe most disorders that do not appear to have identifiable neurological causes has changed from *minimal brain dysfunction (MBD)* to *hyperkinetic syndrome of childhood.* Subcategories of problems identified under this umbrella have included learning disabilities, specific learning disability, attention-deficit disorder, attention-deficit hyperactivity disorder, developmental coordination disorder, dyspraxia, and somatodyspraxia.

In the newest version of the *DSM-IV*, developmental coordination disorder is classified by itself as a motor skills disorder. It is a problem frequently referred to physical therapy in school-aged children. Attention-deficit hyperactivity disorder is another disorder that may have motor consequences. These and learning disorders are the major categories that will be addressed in this section. Children whose problems fall into one of these categories may also have problems in another. For instance, a child with a learning disability may also have a developmental coordination disorder.

Learning Disabilities

Academic education has become important for persons from all socioeconomic levels as jobs that do not require academic skills become fewer and jobs that do require academic skills become more prevalent. Children who used to be dismissed from school because they had "no aptitude" are now expected to succeed in school. Teachers and administrators are more familiar with diagnosing and addressing children's learning problems and are less apt to label the children "lazy" or "stupid." They recognize that there is an underlying cause of the disability, and fault cannot be attributed to the child or family. Since the Education of the Handicapped Act, also known as Public Law 94-142, was passed by the legislature in 1975, all school districts have been required to provide an appropriate education to children with disabilities, including those with learning disabilities.

The Individuals with Disabilities Education Act (IDEA), also known as Public Law 101-476, defines a child with a learning disability as someone who does not achieve academically commensurate with age and ability levels in one or more of the following areas: oral expression, listening comprehension, written expression, basic reading skills, reading comprehension, mathematics calculation, or mathematical reasoning. This discrepancy cannot be due to a visual, hearing, or motor handicap; mental retardation; emotional disturbance; or environmental, cultural or economic disadvantage (Bateman, 1996).

Incidence and cause. The incidence of learning disabilities varies depending on the specific definition given, but it may be up to 10% of school-aged children (National Information Center for Children and Youth with Disabilities, 1993). Usually the cause of learning disabilities is unknown. Therefore the term *learning disability* should be applied only after all other causes for the academic difficulties have been ruled out. Boys are seven times more likely than girls to be diagnosed with a learning disability, with 10% of all boys likely to have some reading difficulty (Smith, Centerwall, & Centerwall, 1983).

Clinical features. Each child with a learning disability is unique and must be evaluated individually. However, two major categories of learning disabilities include (1) those that involve difficulty with basic academic skills, such as reading, writing, spelling, arithmetic, and language (both comprehension and expression) and (2) those that involve skills that surround the

learning of academic skills, such as persistence, organization, impulse control, social competence, and coordination (Selikowitz, 1993). Children may have difficulties in any one or in several of these areas.

The defined fields of learning disorders in the *DSM IV* include reading disorder, mathematics disorder, disorder of written expression, and learning disorder, not otherwise specified. Many other terms exist to describe these disorders, however. Some of them are described here.

The term *specific learning disability* can be defined as "an unexpected and unexplained condition, occurring in a child of average or above average intelligence, characterized by a significant delay in one or more areas of learning" (Selikowitz, 1993). Of the children with a specific learning disability 75% to 80% have difficulty with language and reading. *Dyslexia,* a term meaning a reading disability, is still commonly used.

Another common designation for children with learning disabilities is problems with *central auditory processing.* These children have difficulty understanding, or processing, what they hear, although hearing acuity is normal. The inability to understand spoken language in a meaningful way can result in an inability to follow directions, the appearance of laziness, distractibility, or even deafness. Other terms used to describe this disability include auditory comprehension deficit, central deafness, work deafness, and auditory perceptual processing dysfunction.

Intervention. Special education teachers are trained in educational techniques to address problems children have with academic skills. Providing a team evaluation of a student who is performing significantly less than age or ability indicate is a necessary first step.

Physical therapy may be involved if the child has problems with coordination, balance, or age-appropriate gross motor skills. Other team members may be from nursing, occupational therapy, special education, regular education, physical education, computer science, and administration.

After the assessments have been completed, the team, including the parents and the child, will write an individual education program (IEP) to help the child set and achieve appropriate

Supportive Practices for Child With a Learning Disability

BOX 10-7

1. A child may become easily frustrated or angry because of a long history of failure. Be patient and supportive.
2. Ask the child to help you understand what kinds of support he or she needs to learn.
3. Allow the child time to process information and generate a response.
4. Use simple sentence structure if needed.
5. Recognize that the child is not stupid but learns in different ways than other children.
6. Ask teachers or parents for ideas on how to structure therapy sessions, present ideas to a child, or elicit cooperation from a child.

educational goals. Support from therapy providers, teachers, and classroom aides to help the child learn new or reinforce weak skills may be described in the IEP. Assistive technology supports to help the child succeed academically, such as computers, special seats, or calculators are described in the IEP. Interventions to help the child learn, such as individualized lesson plans, and structuring the environment or academic work so the child can be successful will be written into the IEP.

Physical therapy will not usually be directly involved with a child with learning disabilities unless there is a motor component to the disability, such as a developmental coordination disorder, mild cerebral palsy, or a head injury. Because children with learning disabilities may be included in groups or in classrooms where therapy is provided, it is important that PTAs be familiar with the problems these children may face. Box 10-7 lists supportive behaviors that may be helpful when working with a child with learning disabilities.

Attention-Deficit Hyperactivity Disorder

Attention-deficit hyperactivity disorder (ADHD) has been in the news recently because of the increasing use of pharmacological treatment for children who are hard to manage in school. All of us remember at least one child, usually a boy, in our elementary school classroom who was very difficult to manage. This child was constantly out of his seat, bothering other students, throwing objects, and talking out of turn. It is unclear whether the incidence of this disorder is increasing or whether the identification of children who can benefit from drug therapy to control their behavior to allow them to learn in school is getting better. A third alternative is that parents and teachers have less tolerance for poor behavior in school and are increasingly clamoring for drugs to treat the unruly.

Incidence and cause. Incidence of ADHD may be as high as 5% to 10% of the school-aged population. The incidence in the United States is higher than other parts of the world, partly because of looser criteria for diagnosis. ADHD occurs more than five times more frequently in boys than girls (Selikowitz, 1993). The cause of ADHD is not well determined but could result from a variety of mechanisms and is probably multifactorial.

Clinical features. Attention-deficit disorder may occur with or without hyperactivity. Criteria for diagnosing ADHD includes whether or not the child has difficulty remaining seated, fidgets with hands or feet, squirms in seat, shifts from one uncompleted activity to another, has difficulty following through on instructions, and often loses things needed for tasks (David, 1995). Children with ADHD are more likely to have reached motor milestones, such as independent sitting or walking, later than their peers.

Intervention. Although the mechanism of ADHD is not known, some medical interventions have proven to be effective for some children. Pharmacological stimulants, such as methylphenidate (Ritalin), have been shown to help children with ADHD organize their behavior. These medications can help children attend longer to academic tasks, learn more appropriate social skills, and decrease their overall activity to a more socially acceptable level. Side effects can include appetite suppression, mood elevation, tachycardia, and hypertension but are usually temporary and have not been shown to have long-lasting adverse

effects (Safer, 1995). The stimulants are usually given in the smallest dose needed to help the child organize behavior. Because the half-life is short (4 to 6 hours), children may be medicated for school only and given a break from the medication in the evenings and at night. The prescription of Ritalin has skyrocketed in recent years, and some concerns have arisen in the popular press about the overdiagnosis of ADHD and related disorders. Other pharmaceuticals, such as tricyclic antidepressants, clonidine, and neuroleptic medications, have not been shown to be effective in children with ADHD.

Interventions as part of a behavior management plan, including setting clear limits, providing natural consequences for positive and negative behaviors, and providing a defined structure to routines and activities, may help the child with ADHD organize behavior. These techniques may be even more helpful in combination with pharmacological therapy.

Children with ADHD may have motor difficulties that require physical therapy consultation or intervention. They may also participate as part of a classroom or group involved in therapeutic activities. The PTA should be aware of the issues and management strategies for helping children with ADHD participate as fully as possible. Box 10-8 lists ideas which may help the PTA work with a child who has ADHD.

Developmental Coordination Disorder

Children sometimes have coordination problems that have led to labels of "clumsy," "developmental clumsiness," and "developmental apraxia" in the past. These disorders are now considered under the classification of developmental coordination disorder (DCD).

By definition, these motor problems are different from those that children experience when they have an identifiable underlying disorder—for example, cerebral palsy, mental retardation, or Down syndrome. The "clumsy child" has been associated with learning disabilities, sensory integration problems, and minimal brain dysfunction. Children may have associated disorders that range between motor, attention, perceptual, and learning disorders.

BOX 10-8

Supportive Practices for Child With ADHD

1. Make sure you get the attention of the child before giving instructions.
2. Be clear in your instructions. Repeat them if needed.
3. Break down tasks to smaller parts.
4. Structure activities in short segments.
5. Be aware of and use behavioral management techniques that have been developed for the child.
6. Provide an area for therapy that is free of distractions.
7. If other children are around, structure the therapy session to include them so as to minimize distractions and maximize opportunity for building social skills.
8. Do not get frustrated when you must continually remind the child to get back on task.

Incidence and cause. The incidence of DCD is difficult to determine because of the many different ways that this disorder has been classified in the past, but David (1995) summed up some research on DCD and related disorders and found the incidence ranging between 4% and 10% of the school-aged population. Because there is no identifiable neurological disorder in children with DCD, the cause of this disorder is unknown. Theories range from a failure of cerebral dominance to disorders in the function of the cerebellum, disorders in neurotransmitter function, poor brain maturation, and disorders in information processing. Causes likely are multifactorial and probably vary between individuals.

Clinical features. The child with DCD may trip frequently, have constantly skinned knees or bruised calves, or demonstrate an awkward gait during walking or running. The child will have difficulty with age-related gross motor skills, such as throwing a ball, catching a ball, running, or jumping. Children with DCD may avoid gross motor activities, such as climbing a jungle gym or slide, because poor coordination leads to fear of gross motor risks. They may have perceptual problems, such as confusion between their left and right or poor handwriting. Poor rhythm indicates problems with timing and coordination. Joint laxity, including scapular winging, poor motor planning, and delayed postural reactions, may be present. Children with DCD may have other "soft" neurological signs, including learning disabilities.

Intervention. Children with DCD may be seen for direct therapy to address specific deficits in gross motor skills. Generally, however, their gross motor skills will be near the level of their peers in quantity but will be lacking in quality. In other words, the child with DCD may be able to jump with both feet leaving the ground but may not be able to participate in jump-roping with peers be-

cause he or she cannot jump repetitively or swing the rope consistently. Direct therapy services may be difficult to justify.

The PT or PTA in the school setting may provide consultation to the classroom teacher, physical education teacher, or coach regarding how to optimize the opportunities for the child with DCD to participate and what activities might help the child develop more functional skills (Box 10-9). Working with teachers to develop gross motor curriculum, especially for preschool and early education environments, may help to avert greater problems later on for the child. The occupational therapist will probably be working with the child on classroom skills, such as handwriting, coloring, or cutting with scissors. The physical therapy provider may consult for posture, including proper chair and desk height, for optimal performance.

Exposure to Environmental Threats

In utero exposure to teratogens, such as alcohol, drugs, and certain viruses, can affect fetal development drastically. In this section, common threats to fetal development, which may result in developmental disabilities, will be discussed. The long-lasting effects of maternal alcohol ingestion, maternal ingestion of street drugs, such as cocaine or heroin, and in utero exposure to cytomegalovirus (CMV) and human immunodeficiency virus (HIV), will be explored. Disabilities resulting from each of these teratogens have predictable patterns, and many will result in motor dysfunction that will require physical therapy treatment.

Fetal Alcohol Syndrome and Fetal Alcohol Effects

Drinking any alcohol during pregnancy can have devastating effects on the unborn fetus. Fetal alcohol syndrome (FAS) is currently the leading cause of mental retardation in the United States (Cook, Peterson, & Moore, 1994). The amount and frequency of alcohol consumption, the developmental age of the fetus, and the genetics of the mother all contribute to the severity of the outcome. The spectrum of effects from maternal alcohol consumption includes FAS, the most severe manifestation, with characteristic facial dysmorphia, and impairment of the central nervous system. Fetal alcohol effects (FAE) are a lesser form of fetal alcohol poisoning exhibiting many of the central nervous system effects but not the physical characteristics of facial dysmorphia. Children with FAE are more common than children with FAS but are more difficult to identify. Therefore the incidence of FAE may be more common than is documented in the literature.

Incidence and cause. The cause of FAS and FAE is very clear—the ingestion of alcohol by a pregnant woman. One in six women will drink enough during her pregnancy to harm her fetus (National Institute on Alcohol Abuse and Alcoholism, 1987). The incidence of FAS is estimated to be 1 to 3 per 1000 births, with FAE occurring more frequently (National Institute on Alcohol Abuse and Alcoholism, 1987). Among women with sociocultural propensity for alcoholism, the incidence rises significantly. For instance, a review of epidemiological studies found that rates of FAS varied between 190 per 1,000 children to 1.3 per 1,000 children in Southwest Indian communities, depending on sociocultural and drinking patterns (May, 1994). The alcohol in the maternal bloodstream goes directly to the fetal

 Use playground equipment outside of regular playground time (for privacy) to work on skills with a child with developmental coordination disorder. Frequently a child will want to be able to swing, climb the jungle gym, or progress on the monkey bars to keep up with peers and so will be motivated to work.

Supportive Practices for Child With DCD

BOX 10-9

1. Include other children in the therapy session for peer support.
2. Develop and use activities that are cooperative rather than competitive.
3. Incorporate rhythmic activities into the session.
4. Use age-appropriate activities to develop specific skills, such as jump-rope, hopscotch, baseball.
5. Be aware that the child may have other developmental problems, such as learning disabilities or ADHD, and follow supportive practices for these developmental problems as well.

bloodstream. The fetal liver is small and immature. The fetus may take days to detoxify a blood alcohol concentration that the mother's liver may handle in hours. Therefore binge drinking is known to be more detrimental to a developing fetus than low-level chronic drinking. Other maternal predictors for FAS/FAE include having more than five drinks on any one occasion and drinking during the first 2 months of pregnancy (Cook, Peterson, & Moore, 1994).

Clinical features. Children exposed to alcohol in utero can have a range of problems that vary from mental retardation and growth retardation to seizures, behavior differences, and learning disabilities. Four specific features are used to diagnose FAS/FAE: (1) history of maternal drinking during pregnancy, (2) central nervous system involvement, including mental retardation or severe learning disabilities, (3) prenatal and postnatal growth retardation, and (4) characteristic facial dysmorphia. Central nervous system involvement can be subtle and include developmental delay, poor motor control, attention deficits or hyperactivity, and muscular weakness. Growth retardation can include low birth weight, failure to thrive, and small or thin stature. Facial dysmorphology is described in Figure 10-13. Characteristic facial features change with age, becoming less noticeable as a child gets older. Other features that may occur with FAS/FAE include strabismus, nearsightedness, malformations of the ears, heart murmurs, liver and kidney problems, retarded bone growth and skeletal defects, increases in upper respiratory infections and middle ear infections, undescended testicles, and hernias (Cook, Peterson, & Moore, 1994; Randall & Riley, 1995).

Whereas features characteristic of FAS may be very noticeable in a preschool-aged child, by the time the child is an adolescent, the facial features are unremarkable. The most common expression of FAS/FAE is the child with low to average intelligence who has difficulty keeping up with peers in school. This child may have subtle facial features that are not obvious as FAS features except to experienced observers. Many children go undiagnosed.

As children with FAS/FAE grow, the characteristics of their disability change. The young child may be thin, small, and weak; have excess energy or distractibility; poorly aligned teeth; and hearing or visual deficits. The child may be emotionally unstable, noncompliant, and may fight or have tantrums. The school-aged child has less observable facial features and exhibits difficulties with academics. Children may be naive and prone to victimization (Dorris, 1989). In adolescence, children with FAS/FAE may continue to have small stature and head circumference, act impulsively, take risks, use time poorly, lie, and have poor planning abilities. Judgment and reasoning abilities are severely affected, and the adolescent will need supervision, which is not usually graciously accepted.

As reflected by the constant alcohol abuse, mothers of children with FAS may have high-risk lifestyles. Many children with FAS live in foster care or adoptive homes. Parents and caregivers may not understand the reasons for their child's behavior, and may be confused about causes of the behaviors and possible treatments.

Intervention. The primary treatment for FAS/FAE is prevention. Once the damage has occurred, a child has permanent disability. Interventions to help the child succeed in school, learn appropriate social skills, and control inappropriate behaviors can make a significant difference in how the older child or adult with FAS/FAE is able to function in society. Medical interventions to control seizures for those children who have them, nutrition consultation to help a child grow, and education for parents and caregivers about FAS/FAE can help provide optimal outcomes. Team interactions by psychologists, nurses, teachers, therapists, and parents to support children with FAS/FAE in educational settings are essential. Physical therapy can play a role with younger children who need help gaining strength and age-appropriate gross motor skills. Emotional support for children with FAS/FAE and their families can help address problems of guilt, self-doubt, and anger that can impede optimal functioning. Most parents feel very guilty for, usually unwittingly, causing their child's disability. If a service provider suspends judgment and interacts with the parent, basing his or her actions in the present rather than the past, trusting relationships can develop that will benefit the child.

Children With In Utero Drug Exposure

Although alcohol has been shown to have the strongest teratologic effect on the developing fetus, other drugs have harmful effects as well. Illicit drugs that could have negative effects on growing embryos and fetuses include stimulants, such as cocaine and amphetamines, heroin and other narcotics, and marijuana. Other drugs that have been shown to affect the growing fetus include tobacco and various prescription drugs. Women who abuse drugs are likely to use multiple drugs during their pregnancies.

Tobacco. Tobacco use has been shown to cause as much as 14% of preterm deliveries in the United States (Cook, Peterson, & Moore, 1994). Spontaneous abortion and fetal death have been associated with smoking during pregnancy. Other problems related to smoking during pregnancy include a higher risk for placenta previa (growth of the placenta over the opening of the cervix), abruptio placentae (early separation of the placenta from the uterine wall), and vaginal bleeding. Any of these conditions can lead to premature labor, premature delivery, or fetal death. Birth weights of children born to mothers who smoke are significantly less than those of children born to nonsmoking mothers (Figure 10-14). From 21% to 39% of low birth weight in children is attributable to maternal cigarette smoking (Wong,

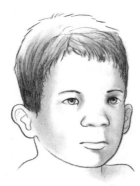

Figure 10-13 Characteristic facial features of a child with fetal alcohol syndrome include microcephaly, widely spaced eyes, narrow eyelids, large low-set ears, short nose, undefined long philtrum (between nose and upper lip), and thin upper lip.

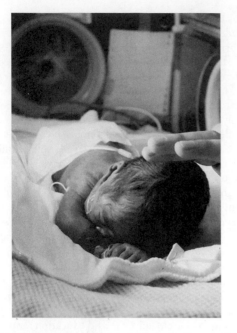

Figure 10-14 Low-birth-weight children are frequently born to mothers who smoked cigarettes.

1995). The birth weight of the infant is proportional to the amount the mother smokes. Other birth defects that have been linked to smoking include cleft palate, heart defects, hernias, and central nervous system abnormalities (Cook, Peterson, & Moore, 1994). Children whose mothers smoke are more likely to die of a respiratory infection or of sudden infant death syndrome (SIDS) during the first year of life. The Health Education Authority reported in December, 1996, that 30% of pregnant women in the United States smoke.

Street drugs. In the 1970s heroin use in the United States increased significantly, causing an increase of births to addicted mothers. Infants were born with severe symptoms of narcotic withdrawal. In the 1980s cocaine use increased as a result of a steep drop in price and the advent of crack, a smokeable form of cocaine. Jittery, inconsolable infants born to crack-addicted mothers made headlines, and public outcry resulted in arrests of addicted mothers, removal of children from the care of addicted mothers, and a punitive rather than rehabilitative attitude. The percentage of infants born to mothers who abused drugs ranges from 3% to 30%, varying between neighborhoods. The incidence is difficult to determine because of the difficulty in ascertaining which mothers used drugs during pregnancy. The effects of multiple drug use on infants is difficult to determine for the same reason.

Effects of the drugs on newborns are well documented. Infants born to mothers addicted to cocaine or heroin are more often born prematurely, small for gestational age, and with significant drug-related behaviors. Infants born addicted to heroin or methadone may demonstrate withdrawal behaviors within the first 48 to 72 hours, or sometimes not until 2 to 4 weeks after birth. Whether or not withdrawal symptoms occur depends on the quantity and regularity of drug use by the mother. Symptoms include irritability, seizures, irregular breathing, twitches, hiccups, crying, stuffy nose, vomiting, and diarrhea. Symptoms usually last from 1 to 3 months. Older children born to heroin- or methadone-addicted mothers are likely to have shortened attention spans, temper tantrums, delayed psychomotor development, visual-motor perceptual problems, and hyperactivity. These problems can persist into school age and may affect the child's adjustment to school.

Infants born to mothers who used cocaine during pregnancy are likely to be irritable, have poor tolerance to handling, have poor state regulation, and feed poorly. They may be hypertonic and hyperactive or lethargic and hypotonic. They may have low birth weight and small head circumference. Defects ranging from genitourinary malformations, intracranial defects, congenital heart malformations, and limb reductions have been reported in cocaine-exposed infants, but a definitive relationship has not been established (Robins & Mills, 1993).

Reviews of the research on long-term outcomes of infants born to cocaine-addicted mothers does not bear out the early fears of long-term disability among these children. Although the research is not conclusive, the effects of prematurity and a chaotic and uncertain environment seem to have a stronger long-term impact on children than in utero exposure to cocaine (Cook, Peterson, & Moore, 1994; Frank, Bresnahan, & Zuckerman, 1996; Robins, & Mills, 1993). This is not to say that mothers should continue their use of illicit drugs. Researchers are careful to point out that long-term effects on self-regulation and learning have not been studied adequately, and subtle disturbances may cause problems in school and in interpersonal relationships in later life. Studies are now underway to look at the effects of in utero cocaine exposure on higher cognitive and interpersonal relations in school-aged children (Pokorni & Stangae, 1996).

Interventions. Overt medical problems, including seizures, respiratory distress, and congenital malformations, are addressed as needed. The infant with cocaine exposure who is oversensitive to environmental stimulation can be handled minimally and kept in a darkened room with external sounds muted to avoid distressing the infant. These interventions may help the infant to learn better regulation of state and to adapt more readily to environmental stimulation.

Physical therapy intervention may include evaluating neonatal behavior using an instrument, such as the Neonatal Behavioral Assessment Scale (NBAS), sometimes called a "Brazelton" after its creator, T. Berry Brazelton, MD. Assessing infant reflexes, muscle tone, ability to interact with caregivers and the environment, and ability to calm himself or herself, with the parent observing, can help foster understanding of the infant's precarious grasp of some of these skills, as well as an appreciation of the skills the infant brings into the world.

Difficulty in calming infants with cocaine exposure can affect bonding between infants and their caretakers. This interruption in bonding can have severe consequences in later development. Teaching caregivers methods to calm hyperstimulated infants, such as swaddling, holding arms and legs in flexion against the body, and minimizing sensory input, such as eye contact and talking, can help them feel more comfortable and capable with these highly irritable infants.

Children With In Utero Exposure to Viral Infections

Pregnant women may be exposed to viral agents that have disastrous effects on their unborn fetus, with or without awareness of their exposure. Although many viral agents can be implicated as teratogens, cytomegalovirus and human immunodeficiency virus are two that are well known and cause very different kinds of problems in the infants and children who become exposed.

Cytomegalovirus (CMV). Most of us have been exposed to CMV at some time in our lives. It may have affected us like a mild cold. Fever, sore throat, swollen glands, and fatigue are the most common symptoms. Many people get no symptoms at all. We catch CMV much like a cold, through personal contact with infected body fluids, such as saliva, blood, feces, or urine. Day care settings and schools are common breeding grounds for CMV, the same as for colds. Once exposed, we develop antibodies, which are detectable in our blood.

Only certain people need to worry about being exposed to this virus; people with compromised immune systems, such as those with HIV, people taking certain drugs, such as those used during chemotherapy or those used for organ transplants, and those unborn children of mothers who have never been exposed to CMV. Only about 7% to 10% of unborn infants whose mothers are exposed to CMV for the first time will develop disabilities as a result of their exposure. The incidence of CMV in newborns is 2 to 20 per 1000 newborns, however, not all will develop disabilities (Batshaw & Perret, 1986).

Children who develop problems as a result of CMV exposure will each have a unique expression, but common symptoms include mental retardation, hearing impairment, and learning disabilities (Figure 10-15). Some children will have physical disability that will usually express itself as hypotonia with delay of age-appropriate gross motor skills.

Children who were exposed to CMV in utero may still be shedding live virus, just as those of us who contract it every day shed live virus for months or years. This is no reason to exclude a child from daycare settings or infant development programs. Proper hygiene, including frequent hand washing and other body fluid precautions, will protect anyone from contracting the virus. Pregnant women who work in day care settings need to be extra careful to follow good body fluid precautions.

> Wash your hands frequently to avoid infections. This may seem so basic that it is not even worth mentioning, but, in fact, almost everyone is not as conscientious as he or she should be. Handwashing makes a huge difference in avoiding colds and flu, as well as other infections. The person just beginning to work with children is likely to be sick frequently during the first year.

Human immunodeficiency virus (HIV). The mechanism of exposure, and the care of children with HIV/AIDS is changing rapidly as new drug therapies are tested and proven. As of September 30, 1996, a total of 7472 cases among children aged less than 13 years had been reported to the Centers for Disease Control and Prevention (CDC) (1996) by state and territorial health departments. More than 80% of these children were black or Hispanic. Because of new treatments, there has been a significant decline of 27% in perinatally acquired AIDS cases from 1992 through 1995.

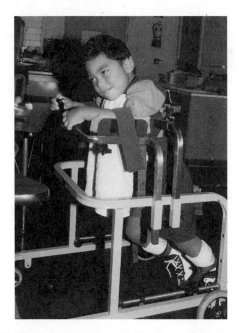

Figure 10-15 Kameron was exposed to cytomegalovirus in utero. He has microcephaly and hypotonia with poor motor control of his trunk and extremities. He has a significant hearing impairment and other medical problems.

Several methods of exposure cause children to become infected with HIV:

- From mother to child during pregnancy or at the time of delivery
- From transfusion with infected blood or blood products
- From mother to the child by way of breast feeding
- From sexual abuse by an HIV-infected person

Although the incidence of HIV and AIDS in the United States was originally fairly isolated in the population of homosexual males and intravenous drug users, the percentage of women with the disease has steadily increased, as it spreads through the heterosexual population. In 1986 women comprised 3% of infected persons, and by 1989, the percentage increased to 11% (Allbritten, 1990). In 1995, 14% of cases of AIDS were women, with women comprising 25% of the newly diagnosed cases (Veterans Administration, 1995). Most of these women are of childbearing age, and many may not realize that they are infected. Ninety percent of the children infected with HIV have been infected from an HIV positive mother.

The first three methods of transmission have decreased significantly since the improved testing of blood and blood products for HIV, starting in the late 1980s and the advent in the early 1990s of zidovudine (ZVD) therapy (formerly called AZT) to reduce perinatal HIV transmission in pregnant women. Before this time, about 25% to 30% of infants born to HIV-infected mothers became infected (Ammann, 1994; National Pediatric HIV

Resource Center, 1992). Transmission of HIV from infected mother to infant has been reduced by two thirds with the advent of ZVD therapy for mother and newborn (CDC, 1996).

Children exposed to HIV in utero may have symptoms at birth, or the symptoms may not appear until several months or years have passed. The median age of diagnosis is 18 months. The new classification system developed by the CDC in 1994 uses two axes to indicate (1) severity of clinical signs and symptoms, and (2) the degree of immunosuppression. This replaces a classification system that relied on symptoms alone. Table 10-2 outlines the classification systems.

Symptoms can include opportunistic infections from weakened immune systems, such as pneumonia, thrush, cytomegalovirus, and mycobacteria infections. Children with HIV are more susceptible to routine childhood illnesses, such as colds, fungal disorders of the skin, ear infections, and chickenpox. Organ system involvement can include the brain and the nervous system. At least 60% of children with HIV show neurological signs, with some authors finding up to 90% showing signs (Belman et al., 1988). Manifestations of central nervous system involvement can be subtle, or more overt as in a progressive encephalopathy. Other organ systems that may be involved include the kidneys, heart, stomach, and intestines. Young children with multiple organ system involvement may have failure to thrive as a first outward manifestation of the disease.

Two clinical paths have been identified for children. An infant who has an opportunistic infection or HIV encephalopathy at presentation will have a poor prognosis. A child with late onset of signs and symptoms, a slow decline of immunosuppression, and who develops lymphoid interstitial pneumonitis/pulmonary lymphoid hyperplasia (LIP/PLH) will have a better prognosis. Different strains of HIV may be responsible for different outcomes. All children with AIDS die, but it is considered a chronic disease rather than a terminal illness, because many children are living longer, into adolescence and beyond. More effective treatments may help children live into young adulthood in the near future. Problems of emerging sexuality, long-term disability, and vocation are issues that need to be addressed for these long-term survivors.

Children who are HIV positive, or have full-blown AIDS, have a variety of symptoms that can be addressed by physical therapy. Younger children may have microcephaly with resultant abnormalities of muscle tone and lack of age-appropriate gross motor skills. Because of frequent illness, developmental skills may not have ever been achieved. Older children and adolescents may have differing degrees of encephalopathies engendering different symptoms, including spasticity, muscle wasting, weakness, and loss of cognitive skills. Atrophy of the brain cells, abnormalities of myelin, disease of vascular systems in the brain and spinal cord, calcifications in the central nervous system, and neoplasias or cancers in the central nervous system are some of the many central nervous system disorders which can occur with HIV/AIDS. Each child should be evaluated individually, and a program planned to help the child learn and maintain functional skills, including self-help, mobility, communication, and academics.

Physical therapy intervention for the child with HIV. Physical therapy may help provide adaptive equipment, including walkers or wheelchairs, to maintain mobility. Exercises to regain or maintain strength and range of motion to perform functional skills can be done at school, home, or in the clinic. Children who are

TABLE 10-2 Classification Systems for Pediatric HIV

| Original pediatric classification system (1987) | Revised pediatric classification system (two axes) | |
	Severity of clinical signs and symptoms	Degree of immunosuppression (based on level of CD4+ lymphocyte counts and percentages for age)
P0: Indeterminate infection (unconfirmed HIV infection—may be seropositive after birth due to an HIV-positive mother)	N: No signs and symptoms E: Vertically exposed (from maternal antibodies)	1: No evidence of immunologic suppression
P1: Asymptomatic infection	A: Mild signs and symptoms	2: Moderate immunologic suppression
P2: Symptomatic infection	B: Moderate signs and symptoms (lymphoid interstitial pneumonia/pulmonary lymphoid hyperplasia (LIP/PLH), plus infections, organ dysfunctions) C: Severe signs and symptoms (all other AIDS defining conditions)	3: Severe immunologic suppression
P3: Unofficial category designating children who change from positive to negative status after 6 months of age, without demonstrating any infection.	SR: "Seroreverters"—those infants who change from positive to negative status after 6 months of age, without demonstrating any infection.	

Examples: A child may be classified under the old system as P0: indeterminate infection, meaning the child was exposed prenatally but has no signs and symptoms of AIDS. Under the new system, a designation of EN1 means that the child was "vertically exposed" through maternal antibodies but has no signs and symptoms and no immunosuppression.

Another child may be classified under the P2 designation in the old classification system, meaning the child has symptomatic infection. Under the revised system, the same child with symptoms may be classified B2, meaning moderate signs and symptoms and moderate immunosuppression. The revised category gives more information.

hospitalized may need help to recover lost skills from long periods of illness.

Sensory Disorders of Childhood

Children with blindness or deafness may be seen by physical therapy for related neuromuscular problems, or for problems directly related to the sensory impairment, including balance or mobility. Children may have multiple sensory disorders involving both vision and hearing. As much as 99% of acquired information and knowledge may be learned using the two sensory modalities of vision and hearing (Hicks & Pfau, 1979). Individuals who have impairments in one or another, or both, need a significantly different habilitation, rehabilitation, or educational program. This can have profound implications for the provision of physical therapy services to children with sensory impairments.

Impaired Vision

Visual disorders can take a variety of forms, but all involve some degree of deficient visual skills. The disorder can be related to the structures of the eye, such as the eye muscles, cornea, retina, optic nerve, and optic chiasma, which make up the neural pathway between the eye and the brain, or visual centers in the brain

itself (Figure 10-16). Visual disorders in children differ significantly in their causes than those of adults who frequently have aquired visual deficits. Congenital disruptions, such as in utero infections (toxoplasmosis and rubella commonly cause visual deficits), malformations of the brain (such as in cerebral palsy), or events occurring after birth, such as trauma, eye infections, tumors, or vitamin A deficiency, cause visual deficits in children.

Disorders involving structures of the eye. To see young children with glasses is not uncommon (Figure 10-17). Children with disabilities have many visual problems that might respond to correction, including refraction errors causing hyperopia (farsightedness) and astigmatism (blurry vision). Glasses are usually used with young children rather than contact lenses, which may be more cosmetically appropriate for adolescents. Glasses will usually be thick and durable to resist the trauma they can be subjected to from young children. Glasses may be strapped onto the head to keep them from sliding down small noses; however, straps should always have an automatic release mechanism to avoid strangling the child should they catch on something. Pediatric disorders that are similar to those of adults include cataracts, glaucoma, and retinoblastoma, a tumor of the retina.

A common disorder of vision in children with cerebral palsy and other developmental disorders is strabismus. This disorder occurs in 3% to 4% of the general pediatric population but in 15% of children who were born prematurely and in 40% of children with cerebral palsy (Nelsen, Calhoun, & Harley, 1991). It usually becomes evident before 3 years of age. Strabismus is a disorder of the muscles of the eye, causing abnormal alignment. Both eyes may turn in, out, or only one eye may deviate (Figure 10-18). This problem may occur continuously or intermittently. This disorder can cause blurring of vision or a double image. The young child will suppress vision in one eye (usually the

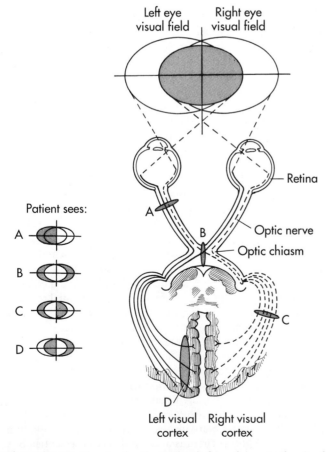

Figure 10-16 The visual pathway travels from the eye to the visual cortex of the occipital lobe of the brain.

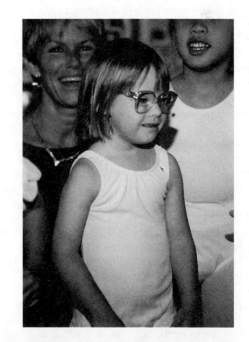

Figure 10-17 Alice, who has Down syndrome, wears glasses to correct an astigmatism causing her vision to be blurry.

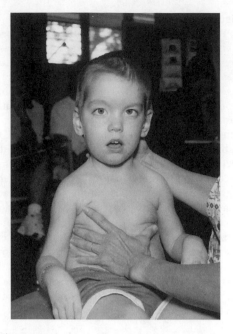

Figure 10-18 Ian has esotropia of the left eye—it turns inward.

weaker) to correct the image. Suppression can become permanent if the vision is not corrected, and vision will be lost in that eye. Correction is obtained through patching the strong eye to force the brain to recognize the image sent by the weaker eye or through surgical correction of the muscles.

High levels of oxygen used to treat a premature infant with respiratory distress can cause a disruption of the development of normal blood vessels in the retina. This disruption may lead to too many blood vessels extending out from the retina and a detachment of portions of the retina, causing partial or complete blindness in one or both eyes. This disease, called *retinopathy of prematurity,* affects 7% of premature infants who weigh less than 2.5 pounds at birth (Batshaw & Perret, 1986). Once the cause of this disorder was recognized, efforts were made to decrease the use of oxygen with small premature infants; however, respiratory needs frequently necessitate the use of oxygen with this population.

Disorders involving the central nervous system. When structures of the eye are intact, yet the child still cannot see, cortical blindness is diagnosed. The problem may lie anywhere in the optic nerve, the visual tract leading the brain, or in the visual cortex of the brain itself. Head injury, brain infections such as meningitis or encephalitis, or anoxia (lack of oxygen to the brain) can cause cortical blindness. Because the nervous system of a child is still developing, visual deficits caused by cortical blindness can change over time. A parent may be the first to notice that a child who previously was thought to be blind now appears to see. The extent of vision is difficult to measure in a young child, especially a child with severe disabilities.

Some children may exhibit visual field deficits. Similar to an adult, a child with brain damage may be born with or develop hemianopsia (unable to see one half of each eye's visual field), tunnel vision (lack of peripheral vision), or lack of central vision (seeing only with peripheral vision). Although difficult to identify, these children may tilt their head to see, turn their head so

they are using peripheral vision, or otherwise hold their head in a unique orientation to visual stimuli. Children may respond intermittently to visual stimuli, depending on where it is presented. Becoming aware of these unique behaviors can help caregivers, therapists, and teachers to present visual stimuli in ways that the child can optimally access.

Children who are blind from birth. Children who are blind from birth and who have no other developmental problems have a different developmental pattern than sighted children. Muscle tone tends to be low, and gross motor milestones are reached later than typically developing children. A child may not sit until 8 months or walk until 2 to 2½ years of age. Gait is wide based to compensate for lack of vision. A child who is blind will reach for objects later than a sighted child, and language and social development will be delayed (Batshaw & Perret, 1986). These delays point out the importance of vision as a source of information to develop language and interactive skills. Blind children may develop self-stimulatory behaviors, such as pressing the eyes, flicking fingers in front of the eyes, or rolling the head, but these behaviors will usually diminish as a child reaches school age. Children who cannot see need help to identify social cues and may never develop the same communicative facial expressions or body language as their sighted peers.

Physical therapy intervention for a child with impaired vision. A child who is blind may have delayed gross motor skills and need help to develop strength and confidence in his or her ability to move. Movement transitions, pulling to stand, cruising, and independent walking can all be facilitated through play. Family members can help identify motivators for a young child, and different strategies, such as assistive technology, voice cueing, and structuring the environment, can increase the child's independence.

With a child who is blind but has no motor deficits, a PT may be involved to assist with mobility skills. Working with the teacher, parent, and others who are with the child during the bulk of the day is essential because methods to help the child learn more independence in mobility should be consistent. Children of different ages and different cognitive abilities need different strategies to learn mobility. Teaching the child about the layout of his or her environment is a beginning step, as well as ensuring that this layout remains consistent over time. For the child who is learning to walk or to explore the environment in an upright position, obstacles, such as throw rugs, rocking chairs with long rockers, or other protrusions into open space that might trip or otherwise impede progress, should be eliminated. *Trailing* is a form of walking when the child "trails" a hand on the wall to assess position in the environment. This method is often used for a young child or for a child with mental retardation (Figure 10-19). For an older child, assistive devices, such as canes, guide dogs, or laser devices to identify obstacles, can be helpful. Each of these devices takes training and practice to use effectively, and a child may choose to use different devices in different circumstances. A therapy provider working with a child who is blind can work with trainers who are skilled in teaching mobility skills to the blind. All states have programs specifically for the blind, and most workers are willing to participate on a team with others who are involved with the child. Adaptation to the child's specific circumstances and needs is essential. Box 10-10 lists supportive practices for interacting with a child who is blind.

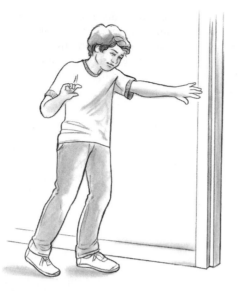

Figure 10-19 A blind child may initially learn to move through his or her environment using trailing or contact of one or both hands with the wall or furniture.

Role of the PTA with a child who is blind or visually impaired. The PTA may work with a child who is visually impaired at home, in school or in the clinic. The child may be receiving therapy that is related directly to the visual impairment, or therapy may be related to another circumstance in the child's life. Because the blind child learns through auditory and tactile means, talking, verbal descriptions, verbal cues, tactile cues, and tactile stimulation should all be used frequently in a therapy session. Toys with auditory feedback can be as simple as a ball with a bell inside. Getting specific information about the extent and quality of a child's vision can help plan how to present visual information to the child, even where to place oneself in relation to the child. For young children with multiple disabilities, the visual capabilities of a child may not be known. In this case, careful ongoing assessment of a child's visual responses during therapy can help all team members be aware of the child's visual skills, which may change over time. Do not assume that a child who has been diagnosed as cortically blind cannot see at all. Continue to provide visual stimulation. The nervous system may remodel to allow the child some vision.

Impaired Hearing

One to two of every 100 children will have some degree of persistent hearing impairment. Sixty percent of children with a hearing loss will have moderate (20%), severe (20%), or profound loss (20%) (Batshaw & Perret, 1986). The timing of hearing loss is important, with at least 90% of children becoming hearing impaired before their third birthday. This is in the "prelingual" phase of life and indicates a poor prognosis for developing speech and oral language. The earlier the hearing impairment occurs, the worse the prognosis for developing speech and language.

Thirty percent of hearing impairment beginning before birth or in infancy is caused by environmental conditions, including prenatal maternal infections, such as rubella, toxoplasmosis or

Supportive Practices for Blind or Visually Impaired Child or Adult

BOX 10-10

1. Use toys that have sound, such as balls with bells inside or toys that make sound when they are moved or rocked.
2. Talk to the child, not the parent or caregiver. A child who is blind needs to learn to respond to social and other conversation just like any other child.
3. Finger foods can help a child learn to self-feed. Mushy or sticky foods may be rejected because a child likes to keep hands clean and the child's hands are sensitive to touch.
4. Children who can see 12 inches away can walk independently.
5. Encourage early walking for strength and independence.
6. Hook and loop fasteners can help a child learn more independent dressing skills.
7. Verbally describe the therapy room, classroom, or other environment where you might be interacting, especially if it is an unfamiliar environment. If it is a familiar environment, describe any differences from usual. This can help the child orient himself or herself.

When interacting with older children and adults who are blind:

8. Offer assistance when traversing streets or uneven ground, but let the person decide how to use your assistance. Let the person take your arm. He or she will walk about a half step behind you to anticipate curbs and other obstacles.
9. Tell the blind person the names of the individuals in the room and their approximate orientation to him or her. Let the person know whether there are children or animals in the room as well.
10. Do not raise your voice. A person who is blind can usually hear as well as anyone else.
11. Words like "see" or "view" are ordinary words with many meanings and are not offensive to a person who is blind.

CMV, postnatal infections, such as meningitis or encephalitis, trauma, exposure to ototoxic antibiotics, and prematurity.

Another 30% of hearing impairment has genetic causes. Genetic syndromes may include hearing loss as one of the symptoms, and some autosomal recessive disorders cause deafness as a primary symptom. Chromosomal disorders may include hearing impairment as part of the disorder. For instance, 60% to 80% of children with Down syndrome will have a conductive hearing loss (because of narrow ear canals) and a high incidence of middle ear infections. The final third of children with hearing losses have unknown causes.

Children with developmental disabilities are likely to have hearing loss related to any of the above causes. Children with mental retardation have three times the incidence of hearing loss as other children (Lloyd & Young, 1969).

Terminology related to hearing impairment. Terminology referring to different types of hearing impairment is inconsis-

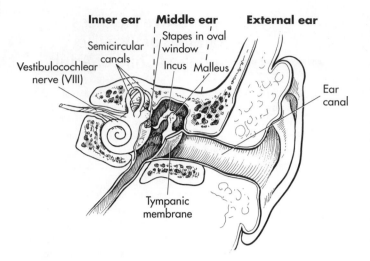

Figure 10-20 The external ear, middle ear, cochlea, auditory nerve, and auditory cortex of the brain make up the auditory system.

tently used throughout the literature. The most common terms and their definitions follow:

Hearing impairment: Any type or degree of hearing loss.

Hard of hearing: A person can understand most speech through aural mechanisms, with or without a hearing aid.

Deaf: A deaf person cannot understand speech aurally and uses primarily visual means for communication.

Deaf community: Deaf also refers to the deaf community, a culturally distinct group of people who use a defined language (American Sign Language [ASL]) to communicate. Members of the deaf community may be hard of hearing, yet choose to use ASL for communication, or may be deaf.

Conductive hearing loss. When problems occur with the structures of the external or middle ear, the resultant hearing loss is called a conductive hearing loss (Figure 10-20). Causes of a conductive hearing loss include repeated ear infections, a build-up of fluid in the middle ear causing poor conduction of sound, or damage to the tympanic membrane. Chronic middle ear infections are the most common cause of a conductive hearing loss. Children at high risk of ear infections include children with Down syndrome because of anatomic considerations and children of certain cultural groups, such as Native American Indians or Eskimos. These children are more likely to sustain hearing loss because of chronic ear infections. Antibiotics to treat infection and/or surgery, such as adenoidectomy or placement of tubes to drain fluid and equalize pressure from the middle ear (myringotomy), can restore lost hearing. Children with a conductive hearing loss are not likely to lose more than 60 decibels of hearing, because their sensorineural auditory mechanisms are still intact. To give you a perspective on what this means functionally, a whisper is at 30 decibels, most conversation occurs at 40 to 60 decibels, and a loud rock concert is at 100 decibels. Another mechanism to conduct sound to the cochlea is the temporal bone itself. The outer and middle ear rely on air conduction

of sound, but the bone also conducts sound, bypassing the outer and middle ear, and going directly to the cochlea.

Sensorineural hearing loss. If the disorder occurs in the cochlea or the auditory nerve, a sensorineural hearing loss results. The range of sensorineural hearing loss is wide, from mild to profound. Table 10-3 lists varying degrees and types of hearing loss with their functional effect and intervention. Causes of sensorineural hearing loss include brain hemorrhage and asphyxia in premature infants and cerebral malformations. Children with persistent fetal circulation have a 25% chance of developing progressive sensorineural hearing loss. Trauma to the cochlea through head injury or exposure to loud noise can cause sensorineural hearing loss. Infections, either sustained in utero or after birth, may result in hearing loss. The antibiotics used to treat infections may be toxic to the cochlea and cause hearing loss in their attempt to treat infections.

The most common maternal infection is CMV. Thirty percent of the infants with observable symptoms, as well as 10% of infants without observable symptoms from in-utero CMV exposure, develop a sensorineural hearing loss. This hearing loss is high frequency and can be progressive. Children with certain disabilities, such as cleft palate, may have a mixed hearing loss, meaning both a conductive and a sensorineural hearing loss.

Intervention. Interventions for hearing impairment are summarized in Table 10-3. Medical interventions include early detection and treatment of ear infections, especially among groups who are at the most risk for developing hearing loss. Surgery to remove adenoids or place tubes to drain fluid and equalize pressure between the middle and outer ear are also common procedures.

Amplification of sound can help children with mild or moderate hearing loss improve their hearing and understanding of conversation. Hearing aids are generally used with even very young children, so that sounds and language can be heard during the prelingual phase when language and communication centers in the brain are being organized. If this time is missed, a child will have much more difficulty using these modalities for communication, or even understanding written and verbal language.

For example, Helen Keller was only 18 months old when she contracted meningitis and lost her hearing and vision. Because she was exposed to language before her illness, with extensive intervention, she was able to learn to use language again in a meaningful way. Most profoundly deaf children are able to use sign language to communicate and can interact meaningfully within the deaf community. They may have considerable difficulty reading and writing, however, because of their lack of exposure to written and oral language in early life.

Other technology can also help children be more independent. An FM system is a radio transmitter and receiver. The teacher speaks into a radio transmitter and the child uses a receiver, which amplifies the teacher's voice and filters out extraneous sounds. This system can help children participate more fully in school. Devices that use light instead of sound to indicate a doorbell or telephone ringing, or vibrations to indicate an alarm clock going off, can be very useful. Service animals or pets can indicate visitors to the house among many other things. Cochlear implants can improve cochlear function to improve hearing.

TABLE 10-3 Effects of Hearing Loss on Function

Hearing level (decibel)	Degree of loss	Type	Missed sounds	Effect	Intervention
16-25	Slight	C, SN	10% speech sounds	Miss fast-paced peer interactions, fatigue in listening.	Hearing aids or FM system, seating in front, antibiotics, myringotomy.
26-40	Mild	C, SN	25%-40% speech sounds, distant sounds, unvoiced consonants, plurals, and tenses.	Miss 50% of class discussion, has problem suppressing background noise.	Seating in front, hearing aids or FM system, language therapy, antibiotics, myringotomy.
41-55	Moderate	C, SN	50%-80% of speech sounds	Articulation deficits, limited vocabulary, learning dysfunction	Hearing aids or FM system, resource help, speech-language therapy, speech reading.
56-70	Moderate-severe	SN or mixed	100% of speech information	Delayed language, syntax, atonal voice, reduced speech intelligibility.	Full-time amplification, special education class, speech-language therapy.
71-90	Severe	SN or mixed	All speech sounds; can hear loud environmental noises	Speech not developed or deteriorates, learning deficits.	Full-time program for deaf, signing or total communication, amplification.
>90	Profound	SN or mixed	All speech and other sounds; feels vibrations	As above.	As above, cochlear implant.

From Anderson, K.L., & Matkin, N.D. (1991). Hearing conservation in the public schools revisited. *Seminars in Hearing,* 12, 340-364.
C, Conductive; *SN,* sensorineural.

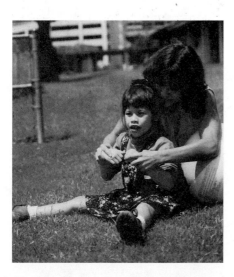

Figure 10-21 Amanda signs "more" to indicate that she wants to play more catch with her friend. Her teacher helps her form the sign.

Speech-language therapy can help a child with a hearing disorder learn to use speech, sign language, or other methods of communication (Figure 10-21). Articulation training can help speech patterns to develop and a child to be more intelligible when using speech. Special education can be a valuable resource for children with hearing impairments to help them gain academic skills.

Methods of communication among deaf children. Many members of the deaf community strongly believe that deaf children should learn to function in a signing world. American Sign Language is the language of the deaf community in the United States. To learn this language well, children need to be in environments where signing is used exclusively. Therefore separate schools where ASL is the language of choice have been developed. Because most deaf children are born to hearing parents, this method of communication may cause communication problems between children and their parents.

Other people believe that deaf children need to focus exclusively on oral language to learn communication skills well enough to function in the everyday world. These people believe that learning lip reading and developing speech skills are essential and advocate not using ASL at all. Children are taught in regular schools, so they can learn to use the same methods of communicating and learning as other children. Children with severe and profound hearing loss may not be able to overcome articulation difficulties, and their speech may not be intelligible to everyone.

Still others take a compromise position and believe that deaf children need skills that can help them interact with the rest of American society where English is the language of choice, but they also need to learn ASL. Advocates of total communication recommend using signing, as well as written and oral language, to develop flexibility in communication strategies. Total communication is usually taught in separate schools where deaf children can interact with other deaf children, and where teaching methods are developed specifically for deaf children, taking into account specific learning problems and issues arising from deafness.

Although there are strong beliefs about which method should be used, there is no right answer to this controversy. The system of communication should be chosen with the needs of the child and family in mind. This is an important decision that families need to make early in the life of their child. Box 10-11 outlines some supportive strategies to use with a person who is deaf.

Role of physical therapy. Because children with disabilities are more likely to have hearing impairments than the general population, physical therapists and physical therapist assistants are likely to work with them. A minimum knowledge of basic signs is useful when working with young children who have any type of language delay and essential when working with a child whose language delay is due to a hearing impairment. Some basic signs are listed in Table 10-4. Young children, or children with motor disabilities, may use adapted signs. A speech language pathologist can be a valuable resource as to which signs a child knows, and what communication methods are being used with a child.

Understanding of the frustration a child feels when communication is difficult, and the isolation that can be felt by not being part of the hearing world can help a therapy provider understand the sometimes challenging behaviors a child may exhibit (Figure 10-22). Temper tantrums, sadness, withdrawal, and noncompliance may all be strategies a child has learned to deal with feelings or may be manipulative behaviors that have a communicative intent. The Applications section in this chapter discusses how to address behavioral challenges that may occur with children who have a hearing impairment.

Some children with hearing impairment may also have impairment of their vestibular apparatus in the inner ear, causing problems with balance. Usually vision and proprioception will compensate to allow balance skills to emerge, but children may need extra help to use these senses to develop effective balance reactions in different positions. Balancing while moving may be more difficult than for a hearing child. Providing extra proprioceptive input by having the child carry heavy toys, giving approximation through the pelvis or shoulders, and emphasizing activities that activate proprioceptive receptors may help a child

Supportive Practices for Hearing-Impaired Child

BOX 10-11

1. Use toys with bright visual appeal.
2. Make sure the child is looking at you when you are talking.
3. Learn the signs that the child knows and use them consistently during therapy. Keep up as the child learns new signs.
4. Encourage the child's early use of hearing aids.
5. Learn to adjust the hearing aids to avoid feedback and ensure they are operating optimally.
6. Encourage early language activities using any means available (computers, toys, books, pictures, etc.)
7. Most hearing impaired children have residual hearing, which should be encouraged by talking, singing, playing music, and using rhythm and vibration during therapy activities.

TABLE 10-4   ## Basic Sign Language for Children

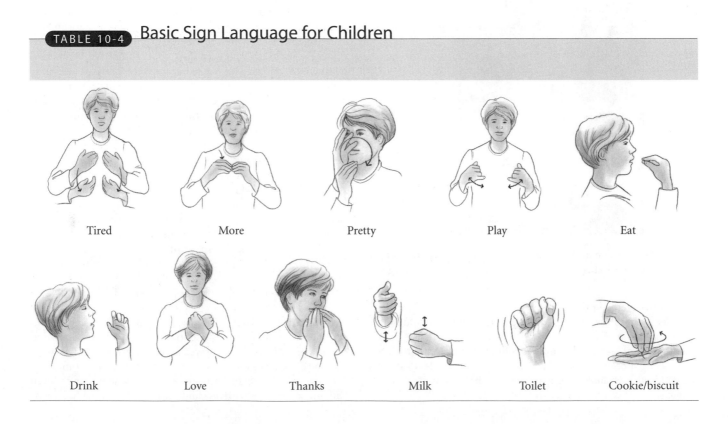

| Tired | More | Pretty | Play | Eat |
| Drink | Love | Thanks | Milk | Toilet | Cookie/biscuit |

become more aware of these sensory inputs. Some activities that emphasize proprioceptive feedback include jumping, marching, stamping, wheelbarrow walking, and pushing activities. Having the child trail a wall or table with one hand while walking or carrying a toy that drags on the ground can give continuous proprioceptive feedback regarding orientation in space. Emphasizing visual input through encouraging visual reference to external objects may also give the child some early skills at orienting in space.

When working with a child who cannot hear, a PTA can rely on other senses to provide sensory stimulation to interest the child, arouse the child, or calm the child down. Brightly colored toys, pictures, and therapy tools can be visually stimulating. Movement in space, such as rocking, bouncing, swinging, or jumping may all be enjoyable and help the child be more alert. Sounds should not be avoided. Talking, signing, and singing to the child can all provide a context for therapy activities. Make sure the child has his or her hearing aid in place and turned on so that sounds that occur during therapy will have the most impact. Rhythm and beat can be felt through other senses (vibration, touch), even in a child who is profoundly deaf.

The Child With Multiple Sensory Impairments

Blindness and deafness may occur together in children with both congenital and acquired disabilities. Frequently, the child with multiple sensory impairments has other disorders that may include mental retardation or physical disability. Because the development of a child with both blindness and deafness is so profoundly affected by the absence of these senses, testing cognition may be very difficult. In a child with multiple disabilities, testing vision and hearing may be difficult as well. Even in a child whose cognition is not affected, development will be very different than a child without disabilities. A child will develop motor skills later, muscle tone will be low, and the child may have less initiative to learn or move around.

The ability to communicate is significantly impaired in children who can neither hear nor see; vision and hearing are the most important sensory modalities to both receive and express communications. Of the remaining senses, touch, smell, and taste, touch is the most functional for developing a communication strategy. Tactile cues can help a child know who is near. Consistently different cues for each person can be one of the first communications a child learns to understand. For example, mother may always touch the child's hair when she approaches, and father may always place his hand on the child's chest. Try developing your own way of approaching a child who is both blind and deaf.

Structuring the environment so it is consistent can help a child make sense out of external cues. Keeping the orientation of furniture consistent in a classroom or home can help a child learn to move independently. Following the same procedures leading to the same activities can help a child learn to anticipate events.

The most effective early strategy for communicating with a child is to use signs that are given tactually. You make the sign into the child's hands so he or she can feel what sign you are making. Always relate the sign immediately to an object or action so the child can associate the meaning, and learn to increase his or her sign vocabulary. Children may have some hearing or vision, so it is important not to avoid these sensory modalities. For children with such a profound communication handicap, the parents, teacher, or speech-language pathologist, those who know the child best, are essential team members in helping others communicate and interact with the child.

The child with a profound sensory disability will feel isolated from other people and may develop behaviors that isolate even further, such as head banging, eye gouging, or other self-abuse. It may be difficult to understand the origin of self-abusive behaviors, but they may represent a search for meaningful sensory input, an attempt to provide any sensory input at all, or a means of communicating.

Physical therapy intervention. Physical therapy may be involved with the child who is blind and deaf because of a primary motor disability or to help a child develop postural and mobility skills. Sensory input and feedback through hand placement and directional forces can help the child modify motor patterns that are not functional or look abnormal. Helping a child develop normal looking posture and movement can be not only functional, but may also allow the child to be more easily accepted by peers. The development of mobility skills using trailing, a cane, or other means to learn the environment and move about in it without assistance can be functional for a child with multiple sensory impairments. Learn what the child likes and dislikes and develop a relationship with the child with consistent communications and interactions. A PTA who works with a child every day and learns more about a child can help team members make decisions about what to teach the child, what kinds of experiences to provide, and what goals may be appropriate for that child.

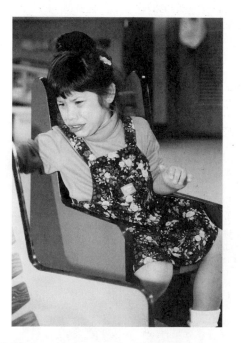

Figure 10-22 Amanda becomes frustrated when she cannot make herself understood.

Positive Behavior Support Interventions

LINDA McCORMICK

Some children with disabilities exhibit physically dangerous and severely disruptive behaviors, such as head banging, self-biting, verbal threats, hitting and kicking, biting, screaming, and overt defiance. These children need and typically receive professional assistance and support from a behavioral specialist, such as a special educator, psychologist, or counselor, and/or a team of professionals (often called a behavior support team). In the past, problem behaviors were viewed as separate from other aspects of the child's life. Intervention focused myopically on decreasing or eliminating the disturbing behavior. The procedures used most often were negative, such as punishment. Current efforts focus on the whole child. First, the reasons *why* the problem behaviors are occurring are determined. Then a behavior support plan is developed to provide the child with assistance, instruction, and support. Especially where children with severe disabilities are concerned, the goal is to change all aspects of what is typically a limited social system in ways that will increase the child's quality of life.

Positive behavior support interventions go by various names: communication-based intervention, nonaversive behavior management, and/or positive/comprehensive behavior support (Carr & Durand, 1985; Koegel, Koegel, & Dunlap, 1996; Meyer & Evans, 1989; Reichel & Wacker, 1993). The commonality among these approaches is the view that problem behavior occurs in response to specific events in the child's environment, that is, the behavior serves a purpose or has a function for the child.

It is beyond the scope of this section to review all the knowledge, skills, and issues involved in dealing with children with significant problem behaviors. This discussion will be limited to reviewing the assumptions and procedures associated with positive intervention approaches. We will outline techniques for functional assessment, briefly describe development of behavior support plans, and suggest some resources for more extensive study of these procedures. First, however, based on the belief that implementation of procedures to prevent problem behavior should take precedence over intervention, we will provide some general strategies to prevent problem behaviors and/or to address them before they escalate to the point of requiring application of systematic intervention procedures.

General Strategies for Preventing or Addressing Behavior Problems
Let Children Know the Rules and Procedures

Whenever possible, children should be involved in developing rules and procedures for the setting. Then they should be taught to follow the rules and procedures. If for some reason a child has not been involved in establishing the rules and procedures, these should be discussed in a calm voice with an explanation for why each is necessary. Rules and procedures should be logical and easy to follow. Whenever a new activity is introduced, it is a good idea to discuss how existing rules and procedures will apply to this new activity. Let children know exactly what the consequences are if the rules and procedures are not followed. It is a good idea to review the rules and procedures *and the consequences* on a regular basis, and it is imperative to consistently follow through if they are not respected (Figure 10-23).

Hold Developmentally Appropriate Expectations

There is always a potential for misbehavior if expectations are not in line with children's developmental abilities. Children misbehave if expectations are too advanced, because they become frustrated. Too few expectations may mean that children are not being challenged. When this is the case, they may misbehave because they are bored.

Let Children Know What Behaviors Are Unacceptable

Proactive management means discussing and rehearsing appropriate ways of behaving in new situations. Usually children know when they behave in unacceptable ways. However, in new situations, they may be unaware of the inappropriateness of their actions. They may be in that particular situation for the first time so they do not know what is expected; or they know what is expected but lack the skills to perform the expected behavior. For example, a child who has never been in a library, hospital, or church may not know that using a loud voice and running are not acceptable in those settings.

Use the "When-Then" Rule

The "when-then" rule, also called "Grandma's rule" or the "Premack principle" (Premack, 1959), states that making a desired activity available to a child contingent on the completion of

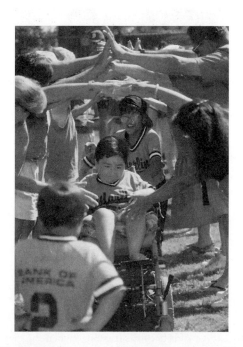

Figure 10-23 Children should be taught the rules and procedures for different environments, including school, community settings, and home situations.

an undesirable activity will increase performance of the undesirable activity. Many of us first experienced this principle when we were told "when you finish your vegetables, then you may have your dessert." This is not bribery. Bribery is providing a reward for performance of an illegal or inappropriate action. Using the "when-then" rule is simply a reminder that a desired activity will be available when the child completes the less preferred activity.

Recognize That Some Situations Are Especially Problematic for All Children

Transition from one activity to another or one place to another is problematic for the majority of children. The child must stop something that he or she is engaged in (possibly a preferred activity) and move to another activity or another location (which may or may not be as enjoyable). Teachers often minimize the potential for disruptive behavior at transition times by providing specific instructions for transition. In addition, they provide opportunities to practice transition behaviors, such as where and how to line up, where and how to put away materials, and how to move quietly to another activity (McCormick & Feeney, 1995). When it is almost time for an activity to end, they give advance notice so that children have time to prepare themselves for the transition. Also, they make a point of stating what the next activity will be. Another situation that is difficult for children is not having any control. Within reason, children should have the opportunity to make choices about what they will do and where and with whom they will do it. Thus, by being flexible and respectful of children's feelings, adults can often avoid having to deal with inappropriate behavior (Figure 10-24).

Provide a Quiet Place and Time for Children to Calm Down and Gain Control

Some children may find themselves overwhelmed with the noise and activity level in a particular setting. Their response to the overstimulation may be inappropriate behaviors, such as hitting, kicking, yelling, and/or running around wildly. What they need is a quiet, less stimulating area where they can calm themselves down. This is not a punishment, but rather an opportunity to "unwind." Children who seem to have a hard time handling very stimulating environments should be taught to recognize when they are "feeling upset inside by all the noise and activity" and to remove themselves to a quiet location.

Recognize the Potential Effects of Environmental Conditions That Are Beyond Children's Control

We need only to reflect on our own behavior when we have an upset stomach, a headache, or a sore throat to recognize the effect that health has on behavior. Children rarely handle pain or feeling sick as well as adults and many cannot talk about how they are feeling. It is important to be sensitive to the possibility that a child's misbehavior may be related to physical discomfort, possibly a low grade infection or a chronic health problem. Other causes of inappropriate behavior (particularly behaviors such as overactivity, short attention span, and irritability) are (1) food or environmental allergies, (2) poor nutrition (no breakfast), and/or (3) stressful conditions at home. Children frequently misbehave at school when they are anxious about home situations, such as parental separation, divorce, illness, frequent arguments, new sibling, or visiting relatives (Figure 10-25).

In conclusion, adults always need to have a plan for managing whatever activities and environments for which they are responsible. The need for a positive behavior support intervention can be avoided by preventing problem behaviors. Wise adults anticipate and prevent problems before they occur.

Positive Behavior Support Intervention

Many positive intervention procedures begin with the assumption that problem behaviors are a form of communication. Some children may not yet have learned adequate language skills to express their needs and feelings. Others have adequate communi-

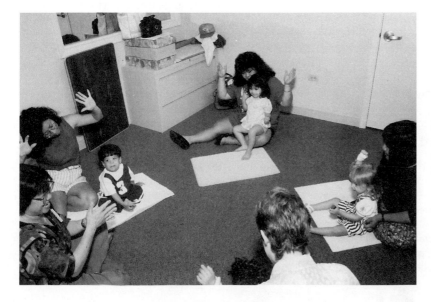

Figure 10-24 Children may need time to adjust to a change of activity or place. Group situations may be especially problematic because some children are ready for a change, while others are not.

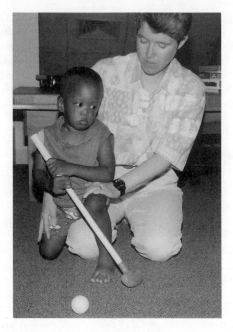

Figure 10-25 Poor behavior may be a result of illness, hunger, or fatigue.

cation skills, but they are not using them because the problem behavior is a more effective means of getting the messages across. Certainly, the problem behaviors are not being used systematically or intentionally to influence others, but they are successful for the child in getting needs met. The behaviors tend to be very successful in enabling their users to gain attention, desired objects or activities, or to escape unpleasant situations.

Carr, Levin, McConnachie, Carlson, Kemp, and Smith (1994) provide a succinct review of the basic assumptions of positive behavior support approaches:

Problem behavior is purposeful. The assumption is that problem behavior is adaptive and purposeful. It is used because it "works" in the sense that it helps the child get his/her needs met. All of us behave for a purpose: what differs is the *form* of the behavior.

Problem behavior cannot be changed unless we can identify what purpose it serves. Because the problem behavior is typically purposeful, it cannot be successfully changed without knowing the purpose. The process of discovering the purpose is called functional assessment or functional analysis.

Intervention must focus on education, not simply problem reduction. Because the problem behavior serves a purpose for the child, the goal of intervention must be teaching new ways of achieving that purpose. Once new strategies are learned, the problem behavior will no longer be needed.

Change requires many interventions. Because problem behaviors occur in many social contexts, including home, school, and community settings, and thus serve many purposes, a single intervention strategy is unlikely to be successful in affecting pervasive change.

Intervention involves changing social systems, not persons. Intervention is not something you do *to* a child, but rather, you do it *with* the child. Just as the problem behavior was learned in transactions with persons in the child's social environment, it can be unlearned and new, more adaptive behaviors can be acquired in the same interactions. Thus intervention should lead to desirable behavior change on the part of everyone involved, the child, and the child's social systems.

Lifestyle change is the ultimate goal of intervention. The goal is to improve the life of the child with disabilities so that he or she can influence others without resorting to inappropriate behaviors. Successful interventions provide children with more opportunities to participate in effective ways.

Recognizing that disruptive, even dangerous, behavior serves a communicative function does not mean that the behavior can be accepted. The child must be provided with appropriate communicative alternatives. First, it is determined through a functional assessment what the child is communicating with the problem behavior. Then the support plan is developed and implemented.

Functional Assessment

The purpose of functional assessment, which is performed by the behavioral specialist and/or the behavior support team, is to collect sufficient information so that an effective behavior support plan can be developed. Functional assessment is undertaken to gain an understanding of the child, the problem behavior(s), the child's environment, and, most importantly, the relationships among the three. It is a process for determining the variables that may be associated with the problem behaviors, specific function(s) of the behavior, and the consequences that may be contributing to its maintenance.

In addition to formulating an operational definition of the problem behavior(s) or class of behaviors of concern, the functional assessment process identifies the variables that predict the occurrences and nonoccurrences of the problem behavior, generates hypotheses about the consequences that are maintaining the problem behavior(s), and verifies the hypothesis. To do this, functional assessment must gather information about (1) environmental variables associated with the problem behavior, (2) the social context for and social reactions to the behavior, (3) possible functions of the problem behavior, (4) the extent of the child's choices and control over environmental events, and (5) extant expectations and teaching strategies (those that have worked and those that have not worked). Box 10-12 provides a sample of the questions that the functional assessment process seeks to answer.

The primary procedures that are used in the functional assessment are direct observations, rating scales, interviews with persons who have daily contact with the child, and functional analysis. In direct observation, observers use a recording procedure to note occurrences of the target behaviors and conditions in effect at the time the behaviors occur. Rating scales are standardized instruments, such as the Motivation Assessment Scale (MAS) (Durand & Crimmins, 1990). The MAS is a 16-question scale that assesses the potential functions of behaviors with regard to four major classes of consequences: sensory reinforcement, escape-avoidance, social attention, and obtaining tangible rewards. Interviews use questions, such as those presented in Box 10-12.

Functional analysis, the fourth procedure, is the explicit manipulation of relevant variables and direct observation to test whatever hypotheses have been generated from the information

BOX 10-12   Questions for the Functional Assessment

- What is the problem behavior?
- Specifically when and where is the problem behavior most likely to occur?
- With whom is the problem behavior most likely to occur?
- Is the problem behavior successful in gaining attention for the child?
- Is the problem behavior successful in gaining access to desired objects and activities?
- Does the problem behavior allow the child to avoid/escape an unpleasant situation?
- Does the problem behavior happen more/less often when the child is involved with difficult tasks?
- Does the problem behavior happen more/less often when the child is involved with long, tedious, repetitive, and/or boring tasks?
- Does the purpose of the problem behavior seem to be to protest something?
- Does the child have appropriate alternative behaviors that serve the same function as the problem behavior?
- Does the child have control over selection of and access to routine daily activities, such as what to wear, when and what to eat, what to play with, what to watch on television, etc.?

- Does the child have meaningful relationships with others?
- Of the strategies that teachers and others have used to address the problem behavior, what has not worked?
- What does the child enjoy doing?
- How could the activities that the child enjoys doing be expanded and restructured to occur more often?
- What are the activities that the child does not enjoy?
- How can the activities that the child does not enjoy be discontinued?
- What kinds of information does the child communicate spontaneously?
- How does the child communicate preferences and choices?
- How does the child gain the attention of others?
- How does the child refuse to participate in activity?
- How does the child reject an object?
- What vocabulary and what mode of communication would better support this child to get what he wants?
- What are the opportunities for making choices throughout the child's day?
- With whom does the child like to spend time?
- When does the child seem to be having a good time with others? With whom?

collected through the other procedures. Its purpose is to provide clear and precise demonstrations of the influence of relevant variables on the occurrences of the targeted problem behaviors. For example, if it is hypothesized that one of the purposes of Amy's problem behavior is to gain attention, then various manipulations might be undertaken to determine whether she is attempting to gain the attention of a specific peer or peers or a specific adult or adults and, if so, who they are. If it is hypothesized that one of the purposes of her problem behavior is to obtain certain objects or activities, then various manipulations are undertaken to verify specifically what objects and activities the child favors. If escape or avoidance is thought to be the purpose of the child's problem behaviors, then manipulations are undertaken to verify the specific people, tasks, materials, or activities the child wants to avoid.

Behavior Support Plan

How long the functional assessment will take is difficult to predict. It should continue until environmental variables that correlate with the problem behavior have been identified and tested. After the functional assessment is completed, the next step is to use the information generated by the functional assessment to plan intervention that is matched to the function(s) of the problem behavior. This plan defines the problem behavior(s), describes what needs to be done to address the problem behavior(s), and provides procedures for monitoring the proposed intervention process. The plan is written in sufficient detail to allow all persons who come into contact with the child to understand what problem behaviors occur, the hypotheses about why the behaviors occur, and what their role is in implementing the plan. It generally describes procedures to (1) reduce the targeted problem behavior(s), (2) improve the child's health and

safety, (3) develop new skills (or strengthen skills already in the child's repertoire), (4) modify and expand the child's activity options so that there is more participation in typical environments, and (5) increase the choices available to the child (Horner, O'Neill, & Flannery, 1993).

Horner, O'Neill, and Flannery (1993) have provided a helpful discussion of the components of a behavior support plan. The first component is a description of the problem behavior(s), which provides a clear description of the context that is likely to elicit the problem behavior and the class of behaviors involved. For example, the problem description might be: "When Timmy realizes that a transition is imminent, he is likely to scream and/or throw whatever objects/toys/materials are within reach." Following the problem behavior statements, the plan usually includes at least a summary of the hypotheses developed through the functional assessment as to why the problem behaviors occur. One approach is to list the problem behaviors and indicate (for each problem behavior) the specific events that are likely to predict its occurrence and the typical consequences for the child.

Another component of the behavioral support plan is a description of ecological support procedures. How can the child's physical settings be altered to affect the problem behaviors? For example, in the classroom, a physical setting alteration would be changing the location of the child's desk or removing a bulletin board next to the child's desk if these variables are thought to contribute to the problem behaviors. The plan also describes changes in the social context. For example, it might describe strategies for increasing interactions with peers and strategies that adults have found useful for building personal rapport with the child.

Many comprehensive support plans also involve examination of medical, health, and safety concerns (e.g., medications, physical prosthetics), as well as consideration of changes in sleep and diet patterns. There may be an overview and analysis of the child's daily activities with special attention to variety, interest, balance between physically active and less active activities, personal control, and opportunities for socialization.

Finally, the support plan lists the specific new skills that the child needs to learn. These are the alternative behaviors identified during the functional assessment (and verified in the functional analysis). The following are some examples of new skills that might be taught: "pointing to pictures of desired activities," "independently accessing snacks," "indicating the need for assistance," "indicating the need for a break," and "indicating a desire to spend some time with a favorite peer." Also, there may be instruction on such skills as taking turns and engaging in a relaxation routine in stressful situations.

The behavior support plan also identifies events that predict the problem behaviors and specify how they can be changed. For example, if the functional assessment has determined that Jason is less likely to engage in self-abusive behavior when he is given a chance to choose the tasks and reinforcers associated with work activities, then his schedule should be arranged so that, in addition to no-choice activities, he has a significant number of activities where he can select among several task and reinforcement options. He can select by pointing to a picture of or naming the tasks. Another example is: The functional assessment has determined that Jessica screams and throws herself on the floor whenever there is deviation from the daily schedule (because she finds uncertainty and unpredictability very aversive). This behavior allows her to escape unpredictable situations and be left alone. The solution might be to spend some time with Jessica each morning constructing a picture schedule and discussing what is going to happen that day. The picture schedule can be reviewed just before each transition.

A behavior plan should also describe how adults should respond to particular child behaviors. Consequences may be manipulated to (1) maximize the positive consequences for appropriate, alternative behaviors, (2) redirect the child to alternative behaviors, (3) minimize the positive consequences for problem behaviors, (4) provide negative consequences for problem behaviors, and/or (5) minimize the health and safety risks created by the problem behaviors. The support plan should describe the basic effect desired and provide detailed scripts for involved adults to use for important and frequently occurring situations.

The last component of the behavior support plan describes monitoring and evaluation procedures. The purposes of these procedures are to determine whether the support plan is resulting in the desired effects, to provide information that may be useful in revising the plan across time, and to provide adults with regular feedback to facilitate implementation of the plan.

Summary

Whether they occur several times an hour or several times a week, month, or year, blatant noncompliance, physical and verbal abuse, and aggressive behavior are reasons for serious concern. These behaviors isolate children from positive social experiences, and they limit both present and future choices. Over time they interfere more and more with the child's ability to achieve the type of outcomes our society values, for example, having friends and moving around freely and independently in the community.

This section has provided only an introduction to what to expect from positive behavior support approaches. Most important

to keep in mind is that these approaches view problem behaviors as the child's means of getting needs met. Functional assessment identifies alternative behaviors (typically, new communication skills) that will accomplish the same functions as do the problem behaviors. Intervention focuses on teaching acceptable alternative behaviors and generally improving the child's quality of life.

EXERCISES

1. Find an agency that serves adults with developmental disabilities. Observe or volunteer there for at least a few hours. Remember that the children we work with today are the adults of tomorrow.
2. Observe or volunteer for at least a few hours in a school or program that serves children with visual or hearing impairments.
3. Look up "universal precautions" and teach your classmates methods to avoid contracting infections from the environment and from children with whom you work.

QUESTIONS TO PONDER

1. Is it better to raise deaf children with American Sign Language (ASL) as a primary language, or using total communication, or using strictly oral communication (talking)? Why?
2. Should punitive consequences like arrest and jail be mandated for women who take drugs or alcohol when they are pregnant? Why or why not?
3. Should HIV testing be required for all pregnant women? Why or why not?
4. If a physical therapy provider does not agree with the lifestyle of a parent, how should he or she address it? (The parent may be homosexual, a drug user, a child or spouse abuser, homeless, etc.) Is it all right to have a colleague provide treatment if you are not comfortable with the parent's lifestyle? Should you tell the parent how you feel? Why or why not?

Annotated Bibliography

Dorris, M. (1989). *The broken cord.* New York: HarperCollins.

> This heart-wrenching true story by the adoptive father of a boy with FAS exposes the typical behaviors of a severely affected child from toddlerhood through adulthood as the father searches for the meaning of his son's behaviors and medical problems. Cultural issues of Native Americans and their use of alcohol blend with the awakening of the medical community to the effects of maternal alcohol ingestion on the fetus. Family experiences of prejudice, discrimination, frustration, and love temper the story of a boy's life and his father's search for answers.

Williams, D. (1992). *Nobody nowhere.* New York: Avon.

> Among the spectrum of individuals with autism, some have skills to communicate and to function in the world. Donna Williams does not have the cognitive disabilities that many individuals with autism exhibit and has been able to go through school successfully, including higher education. In this book she recounts her experiences growing up as a child with autism. Her history is unique because her family is not typical, and her experiences are unique because Donna is not typical either. Her descriptions of the reasoning and feelings behind her "autistic" behavior and her struggles with relationships and physical touch bring some understanding to those of us who do not experience the world in the same way. This book can begin to help us appreciate the significant differences that shape the behavior of individuals with autism.

References

Allbritten, P. J. (1990). *Children with HIV/AIDS: A source book for caring.* Newark, NJ: National Pediatric HIV Resource Center.

Aman, M. G., Hammer, D., Rojahn, J. (1993). Mental retardation. In T. H. Ollendick & M. Hersen (Eds.) *Handbook of child and adolescent assessment.* Boston: Allyn & Bacon.

American Psychological Association (1995). *Diagnostic and statistical manual of mental disorders* (4th ed.). Washington, DC: Author.

Ammann, A. J. (1994). Human immunodeficiency virus infection/AIDS in children: The next decade. *Pediatrics, 93*(6): 930-935.

Baroff, G. S. (1986). *Mental retardation: Nature, cause and management* (2nd ed.). New York: John Wiley.

Bateman, B. (January/February, 1996). Legal definitions and the juvenile delinquency-learning disability linkage. *LDA Newsbriefs,* 37-38.

Batshaw, M. L., & Perret, Y. M. (1986). *Children with disabilities: A medical primer.* Baltimore: Paul H. Brookes.

Belman, A., Diamond, G., Dickson, D., Horoupian, D., Llena, J., Lantos, G., & Rubenstein, A. (1988). Pediatric acquired immunodeficiency syndrome: Neurologic syndromes. *American Journal of Diseases of Children, 142,* 29-35.

Bolton, P., & Rutter, M. (1990). Genetic influences in autism. *International Review of Psychiatry, 2,* 67-80.

Carr, E. G., & Durand, V. M. (1985). Reducing behavior problems through functional communication training. *Journal of Applied Behavior Analysis, 18,* 111-126.

Carr, E. G., Levin, L., McConnachie, G., Carlson, J. I., Kemp, D. C., & Smith, C. E. (1994). *Communication-based intervention for problem behavior.* Baltimore: Paul H. Brookes.

Centers for Disease Control and Prevention. (1996). *AIDS among children– United States, 1996* [On-line]. Available: www3.medscape.com/Clinical/other/MMWR/1996/1996/nov/4546/4546.

Cook, P. S., Peterson, P. C., & Moore, D. T. (1994). Hazards of prenatal exposure to alcohol, tobacco, and other drugs. In U. S. Department of Health and Human Services, Office for Substance Abuse Prevention (Ed.). *Alcohol, tobacco, and other drugs may harm the unborn.* (Publication No. ADM90-1711). Washington, DC: US Government Printing Office.

David, K. S. (1995). Developmental coordination disorders. In S. K. Campbell (Ed.) *Physical therapy for children* (pp. 425-458). Philadelphia: WB Saunders.

Dorris, M. (1989). *The broken cord.* New York: Harper Collins.

Durand, V. M., & Crimmins, D. B. (1990). Assessment. In V. M. Durand (Ed.), *Severe behavior problems: A functional communication training approach* (pp. 31-82). New York: Guilford Press.

Dykens, E. M., Hodapp, R. M., & Leckman, J. F. (1994). *Behavior and development in fragile X syndrome.* Thousand Oaks, CA: Sage Publications.

Frith, U. (1991). Asperger and his syndrome. In U. Frith (Ed.). *Autism and Asperger syndrome.* New York: Cambridge University Press.

Frith, U. (1993). Autism. *Scientific American, 6,* 108-114.

Gillberg, C., & Coleman, M. (1996). Autism and medical disorders: A review of the literature. *Developmental Medicine and Child Neurology, 38,* 191-202.

Grossman, H. J. (Ed.). (1983). *Manual on terminology and classification in mental retardation.* Washington, DC: American Association of Mental Retardation.

Hagerman, R. J. (1987). Fragile-X syndrome. *Current Problems in Pediatrics, 17,* 621-674.

Hicks, W., & Pfau, G. (1979). Deaf-visually impaired persons: Incidence and services. *American Annals of the Deaf, 124,* 76-92.

Horner, R. H., O'Neill, R. E., & Flannery, K. B. (1993). Effective behavior support plans. In M. E. Snell (Ed.), *Instruction of students with severe disabilities* (pp. 184-210). New York: Merrill.

Koegel, L. K., Koegel, R. L., & Dunlap, G. (1996). *Positive behavioral support: Including people with difficult behavior in the community.* Baltimore: Paul H. Brookes.

Kolb, L. C., & Brodie, H. K. H. (1982). Mental retardation. In L. C. Kolb & H. K. H. Brodie (Ed.). *Modern clinical psychiatry (10th ed.).* (pps. 715-744). Philadelphia: WB Saunders.

Levine, M. D., Carey, W. B., Crocker, A. T., & Gross, R. T. (1992). *Developmental behavioral pediatrics (2nd ed.).* Philadelphia: WB Saunders.

Lloyd, L. L., & Young, C. E. (1969). Pure-tone audiometry. In R. T. Fulton & L. L. Young (Eds.). *Audiometry for the retarded with implication for the difficult-to-test* (pp. 1-31). Baltimore: Williams & Wilkins.

May, P. A. (1994). The epidemiology of alcohol abuse among American Indians: The mythical and real properties. *American Indian Culture and Research Journal, 18*(2),121-143.

McCormick, L., & Feeney, S. (1995). Modifying and expanding activities for children with disabilities. *Young Children, 50*(4), 10-17.

Meyer, L. H., & Evans, I. M., (1989). *Nonaversive intervention for behavior problems: A manual for home and community.* Baltimore: Paul H. Brookes.

National Information Center for Children and Youth with Disabilities. (1993). *General information about learning disabilities.* (Fact Sheet Number 7). Washington, DC: Author.

National Institute on Alcohol Abuse and Alcoholism. (1987). *Program strategies for preventing fetal alcohol syndrome and alcohol-related birth defects* (DHHS Publication No. ADM87-1482). Washington, DC: US Government Printing Office.

National Pediatric HIV Resource Center. (1992). The child with HIV. *Getting a head start on HIV.* New York: Author.

Nelsen, L. B., Calhoun, J. H., & Harley, R. D. (1991). *Pediatric ophthalmology (3rd ed.).* Philadelphia: WB Saunders.

Nordin, V., & Gillberg, C. (1996). Autism spectrum disorders in children with physical or mental disability or both. 1: Clinical and epidemiological aspects. *Developmental Medicine and Child Neurology, 38,* 297-313.

Palmer, F. B., & Capute, A. J. (1994). Mental Retardation. *Pediatrics in Review, 13*(12), 473-479.

Pokorni, J. L., & Stange, J. (1996). Serving infants and families affected by maternal cocaine abuse: Part 1. *Pediatric Nursing, 22*(5), 439-445.

Powers, M. D. (1989). What is autism? In M. D. Powers (Ed.). *Children with autism: A parent's guide.* Rockville, MD: Woodbine House.

Premack, D. (1959). Toward empirical behavior laws. *Psychological Review, 66*(4), 219-233.

Randall, C. L., & Riley, E. P. (1995). Pattern of malformation in offspring of chronic alcoholic mothers. *Alcohol Health and Research World, 19*(1), 38-39.

Reichel, J., & Wacker, D. P. (Eds.). (1993). *Communicative alternatives to challenging behavior: Integrating functional assessment and intervention strategies.* Baltimore: Paul H. Brookes.

Robins, L. N., & Mills, J. L. (1993). Effects of in utero exposure to street drugs. *American Journal of Public Health, 83*(Suppl.), 9-31.

Safer, D. J. (1995). Major treatment considerations for attention-deficit hyperactivity disorder. *Current Problems in Pediatrics, 25,* 137-143.

Selikowitz, M. (1993). *Dyslexia and other learning difficulties: The facts.* New York: Oxford University Press.

Smalley, S. L. (1991). Genetic influences in autism. *Psychiatric Clinics of North America: Pervasive Developmental Disorders, 14*(1), 125-141.

Smith, M. M., Centerwall, W. R., & Centerwall, S. A. (1983). Learning disability. *Introduction to your child* (No. 19). Loma Linda, CA: Light for the Way.

Szatmari, P. (1991). Asperger's syndrome: Diagnosis, treatment, and outcome. *Psychiatric Clinics of North America: Pervasive Developmental Disorders, 14*(1), 81-94.

Veterans Administration. (1995). *VA Bureau of STD/AIDS Surveillance Quarterly, 3,* 28-29.

Wong, D. L. (1995). *Whaley and Wong's nursing care of infants and children* (5th ed.). St. Louis: Mosby.

PART FOUR

Medical Disorders of Childhood

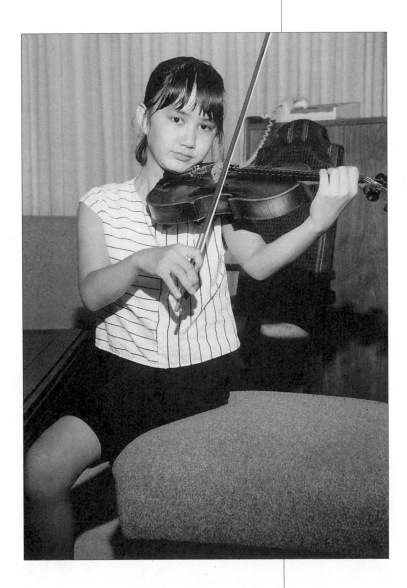

11

Neonatal Disorders

CASE STUDY   Matthew, A Boy Born Prematurely

Matthew lay asleep on his parents' bed, his head and trunk propped on a C-shaped pillow and his bottle of water fallen to the side. His mother lay beside him watching television, and his father sat at the computer across the room, surfing the Internet and keeping an ear out for the late night news on television. Mahina, a small dog with curly white fur, lay next to Matthew.

Matthew's eyes opened when Mahina licked him on the cheek, and he stretched and arched his back as he looked over to see his mother. She was engrossed in the news, so Matthew returned his attention to Mahina. He was able to reach his hand to her belly and grasp a handful of white fur. Mahina licked his cheek again and settled in closer with her head resting next to Matthew's stomach. Matthew giggled aloud and wiggled glee-

fully, kicking his legs and arching his back as he played with Mahina.

"Matthew, are you awake?" asked his mother, leaning over and scooping him up. "It's time for you to go to sleep in your own bed." She carried him over to his dad to get a kiss goodnight and settled him in his crib at the end of their bed. Matthew clutched his bottle with both hands, sucking intermittently until he fell asleep. Mahina moved over to sleep at the foot of the bed by Matthew's crib. She carefully licked her belly where the skin showed a little pink and nosed a tuft of white curly hair that lay on the bed beside her, having fallen out of Matthew's hand as it relaxed in sleep. She sighed and opened one eye watchfully whenever Matthew stirred.

Birth History and Hospital Stay

Dave was working late on the night that Nancy's water suddenly broke (Figure 11-1). He had worked most of the night before, as well as all day, trying to complete an important project for the bank. He rushed home to take Nancy to the emergency department and waited anxiously as the doctors gave her terbutaline to stop the contractions and steroids to facilitate the infant's lung maturation. She was only 26½ weeks into her pregnancy. It was doubtful whether an infant born this early could survive.

The pregnancy had been difficult already with elevated alpha-fetoprotein (AFP) levels in Nancy's blood, which indicated possible problems with the pregnancy such as a genetic or a neural tube defect. An ultrasound at 16 weeks' gestation showed a tumor in her uterus besides the fetus that was Matthew. The doctor felt that the tumor might have been a second fetus that was not viable and may have caused the elevated AFP. The ultrasound had ruled out any visible problems with the infant, but the young parents were worried.

Nancy's contractions were finally stabilized; and although they were still occurring, they were weaker and not as close together. The nurses felt that she was stable enough for Dave to go home and get some rest. After Dave left, Nancy felt thirsty. She was given some ice chips and promptly vomited. The muscle contractions from vomiting caused a placental separation, and an immediate, emergency cesarean section was done to save the infant.

Matthew was born weighing 2 pounds, 10 ounces, and he was 16½ inches long. He was pale and limp at birth; his heart rate was less than 100 beats per minute, not fast enough to send adequate oxygen to his brain. He needed oxygen right away, and the doctors immediately put a tube through his mouth into his lungs to help him breathe. His lungs were not mature enough for him to breathe easily on his own. Twice that first night he needed strong intervention to keep him alive as he stopped breathing. A mechanical ventilator pumped air into his lungs.

When Dave arrived at the hospital the second time that night, Matthew was already lying on a warming table, with tubes into his arm and leg as well as the ventilator tube in his mouth. Because he was so small, he had an isolation mask, instead of a diaper, covering his bottom. Bright lights were focused on him so the staff could see him well. With the overhead lights turned off in the neonatal intensive care unit (NICU) because of the late

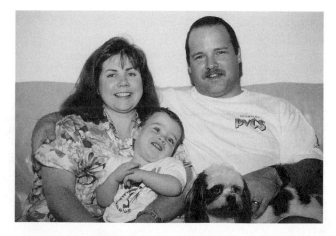

Figure 11-1 Family portrait.

hour, Dave felt that the experience of seeing his new son was surreal. The infant was a small bundle of skin and tubes in bright light fading away to darkness on all sides. Matthew did not look human to his dad.

Nancy was still in the recovery room, recovering from the general anesthesia she needed for the emergency cesarean section. Dave tried to describe Matthew to her after she woke up, but Nancy wanted to see him for herself. The nurses told her that if she took painkillers for her own pain, she would not be alert enough to go and see her son; so she refrained from taking them. Dave wheeled her into the NICU in a wheelchair on the afternoon of her first day in the hospital. The infant was still less than 24 hours old.

Nancy was shocked at how small he was, but she ached to hold him. The best she could do was to stroke his arms and legs and put her finger into his hand. His eyes stayed closed and he breathed steadily to the rhythm of the ventilator. His skin looked translucent. Yet at times he moved his tiny limbs, flailing them about with his fingers open. Nancy was relieved to see that he had all of his toes and fingers and that he was moving all of his arms and legs.

Nancy soon recovered enough to go home, but Matthew stayed in the NICU for 3 more months. During his second week of life, his nurse suctioned out a blood clot from his lungs. This signaled a turn in his health, and he fought a tough battle to stay alive. He was placed on an oscillating ventilator, which caused less pressure to his lungs as it blew the air in so Matthew could get the oxygen he desperately needed. Every day a new crisis arose that required some sort of intervention: a new drug, a new tube, a new machine.

After a few weeks Nancy returned to her job as a nuclear medicine technologist for another hospital, and Dave went back to work, too. They spent every evening at the hospital with Matthew, watching over him, talking to him, and finally, holding him. Mahina, a white dog with black spots and their only other family member, was very lonely at home. Their life took on a weird kind of rhythm filled with work, the hospital with its fluorescent lights and muted sounds, and brief periods of sleep at home.

Dave kept his sense of humor during most of their experience in the NICU. He drew eyes on the mask that Matthew wore over his eyes as he lay under the lights that were treating him for jaundice. He even drew eyes on the isolation masks that Matthew used for his first diapers. He and Nancy developed relationships with the nurses and doctors who were caring for Matthew, and they grew to respect most of them. A few personality conflicts arose; once Dave became so angry at a nurse he felt was being rough and inattentive with Matthew that he requested she not be allowed to take care of him again. The nursing administrator respected his request.

Early in Matthew's NICU stay Dave and Nancy were approached by Jane, a nurse who said that she would like to be Matthew's primary nurse. She would take care of him most days that she was working and would be the liaison between Dave and Nancy and the staff in the NICU. They liked Jane and agreed to have her be his primary nurse. That relationship was an important one and helped provide some stability during the months that Matthew recovered and grew enough to go home. Even so, Dave and Nancy felt that a support person for parents would have helped them in the NICU. It was a strange and alien environment in which to first develop a relationship with their son.

Besides getting to know him and his personality, needs, and temperament, they had to also learn his medical care. Interacting with so many people while trying to assimilate so much information was difficult. During the months they spent there they felt ill equipped to cope with difficulties that ranged from interpersonal conflicts, conflicting information provided by staff, uncertainties regarding the decisions they had to make concerning his medical care, and incredible fatigue and disorientation related to the lack of privacy in their lives and the long hours they spent at the hospital.

For his last few weeks in the hospital Matthew was moved to the intermediate nursery. His medical needs had stabilized, and although he still needed oxygen, he mostly needed to gain size and strength so he could go home. The intermediate nursery was another adjustment for Nancy and Dave. The nurses were less communicative about Matthew's medical status. Athough they were able to provide the care he needed, they had trouble answering some of the questions Matthew's parents asked. There was no primary nurse to help communicate with the physicians and other staff.

When Matthew was still in the NICU, he was seen by both a physical therapist (PT) and an occupational therapist (OT), who evaluated him for developmental skills including motor control, relating to his environment, muscle tone, and organization of his movements. The PT became Matthew's primary therapist and worked with the OT to develop a program to help Matthew develop his feeding skills, organize his movements, and relate to his environment. She taught Dave and Nancy how premature infants respond differently from term infants to environmental stimuli and helped them recognize how Matthew was communicating his needs. She taught them activities that they could do to help Matthew develop skills as he grew, including positioning him, holding and carrying him, interacting with him, and doing exercises with him.

When Matthew had been in the hospital almost 3 months, he was ready to go home. Although he was almost 3 months old, he was not quite at his originally projected birth date! The PT and OT performed final evaluations to assess his development and determine whether he needed more follow-up. He also was given an audiological screening test called an ABR, which is routine for all newborns and especially important for premature infants taking antibiotics that can potentially damage their hearing. It was becoming clearer that his movements were not as smooth and organized as they might have been. The therapists recommended that he receive services at home to monitor his development and that his parents continue to receive teaching to help them interact with Matthew in ways that would promote his developmental skills. He also failed his ABR test, which could mean that he had a severe or profound hearing loss in one or both ears. Matthew was to take another audiological test when he was 6 months old.

Matthew continued to need supplemental oxygen all of the time. His lungs had been damaged by the high pressures needed to give him enough air through the ventilator when he was so small. As he grew, his lungs would grow and the scarring would become smaller in relation to the total size of his lungs. But for now he needed a tube under his nose, which was hooked around his ears and attached to a large green oxygen tank. The tank was mounted on wheels and was heavy and bulky.

Matthew at Home

Mahina was thrilled when Matthew came home. She finally had her family back with her. She soon learned that life revolved around Matthew's needs and would "notify" Nancy or Dave if Matthew stirred in his crib or cried. When Matthew slept on a blanket on the couch or the floor, Mahina curled up next to him and kept a watchful eye.

Nancy took 6 months off from her job to care for Matthew when he came home and to allow their life to settle as a family at home. She learned to manage the oxygen tank, as well as Matthew, on shopping trips and doctor visits. Therapy services were provided at home for Matthew because he was considered medically fragile, and an OT and PT alternated visits once per week. The therapists taught Nancy correct positioning for Matthew and activities to help him learn to roll over, reach for toys, and push up onto his arms when he was on his stomach. He had trouble holding his head up; his movements were still more jerky than other babies, but he was very alert and had a wonderful smile. He followed everything with his eyes and laughed out loud. When he was 9 months old, he was diagnosed with cerebral palsy, which affected all four of his limbs and his trunk.

At 6 months old Matthew's hearing test was still abnormal. No one could tell his parents how much he was able to hear. Nancy and Dave began to learn sign language. They were able to borrow a series of videotapes to watch in the evenings and began to use signs with Matthew at home. After reviewing the literature and talking with professionals and people who were deaf, they decided to bring up Matthew using American sign language (ASL) to communicate, rather than teaching him lip reading and oral communication alone.

When Nancy returned to work, she made an effort to find a sitter who understood some of Matthew's needs. She found a woman who is hard of hearing herself. Not only that, but she has three children who are deaf or hard of hearing, and her husband is deaf. Mrs. Lee's family members use sign language to communicate, and she promised that she would use sign language with Matthew. She has been an important resource for Nancy and Dave, helping them understand some of the issues related to deafness for a young child.

When Matthew was 15 months old, he was weaned from the oxygen. His parents were relieved to relinquish the giant green oxygen bottle. When he was 16 months old, his hearing test revealed a profound hearing loss in both ears. He seemed to be able to hear some sounds in low frequency ranges. Dave changed the way he talked to Matthew and pitched his voice low. Matthew was also fitted for his first hearing aids, which he acquired when he was 18 months old (Figure 11-2).

Matthew is now 20 months old. He started to attend a weekly infant development program on Saturdays for therapy services once his mother returned to work. He goes for 2 hours; the first hour is spent in an individual therapy session, which alternates between occupational therapy, physical therapy, and speech-language services. (See Box 11-1 for a summary of his recent physical therapy evaluation, including recommendations by the physical therapist for exercises and adaptations at home and at the sitter's house.) Matthew's second hour at the infant program is spent in a group session with other children ranging in age from 1 to 3 years. Although a teacher runs the group session, therapists spend time one-on-one with the children. Matthew receives therapy from one of the other therapists in the context of the group activities. He loves the other children; although he is usually tired by the time the group session begins, he pays rapt attention to all that is happening around him. Matthew has an individualized family support plan (IFSP) that was developed for him based on needs that his parents expressed. See Table 11-1 for sample goals and objectives in his IFSP.

On a regular work day Matthew usually wakes up first. He sleeps in a crib in his own room except when there are house guests, then his crib is moved to the foot of his parents' bed. He plays quietly in his crib until he sees someone moving. His mother, who needs to be at work early, slips out of bed quietly so Matthew does not see her. She has been known to crawl the short distance to the bathroom. If Matthew sees her, he will cry until someone comes and plays with him.

After Nancy leaves for work, Dave wakes up and gets ready for work. He gets Matthew up and dressed. While he prepares breakfast, he leaves Matthew playing on the floor in the living room. Matthew has learned to scoot on his back and can scoot himself all the way to the kitchen to be with his father. Mahina watches Matthew carefully. Once, when Mahina was barking to get his attention, Dave found Matthew half way out the screen

---

BOX 11-1 Physical Therapy Evaluation Summary: Matthew

Social and Medical History
Addressed in the Case Study.

Range of Motion
Passive range of motion is full with active movement of his lower extremities, primarily in hip and knee flexion and hip abduction.

Muscle Strength, Tone, and Bulk
Muscle tone is low proximally with distal hypertonicity seen with effort. Matthew tends to arch his trunk and pull his lower extremities into hip and knee flexion and hip abduction with effort. Muscle strength is difficult to assess because his movements are influenced by abnormal muscle tone; but strength appears generally in the fair to good ranges, especially in his upper extremities with lower strength in his lower extremities. Strength is poor to fair in his trunk. He can use extensor tone in his trunk functionally although movement is poorly graded. Muscle bulk appears appropriate for his age.

Reflexes and Developmental Reactions
Matthew continues to be influenced by the asymmetrical tonic neck reflex to both sides, although he can move out of it for functional skills such as reaching and rolling. He continues to have a plantar grasp reflex bilaterally. Other primitive reflexes do not seem to influence his movement patterns. He demonstrates balance reactions in supine and prone positions, even though he demonstrates insecurity when his balance is challenged. He cannot yet sit or stand without significant support.

Developmental Skills
Matthew is most functional in a supported sitting position. When given adequate support for his trunk, he is able to briefly hold his head in midline and turn it to both sides. Without enough trunk support, he cannot resist gravity and falls forward or to either side. His spine already has a forward C-curve, but it can straighten to neutral when Matthew arches. When supported, he also can reach with either arm and grasp toys or food in front of him or to the side. He is able to get the objects to his mouth, but he has trouble releasing his grasp. Upper extremity movements are jerky and poorly graded. On the floor he can roll prone to and from supine by arching his trunk and neck. He can scoot backwards on his back at least 30 feet. In the prone position he can hold his head up 45 degrees for 1 to 2 minutes; he tends to arch his body to maintain this position. He can reach for a toy with a poor weight shift. He takes full weight through his legs in supported standing for a few minutes, but he needs support for his trunk and head. In supported standing his legs and arms tend to be extended and adducted. He is beginning to take steps in this position. He tolerates standing in a standing frame with trunk support for only 10 minutes and needs frequent repositioning for his head and upper trunk.

Recommendations
1. Matthew should continue standing daily at home to develop trunk and neck strength and control; to assist in the function of kidneys, lungs, and bowels; and to assist in the developmental shaping of his acetabulum and femoral head and neck bilaterally. Increase standing time to 30 minutes as tolerated.
2. Provide adaptive positioning for his high chair and stroller for additional trunk support to allow Matthew to sit up and access the world visually and to encourage interaction with objects and people.
3. Ensure adequate adaptive positioning at the babysitter's house so Matthew can interact with the other children at their level.
4. Assist in planning for Matthew's transition to the preschool setting to ensure that the supports he needs are in place.
5. Continue direct therapy at least weekly to help Matthew develop and coordinate his muscle control for functional skills, such as independent mobility (rolling or scooting), more upright mobility (hands and knees), and play (reaching, sitting, movement transitions).

Long-term goal
Matthew will have independent mobility and functional skills to access play, social opportunities, educational opportunities, and perform age-appropriate, self-care skills.

Short-term objectives (due in 6 months)
1. Matthew will sit up without support for 5 seconds.
2. Matthew will reach for a toy in unsupported sitting without falling.
3. Matthew will maintain a hands-and-knees position for 3 seconds as he moves to and from a supported sitting position.
4. Matthew will tolerate standing in stander or other alternative support for 30 minutes while interacting with others.
5. Matthew will move forward 15 feet independently using scooting, rolling, or other means.

door onto the patio. Somehow he had slid the door open and gotten himself outside!

Matthew sits in his infant walker to eat breakfast. The sides are high and provide enough support to sit more upright than he can in his high chair. Dad feeds him pureed food with a spoon, and Matthew grabs small pieces of soft toast to stuff into his mouth (Figure 11-3). He has a hard time releasing his grip to get the toast out of his fingers, so he uses munching and sucking to get the toast into his mouth. Sometimes he chokes when the food goes straight down his throat. Dave helps him move the food to the side of his mouth where he has more control of it. When Dave uses the sign for milk, Matthew eagerly looks for his bottle. He becomes upset when Dave takes a minute to obtain it from the kitchen. Matthew lies on the floor on a crescent-shaped pillow to drink his bottle, while Dave washes up. Matthew can grasp his bottle with one or two hands and hold it himself. He uses a bottle with a split trunk, which is easier to grasp. If he loses the nipple, Dave helps him get it back into his mouth (Figure 11-4).

After breakfast Matthew is strapped into his carseat, and Dave takes him to the sitter's house. Matthew enjoys being at Mrs. Lee's house, because there are other children to watch. He watches the manual communication between Mrs. Lee and her children and the oral communication between the children who are there just for the day. Mrs. Lee puts Matthew's hearing aids in, and he grabs them and pulls them out again. He does not like to have anything in his ears. Mrs. Lee has explained to Nancy and Dave that this is normal behavior for a small child. Her children also had difficulty in keeping their hearing aids in for more than brief periods of time until they were 3 years old. She told Nancy

that one of her children used to take out her hearing aids on the bus to school and give them to the other children. Luckily, Mrs. Lee always reacquired them from the concerned parents of the other children.

In the early afternoon Nancy stops by Mrs. Lee's house to pick up Matthew on her way home from work. He has usually napped for a few hours after lunch and is sometimes still sleeping. Mahina is happy to see them come home and leaps and dances for attention. Nancy takes Mahina out for a walk/run, putting Matthew in the three-wheeled "jog stroller," and tying Mahina's leash to the handle. This method provides exercise for all.

TABLE 11-1	Individual Family Support Plan*
Goal	**How goal will be addressed**
Matthew will eat by himself.	Matthew will receive occupational therapy once per week.
Matthew will communicate with others.	Matthew will receive speech-language therapy once per week.
Matthew's health needs will be met.	The infant development program will communicate regularly with Matthew's physician(s) regarding his progress.
Matthew will sit up by himself and hold up his head.	Matthew will receive physical therapy once per week.
Matthew will be able to play better with toys and with peers.	Matthew will receive physical therapy and occupational therapy and will be followed by a special educator with specialization in the 0 to 3 year age group. He will participate in a group activity once per week with other children from 2 to 3 years old.

*These objectives were generated by Dave and Nancy when they first started at the infant program. By law an IFSP must reflect the family's goals for their child. Individual discipline goals are integrated into the IFSP or are written separately in the discipline reports after being discussed and agreed to by the family.

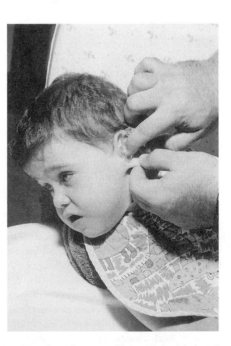

Figure 11-2 Matthew does not like to have his hearing aids inserted. Although he has difficulty with gross and fine motor skills, he can reach up very quickly to remove them. His parents try to distract him so that he will wear them as much as possible. They want him to learn to differentiate sounds while he is young.

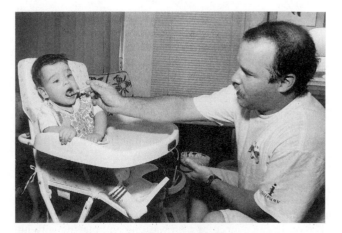

Figure 11-3 Matthew is a good eater. He uses both hands to hold himself upright in his high chair while his father feeds him.

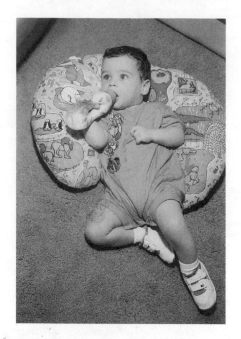

Figure 11-4 Using a bottle with a split trunk allows Matthew to grip it independently. The crescent-shaped pillow is ideal for positioning on the floor. It keeps his arms forward and helps him hold his head in midline.

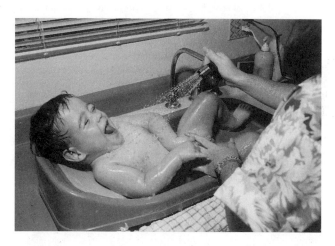

Figure 11-5 Bath time with Mom is fun. Soon Matthew will outgrow this infant bathtub, and his parents will need to find an alternative for bathing him.

After playing for a few hours, Matthew is bathed in a plastic infant bathtub, which sits easily in the double sink in the kitchen. He enjoys splashing in the water, but he does not like his hair washed. Although he has actually outgrown the infant tub, it is convenient for his mother, who does not want to hurt her back leaning over the bathtub. It provides adequate support for him so his mother can concentrate on washing and playing with him rather than trying to support a slippery wet body (Figure 11-5).

He eats dinner sitting in his high chair with an added plastic

---

pommel to keep him from sliding out the front. His mother props towels beside him to try to keep him upright. He tends to lean to either side, even with the towels. His father feels that Matthew should not be given support all the time in the high chair because he should learn to use his own muscles to sit up straight. Matthew is able to sit up himself briefly, but he soon falls back to the side when he tries to use his arms to feed himself. (See Box 11-2 for a list of adapted supports that Matthew uses in his daily life.) His parents have been successful at using many of the devices commercially available to infants and toddlers to give Matthew the support he needs, but he is beginning to grow out of some of them.

By the time his father comes home from work, Matthew is fed and washed and eager to play. He sits back in his high chair and finger-feeds himself some rice while his parents eat their dinner. Sometimes they go out to a restaurant, and Matthew is usually content to stay in his stroller while his parents eat.

After dinner Dave puts Matthew up in a stander that was loaned to them by the infant development program (Figure 11-6). The PT came to the house to teach them how to use it, and Dave was able to help adjust it for Matthew. While standing, Matthew likes grabbing at the puppet glove Dave has on his hand and shrieks with glee when it wiggles in his grasp. Nancy and Dave plan a grocery shopping trip for the next day. Because Matthew cannot sit in the grocery cart by himself, shopping with both parents is easier. One can push Matthew in his stroller, and the other can push the grocery cart. Nancy tried a terry wrap to help hold him up in the grocery cart, but it did not provide enough support. They also talk about going to the beach the upcoming weekend. Matthew likes the beach, but he does not like to touch the sand. He enjoys going in the water, though, and Dave or Nancy takes him in the ocean when the water is warm enough.

When Matthew starts complaining after about 15 minutes in the stander, Dave takes him out. Nancy's beeper goes off, and she goes to the phone to call work while Dave changes Matthew's diaper and puts on his pajamas. Matthew enjoys playing hide and seek with a cloth and giggles when his dad puts the pajamas lightly over Matthew's face. Matthew becomes concerned when

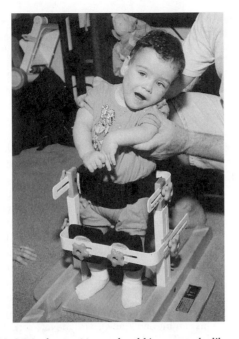

Figure 11-6 Matthew at 20 months old is not sure he likes standing. With sturdy shoes to support his feet and an extension with a strap to support his upper trunk, he has been able to start standing in the stander up to 10 minutes while a family member plays with him.

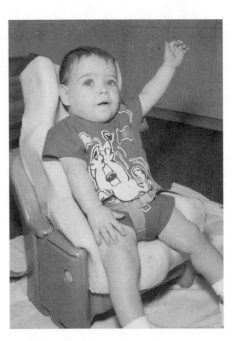

Figure 11-7 In this customized foam seat, Matthew can hold his head and trunk up against gravity. He can also use his arms for functional skills, such as waving or playing with toys, in this position. He continues to use distal "fixing" for stability, as evidenced by the extension of his legs when sitting on the seat.

Dave approaches him with a new, unfamiliar stuffed toy. His hands come up, and he turns his face away as the toy comes closer. When he starts complaining loudly, Dave tosses the toy away and picks up Matthew to comfort him. Matthew is only comfortable with certain stuffed toys; others scare him until he gets used to them (Figure 11-7).

Nancy comes back from the phone, relieved. She does not have to go in to work this time. She scoops up Matthew from the floor and lifts him high above her head. Matthew grins widely and looks down at his mother and father, who are both enjoying his delight. Nancy carries Matthew into the bedroom, while Dave finishes the dishes. She blocks Matthew onto their bed with pillows so he can play and settles down to read. Soon Dave joins them, turning on the evening news as he sits down at the computer to check his e-mail. Mahina settles down on the bed near Matthew.

BACKGROUND AND THEORY

Physical therapist assistants (PTAs) do not work with medically fragile infants, such as premature infants with acute medical issues. The draft position paper on PTAs in pediatrics from the Pediatric Section of the American Physical Therapy Association (APTA) specifically eliminates this area of practice from the scope of the PTA, stating that the advanced assessment and handling skills of the physical therapist are needed with this very fragile population (Pediatric Section of the APTA, 1996). Even among physical therapists, only those with specialized training can treat premature infants and work with families in the neonatal intensive care unit (NICU). This training usually occurs on the job from a peer or supervisor who is proficient in the skills needed. Most rehabilitation departments in medical facilities that have NICUs have developed a skills checklist or training protocol based on the competencies developed by the Pediatric Section of the APTA for therapists working with premature infants. Physicians, nurses, respiratory therapists, and other personnel who work with this population also usually receive specialized training to work with these infants and their families.

PTAs do, however, work with these children once they become medically stable and are discharged from the NICU. Some of the problems the infants have that may result from a premature birth or a medical illness may continue to affect the child, even after discharge from the hospital or enrollment in an infant development program. The goals of this chapter include familiarizing the PTA with some of the problems premature infants face and how these problems might express themselves in infants who are older and more mature.

The experience of living for weeks, months, or sometimes even longer in the NICU may affect an infant's social responses, language, or sleep cycles. The family is likely to be profoundly affected by their experience in the NICU, may refer to their positive and negative experiences, and may expect the PTA to understand their feelings and emotions. The PTA should be aware of the environment of the NICU and of current theories of how to optimize the development of a premature infant. Knowledge of specific language and acronyms surrounding these infants can help the PTA be more effective in working with families and medical professionals who treat premature infants.

> ☀ Family members of a child you are working with may be able to provide a unique viewpiont of the disease or disability affecting their child based on personal experience, especially as it relates to their own child. They may have recent literature about the condition that they would be willing to share.

The Case Study of Matthew demonstrates some of the issues surrounding working with a child born prematurely. Matthew was born at 26½ weeks of gestation. He has cerebral palsy and is deaf. He attends an infant development program and receives physical therapy, occupational therapy, and speech-language therapy. The effects of his prematurity continue to have a strong influence on his development and affect how his parents and caregivers think about his future. Andrew, the child featured in a Case Study in Chapter 7, was also born prematurely. Compare and contrast the early experiences of these two children to find substantial differences and similarities in their history and development and in the experiences of their families.

Children born prematurely cannot nipple like infants born at term. Feeding problems may ensue from abnormal experiences, as well as potential abnormal neuromuscular development resulting from neonatal problems. Although feeding is generally seen as the province of the OT, when working with young children, a transdisciplinary approach is generally taken, with each discipline supporting the other's goals. The Applications section on feeding (p. 368) outlines the development of feeding and language skills and offers practical advice on how to help children progress between different feeding skills. Feeding can be an excellent opportunity to integrate other developmental goals, such as language and social skills. What types of food to give children, how to advise parents, how to understand some of the problems seen, and practical advice on how to address specific problems are presented in case scenerios.

Many young children continue to have respiratory effects from their prematurity. The special section on chest physical therapy presents practical suggestions for helping a child achieve optimal respiratory health. Chest physical therapy is sometimes performed by physical therapy and sometimes by respiratory therapy; it is usually carried out by the family once the infant returns home. It is a skill that we should all possess and of which we should be aware, no matter which discipline is responsible for its implementation.

History and Environment of the NICU

The neonatal intensive care unit (NICU) is usually a bustling place. Incubators, or isolettes, look like huge glass boxes on wheels and stand at intervals. Each one is affiliated with at least one intimidating-looking machine that emits beeps or bells.

Medical staff peer into the boxes, adjust the machines, and write busily in patient charts. In NICUs that keep up with "best practices," blankets are draped over the incubators to mute sounds and lights, trash cans are padded, and voices and lights are lowered. NICU staff wear scrubs or other hospital dress. Parents are dressed in street clothes. Other NICU environments are loud and bright places 24 hours a day as staff bustle around to address medical emergencies and take care of infants. In some facilities staff and parents must don gowns and masks.

Harrison and Kositsky (1983) summarized the development of neonatal care, which began in France and expanded to the United States in the 1920s. In the late 1800s Dr. Tarnier of Paris designed an incubator for premature infants and with his colleague, Pierre Budin, began the science of neonatology, the study of the special needs and problems of premature infants. His student, Martin Couney, exhibited premature infants in their incubators at fairs throughout Europe as a way to make money. The money was used to care for the infants and to support the staff. Couney and his exhibit traveled throughout Europe and the United States for almost 30 years. Although his efforts saved many infants, they offended many people along the way. Couney finally settled his exhibit on Coney Island in New York. Although much criticism was leveled at his exploitative practices, Martin Couney's methods of supporting premature infants caught on and helped establish premature nurseries in hospitals across the country. The first was in Chicago's Sarah Lawrence Hospital in 1923 (Harrison & Kositsky, 1983).

Interventions evolved as new information and technology became available. Initially the treatment priority for premature nurseries was temperature control. Oxygen and antibiotic therapy were introduced in the 1940s. Although side effects of these treatments are serious and include eye and ear damage, the consequences of withholding them increases infant mortality. High levels of oxygen cause retinopathy of prematurity (ROP), and high amounts of mycin types of antibiotics are toxic to the inner ear, causing deafness.

Parents were often isolated from their infants, with the idea that minimal handling and stimulation were desirable for the infant. Only in recent decades have the importance of involving parents in the care of their premature infants and regulation of the NICU environment been recognized as beneficial.

Outcomes for Premature Infants

In the early days of caring for premature infants, those less than 1500 g were considered extremely fragile, and of those who survived, more than 50% had serious disabilities (Harrison & Kositsky, 1983). Physical and occupational therapy evaluations and care were routinely given to all infants less than 1500 g. Medical care has improved significantly, and outcomes are more favorable for infants who weigh between 1250 and 1500 g at birth. In recent years many hospitals have revised policies and procedures so that routine referrals for developmental screening and intervention occur only for infants below 1250 g birth weight. The survival rates and outcomes for very low birth weight (VLBW) infants, those below 1500 g, have improved significantly. The rate of disability among VLBW survivors is generally 25% (Escobar, Littenberg, & Petitti, 1991; Halsey, Collin, & Anderson, 1996). The extremely low birth weight (ELBW) infant weighs less than 1000 g at birth. The survival rates of these very small infants have also significantly improved in the past two decades, from 20% in the late 1970s to almost 50% in the late 1980s. Unfortunately, the rate of neurosensory impairments has remained nearly the same ranging from 19% to 22% (La Pine, Jackson, & Bennet, 1994).

Prematurity

Incidence and Cause

For a variety of reasons the survival rate for infants born prematurely is improving (Hack & Fanaroff, 1986 and 1989; La Pine, Jackson, & Bennet, 1994). Physicians are better able to control premature labor, allowing infants to more fully develop in the womb. Advanced medical technology and knowledge provide efficient techniques for managing the problems of prematurity. Just 10 years ago an infant born at 28 weeks' gestation was considered very high risk with little chance of survival. Now infants as young as 22 and 23 weeks of gestational age have a good chance of surviving (Figure 11-8).

The incidence of births occurring before 37 weeks is 50.4 per 1000 deliveries (Harlow, et al., 1996). At least 250,000 premature births occur each year in the United States, with approximately 40,000 of these infants in the very low birth weight (VLBW) category, below 1500 g of weight (Semmler, 1989). The number of NICUs has risen from an average of less than one per state in the 1960s to a current average of over 50 per state. NICUs are organized into regional care units, which respond to needs in specific geographic regions; they pool knowledge and resources to provide the most up-to-date care.

Factors contributing to premature births vary and in many cases are unknown. Maternal factors include eclampsia (a serious disease of high blood pressure that causes fluid retention, seizures, coma, and death if untreated), placenta previa (the placenta grows low in the uterus and partially or completely covers the cervix), abruptio placentae (the placenta separates prematurely from the uterine wall), incompetent cervix (the cervix opens too early), abnormal uterine shape, and infection or other illness that may precipitate a preterm labor. Fetal factors, such as congenital deformity, multiple pregnancy, and fetal infection, may also precipitate an early delivery. Although all women are

susceptible to premature labor, it occurs more frequently in women who have inadequate or no prenatal care, poor nutrition, and low socioeconomic status. Premature infants are more frequently born to African-American women than Caucasian women, and to Caucasian women more frequently than Asian-American women. African-American infants born prematurely do better than Caucasian infants, probably as a result of faster in utero maturation in African-Americans. Girls who are born prematurely have a better outcome than boys, in general, probably for the same reason. Each infant is unique, however, and individual differences may have a greater effect on outcome than ethnicity or gender.

Clinical Features

The premature infant looks very different from the term infant. Physical characteristics vary depending on the gestational age of the infant, illness, presence or absence of genetic or other disorders, and other factors. In general, the preterm infant has less body fat and less muscle tone and is physically smaller than the term infant. The premature infant also is less able to regulate body states (e.g., fussy, crying, quiet alert, sleeping) than the term infant (Figure 11-9). Table 11-2 outlines some significant features of preterm development. Specific terms are used to describe problems related to prematurity. Although many of these are described in the text, the glossary in Box 11-3 defines acronyms frequently used with premature infants.

The preterm baby, besides obvious physical and behavioral differences from the term baby, has less maturation of organ systems causing significant risks of medical problems that can be life threatening. The interaction between immature behavioral and state regulation with immature organ systems poses further threat to the premature infant. Some of the issues a small infant may face are problems with temperature regulation; regulating the rhythm of breathing, swallowing, and sucking; remembering to breathe; jaundice; and infections. Additional problems can include respiratory complications, heart problems, bleeding into the brain, poor function of the gastrointestinal system, and eye or ear damage resulting from medical interventions. Although they are discussed individually below, many of these problems of prematurity are associated. For instance, the stress of respira-

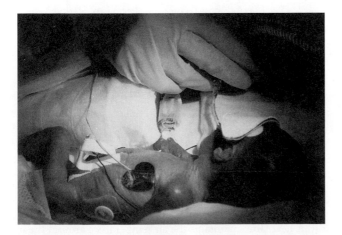

Figure 11-8 At 22 weeks of gestation, this infant has an improved chance of survival as a result of advances in medical care.

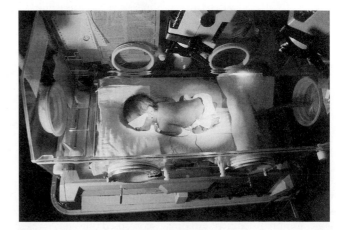

Figure 11-9 The premature infant is smaller and has less fat and lower muscle tone than a term infant.

TABLE 11-2 Characteristics of Premature Infants

Factor	Very premature (25-30 weeks)	Moderately premature (31-36 weeks)	Almost term (37-38 weeks)	Term (39-42 weeks)
Muscle tone	Extremely hypotonic, floppy	Hypotonic; some beginning flexor tone can be felt and seen at rest	Moderate flexor tone at rest	Strong physiological flexion
Posture	Lies with all extremities in full extension	Lies with all extremities in moderate extension	Lies with some flexion of extremities	Strong flexion of all extremities
Facial features	Well defined, except ears have no cartilage formation and can be folded	Well defined; ear cartilage is beginning to form	Well defined	Well defined
Hair and nails	Early hair, called lanugo, forms over most of body; healthy scalp hair	Has fingernails and toenails	Lanugo and much of scalp hair may fall out; fingernails and toenails may need trimming	Lanugo and much of scalp hair may fall out; fingernails and toenails may need trimming
Genitals	Poorly developed. Females: outer labia do not cover inner labia and clitoris. Male: scrotum small and smooth; testicles undescended	Still undeveloped. Females: outer labia do not cover inner labia and clitoris. Male: scrotum small and smooth; testicles undescended	More fully developed. Female: outer labia cover inner tissues. Male: testicles may descend to fill scrotum	Fully developed
Skin	Thin, translucent with wrinkles; veins apparent; dusky red color at birth	Still thin but more opaque; more fat under skin but still somewhat wrinkled	Opaque, healthy layer of fat under skin	Opaque, chubby appearance
Head shape	Skull bones thin and malleable; exposed to gravity and uneven pressure, head often becomes elongated and flattened	Skull bones thin and malleable; exposed to gravity and uneven pressure, head often becomes elongated and flattened	Skull bones thicker in older premature infant; head shaping is not as typical of earlier premature infant	Skull bones shaped by more even pressure of uterus, so are relatively round
Movements	Jerky, unorganized	Jerky and unorganized but better controlled than in very premature infant	Movements more controlled; less excursion than in premature infant	Movements smooth most of time
Behavior	Poor state control; overwhelmed by sensory stimuli	Poor state control; beginning habituation to aversive or repetitive stimuli	Emerging state control; can calm self sometimes	Variable state control; may be able to calm self
Sleep	Sleeps most of time; sleep characterized by restlessness	More quiet sleep; still sleeps most of time	Brief periods of wakefulness; sleep mostly quiet	Periods of alert wakefulness; sleep mostly quiet

tory complications can be related to an intraventricular hemorrhage; and deafness may be caused by strong antibiotics used to treat an infection. Many of the problems of prematurity have effects that can last into childhood and much later.

When the infant is born, a developmental assessment is performed; this defines the gestational age of the infant based on muscle tone, reflexes, and behavior. Different developmental assessments are used in different medical centers, but the Dubowitz is a common instrument. An Apgar score, used universally, is also tabulated at 1 and 5 minutes after birth. The Apgar scores the infant's heart rate, respiratory effort, muscle tone, reflex irritability and color, arriving at a score for each time interval. Most infants will have a lower score at 1 minute and a higher score at 5 minutes; although a score of 10 is possible, the highest score seen is usually 9. Table 11-3 outlines Apgar scoring. The Apgar score may be prognostic of the child's future functioning, with low scores indicating the potential for greater problems; however, it is not always an accurate prognostic indicator.

Initially the premature infant is placed on a warming table or tray. A heat lamp maintains the air temperature around the infant, and open sides allow medical personnel unlimited access (Figure 11-10). The more stable premature infant is assisted with

BOX 11-3 Frequently Used Acronyms Related to Prematurity

Size of Infants

SGA — Small for gestational age. Infants who are below the 10th percentile for infants the same age. Infants with various problems or exposures including Down syndrome, fetal alcohol syndrome, maternal cigarette smoking, multiple delivery, or poor intrauterine nutrition for various reasons may be SGA.

LGA — Large for gestational age. Infants who are above the 90th percentile for infants the same age. Infants born to mothers with diabetes are at risk for being LGA

AGA — Appropriate for gestational age. Infants between the 10th and 90th percentiles of weights for infants the same age are AGA.

IUGR — Intrauterine growth retardation. Infants who are smaller than normal for gestational age. Some centers use this term interchangeably with SGA; others use IUGR as meaning smaller than the typical SGA infant.

LBW — Low birth weight. Infants below 2500 g (5 pounds, 8 ounces).

VLBW — Very low birth weight. Infants below 1500 g (3 pounds, 5 ounces).

ELBW — Extremely low birth weight. Infants below 1000 g (2 pounds, 3½ ounces).

VVLBW — Very very low birth weight. Means the same as ELBW.

Disorders of Prematurity

NEC — Necrotizing enterocolitis. A disease of the immature intestinal tract where the intestinal wall becomes infected and dies.

RDS — Respiratory distress syndrome. Respiratory distress caused by a lack of surfactant (substance that helps keep lung tissues expanded) in immature lungs.

HMD — Hyaline membrane disease. The same as RDS.

BPD — Bronchopulmonary dysplasia. An advanced lung disease in infants caused by damage to lung tissues from mechanical ventilation.

CLD — Chronic lung disease. Means the same as BPD.

PDA — Patent ductus arteriosis. The ductus arteriosus, which shunts blood from the aorta to the pulmonary artery (past the lungs) in the fetus, sometimes fails to close in the premature infant, causing blood to bypass the lungs, resulting in decreased oxygenation to the blood and tissues.

Procedures or Equipment

CPAP — Continuous positive airway pressure. A form of mechanical ventilation to assist the child's own respiratory efforts.

PEEP — Positive end-expiratory pressure. A mechanical assistance for the child's own respiratory efforts.

ECMO — Extracorporeal membrane oxygenation. An advanced treatment for respiratory diseases involving oxygenation of the blood outside the body.

---

temperature regulation using the controlled environment of the incubator or Isolette. Portholes allow handling of the infant, adjustment of monitoring devices, and changing of diapers. The incubator also allows for controlled delivery of oxygen or lights to treat jaundice (Figure 11-11).

Respiratory problems of prematurity. Respiratory distress syndrome (RDS), also called hyaline membrane disease, is caused by insufficient amounts of surfactant in the immature lungs and can be a major hurdle for premature infants. RDS is the most common cause of respiratory distress in infants. Surfactant is a substance secreted by the lungs, which allows the small air sacs called alveoli to remain open and thus available for oxygen transfer. Premature infants have inadequate amounts of surfactant, resulting in poor inflation of the lungs and poor oxygenation of the blood and tissues. Several treatments are available for RDS, some beginning before birth. The mother in imminent danger of premature labor is given the steroid betamethasone (Celestone), which helps the unborn infant's lungs mature. Optimally, the drug should be given 72 hours before birth. Some deliveries cannot be delayed 72 hours after administration, and other infants develop RDS even after administration of the drug. Other infants are born so precipitously that the drug cannot be given at all.

Administering surfactant to infants with RDS is a recent intervention that has made a significant difference in the outcomes of infants with this disease. Surfactant is administered directly

TABLE 11-3 Apgar Scoring

Sign	0	1	2
Heart rate	Absent	Less than 100 beats per minute	Greater than 100 beats per minute
Respiratory effort	Absent	Irregular or slow	Good, strong cry
Muscle tone	Extremely hypotonic, limp	Some flexion of extremities	Normal physiological flexion
Reflex irritability (response to nasal suctioning or foot slap)	None	Grimace	Cry or sneeze
Color	Blue, pale	Body pink, extremities blue or pale	Pink color throughout

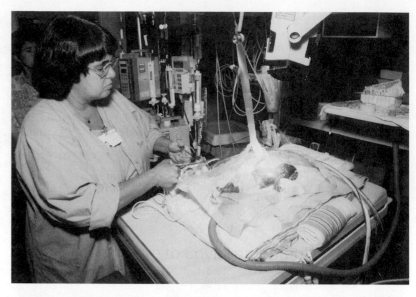

Figure 11-10 The warming table helps an infant maintain body temperature and allows optimal access for medical procedures.

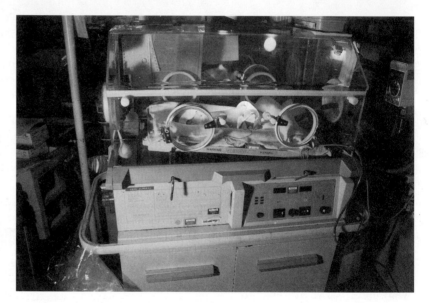

Figure 11-11 The Isolette, or incubator, allows a more controlled environment for the premature infant.

into the lungs through the endotracheal tube, usually in several doses. Other interventions include administration of oxygen, mechanical ventilation, and extracorporeal membrane oxygenation (ECMO) for those infants with severe RDS. ECMO is a technique of bypassing the lungs to oxygenate blood outside the body, thus allowing damaged lungs to rest and mature. It is only available at certain centers, is very expensive, and is not always successful in the very sick or very young infant.

Those children who need ventilatory assistance run the risk of developing *bronchopulmonary dysplasia (BPD),* a more serious respiratory condition that can lead to continued respiratory problems throughout childhood. Infants who need mechanical ventilation are often subjected to high ventilatory pressures, which cause damage to immature lung tissue. Fibrotic or inelastic tissue can be caused by scarring, alveolar collapse, or fibrosis between the alveolar sacs. Hypertrophy of muscles in the bronchioles can cause decreased airway diameter, which further in-

hibits air circulation in the lungs. Other factors leading to BPD include high levels of oxygen and poor drainage of fluids resulting from the endotracheal tube placement. BPD is treated by oxygen administration, antibiotics to control infections, and breathing treatments with drugs to dilate the bronchioles. Steroid therapy has been shown to decrease the severity of BPD in some cases (Abman & Groothius, 1994). Alternative types of ventilators, such as high frequency oscillation ventilators, can decrease the barotrauma that can lead to BPD.

A range of problems may continue throughout childhood that are related to early respiratory distress. Children who have had RDS may have an increased incidence of respiratory infections during childhood. Children with BPD usually have chronic lung problems, including repeated infections, which can affect their respiration until late childhood or early adolescence (Abman & Groothius, 1994). Some children need to receive therapy services at home to decrease their exposure to illness carried by

While doing chest physical therapy, sing a song in rhythm to the percussion. If you are not comfortable singing, you can use taped music, such as aerobics tapes, with varying speeds and rhythm. There is no rule that the percussions need to be regular; you can use complex and interesting rhythms that both you and the child may enjoy.

other children. Many children with BPD go home from the hospital on supplemental oxygen and require close respiratory surveillance. Their endurance is limited by respiratory capacity. Some children with severe BPD may need ventilatory support for months or years and may go home using a ventilator for respiratory support at night or during the day.

Pulmonary hypertension and cardiac hypertrophy are other problems that may persist beyond infancy and that are related to early respiratory disease. Transitory hypertonicity is sometimes seen in infants with BPD and may be related to the extra effort of breathing. Transient high muscle tone usually normalizes by the time the infant is walking. Infants with BPD may have related neurodevelopmental problems, including cerebral palsy, that cause changes in muscle tone that are not transitory. The incidence of cerebral palsy is higher for children who have had BPD than for the general population of premature infants, probably because of the stress related to severe lung disease.

Cardiac problems of prematurity. During fetal circulation the blood has no need to pass through the lungs to become oxygenated because the placenta is the organ responsible for this task. The ductus arteriosis shunts the blood between the main pulmonary artery and the descending aorta to bypass the fetus's developing lungs. It usually closes shortly after birth; but in up to 65% of premature infants weighing less than 1750 g (4 pounds) it remains open for at least several hours and sometimes longer. This may be as a response to decreased levels of oxygen or other chemical changes; no one is really sure. This condition is called *patent ductus arteriosus (PDA)*.

The effects of a PDA on a child with RDS is that less oxygenated blood is available because some blood bypasses the lungs, going straight from the pulmonary artery to the aorta, and then back to the heart. This is called *persistent fetal circulation* because it is the same circulation pattern as a fetus. As the child grows and the lungs become more mature and have greater expansion, different thoracic pressures may divert blood in the opposite direction, from the aorta into the pulmonary artery. This causes too much blood to go to the lungs and further decreases the amount of oxygenated blood going to the tissues. In addition, the heart and lungs may become overworked. The infant will develop problems related to the PDA including poor progress weaning from the ventilator, poor growth, or need for more supplementary oxygen. The ductus arteriosus needs to be closed to allow blood to fully circulate to the lungs and tissues and to relieve the strain on the heart and lungs.

The drug indomethacin is the treatment of choice for PDA. One or two doses of this drug facilitates closure of a PDA in most children. One side effect of indomethacin is increased bleeding, potentially causing problems for children who are at risk for bleeding into the brain; however, indomethacin is fairly safe overall. Some children may need surgery to ligate or tie off the ductus. The surgery is fairly safe and is tolerated well. The PTA may see a scar on the left side of the child's chest indicating that this surgery was performed. Most children have no sequelae from a PDA.

Intracranial hemorrhage. Many premature infants sustain bleeding in the brain, called intracranial hemorrhage (ICH). Other names for bleeding in the brain include intraventricular hemorrhage (IVH), subarachnoid hemorrhage, and subependymal hemorrhage; each term indicates the part of the brain or tissue where the bleeding occurred. The most common type of bleeding in premature infants is the intraventricular hemorrhage, bleeding into the ventricles of the brain. Children with a subarachnoid hemorrhage, bleeding on the surface of the brain, have a better prognosis than those with an IVH.

The causes of IVH are not entirely clear; however, low oxygenation to the brain as a result of respiratory distress and poor structural support for blood vessels around the ventricles because of immaturity are thought to play a part. Changes in the blood pressure of infants during the birth process and stress caused by asphyxia, too much handling, and invasive medical procedures are also thought to be possible contributors to this problem.

This complication of prematurity is potentially the most devastating, because it can cause brain damage with resulting neurological deficits including cerebral palsy. Approximately 40% to 45% of the children under 1500 g at birth sustain an IVH (Hack, et al., 1991). The severity of IVH is categorized from grade 1 (smallest) to grade 4 (largest). A grade 1 bleed is also called a *subependymal hemorrhage*, meaning a bleed into the subependymal tissues around the ventricles. A grade 2 bleed involves some bleeding into the ventricles themselves. A grade 3 bleed fills the ventricles with blood and pushes out against surrounding tissues, and a grade 4 bleed forces blood from the dilated ventricles back into the tissues surrounding the ventricles. Children with a grade 4 bleed almost always have neurological damage, but children with grades 1 through 3 have a more optimistic prognosis.

Approximately 40% to 60% of children with an IVH sustain some type of neurodevelopmental abnormality identified within the first 3 years of life (Selzer, Lindgren, & Blackman, 1992). Other children without a measurable form of neurological abnormality in the first 3 years may have other signs of neurological problems later in life, especially as they reach school age and are expected to perform in the school environment. More severe bleeds are associated with increasing neurological damage. One consequence of IVH is spastic diplegic cerebral palsy, the most common type of cerebral palsy seen in premature infants (Figure 11-12).

Bleeding into the ventricles can cause a blockage of the normal flow of cerebrospinal fluid around the brain, called *hydrocephalus*. This fluid typically flows through the four ventricles of the brain and around the outside of the brain and spinal cord. These areas are contiguous with one another, and if a blockage occurs, the fluid backs up in the ventricles and causes them to expand and push into the surrounding brain tissue. To treat this condition, a thin tube called a *shunt* is inserted into the ventricle and threaded under the skin of the head and neck to the heart or the abdomen to provide a route for the cerebrospinal fluid to be reabsorbed. It may be called a *ventriculoperitoneal* or a *ventricu-*

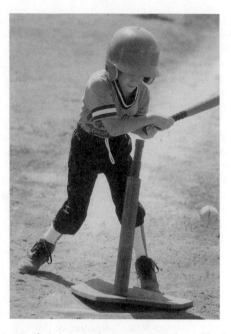

Figure 11-12 Christian was born prematurely and had a grade 3 intraventricular hemorrhage, leading to a diagnosis of spastic diplegia. He enjoys playing baseball with his friends on the weekends.

loatrial shunt, depending on the endpoint. The shunt relieves pressure in the ventricles and preserves brain tissue.

Some factors have been found to protect premature infants from ICH, including antenatal steroid administration, African-American maternal race, female gender, increasing gestational age, heavier birth weight, and maternal history of preeclampsia or hypertension (Shankaran, Bauer, Bain, Wright, & Zachary, 1996). Controlling the NICU environment is thought to reduce infants' stress and has been shown to promote better weight gain, decreased time needed with mechanical ventilation, and decreased supplementary oxygen requirements (Als, et al., 1994). It may also contribute to a decrease in ICH.

The older child who has had an IVH may have cerebral palsy, particularly spastic diplegia, although the specific manifestations of neurological damage varies. Other neurological problems may be more global, resulting from the bleed itself or from hydrocephalus that was caused by an IVH. A child with a shunt has a bump under the scalp just behind and above one ear. The drainage tube for the shunt can usually be seen traveling under the skin down the side of the neck and over the chest; a small scar resulting from the incision made to help guide the tube placement can be seen on the abdomen.

The PTA should be alert for signs of shunt malfunction including lethargy, irritability, or a change in behavior. A further discussion of shunts is included in Chapter 5 for the child with spina bifida. Awareness of the potential problems is important because a shunt malfunction can cause increasing neurological damage and can lead to death. If a shunt malfunction is suspected, immediate medical attention is imperative.

Necrotizing enterocolitis. Necrotizing enterocolitis (NEC) is unique to premature infants and was first recognized in the 1960s when greater numbers of smaller premature infants were surviving. Parts of the intestinal wall become inflamed and begin to die, causing symptoms of pain, infection, and poor nutrition. The cause of NEC is not clear, but disruption of circulation to the intestines is thought to allow bacteria to proliferate and cause infection. Circulation to the intestines can be impaired because of immaturity, stress, or other factors. If the intestinal wall perforates, the infection can spread throughout the abdominal cavity, causing more severe illness and threatening life. Infants who are given formula rather than breast milk are thought to be more at risk for this disease; however, infants who have been given only breast milk or those who have had no oral feedings at all also develop the disease.

Treatment includes giving antibiotics to fight infection, suctioning with a nasogastric tube to decrease the pressure in the intestines, and providing nutrients through intravenous routes. If the disease progresses, surgery may be necessary to remove the damaged portion of the intestines. A colostomy, jejunostomy, or iliostomy may be required to divert intestinal contents away from recovering tissues.

The older child who has had NEC as an infant may have residual feeding problems. Some children need an ostomy with an external bag on the abdomen to collect fecal contents or just an opening (stoma) on the abdomen where fecal contents empty into a diaper. Other children may have a scar indicating where surgery occurred. Most children with an ostomy have surgery to reconnect the bowel after it recovers to redivert fecal contents along their normal route.

Retinopathy of prematurity. The infant exposed to high levels of oxygen for prolonged periods may develop abnormalities in the retina of one or both eyes. Because of immature vascularization, oxygen causes a proliferation of blood vessels in the retina, which can cause visual impairment or blindness. A further description of this condition is found in Chapter 10. The PTA may work with children who have visual impairments or blindness as a consequence of their prematurity.

Hyperbilirubinemia. Children with immature liver functions may have difficulty handling the high concentrations of bilirubin, a breakdown product of red blood cells, which is characteristic of newborns. All newborns are susceptible to this complication, but premature infants have particular susceptibility because of their immaturity. The inability to excrete enough bilirubin can cause hyperbilirubinemia and result in jaundice, or icterus, characterized by a yellow cast to the skin and tissues. If bilirubin is allowed to increase to toxic levels, it can be deposited in the brain, especially in the basal ganglia and hippocampus, a condition called *kernicterus* or *bilirubin encephalopathy.* Damage to these and other centers in the brain can cause athetoid cerebral palsy, mental retardation, sensorineural hearing loss, or other neurological symptoms.

Because physicians are aware of the dangerous effects of kernicterus, treatment is initiated early to help rid the body of high levels of bilirubin. Light is one method of breaking down this substance, so phototherapy is the most commonly used treatment. Children are placed under or near banks of fluorescent lights with as much skin exposed as possible. Eyes and genitals are protected using opaque patches, masks, or small diapers (Figure 11-13). Advanced methods of applying phototherapy include using fiberoptic light, which is piped into blankets underneath or wrapped around children. This method may be particularly effective for home phototherapy treatment; it allows for more natural parent-child interaction and improved temperature regulation.

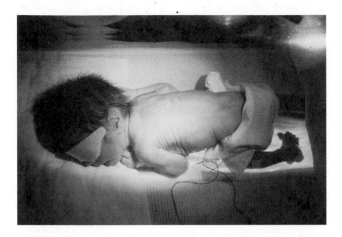

Figure 11-13 This infant is being treated for hyperbilirubinemia through phototherapy to break down the high levels of bilirubin. He is lying on a light source, and lights are being directed at him from above.

If phototherapy is not effective in decreasing bilirubin concentrations, blood transfusions can replace red blood cells and decrease concentrations of bilirubin. Treatment with phenobarbital to break down bilirubin may be used in extreme cases, but this is not as effective as other methods.

Most children with hyperbilirubinemia are treated successfully, and the PTA would normally see no sequelae in the older child. Children who develop kernicterus, however, may have particular patterns of neurological damage, such as athetoid cerebral palsy, which are not common from other mechanisms of neurological insult.

Apnea and bradycardia. Children with immature respiratory regulation may "forget" to breathe (apnea), with resultant slowing of the heart rate (bradycardia). This is sometimes called "A's and B's" in the jargon of the NICU staff. It is characteristic of young premature babies and of some older premature infants who are medically stable but need to grow and acquire more weight before going home ("feeders and growers"). In the NICU heart rate and respiratory rate are constantly monitored, and an alarm sounds if the infant's heart rate drops below a threshold level. Sometimes the sound of the alarm stimulates the child to begin breathing. Nurses are also trained to stimulate the infant by flicking the feet or gently moving the infant to encourage breathing. If these episodes of apnea and bradycardia continue until the child is ready to go home, the family may use a monitor at home to protect against sudden infant death syndrome (SIDS). The monitor may be used only for naps and nighttime sleeping or all the time. Parents using a monitor are generally trained in cardiopulmonary resuscitation (CPR) and in the care and use of the monitor. Some children need monitoring only for a few weeks; others may have episodes of apnea and bradycardia that require monitoring for months after going home.

The PTA may encounter an apnea monitor if a child is seen for therapy in the home. Learning how to assess whether an alarm is an artifact of movement or indicative of a problem is important. Parents should teach the therapy provider how to silence the alarm if it should sound. The alarm can be turned off completely for the therapy session because the therapy provider is with the child to monitor vital signs. If a child needs the monitor, turning the alarm function back on after therapy is finished is very important.

Interventions in the NICU

Attention to the environment of the NICU is essential for the optimal health of the premature infant. Because the primary efforts in this environment are to preserve the health of the child, attention has not traditionally been paid to the developing relationship between the parents and the infant, behavioral aspects of the child's maturation and recovery from medical conditions, or assisting the child to preserve normal sleep/wake cycles. The NICU is traditionally loud, bright, and busy, with emphasis on medical assessment and treatment.

Research over the past few decades has demonstrated that loud noises, bright lights, and insensitive handling may contribute to medical problems in these small infants. Decreased oxygenation levels, fluctuations in heart or respiratory rates, and crying causing higher intracranial pressures have all been observed in premature infants in response to noises, lights, and handling in the NICU.

Emphasis in many hospitals has changed toward directing the environment for the optimal growth and development of the child. This includes promoting a night/day schedule with lights dimmed at night; fostering caring relationships and bonding of infants and parents; decreasing light and noise levels at all times; and grouping handling and medical procedures to minimize disturbance and maximize sleep times (Als, et al., 1994). These efforts have also directed the way physical therapy may be provided for premature infants.

Physical therapy intervention in the NICU. Physical therapy intervention for the premature infant changes according to the medical stability and gestational age of the infant. Common interventions include promoting proper positioning, including the emphasis on physiological flexion, teaching parents methods of assisting the behavioral and motor skills acquisition of infants, handling to provide experiences to help the child develop appropriate skills, and continual assessment of the clinical neuromotor status of the infant. In the NICU a transdisciplinary approach is most often used, with many occupational and physical therapists working closely in teams. To minimize the number of people handling the infant and interacting with parents, a primary therapist who will provide all of the interventions to the family and infant may be chosen. This therapist may cross traditional boundaries of occupational and physical therapy to work with feeding, positioning, gross motor skills, and fine motor skills, with consultation from other team members as needed.

Positioning is initially designed to promote normal physiological flexion, even in the very small infant. The premature infant has significantly less flexor tone than a term infant and is exposed to gravity, handling, and flat mattresses without the benefit of the close-fitting uterus to promote a flexed posture. With a minimum of handling the therapist or nurse can help the infant sustain a flexed posture, even on a flat mattress. Figure 11-14 demonstrates some positioning techniques.

Parents are usually anxious to begin handling their premature infant. They may be uncomfortable, however, not knowing how to optimally stimulate their infant or even how to interact with the infant. The nursing staff usually promotes parent-child inter-

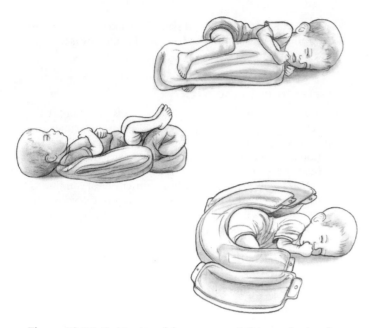

Figure 11-14 Positioning of the premature infant emphasizes flexion to promote developmentally appropriate muscle tone.

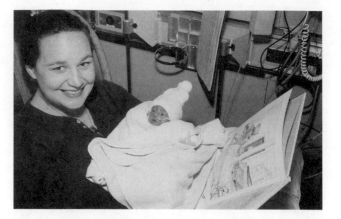

Figure 11-15 This infant is in an alert state and is ready to respond to his mother's interactions.

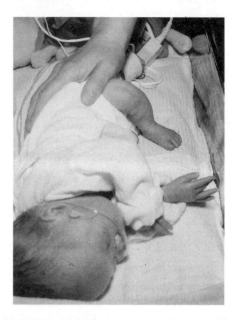

Figure 11-16 This weight-bearing activity for the medically stable premature infant is thought to mimic sensation that the infant might have experienced while in utero.

action by helping the parent hold or touch the infant as soon as possible. The therapist can help the parents learn basic communication strategies with their premature child. Most parents can easily recognize and respond to signs that the infant is ready for interaction. These may include an open, alert expression, pursed lips, and a steady gaze (Figure 11-15). Obvious signs that the infant is stressed include crying, arching, and turning away. Not so obvious signs that may also indicate that the infant is overstimulated or needs a break include hiccups, sneezing, holding an arm straight out as if saying "Stop," or change in skin color. Being sensitive to these signs can help a baby avoid stress and can help parents feel that they are more effective at communicating with their child. This interaction can facilitate the bonding process and encourage positive relations between parents and child.

Therapists also help parents recognize strengths or needs of their child in areas of state regulation, awareness of environmental sounds or sights, and tuning out stressful stimuli. Informed parents are more sensitive to helping their child develop these important skills.

Provision of therapy services to the child in the NICU usually focuses primarily on parent teaching, with some direct intervention with the infant as he or she gets stronger. Research has shown that parent teaching has a greater impact on the development of a child born prematurely than direct therapy services.

Parent teaching and direct therapy services can also focus on physical interactions with the baby. Some interactions that are believed to help the infant mature include providing sensations that the baby might have experienced in utero had the birth not been early (Deiriggi, 1990, Korner, 1986). These may include environmental interventions, such as a waterbed and audiotapes of parents' voices. Provision of physical sensations, such as weight bearing through the feet and hands (as though the infant were kicking in utero) or vestibular input, such as rocking, can also be helpful (Figure 11-16). As the infant grows, beginning skills in moving against gravity can be facilitated, including head

control in supported sitting. Because the premature infant tends to develop extensor strength and control before that of flexor muscle groups, activities to promote flexion of the neck, trunk, and extremities are encouraged.

Provision of sensory experiences that infants may have felt in utero can help infants organize their behavior and movements. This can include holding arms and legs in flexion, gentle massage, wrapping or bundling the child in blankets, carrying the child in a front backpack, and skin-to-skin contact with a parent. Medical personnel should approve these activities because of the need to closely monitor and treat the infant for medical conditions. Any interventions are dependent on the infant's medical stability and readiness for handling. Physical therapy interventions and parent teaching usually occur just before or after feeding to allow the infant maximum sleep time. Many of the interventions described are also suitable for older infants who need help in developing motor and behavioral organization and skills.

Feeding is an area of intervention in the NICU that may have special emotional overtones for parents. Tiny infants do not have the strength or endurance to suck their food through a nipple, so they are fed using the gavage method. A thin tube is snaked through the nostril and down into the stomach, then the mother's breast milk or infant formula is poured slowly through the tube. Parents can be taught to provide face-to-face interaction with the child, to help the baby suck on something during the feeding, and to provide other sensory stimuli, such as touch or stroking, that will make this a positive experience for parents and child. As the baby becomes stronger, he or she may be allowed to nipple small amounts. The mother may choose to breastfeed or use a bottle. Because of poor strength, endurance, and sensorimotor organization, the premature infant may need more help and time to learn to effectively nipple feed than a typical term infant. The therapy provider in the NICU is in a position to help the parents and the infant learn nippling skills. Feeding problems may persist in the older child because of poor strength, endurance, negative experiences with tube feeding, or poor neuromuscular coordination from immaturity or cerebral palsy. The PTA may assist with feeding skills after an infant is discharged from the hospital. A team effort involving the occupational therapist, nutritionist, physical therapy provider, the parents, nurse, and the physician is essential in managing a feeding problem.

> Ask family members what foods their child likes and what foods the family normally eats at home. Ask how they feed their child at home. You may learn about new foods and gain a better understanding of the difficulties a family faces with a child who has an eating disorder.

The experiences of the NICU can be quite intense, both for the parent and the child. Although efforts are made to promote behavioral adjustment of the infant, in the world of medical crises, this may not always be possible. The child may have difficulty adjusting to life at home, especially sleeping for longer blocks of time, and tolerating absence of excessive sound and light; and the parents may find themselves emotionally exhausted after the child comes home. Therapy providers should support parents and infants during this period of adjustment by encouraging discussions about their experiences, allowing long silences, or providing information.

Other Neonatal Problems

Common problems related to neonates, such as hip dysplasia (Chapter 4), cardiac defects (Chapter 12), and jaundice (this chapter) may require physical therapy treatment. Other problems that may generate referral to physical therapy in the neonatal period or need for continued services in the infant or toddler years include inguinal hernia, gastroesophageal reflux, and meconium aspiration syndrome. These problems may also be associated with other developmental problems and are addressed in this section.

Meconium Aspiration Syndrome

The first stool of the newborn is called *meconium* and has a greenish black color and a thick, tarry consistency. This stool is made before birth from amniotic fluid swallowed by the fetus. Stress to the fetus, such as from anoxia or hypoxia, can cause relaxation of the anal sphincter and stooling of the meconium. When stooling occurs before or during the birth process, the meconium stains the amniotic fluid around the infant. A small percentage of infants with stained amniotic fluid aspirate the meconium into their lungs, causing respiratory distress that ranges from mild to severe, known as meconium aspiration syndrome (MAS).

Incidence and cause. Approximately 9% to 20% of all infants are born with meconium-stained fluid (Houlihan & Knuppel, 1994). Estimates regarding the number of these infants developing MAS vary according to geographical area and particular study. They range from 4 to 11 per 1000 live births in South Africa (Adhikari & Gouws, 1995), to 5.3 per 1000 live births in Hawaii (Sunoo, Kosasa, Nakayama, & Hale, 1993), to 1.8 per 1000 live births in Texas (Hernandez, Little, Dax, Gilstrap, & Rosenfeld, 1993), to 1.3 per 1000 live births in Finland (Erkkola, Kero, Suhonen-Polvi, & Korvenranta, 1994).

Meconium staining is thought to be caused by fetal distress, occurring either before or during the birth process. Infants born by cesarean section, those with an Apgar score lower than 4 at 1 minute, history of fetal tachycardia (high heart rate), and those with a need for deep suctioning or intubation are at higher risk for developing MAS than infants without these problems. Infants with a gestational age of greater than 41 weeks are also more at risk of developing this syndrome.

Clinical features and treatment. Infants with MAS develop respiratory distress, which requires medical support and usually includes the need for supplemental oxygen and intubation. The meconium not only obstructs the infant's airways and causes injury to the sensitive epithelium of the respiratory tract, but it can also interfere with surfactant function. Surfactant replacement therapy has been effective in improving oxygenation and reducing the hospitalization time of term infants with MAS (Findlay, Taeusch, & Walther, 1996).

For infants with severe respiratory distress who are intubated, paralytic drugs such as pancuronium bromide (Pavulon) or curare may be used to prevent the infant fighting against the ventilator. These medications may cause lingering hypotonia, sometimes for weeks or months after discontinuation. Physical therapy may work with infants with MAS for positioning in the neonatal period and for strengthening and developmental activities as the child grows stronger. The child with MAS may sustain brain damage related to severe respiratory distress. Physical therapy provides neurodevelopmental intervention for these children.

Gastroesophageal Reflux

Incidence and cause. Infants with frequent regurgitation, emesis, poor weight gain, irritability, frequent respiratory infections, or recurrent apnea may have gastroesophageal reflux (GES). Stomach contents back up into the esophagus, causing irritation to the esophagus and the potential for aspiration into the lungs. Infants with scoliosis, neurological disability, hiatal hernia, and cystic fibrosis are at particular risk for this problem.

It was previously believed that chronic low tone of the lower esophageal sphincter caused GES, but current opinion is that it is caused by transient or inappropriate relaxation of the sphincter (Wong, 1995). High abdominal pressures, such as those caused by coughing, can also contribute to GES.

One out of every 300 to 1000 children have GES to some extent. Most infants grow out of GES by the time they are 18 months of age with no sequelae, and their symptoms are managed by drugs and positioning. Forty percent of children with GES may have continued problems with reflux and require more aggressive intervention, including surgery later in childhood.

Treatment. Medical intervention with drugs including metoclopramide (Reglan) or bethanechol (Urecholine) can decrease symptoms. Although thickening food with rice cereal or commercial thickening agents may reduce the incidence of emesis, allow for quieter sleeping, and decrease irritability, it may not decrease the actual incidence of GES. Positioning infants to decrease the physical excursion of stomach contents into the esophagus can also be effective. Appropriate positioning usually includes a 30-degree angle of the sleeping surface, with the infant in the prone position. Flat prone positioning has been shown to be equally effective as a 30-degree tilt. Upright or supine positioning has not been shown to be effective in preventing reflux.

In some hospitals or outpatient clinics infants are referred to physical therapy for loan or purchase of a 30-degree wedge and parent instruction for positioning. Infants who are mobile can easily slide down a tilted surface, so a makeshift or commercially available harness may be necessary to maintain the position (Figure 11-17).

The PTA may see older children with neurological disorders who have GES continuing beyond the neonatal period. Appropriate roles include scheduling therapy before meals so that a child can remain still when he or she has a full stomach; avoiding head down positions during therapy; and participating in the team process of advising parents regarding nutrition, activity level, and consistency of food.

Hernia

A hernia is a weakness in the abdominal wall where fluid, intestine, or other abdominal contents may protrude. Premature infants are at particular risk for developing hernias because of immaturity and muscular weakness. Hernias are not life threatening unless a loop of

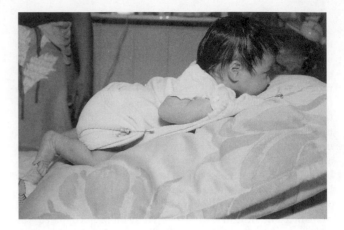

Figure 11-17　The baby blanket can be brought up between the legs of a small infant and pinned to the mattress or sheet to make a simple harness for an infant with gastroesophogeal reflux.

intestine becomes stuck outside the stomach wall and causes the intestine to become blocked. This condition is called *incarceration,* or *strangulation,* and requires emergency surgery to repair.

Umbilical hernia. A protrusion or lump around the umbilicus (belly button) is an umbilical hernia. The hernia may be more prominent when a child cries, stands up, or becomes angry because of increased abdominal pressure forcing fluid or tissue into the opening. An umbilical hernia is not medically treated unless it becomes incarcerated or strangulated; it usually disappears by 2 years of age.

Inguinal hernia. Inguinal hernia is much more common in boys than girls. In the premature male infant the testes may not have descended into the scrotal sac by the time of birth. After they descend a persistent opening in the abdominal wall may allow fluid or a loop of intestine to enter the inguinal canal and/or the scrotum. It usually becomes apparent when the infant is 2 to 3 months old, but it may not become a problem until later in childhood. A swelling or mass can be palpated in the inguinal area and/or in the scrotum. The inguinal hernia is treated surgically as an elective procedure when the infant becomes large enough to tolerate the anesthesia. Some surgeons wait until the child is a toddler or even school-aged to perform this surgery.

Oral Motor Development—The Basis of Feeding and Expressive Speech Development

APPLICATIONS

NANCY B. ROBINSON

For most infants and toddlers the basic skills for talking, eating, and drinking occur in a steady, developmental progression within the second year of life. The underlying "oral motor" mechanism of these children is intact. By about 18 months of age most children who are developing normally have moved from the suckling patterns of early infancy to chewing soft pieces of table food, such as scrambled eggs, tofu pieces, and small bites of crackers. Children who are born with physical disabilities may have impaired or delayed abilities to drink liquids and to eat

solid foods. Just as children with physical disabilities have a wide range of physical development and mobility, a wide range of ability and function also exists in their oral motor skills. By nature of the innervation of cranial nerves to the small muscles in the mouth, jaws, tongue, and throat, oral motor development is considered a specialized case of fine motor development. The extent of oral motor ability may be related to the child's musculoskeletal impairment. For example, a child with paraplegic involvement of the legs may exhibit very little oral motor involvement and show normal oral motor function resulting in normal eating, drinking, and speech skills. In another case a child with involvement of upper and lower limbs may show limited head and neck control with concomitant limitations in lip, tongue, and jaw movements that affect feeding and speech development.

Understanding oral motor development and its relationship to supporting the development of feeding and speech is critical to optimize each child's ability to attain oral motor functioning that supports nutritional intake and verbal skills. An overview of the progression of normal oral motor development in infants is discussed in this section as a foundation for understanding the sequence and stages of increasing control and mastery over the oral motor mechanism. Additionally, the relationship of oral motor functions to the development of feeding and speech skills and the cooccurrence of motor abilities that emerge in the first year of life are discussed. A guide for functional assessment of feeding skills is provided to assist the practitioner in observing the development of feeding behaviors. Finally, specialized problems and strategies to support improved oral motor functioning are presented.

Role of the PTA

The PTA plays a unique role on the team of a child with a motor disability. Provision of regular services to a child in the home or school may allow the PTA to become a confidant of the parent or teacher, a routine observer of the childs skills, or an observer of problems of which the rest of the team is unaware. The role of a physical therapy provider as a team member is to be aware of the child and his or her needs as a whole and to bring concerns and suggestions to the family and other team members. Feeding and language skills acquisition are directly related to gross motor skills, and the PTA should be aware of basic concepts and interventions related to these skills. Direct physical therapy intervention should support the goals of the family and the team related to feeding, language, and gross motor skills. Specific skills that the PTA may bring to the team and child may include positioning, knowledge and use of adaptive equipment, management of abnormal muscle tone, and specific strategies related to movement and stability of the child during functional tasks.

Oral Motor Mechanism

Before describing the role of oral motor development in the development of feeding and speaking skills, an understanding of the structure and function of the oral motor mechanism itself is important. The critical structures in the oral motor mechanism include the jaw, lips, tongue, palate, pharynx, and larynx. A further point that requires clarification is the difference between the oral motor mechanism of the adult and the child. The adult oral structures form an inverted L; the child's oral structures are open and flat in a nearly horizontal plane. With maturation and growth the oral mechanism achieves finer muscle control and coordination.

The oral motor system is primarily designed to support life functions, which include respiratory and protective functions that prevent inhaling foreign particles into the lungs. The struc-

ture of the oral motor mechanism is designed for multiple and discrete functions, which include both involuntary reflexes and volitional movements in eating and speaking. It is important to realize that life-support functions take priority over voluntary functions. Protection of the respiratory system, including the *gag reflex* to prevent inhaling foreign objects, takes precedence over eating, drinking, and speech.

Developmental Stages

In addition to maturation of the oral motor mechanism, learning takes place through repeated actions and behaviors that include involuntary and voluntary functions of the oral motor mechanism. The emergence of feeding and verbal skills can be categorized in several stages:

1. Suckling and sucking in newborns
2. Exploration by mouth
3. Discovering taste for food
4. Biting and chewing food
5. Transitions to cup drinking

Suckling and Sucking in Newborns

Suckling and sucking are feeding patterns typically found in newborn infants. Structures that play critical functions in suckling and sucking are the upper and lower jaw, cheeks, tongue, and palate. Initially muscles of the tongue, lips, and soft palate assist in raising and lowering these structures in a vertical motion. Although muscle movement is primarily limited to up and down motions, *buccal pads,* or fat pads in the cheeks, combine with lip and jaw closure to provide stability for early sucking. The tongue typically fills the oral cavity in the newborn and normally has a short, broad shape. Taste buds *(papilla)* are present on the top *(dorsum)* of the tongue. The infants primary oral motor accomplishment at this time is the achievement of a coordinated suckling-swallowing-breathing process. The infant masters the ability to move and swallow liquid in a coordinated sequence of mouth closure, tongue pressure on the nipple, tongue shortening and broadening, and restriction of the pharynx before pausing for breath. The entire sequence takes less than a second, but it represents a major milestone in the ability to suck and swallow liquids. Infants also produce open vowel sounds and "flat" crying sounds during this stage, related to the open and flat position of the oral mechanism.

Exploration by Mouth

Between three and five months of age the infant begins to have more control of lips, tongue, and jaw movements. Reflex patterns lessen. However, new foods and textures can still trigger the gag reflex. More active sucking is observed in combination with suckling; infants begin to enjoy mouthing objects and toys. Up and down *(phasic)* movements of the jaw are observed. These movements are precursors to more mature "munching" seen as older infants begin to chew foods. Differentiated cries for hunger, pain, anger, and fussing are related to the infant's increasing degree of muscle control over shape of the oral cavity. Increased vocalization is also observed with increased lip and tongue control. As closure of the soft palate is achieved because of greater muscle control, decreased nasal quality in the voice is also observed.

Discovering Taste for Food

At 6 months there is discovery of the taste for food. Many feeding and vocal skills emerge concurrently with this discovery. Examples of maturing oral motor skills include a lessened gag response and greater tolerance of new tastes and textures. Long, coordinated sequences of sucking, swallowing, and breathing are found. The beginning of cup drinking emerges during this stage, observed as a suckle pattern and accompanied by frequent loss of liquid and episodes of choking, as the infant learns to manage increased quantities of liquid from the cup. Infants begin to anticipate feeding with an open-mouth posture upon the sight of food, showing recognition and understanding of the feeding routine. Spoonfeeding becomes more mature, as the lower lip comes up under the spoon and upper lip down to scrape food off the spoon. Food is moved back and forth in the mouth in a sucking pattern. Chewing emerges in an up-and-down motion, which is the beginning of munching. Tongue movement is side-to-side (Figure 11-18). Facial expressions show likes and dislikes. Babbling becomes more prolonged and controlled with repeated sound sequences and variation in pitch, intonation, and loudness. Infants are also gaining control over large muscles that are involved in sitting, crawling, and moving between positions. Front and back consonants made with the tongue, such as /d/ and /g/, begin to emerge related to improved tongue control.

Biting and Chewing Food

Biting and chewing food are observed at 7 to 9 months in the typically developing infant. Cup drinking and improved lip control for drinking are also observed with the bottom lip up under the cup and sucking of liquid when the cup is held in the mouth. Coughing and choking still occur when too much liquid is given.

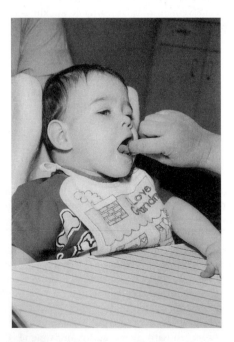

Figure 11-18 Matthew, who has cerebral palsy, is learning to move food around in his mouth at age 15 months. Food is placed in the side of his mouth so that he can better control it.

The mouth is opened for spoonfeeding; the lower lip comes up under the spoon and the upper lip comes forward, down, and inward to remove food from the spoon. Some gagging still occurs when new textures are presented. An up and down chewing motion *(phasic bite)* continues and is now applied to hard solids. "Melting" of soft solids, a new eating strategy, is accomplished with closed lips until the food bite is broken off. Biting on fingers and other objects may be observed to relieve teething discomfort. Sucking on fingers is observed to organize and calm the infant. Long strings of repeated sounds and variations of consonants and vowels, called *reduplicated babbling* and *variegated babbling,* are observed. Increased lip and tongue-tip consonants are observed (m, b, p, t, d and n). Differentiation in nasal/oral sounds are also found in the same place of articulation (m/b, n/d).

Transition to Cup Drinking

Around 10 to 12 months the infant may begin to be weaned from the bottle or breast. Improved cup-drinking skills of jaw and lip control are also found with the tongue and lower lip protruding. Finer control of the upper lip downward while drinking from a cup is also observed. Infants and toddlers at this stage show mature eating patterns, opening the mouth and leaning forward to spoonfeed, closing lips on the spoon, bringing lips inward to clean off food from the spoon, and using neck flexion to assist in lip closure. Food is swallowed using sucking and suckling, tongue protrusion, and elevation. Controlled, sustained biting, such as on a soft cookie or cracker, can also be observed at this stage. Chewing occurs with a mixture of up/down and diagonal rotary jaw movements. Food is moved from the center to the sides of the mouth with tongue motion that is side-to-side in the mouth, called *tongue lateralization.* The child also begins to produce consonants called *fricatives* (s, f, sh) in combination with vowels that require finer muscle control of tongue, oral cavity, lips, and jaw. The child begins to use real words to communicate.

Functional Assessment

Observation of oral motor development in the context of feeding behaviors is an excellent "window" to the coordination of oral motor structures related to speech and feeding. A functional assessment guide was developed and is shown in Figure 11-19. The assessment guide assists interventionists and care providers in assessing the functional abilities of children of physical disabilities, such as cerebral palsy which may affect the oral structures, and in developing appropriate intervention and support strategies for improved nutritional intake and oral motor function. The guide can be used to gain information about individual strengths and needs for support with children with disabilities and reported feeding problems. For example, parents who identify feeding as an area of concern for their children may complete the items with a therapy provider as a means to further define specific areas that are demonstrated consistently and areas in which the child requires more support and intervention. Furthermore, members of the intervention team, such as the physical therapist, speech-language pathologist, nutritionist, occupational therapist, and certified occupational therapy assistant or physical therapist assistant, can use the second part of the

Part 1: Oral Motor Skills

Skill	Demonstrated Consistently	Demonstrated Inconsistently	Demonstrated With Support	Not Observed	Notes
1. Sucks liquid from breast or bottle with lips closed firmly on nipple					
2. Sucks liquid from bottle or breast with regular pauses to breathe and with no gagging or choking					
3. Sucks pureed food from a spoon with lips and tongue					
4. Sucks liquid from cup with very little spilling					
6. Swallows liquid from cup without gagging and choking					
7. Opens mouth when food or drink is presented					
8. Swallows cooked, mashed foods with some lumps (bananas, rice, cereal, yams)					
9. "Munches" soft foods or cookie with up-and-down movement of tongue, lips, jaw					
10. Bites hard cookie or fruit with firm closure of lips and teeth					
11. Finger feeds self small bits of soft, cooked tofu, eggs, cheese, rice					
12. Chews ground and mashed food with side-to-side movement of tongue and jaw					
13. Drinks without spilling from cup with lower and upper lip closed on edge of cup					
14. Feeds self with spoon or finger foods for entire meal					

Part 2: Oral Motor Patterns and Needs

Pattern	Summary of Patterns	Primary Needs/Goal Areas
Head control		
Lip/cheek movement		
Tongue movement		
Jaw movement		
Food preferences and sensitivities		
Nutrition/dietary needs		
Positioning		
Adaptive feeding equipment		
Family/caregiver support in feeding		
Swallowing/oral structures		

Figure 11-19 Functional assessment guide for oral feeding patterns.

assessment guide to target areas for intervention as part of a team assessment that is based on family concerns and family input.

Special Problems: Hypertonicity (High Muscle Tone)

Children with physical disabilities often exhibit difficulties that are related to overall positioning and muscle tone in their oral-motor functions, such as chewing, swallowing, and speaking. The roles of the physical therapist and physical therapist assistant are critical to identify optimal positioning and supports for children with physical disabilities to succeed in learning to eat, drink, and vocalize. Specific examples of some of the most common relationships found between oral motor functioning and physical disabilities are described in this section.

Head and Jaw Extension

Increased muscle tone and extension patterns throughout the upper and lower limbs can contribute to certain motor patterns in children, such as head and jaw extension or thrusting of the head out and backward. A sitting position with hip extension and posterior pelvic tilt can contribute to overall increase in body extension. The extension pattern can extend to the upper body, shoulders, neck, and head, contributing to the outward and backward thrusting of the lower jaw and head in attempting to eat or control oral motor movements in speaking. Other possible contributing factors that are related to jaw and head thrusting in the oral motor mechanism include the following:

- Startle reflexes or overstimulation in the environment can elicit a reflex pattern, causing the individual to extend head, neck, and jaw and to retract arms at the shoulders.
- Respiratory stress may contribute to an "open-mouth" posture with neck extension as the child strives to maintain an open airway.
- Poor ability to maintain muscle contraction may result in jaw instability. The necessary co-contraction of the temporomandibular joint may be limited or lacking, resulting in a jaw thrust pattern to create stability for an open-mouth posture.
- Oral hypersensitivity may be present. Contact of teeth, gums, or tongue with food or eating utensil may elicit an avoidance response or extension reflex.
- Neck hyperextension is present, contributing to jaw thrust.
- Decay in teeth and gums may cause discomfort and difficulty in closing the mouth or jaw.
- Dislocation in cervical spine or jaw joint may cause structural or neurological problems related to oral motor function.

Case Study 1: Celina

Celina is an 8-year-old who lives with her mom, brother, and aunt in a rural area. Her grandparents live nearby, and she stays with her grandmother during the day when her mom is at work. Celina was born with cerebral palsy; she has high muscle tone throughout her body. She has learned to sit by herself with pillows to help support her. The tightness and extension of mus-

cles throughout her body make it more difficult for her to control her neck, head, and oral motor structures. When she is sitting, Celina has difficulty keeping her head forward; when she tries to move her hands and arms, her neck often extends backward. Her extended neck and high muscle tone also contribute to forward extension of her jaw muscles and an open-mouth position. When her grandmother tries to feed Celina, she opens her mouth suddenly and thrusts her head back, away from the food. Feeding Celina is a difficult and time-consuming event for her grandmother and other family members. The role of the intervention team will be to assist the family to identify strategies to improve the overall situation.

Some of the initial questions that can be explored relate to the functional assessment guide, referred to previously. The team will address the following assessment questions with Celina's family:

1. What are Celina's typical oral motor patterns and feeding skills?
2. What types and textures of foods are currently provided to Celina?
3. What are Celina's communication signals that she is hungry and wants to eat or drink?
4. What positions are found to be most comfortable for Celina and for her grandmother during feeding time?
5. How effective are the positions used for feeding to assist Celina to eat foods and to drink liquids?

Through more information and assessment with Celina and her family, the team will gather a comprehensive picture of Celina's current oral motor development, her feeding, and communication skills related to the feeding situation. In addition, her family can demonstrate ways that they have attempted to position Celina most effectively and begin the problem-solving process with the team to increase the overall pleasure and comfort of feeding for Celina, her grandmother, and other family members. Celina's nutritional intake, eating, drinking, and communication skills will also be assessed through the intervention process.

Intervention Strategies

After the assessment with Celina and her family the intervention team identified more specific areas of concern and developed several intervention strategies with her family members. Celina's grandmother reported her concerns that Celina "asked" to eat through single words such as *eat, juice, cookie,* etc. and yet seemed to "refuse" food by thrusting back her head. Many nutritious foods were presented in soft, mashed textures and Celina swallowed most foods willingly. The greatest difficulty for her grandmother and mother was described as getting her to take the food from the spoon. Her grandmother reported that placing her arm behind Celina's shoulders helped to keep her head forward. However, this became tiring and difficult to maintain for long periods. Working together with Celina's grandmother and her mother, the team developed the following adjustments to assist Celina and her family during mealtime:

1. Improve sitting posture for Celina to align her trunk and pelvis with her shoulders forward. Elongation of the neck and forward tucking of the chin were also recommended. Exploration of appropriate seating is a gradual process and

team members will construct a model chair from cardboard, pillows, foam and "no-cost" materials before purchasing or constructing a more permanent piece of equipment. Features of the seating device for Celina require the following:

- Hips must be supported to maintain angle of less than 90 degrees to reduce the extensor thrust at her hips and trunk.
- Posterior head support is needed to guide her head and neck into slight flexion while eating.
- A lap tray will be provided for upper-extremity support and feeding at school. The family will use a chair pulled up to the table to allow Celina to eat with them.

2. Before a seating support or adapted chair is completed, interim or alternate positioning at home on the couch, chair, and floor can be explored to find comfortable and supported positions for Celina.
3. Provide a calm and relaxing environment for feeding to reduce Celina's distractions and potential reactions to noises, which may contribute to her thrusting her head backward suddenly. Quiet music with a regular, moderately slow beat can help to provide a calm environment for the child and caregivers.
4. Provide many opportunities for Celina to communicate when eating and drinking by pausing for her to look at the food before offering it to her, presenting food within her visual range, and waiting for a request or response.

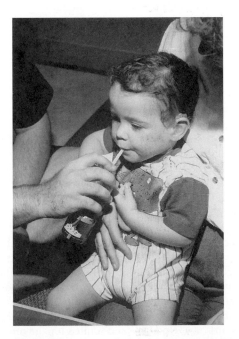

Figure 11-20 Matthew has underlying hypotonicity. Positioning to keep his head forward allows him to close his mouth over the straw and drink. Using a straw helps him practice good lip and jaw closure for other eating tasks.

Special Problems: Hypotonicity (Low Muscle Tone)

Children who exhibit low muscle tone throughout their extremities, trunk, head, and neck may show limited head control and limited movement of lips, tongue, and jaw for feeding and drinking liquids. The challenges and special problems of children with hypotonicity require careful attention to positioning; physical supports including adapted chairs; special feeding equipment such as bowls with lips and built-up spoons; and foods that are introduced to promote sucking, chewing, and swallowing a progression of food textures. Some children with low muscle tone or hypotonicity are at increased risk of choking and aspirating food and liquids because of swallowing difficulties. If a child exhibits low muscle tone that affects head control, the support provided for seating, upper trunk, neck, and head to maintain forward and balanced placement of the head and neck for eating and swallowing is of special importance (Figure 11-20). Possible contributing factors that are related to low muscle tone in children including the following:

- Damage to the facial and/or trigeminal nerves can result in weakness or paralysis of the facial muscles.
- Low muscle tone may create appearance of asymmetry in child's face if there is more nerve impairment on one side of the face.
- Low muscle tone may contribute to an "open-mouth" posture with mouth-breathing and a low-forward tongue position.

Case Study 2: Sarah

Sarah is 6 years old; she lives with her mother, father, and three older brothers. Her mother stays home with Sarah, while her brothers attend school. Sarah had meningitis when she was 4 months old. She appears to understand most of the words spoken to her by her family because she smiles and laughs in response. Feeding Sarah is very time consuming because she has difficulty chewing and swallowing food. Sarah's muscle tone is generally low in her face, neck, and upper body. Her mom holds Sarah in her lap when feeding her in an upright position. Even with the support from her mom, however, she has difficulty in chewing soft foods when they are placed in her mouth. She demonstrates the skill to open her mouth to receive food and "munches" the food slowly. She seems to tire easily and stops munching after a few tries. Food either remains in her mouth or is spit out.

As described previously, the concerns involved in Sarah's oral motor development and current abilities to chew and swallow food are related to low muscle tone throughout her extremities and fine muscles of the neck, jaw, lips, and tongue. Specific questions to address in assessment with Sarah are similar to those presented in Case Study 1 and include the following:

1. What are Sarah's typical oral motor patterns in biting, chewing, and swallowing foods?
2. What textures of foods are provided most often, and what is easiest for Sarah to chew and swallow?
3. How does Sarah indicate that she is hungry, ready for a bite of food, sip of liquid, or her preferences in foods?

4. What position is Sarah's mother using most often to feed her, and what position is most effective for Sarah to keep her head balanced and slightly forward?

Through observation of a meal session with Sarah and her mother, the team will gather a comprehensive picture of Sarah's current abilities to chew and swallow and the types of positioning and support that are most effective. In addition, the family can provide information regarding Sarah's daily intake of foods including the range of textures, liquids, and nutritional value provided. A nutritionist with background in pediatric and developmental nutritional needs for children with disabilities is an important team member in all cases when children exhibit feeding and oral motor problems.

Intervention Strategies

After the assessment the team, Sarah, and her parents discussed observations and identified strengths and needs in Sarah's oral motor and feeding skills. After reviewing the record of Sarah's daily intake of food with the nutritionist, Sarah's mother said that she did not want Sarah to choke on any lumpy or chewy foods. The therapists then demonstrated strategies to assist in chewing and swallowing with Sarah's parents. Sarah's mom was encouraged to present finger foods to Sarah and to practice with a variety of foods in small bites, such as yams, tofu, scrambled eggs, and graham crackers. Following practice at home, Sarah's mom reported that Sarah handled the small bites well without choking. In addition to suggesting a greater variety of foods, the team worked with Sarah's parents to identify physical support needed for her to maintain seating posture with her head upright. With Sarah's parents the team developed a plan to support her eating, drinking, and oral motor skills during mealtimes:

1. Finding the appropriate sitting posture and seating equipment for Sarah was recommended as a first step because of her difficulty sitting upright with her head up for long periods. A slightly tilted chair with approximately a 90-degree angle between the seat and back with full support for her feet, hips, trunk, and head was found to be helpful in enabling Sarah to eat comfortably with her head upright and with minimal expenditure of energy. Her head was supported in slight flexion to encourage swallowing.
2. To stimulate Sarah's muscle tone before mealtimes, the therapist on the team recommended movement games for large and small muscle activity. Controlled, repeated movement was found helpful for increasing muscle tone in Sarah's legs and arms. A musical activity with dance movements was recommended for Sarah and her family to use at school and at home before mealtimes.
3. To stimulate muscle tone and sensory input to Sarah's oral motor structures (lips, jaw, tongue, and cheeks), some rhythmic music can be continued during mealtime. A regular, up tempo, steady beat that is age and culturally appropriate for Sarah's family may be helpful. However, exploration and observation of Sarah's responses are critical to identify effective music and rhythmic tempo.
4. Explore a variety of soft/firm foods in small bites, such as well-cooked potatoes, peas, scrambled eggs, yams, and muffins, that increase nutritional intake and opportunities for chewing and swallowing firmer foods.

5. Support for stimulating chewing and swallowing with Sarah includes several techniques, including physical cues and firm pressure applied under the chin or actual assistance to move the lower jaw up and down. Each of these techniques requires individual training and demonstration by a therapist and practice by the family members.
6. Because Sarah demonstrates difficulty with lip closure and swallowing, allowing her to practice drinking with a straw can be helpful. At first a squeeze bottle with a plastic tube can be used to squeeze a small amount of favorite liquid (thin liquid at first) into the child's mouth. Gradually the amount of liquid squeezed is reduced and the liquid is thickened to increase lip closure and sucking activity.
7. As with Case Study 1, the family was encouraged to provide many opportunities for Sarah to communicate when eating and drinking by pausing for her to look at the food before offering it to her, presenting food within her visual range, talking with her about the food, and waiting for a request or response.

Special Problems: Exaggerated Tongue Protrusion

Children with physical disabilities may have high or low muscle tone or a combination of both. Forward tongue protrusion, which is exaggerated and interferes with eating and drinking, may occur with either high or low muscle tone. In the case of high muscle tone tongue protrusion is most often observed as a *tongue thrust*, a forceful protrusion of the tongue beyond the lower lip, which makes eating and swallowing difficult. Low muscle tone more often contributes to *exaggerated tongue protrusion* during the regular in-out movement of the tongue in swallowing, in which the tongue extends beyond the lower border of the gums and lips. Possible contributing causes that are related to tongue thrust and exaggerated tongue protrusion include the following:

- In the case of tongue thrust, backward extension of the head and neck (*neck hyperextension*) often creates an exaggeration of extensor patterns in the mouth. High muscle tone and extension patterns in larger muscles of the shoulders and hips also contribute to extension patterns in the smaller oral motor structures of tongue, lips, and jaw such as a tongue thrust.
- Low muscle tone can contribute to exaggerated tongue protrusion because of the limited activity of retraction muscles in the tongue and limited co-contraction in the upper and lower jaw joint (*temporomandibular joint*). The forward appearance of the tongue and open-mouth posture, in the case of low muscle tone, is not limited to the tongue but part of a generalized pattern in fine and large muscles.
- Tongue protrusion caused by low muscle tone can contribute to limited tongue mobility and lateralization, meaning that the child will have difficulty moving food from side-to-side and from back-to-front in the mouth.
- Forward tongue posture and limited tongue mobility as a result of low muscle tone is often related to increased tooth decay and gum problems in older children because of the tendency of food to collect in the oral cavity under the tongue or around teeth.

Case Study 3: Sachi

Sachi is 5 years old; he lives with his mother, grandmother, aunt, and cousins in a large family home. Sachi was born with Down syndrome and has delayed development in learning to walk, communicate, and feed himself. His muscle tone is generally low and his mouth, lips, and tongue muscles appear soft and relaxed. Sachi shows the ability to hold his head up, walk, and to feed himself small bites of food from his plate. His family is proud of Sachi's progress in the past year because he does many things for himself. One problem area continues to be in his eating and drinking. He tries very hard to drink his water, juice, and milk from a cup. However, even with help from his mother and grandmother, Sachi extends his tongue forward and spills a lot.

Key questions to ask in further assessment and identification of Sachi's strengths and needs for intervention include these:

1. What is Sachi's daily nutrition and range of food types and textures?
2. What types of cups and liquids are provided, and what is the thickness of each type of drink provided to Sachi?
3. How does Sachi communicate to his family when he is hungry or thirsty and what foods and drinks he wants?
4. How is Sachi seated or positioned for feeding and drinking, and how effective are different seating arrangements?
5. What strategies does Sachi use to swallow liquids, and how do family members try to assist him?

Based on observation of Sachi during mealtime either at home or school, the team can identify possible strategies to assist Sachi and his family in his eating and drinking skills.

Intervention Strategies

Observation of Sachi's use of a cup showed that he tended to "bite" the edge of the cup with his tongue protruding under the cup edge when drinking. Through experimenting with a variety of cups, including a small tumbler with a cut-out space for his nose, and thickened liquids, the team developed alternatives to assist Sachi and his family at mealtimes.

1. Identify appropriate seating and support for Sachi to participate in mealtimes with his family. As Sachi's family routinely sat on the floor around a small table, a small chair was adapted to support Sachi to sit facing forward on the same level as other family members. With his mother, grandmother, and aunt all in proximity, each person could assist him to pour small amounts of liquid in his cup and to present the cup directly in front of him, thus further assisting Sachi to face forward and to sit upright during mealtimes.
2. To increase chewing of different textured foods, an increased variety and choice of foods was recommended based on discussion with Sachi's family. Firm textures such as small slices of apples, dried fruits, other cut-up fruits, chunks of cheese, and chopped bites of fish were planned with his family. Since Sachi's family did not eat other meats (chicken or beef), a range of alternative foods was planned with the nutritionist.
3. His family reported that Sachi tended to become distracted at mealtimes and leave the table, so other distractions and activities were minimized. For example, TV watching was postponed until after the meal, and toys were put away before dinner, when possible.

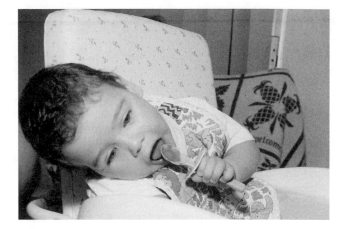

Figure 11-21 Allowing a child with a disability to feed himself part of his meal may take longer but encourages development of independent skills.

4. To assist Sachi in increasing his ability to swallow liquids with less tongue protrusion, a variety of strategies were recommended, including the following:
   - Use of a small, cut-out tumbler will allow Sachi to have success with a small amount of liquid and avoid having to tip his head back to swallow.
   - Use of thickened liquids, such as liquid yogurt and blended fruit milkshakes, are easier for Sachi to swallow than thin liquids.
   - Cold liquids are more stimulating for his oral motor structures than liquids at room temperature.
   - Physical assistance for Sachi to place the cup on his lower lip with gentle, but firm pressure will help to bring his lower lip down and close on the cup to "suck" liquid, rather than using his tongue to obtain liquid.
   - Straw or tube drinking can also be helpful to stimulate lip closure and increase muscle activity related to tongue protrusion in the case of low muscle tone, as previously described in Case Study 2.

• • •

The problems and intervention strategies outlined in the above cases are examples of three types of feeding problems that occur often in children with high and low muscle tone associated with physical and developmental disabilities. Consultation with professionals in a team format is indicated in all cases. Most often, the practitioner will encounter a combination of the problems illustrated in which one or more problems will occur in the same child who may have combined patterns of high and low muscle tone (Figure 11-21). Assessment and intervention must be highly individualized with input from family and team members to identify a range of alternative strategies to increase skills related to feeding and oral motor development for the child. The role of the physical therapist assistant is critical to identify family concerns, problem-solve with all team members, assist in developing and implementing intervention strategies, and offer specialized knowledge regarding positioning, adaptive equipment, and handling strategies for the child with high or low muscle tone.

APPLICATIONS   Chest Physical Therapy

CLARK E. RATLIFFE

Six-year-old Johnny is getting ready for bed. He bathes mostly by himself with help only for washing his hair. He is proud that he is almost independent in this task and is often heard to say "I can do it myself!" His mother lets him play in the water for awhile but soon encourages him to hurry. She knows that about 1½ hours of treatments and bedtime rituals have to be completed before Johnny will be able to actually go to sleep.

After saying goodnight to the rest of the family, Johnny goes with his mother into his bedroom. As he walks in, he grabs his favorite pillow and hands it to his mother who places it on her lap as she sits on the bed. Johnny automatically climbs on her lap and leans slightly forward, ready for his third bronchial drainage treatment of the day. His mother starts percussing his shoulder with a cupped hand, making a hollow popping sound, as she starts what will be a 40-minute to 1-hour process. They quietly talk to each other as the treatment continues. Every 5 to 10 minutes Johnny is encouraged to self-induce a deep and productive cough and spit out the thick mucus that results. This often leads to an exhausting coughing spasm that can last for several minutes. He then moves to the next position without prompting from his mother. He is very familiar with the usual sequence of bronchial drainage positions because every day of his life has been punctuated with this ritual. He cannot remember a time in his life that someone was not pounding on him and making him cough up "junk."

As his mother continues the treatment, she reflects to the time when Johnny was 8 months old and the diagnosis of cystic fibrosis entered their lives. She remembers when the person from the physical therapy department first taught her to do chest physical therapy and how difficult it had seemed at the time. Now, it is just part of her life with Johnny and comes easily to her. Still, she wishes it did not take so very much time and that it was easier for Johnny.

Importance of Respiratory Management

The maintenance of respiratory function is obviously necessary for life. It is the first physiological function that is assessed in any emergency situation. Health care professionals are always taught in their cardiopulmonary resuscitation (CPR) certification courses to remember the "ABCs," which stands for airway, breathing, circulation (Chameides, 1990). Notice that two thirds of this admonition relates to respiratory function. This is particularly true for children because respiratory insufficiency is the most frequent cause of critical illness in children. A little over 60% of all pediatric admissions have a respiratory component. Fortunately, most respiratory problems are manageable by present techniques; and chest physical therapy (CPT) is an important, sometimes essential, adjunct to other medical treatments. Depending on the institution, CPT is done by physical therapy, respiratory therapy, or nursing. To provide good respiratory care, it is necessary to understand some basic respiratory anatomy and physiology and ways in which children's respiratory systems are different than those of adults.

Respiratory Tract Structure and Function

Respiration should be thought of as the delivery of oxygen and removal of waste products at the cellular level. The respiratory system delivers oxygen to the circulatory system and simultaneously removes volatile waste products of cellular respiration. It is important to remember, therefore, that the most fundamental function of the respiratory system is *not* to simply pull air in and out of the lungs; rather, it is to work in consort with the circulatory system to make the fuel of life, oxygen, available to each cell in the body.

Although there are a number of "lesser" functions of the respiratory system, such as air filtration and heat and water loss, there are three main ones to consider. The first of these is to provide a continuous supply of oxygen to the blood, which the circulatory system delivers to tissues. The second function of the respiratory system is the removal of carbon dioxide (CO_2), an indirect by-product of cellular respiration, from the circulatory system. The removal of CO_2 plays an important role in the body's maintenance of acid-base balance, which is the third major function of the respiratory system. The respiratory system participates in acid-base regulation by manipulating CO_2 excretion in an attempt to keep the body as close to a pH of 7.40 as possible. It is not actually CO_2 that makes the body more acidic or basic, but carbonic acid (H_2CO_3). CO_2 and water are the breakdown products of carbonic acid, which is called a *volatile acid* because it can be excreted by the lungs.

Looked at another way, the more CO_2 the body gets rid of by breathing fast, the more carbonic acid is broken down and the more basic (pH over 7.40) the blood becomes. Conversely, if a person is unable to excrete CO_2 because there is a problem with the respiratory system, then CO_2 starts to build up. This drives the equation in the opposite direction, and more carbonic acid is produced by combining CO_2 and water. The result is more acid in the body, making the pH lower than 7.40. The normal range of pH in the body is 7.35 to 7.45. When the pH is lower than 7.35, the body is acidotic; when the pH is higher than 7.45, the body is in a state of alkalosis. The body functions most efficiently in this narrow range of pH. If it is outside these limits for an extended time, cell chemistry is disrupted to the extent that cell death may occur.

Chest physical therapy (sometimes called chest physiotherapy) is a treatment that is designed to mobilize and clear obstructive secretions, as in Johnny's case. His disease, cystic fibrosis, is a multisystem genetic disease that is characterized by abnormally thick respiratory secretions (White, et. al., 1995). These secretions become so thick that they block the air getting to the alveoli, where gas exchange can take place. As a result, Johnny's lungs can easily become so blocked with mucus that he is unable to provide enough oxygen for his cells or excrete enough carbon dioxide to prevent him from getting acidotic. A chest physical therapy treatment at this time could mobilize enough secretions that he is able to exchange adequate amounts of oxygen and carbon dioxide, thus maintaining his acid-base balance and tissue oxygenation.

Functional Components of the Respiratory System

Pump

In general functional terms, the lungs act as a "bellows" mechanism, moving air in and out of the lungs. The medulla, the brain's respiratory control center, modulates the rate and depth of breathing in response to systemic levels of oxygen and carbon dioxide. After determining whether the body needs more or less oxygen or carbon dioxide, the medulla sends "instructions" for an appropriate respiratory rate to the respiratory muscles through the spinal cord, peripheral nerves, and neuromuscular junctions. An injury or disease process, such as head trauma or spinal cord injury, may impair these neurotransmissions and thus decrease the ability of the body to respond to the medulla's instructions. The respiratory muscles, which include the diaphragm and accessory muscles, generate the work of breathing. They move supporting structures, such as the ribs and connective tissues, to accomplish the "bellows" function.

The components of respiratory anatomy in children have some important differences from those in adult anatomy. The ribs transverse the chest from the sternum to the spinal column more horizontally rather than sloping downward as in adults. This distinction results in a chest wall diameter that is almost at its maximum even when relaxed. Also this more perpendicular orientation of the ribs relative to the sternum and spinal column tends to decrease the mechanical efficiency of respiratory muscle function during the first years of life because intercostal muscles do not have the leverage needed to lift the ribs effectively. Infants, therefore, cannot move very much air by increasing their chest wall diameter but must rely almost entirely on diaphragmatic breathing (Wong, 1995). Additionally the supporting structures such as ribs, cartilage, and bronchioles are softer and more compliant in young children. Chest wall compliance is significant when the need exists to increase the work of breathing. If there is too much resistance, the chest wall starts to deform and even partially collapse, causing retractions. Retractions can be observed in the intercostal, suprasternal, clavicular, or subcostal areas in children with respiratory distress (Figure 11-22).

Airways

Airways are the conduits for the delivery of gas in and out of the lungs. The upper airway is composed of the nose, mouth, pharynx, and larynx. It should be remembered that infants are obligate nose breathers and their nasal passages are very small. This factor results in significantly higher airway resistance, in general. Anything that further narrows these small passages, such as mucus, can dramatically affect children, especially infants.

The lower airways are made up of the trachea, bronchi, and bronchioles. The trachea divides at the carina into the right and left mainstem bronchus. These continue to divide in successive generations, or bifurcations. The right side divides into three lobar branches leading to the upper, middle, and lower lobes. The left side divides into two branches leading to the upper and lower lobes. All of the bronchi have a wrapping of smooth muscle and are internally lined with a mucous membrane of ciliated epithelium and supported by cartilage. Ciliated epithelium is a type of epithelium that has cilia, or mobile hairs, which move in a rhythmic pattern and facilitate movement of mucus out of the bronchial tree (Figure 11-23).

The airway cartilage in children is very soft and pliable. Also the smooth muscle wrapping is almost entirely absent in infants less than 1 year. Infants have very delicate airways that are not as reactive to stimuli as adults. During deep suctioning, when a

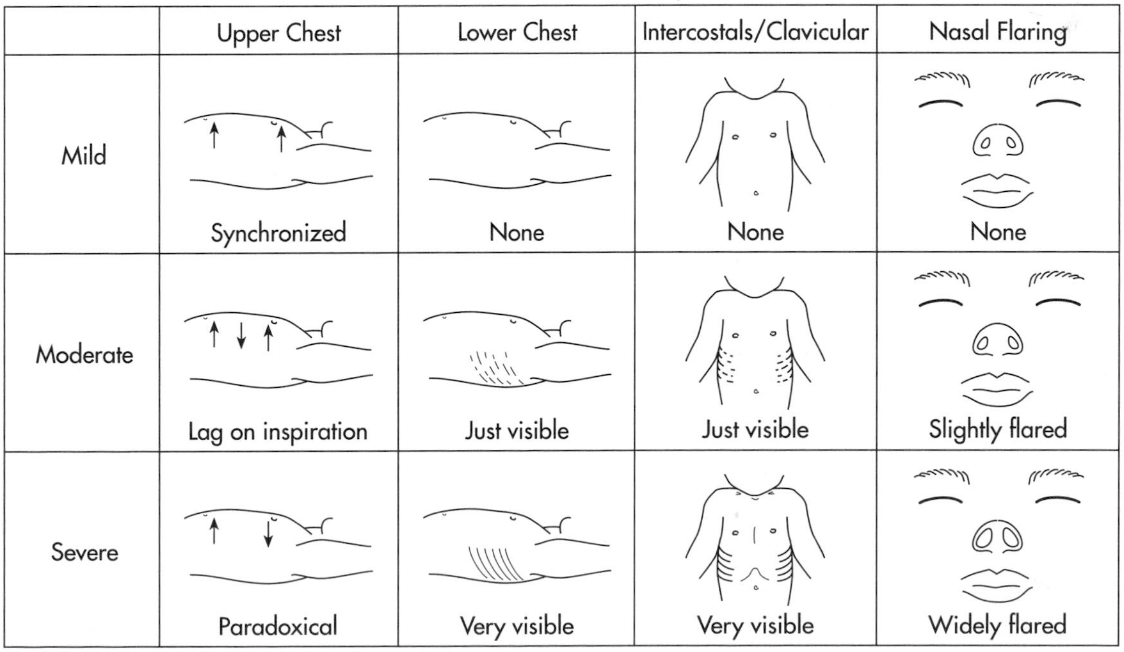

	Upper Chest	Lower Chest	Intercostals/Clavicular	Nasal Flaring
Mild	Synchronized	None	None	None
Moderate	Lag on inspiration	Just visible	Just visible	Slightly flared
Severe	Paradoxical	Very visible	Very visible	Widely flared

Figure 11-22 Respiratory retractions.

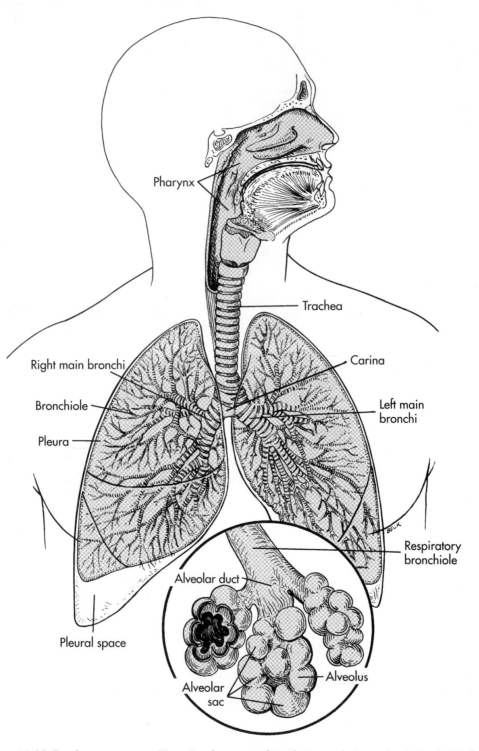

Figure 11-23 Respiratory anatomy. (From Lueckenotte, A. [1966]. *Gerontologic nursing.* St. Louis: Mosby.)

catheter is passed into the trachea, an infant would be more likely to sustain damage to the bronchioles. An adult would be more likely to have bronchospasm from the stimulation.

Gas Exchange Units

All generations of bronchioles down to about the 24th level are conducting airways and do not participate in actual gas exchange. Beyond this alveoli begin to appear and gas exchange finally begins to take place. The gas exchange units are the air sacs or alveoli and their surrounding capillaries. This alveolar/capillary interface performs the actual exchange of oxygen and carbon dioxide by simple diffusion.

As children grow, their alveolar surface area steadily increases. At 12 years, for instance, about nine times more alveoli exist than at birth. In addition, each alveolus increases its surface area over time.

Because of their smaller area for gas exchange, infants are at greater risk for problems from obstruction of airways or atelectasis. Blocked airways or fluid-filled alveoli, therefore, quickly lead to underoxygenation (hypoxia) if too many alveoli become unable to participate in gas exchange. This process tends to happen much more quickly in children than adults because of their lack of "reserve" alveolar surface area.

Because of their narrow airways, children are particularly susceptible to an increase in airway resistance. An increase in airway resistance is like having to breathe through a straw. If you were to do this, you would quickly notice yourself feeling very uncomfortable because of the amount of work required to maintain your oxygenation. The resistance to air movement is inversely proportional to the radius of the airway (Nichols, 1987); in other words, the narrower the airway, the higher the resistance. In fact, airway resistance increase is inversely proportional to the radius of the airway to the fourth power, which is a tremendous increase. For example, if an infant's airway diameter is 4 mm and has a 1 mm layer of mucus, the cross-sectional diameter is decreased by 75% and the resistance is increased by a factor of 16. By contrast, if the same airway in an adult airway is 8 mm in diameter with the same 1 mm of mucus, the cross-sectional diameter is decreased by 44% and the resistance would increase by a factor of only 3 (Cote & Todres, 1986; Hazinski, 1992). This increase in resistance leads to a significant increase in the work of breathing, which can in turn lead to muscle weakness, fatigue, and general respiratory failure. Chest physical therapy is a technique that facilitates the clearance of mucus from the airway. It can be very helpful in decreasing a child's work of breathing and staving off respiratory failure.

Chest Physical Therapy

The object of chest physical therapy is to promote the movement of mucus out of the bronchial tree and decrease atelectasis. Several techniques including percussion, vibration, squeezing, postural drainage, coughing, and deep breathing exercises are incorporated in CPT. Devices, such as vibrators and incentive spirometers, can be used to facilitate and supplement CPT. Research has not supported the efficacy of most of these modalities. Postural drainage, however, has been shown to be of benefit (Kyff, 1987). Further research may confirm anecdotal consensus that all of these modalities are useful. PTAs will find them all used commonly in practice.

Percussion

Percussion is the most common technique used with CPT. It is commonly used by respiratory therapists, nurses, physical therapists, and physical therapist assistants, as well as family members. The patient is placed in a postural drainage position (Figures 11-24 and 11-25) to facilitate the movement of mobilized mucus out of alveolar areas toward central bronchial locations where it can be coughed up. The practitioner percusses the patient's chest firmly with tightly cupped hands. The force used should be based on the size of the child and should not cause discomfort when performed over light clothing. Sometimes the use of a light towel in addition to clothing to protect the skin is helpful. Care should be used, however, not to use too much padding because this decreases the effectiveness of the CPT. When performed properly, a loud popping sound occurs as the cupped hand hits the chest wall. This is the sound of air popping out of the cupped hands. The trapped air cushions the blow and prevents what would otherwise be a painful slapping sensation. The cupped hands allow the practitioner to apply more force without discomfort, thereby mobilizing more mucus (Figure 11-26). Because most adult hands are too big to provide localized percussion on infants, a small mask or percussion cap can be used. If a mask is used, a circular type with the end plugged to prevent air escaping is best. Percussion caps are manufactured specifically for this purpose.

Vibration

Vibrators can be used in conjunction with CPT or alone. A vibrator should be used alone only when the child is unable to tolerate percussion. Because a vibrator is less traumatic, it is also probably less effective but may provide some benefit. This technique is used most in the neonatal intensive care environment where the patients are very fragile and often do not tolerate percussion. A vibrator, or any other electrical device used in an oxygen-rich environment, such as an O_2 tent or hood, should be checked to ensure that no fire danger exists.

Squeezing

Squeezing is a technique that can facilitate movement of mucus up the bronchiole tree to where it can be coughed up by the child. It is accomplished by asking the child to take a deep breath and then exhale rapidly. During the rapid exhalation the practitioner applies pressure to the sides of the chest, thus increasing the expiratory pressure. This action may move mucus and usually precipitates a deep and productive cough. Remember that infants do not have a very reactive airway, so a cough is more likely to be stimulated in older children than infants. For this reason and because they cannot cooperate with the deep breathing, squeezing is not very effective on infants.

Coughing and Deep Breathing

Children are always encouraged not to suppress coughing, which is an important pulmonary hygiene function. Care should be

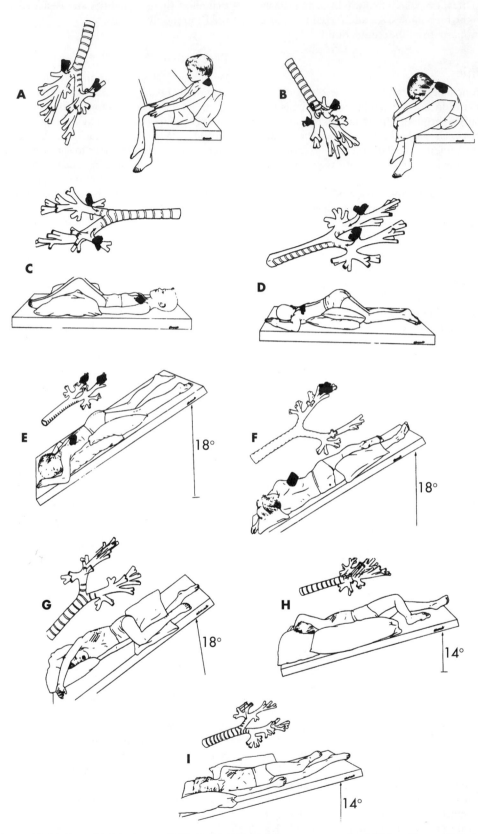

Figure 11-24 Bronchial drainage positions for all major lung segments in children. (From Chernick, V. [Ed.]. [1990]. *Kendig's disorders of the respiratory tract of children* [5th ed.]. Philadelphia: W. B. Saunders.)

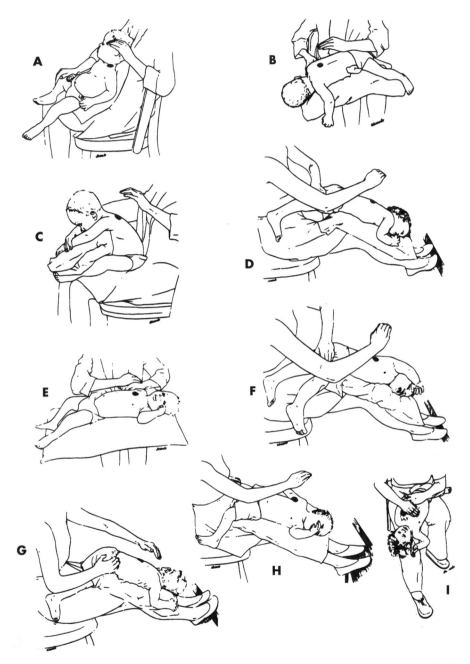

Figure 11-25 Bronchial drainage positions for all major lung segments in infants. (From Wong, D. L. [1995]. *Whaley and Wong's nursing care of infants and children* [5th ed.]. St. Louis: Mosby.)

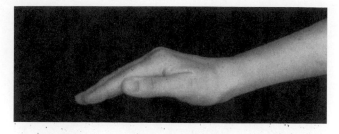

Figure 11-26 The proper hand position for chest physical therapy. From Wong, D. L. [1995]. *Whaley and Wong's nursing care of infants and children* [5th ed.]. St. Louis: Mosby.)

taken, however, not to wear out a child with ineffective coughs. One productive cough is much more effective than many small, dry coughs. One very effective way to help stimulate mucus movement and a productive cough is to have the child take some deep breaths followed by a cough at the end of the last deep breath. This method can be done in each of the postural drainage positions to good effect. Many practitioners use the squeezing technique at this time as well. Deep breathing exercises can also be used to move mucus. These exercises should be fun, creative, and developmentally appropriate.

While many different kinds of incentive spirometers are manufactured to give feedback on inspiratory and/or expiratory effectiveness, most are targeted at adults and would work best for older children and adolescents. More entertaining approaches, such as using a straw to blow ping-pong balls, bits of paper, or cottonballs around a table, can be used for younger children. With a little thought various kinds of "hockey" games for the straw-blowing technique can be devised to maintain interest. Blowing bubbles can be quite fun and interesting for many ages, but this technique requires very little breath pressure and is best used as a first or beginning exercise.

One word of caution: Special care should be taken when using balloons. At first thought blowing up balloons may seem to be a fun way to stimulate forceful deep breathing; in fact, it probably requires too much pressure. There are reports of pneumothorax in normal healthy adults being caused by blowing up balloons (Mumford, 1996). Also, because balloons accounted for 29% of all choking deaths associated with man-made products in children less than 14 years of age between 1972 and 1992, introducing a balloon as a play object is probably not wise (Stenson, 1996).

Contraindications and Guidelines

A number of conditions exist in which CPT is contraindicated. When children have pulmonary hemorrhage or embolism, percussion can damage delicate lung tissue. Children with increased intracranial pressure should not be moved around very much and should never be placed in a head down position. Children with minimal cardiac reserves may not be able to tolerate the significant energy expenditure required for CPT. Also, any child with osteogenesis imperfecta, which is characterized by brittle bones or severe osteoporosis, is not a candidate for CPT because of the risk of broken ribs.

Sutton (1988) suggests the following guidelines for the time when CPT is most useful and effective: (1) CPT is not very useful in the uncomplicated postoperative patient and with most

pneumonias. (2) In general, percussion with deep breathing and squeezing leading to a productive cough are more effective than percussion alone. (3) Finally, bronchodilators before CPT have been shown to greatly increase its effectiveness. It is important to coordinate the CPT treatment with the medication schedule.

Summary

Although the effectiveness of CPT, except postural drainage, is not well supported in the literature, health professionals commonly practice all of the modalities discussed in this section. Perhaps part of the reason the research is sketchy regarding CPT results from the wide variation in patient condition, circumstance, and therapist technique. It is important, therefore, to be meticulous in performing these procedures. Take the time necessary to move the child through all the drainage positions (see Figures 11-24 and 11-25) while percussing and/or vibrating with appropriate technique. This is one procedure that cannot be rushed.

Finally, CPT can be a quiet and intimate time spent with the child. For instance, Johnny's mother, who we met at the beginning of this section, uses CPT time to read Johnny stories. She props a book on a support stand so she has both hands free. For the pediatric health professional this kind of time spent with children is precious indeed.

EXERCISES

1. Interview a family of a child born prematurely about their experiences in the NICU and with service providers after their child has come home. Present an inservice to your classmates about this "case study." You may be able to identify a family through the nearest pediatric physical therapy center (hospital, school, infant development program).

2. Think of three ways that a physical therapy provider can be helpful in improving a child's feeding and language development. Share these ideas with your classmates and generate more ideas. Which ideas are "common sense," and which ideas use specialized knowledge? Which methods would you feel comfortable teaching to family members?

3. Practice the sequence of positions for postural drainage while performing chest physical therapy techniques on a classmate. Switch roles so you can experience the techniques. Share your experience with your classmates, and generate a list of aspects of which to be aware (e.g., how much padding to use and how does it feel when percussion or vibration is too soft, too hard, etc.).

QUESTIONS TO PONDER

1. Should extremely premature infants be saved? Is the cost versus risk benefit worth it? Should all infants be saved regardless of the cost versus risk benefit? Try to look at this issue separately from your own religious beliefs.

2. Should physical therapy providers be responsible for integrating language and feeding into physical therapy treatments? Why or why not?

3. In many parts of the country chest physical therapy is done by respiratory therapists. What should the relationship be between physical therapy and respiratory therapy?

Annotated Bibliography

Harrison, H., & Kositsky, A. (1983). *The premature baby book.* New York: St. Martin's Press.

> Written by a parent and a registered nurse, this book focuses on the parent perspective. Although some of the medical information presented here is now outdated, the parent perspective gives an excellent flavor of the experience of having a child in the NICU. Neonatal problems are explained in basic terms, and many stories of children and their families add depth to the text. As with some of the other books reviewed here, it is hoped that a more recent edition will be forthcoming. Regardless of its limitations, this book continues to be helpful in understanding the NICU experience.

References

Abman, S. H., & Groothius, J. R. (1994). Pathophysiology and treatment of bronchopulmonary dysplasia. *Pediatric Clinics of North America,* 41(2): 277-315.

Adhikari, M., & Gouws, E. (1995). Meconium aspiration in South Africa. *South African Medical Journal,* 85: 891-893.

Als, H., Lawhon, G., Duffy, F. H., McAnulty, G. B., Gibes-Grossman, R., & Glickman, J. G. (1994). Individualized developmental care for the very low-birth-weight preterm infant. *Journal of the American Medical Association,* 272(11): 853-858.

Pediatric Section of the American Physical Therapy Association. (February, 1996). *Utilization of physical therapist assistants in the provision of pediatric physical therapy (draft).* Author.

Chameides, L. (1990). *Textbook of pediatric advanced life support.* Dallas, Texas: American Heart Association.

Cote, C. J., & Todres, I. D. (1986). The pediatric airway. In J. F. Ryan, I. D. Todres, C. J. Cote, & N. Goudsouzian (Eds.). *A practice of anesthesia for infants and children.* New York: Grune & Stratton.

Deiriggi, P. M. (1990). The effects of waterbed flotation on indicators of energy expenditure in preterm infants. *Nursing Research,* 39: 436-442.

Erkkola, R., Kero, P., Suhonen-Polvi, H., & Korvenranta, H. (1994). Meconium aspiration syndrome. *Annals of Surgery and Gynecology Supplement,* 208: 106-109.

Escobar, G. Littenberg, B., & Petitti, D. (1991). Outcomes among surviving very low birthweight infants: A meta-analysis. *Archives of Disability in Children,* 66: 204-211.

Findlay, R. D., Taeusch, H. W., & Walther, F. J. (1996). Surfactant replacement therapy for meconium aspiration syndrome. *Pediatrics,* 97: 48-52.

Hack, M., & Faranoff, A. A. (1986). Special report: Changes in the delivery room care of the extremely small infant (750 grams): Effects on morbidity and outcome. *New England Journal of Medicine,* 314: 660-664.

Hack, M., Horbar, J. D., Malloy, M. H., Tyson, J. E., Wright, E., & Wright L. (1991). Very low birth weight outcomes of the National Institute of Child Health and Human Development Neonatal Research Network. *Pediatrics,* 87: 587-597.

Hack, M., & Faranoff, A. A. (1989). Outcomes of extremely-low-birth-weight infants between 1982-1988. *New England Journal of Medicine,* 321: 1641-1647.

Halsey, C. L. Collin, M. F., & Anderson, C. L. (1996). Extremely low-birth-weight children and their peers: A comparison of school-age outcomes. *Archives of Pediatric and Adolescent Medicine,* 150: 790-794.

Harlow, B. L., Frigoletto, F. D., Cramer, D. W., Evans, J. K., LeFevre, M. L., Bain, R. P., & McNellis, D. (1996). Determinants of preterm delivery in low-risk pregnancies: The RADIUS study group. *Journal of Clinical Epidemiology,* 49: 441-448.

Harrison, H., & Kositsky, A. (1983). *The premature baby book.* New York: St. Martin's Press.

Hazinski, M. F. (1992). *Nursing care of the critically ill child,* (2nd ed.). St. Louis: Mosby.

Hernández, C., Little, B. B., Dax, J. S., Gilstrap, L. C. 3d, & Rosenfeld, C. R. (1993). Prediction of the severity of meconium aspiration syndrome. *American Journal of Obstetrics and Gynecology,* 169: 61-70.

Houlihan, C. M., & Knuppel, R. A. (1994). Meconium-stained amniotic fluid: Current controversies. *Journal of Reproductive Medicine,* 39: 888-898.

Korner, A. F. (1986). The use of waterbeds in the care of preterm infants. *Journal of Perinatology,* 6: 142-147.

Kyff, J. V. (1987). Current thoughts on chest physical therapy. *Respiratory Management,* 17(6): 70-73.

La Pine, T. R., Jackson, J. C., & Bennet, F. C. (1994). Outcome of infants weighing less than 800 grams at birth: 15 years experience. *Pediatrics,* 96: 246-250.

Mumford, A. (1996). Case report. *British Medical Journal,* 313(7).

Nichols, D. G., In M. C. Rogers. (Ed.), (1987). *Textbook of pediatric intensive care,* (Vol. 1). Baltimore, MD: Williams & Wilkins.

Selzer, S. C., Lindgren, S. D., & Blackman, J. A. (1992). Long-term neuropsychological outcome of high risk infants with intracranial hemorrhage. *Journal of Pediatric Psychology,* 17(4): 407-422.

Semmler, C. J. (1989). *A guide to care and management of very low birth weight in infants: A team approach.* Tucson, Az: Therapy Skill Builders.

Shankaran, S., Bauer, C. R., Bain, R., Wright, L. L., & Zachary, J. (1996). Prenatal and perinatal risk and protective factors for neonatal intracranial hemorrhage. *Archives of Pediatric Adolescent Medicine,* 150: 491-497.

Stenson, J. (Jan 11, 1996). Balloons and kids can be a deadly combination. *Medical Tribune.*

Sunoo, C. S., Kosasa, T. S., Nakayama, R. T., & Hale, R. W. (1993). The incidence of meconium aspiration in Hawaii. *Hawaii Medical Journal,* 52: 290-293.

Sutton, P. P. (1988). Chest physiotherapy: time for reappraisal. *British Journal of Diseases of the Chest,* 82:127-137.

White, W. R., Munro, C. L., Pickler, R. H. (Nov/Dec 1995). Therapeutic implications of recent advances in cystic fibrosis. *Maternal Child Nursing,* 20:304-308.

Wong, D. L. (1995). *Whaley and Wong's nursing care of infants and children* (5th ed). St Louis: Mosby.

Medical Disorders

CASE STUDY   Caroline, A Teenager Recovering From Cancer

Caroline finished tuning her viola. She looked around her. Some members of the orchestra were tuning their instruments. Others were talking quietly, waiting for the orchestra director to begin the rehearsal. She carefully kicked her crutches a little further under the chair and shifted her weight so that her leg was stable. When her buttock was on the edge of the chair and her leg was diagonally out from the chair, she felt the most stable (Figure 12-1). She arranged her sheet music on the stand in front of her and smiled at the girl playing first-chair viola. The girl was 2 years older than Caroline and had been playing for 4 years to Caroline's 3 years.

During the last 3 years Caroline had missed orchestra rehearsal often, but that was over now. She intended to attend every rehearsal from now on. Maybe in a few years Caroline could make first chair. The orchestra director coughed and opened his music. With her back held erect, Caroline moved her viola up to her chin and poised her bow, her eyes on the director.

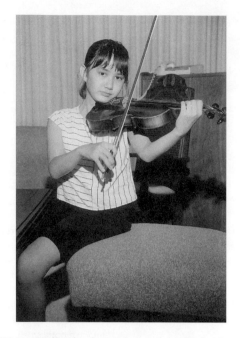

Figure 12-1 Caroline has been playing the viola for 3 years. After her amputation she had to adjust her sitting balance for playing.

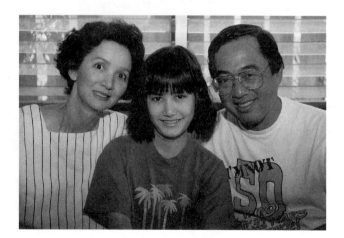

Figure 12-2 Family portrait.

Early Childhood

Caroline was the second child of George, a business executive, and Sheila, a part-time teacher (Figure 12-2). Caroline's infancy was uneventful. She had an older sister Lianne, 5 years her senior, who loved having a baby sister. Caroline sat up, crawled, and learned to walk at the usual times. When she was 2 years old, she developed a lump in her left buttock. It was a solid lump, not painful, or even very pronounced; but her parents took her to see her pediatrician. After an initial period of tests, her parents were shocked when she was diagnosed with fibrosarcoma. The tumor was in her gluteus maximus muscle. This was a traumatic period of time for Caroline's family.

Surgery to remove the tumor was successful. The surgeons felt they had removed the entire tumor with a clear margin of undiseased tissue all around it, along with most of Caroline's gluteus maximus muscle. Although the tumor had been caught early, at stage 1, the biopsy result showed that it was malignant. During the early 1980s the protocol for this type of tumor at stage 1 was for radiation only, no chemotherapy. So at 2 years old Caroline underwent radiation therapy to her left hip and buttock.

In the years that followed her parents noticed many problems related to Caroline's early cancer surgery and subsequent radiation treatments. Caroline's left leg was growing more slowly than her right, and she had a clear leg length discrepancy by the time she was in kindergarten. She wore a lift on her left shoe, and her mother had to buy two pairs of shoes for Caroline because her feet were such discrepant sizes. Her left leg was noticeably smaller than her right with muscle atrophy in all muscle groups. Caroline compensated with her stronger right leg, causing even more asymmetry.

Caroline developed significant pain in her left hip and groin when she was 7 years old. This was finally diagnosed as a stage 1 slipped capital femoral epiphysis. Her physician felt that the slipped epiphysis was caused by the radiation she had undergone when she was a toddler. Caroline had surgery to pin her left hip; although she did not need a cast, Caroline used crutches for 1 month while the bone healed.

Because of her difficulties with mobility and weakness in her left leg specifically, as well as generalized weakness, Caroline qualified for special services in school under Section 504 of the Rehabilitation Act of 1973. She also had a slight hearing impairment unrelated to her cancer that needed to be addressed by the school. Although she continued in her regular education setting, support of the special education staff allowed her to have extra time moving between classrooms, extra help in school if she needed it, and help with her gross motor skills. Her individualized education program (IEP) plan was developed by herself, her parents, teachers, and therapists. Special education staff worked with her to adapt situations so she could be more successful in school.

Caroline had one-on-one support from an adaptive physical education teacher twice per week. Ideally, this occurred while her class was receiving regular physical education activities. In reality, she had to accommodate to the schedule of the adaptive physical education teacher who was not usually available during that time. Therefore she missed some academic work. Through activities such as tennis, Bocce ball, and games using a scooter board she was able to work toward strengthening her trunk and upper body. The physical therapist (PT) consulted with the adaptive physical education teacher to ensure that the activities addressed Caroline's specific needs.

Through this period of time Caroline's family worked together to support each other. Caroline had developed a close relationship with her older sister, Lianne. She also had friends from school and from church. Her family members, especially her father, were very active in their church. Caroline became active in other extracurricular activities as well, including learning to play the viola when she was 10 years old.

A New Cancer

When Caroline was 11 years old and in the fifth grade, her left hip, which had always been weak and painful, started bothering her more. X-ray examination showed a "shadow." A biopsy result eventually led to a new diagnosis of chondrosarcoma and osteosarcoma, cancer of the cartilage and bone. Unfortunately, this new cancer was in her left femur, her pelvis, and even her sacrum. The complicated surgery needed to resect the cancer could not be done in the isolated geographic area where they lived, and the family were referred to a large city hospital to consult experts. They elected to go to New York City, several thousands of miles away from home, so they could consult physicians who treated this type of cancer relatively frequently.

Caroline's parents were devastated with the news of her new cancer and debated how much to tell their young daughter. The diagnosis was made in November, and surgery was scheduled for February in New York. They did not tell Caroline the extent of the surgery she would need until closer to the date of the actual surgery, after she had completed her first treatment of chemotherapy, in January. They felt that she could better accept what was to happen to her in stages. She knew that she would undergo surgery for her cancer in New York but did not know that her entire leg and half of her pelvis would be removed until a few weeks before going to New York.

Anticipating her first round of chemotherapy, Sheila suggested that Caroline get her ears pierced. She would not have the opportunity again until after the full year of chemotherapy had ended because of the risk of infection. They also began to plan how to address her chemotherapy-related hair loss. They decided that Caroline would use a wig and that they would buy it before her chemotherapy started so she would have it available right away. Caroline did not want anyone to see her without her hair. It was important to her that she look as normal as possible. Wigs for children were hard to find, and Caroline and her mother struggled to find something appropriate. Finally the oncology staff at the hospital referred them to a wigmaker. They were able to get a wig made that duplicated Caroline's own hair.

Caroline and her parents spent 3 weeks in New York that first trip. Caroline wanted one of her parents to stay at her bedside all the time in case she needed anything. She stayed at the hospital, but her parents paid for a hotel room even though they were hardly there. It was very expensive. Lianne stayed home with relatives so she would not miss school. George and Sheila made sure that they called her frequently so she could stay involved and support her sister. Being apart was difficult for all of them.

Before her surgery Caroline and her parents met with a rehabilitation specialist, a nurse who had a below-knee prosthesis herself. She talked about life after surgery, what would happen, and what Caroline might experience. They talked about being fitted for a prosthesis and what would be involved in learning to use it. They discussed chemotherapy, what would happen, how Caroline might feel, and how long it would last. She was also shown a video about amputations that included a section on hemipelvectomy. These conversations and the videotape were reassuring to Caroline.

The surgery went well. The surgeons resected her pelvis all the way up to the vertebrae, which was more than had been originally anticipated. They felt they had been able to get all the cancer cells with a clear margin.

Caroline was glad to be away from home after the surgery. Although she appreciated the support of friends and relatives, she needed time to rest without having people constantly around. There was time enough for that after they got home. She found that she was very tired most of the time in the few weeks after her operation.

Shortly after her surgery, while still in New York, Caroline and her parents met with a prosthetist. He explained to them that he was a specialist who made custom prosthetic limbs for people who had amputations. The family decided to work with the prosthetist from New York because prosthetists at home were not familiar with the technology needed to make a socket for someone with a hemipelvectomy. On this trip Caroline was able to watch videos about the type of prosthesis she would get and met others who had hemipelvectomies who were successfully using prostheses. She had to wait a few months to be molded for her own prosthesis, until she had a long enough gap between rounds of chemotherapy to travel to New York again.

Caroline went through one round of chemotherapy before returning home, where she underwent several more rounds. It seemed there was always another round of chemotherapy to go; it would never end. The entire protocol lasted for 1 year.

Caroline and her parents realized how much she needed physical therapy services after they returned home from their first trip to New York. Caroline's bedroom was upstairs, and she was too weak to walk up the stairs using the crutches. Her parents moved a temporary bed downstairs for her and obtained physical therapy services for her at the local children's hospital. She worked with a PT twice per week for 2 months. Some of the activities included strengthening exercises with weights, balance activities using a balance board, and stretching to keep her flexible. She was able to get strong enough and develop more confidence so she could do more things for herself, including finally being able to go up the stairs!

Crutches became the means for Caroline's mobility. She had a clean indoor pair and an outdoor pair that could get dirty. She used both axillary crutches and forearm crutches, but she found that the forearm crutches were lighter and more convenient. When she used her hands while standing, the forearm crutches balanced easily on her arms, whereas the axillary crutches frequently fell over with a clatter when leaned against her body or the wall.

In April Caroline and her parents returned to New York to get her prosthesis made. This time there were openings at the Ronald McDonald House in the city, and the family could stay there much more reasonably than at a hotel.

Getting a prosthesis was a lot of work! Caroline found herself doing exercises to strengthen her abdominal muscles, her right leg, and her arms. A prosthesis was molded right away, and Caroline received it within a week. The prosthesis had a molded "shelf" for her to put her stump and a belt and lacing system to keep the device strapped firmly to her waist so it would not move around. Caroline learned to use her abdominal muscles to bring the prosthesis through in the swing phase of gait and relied heavily on her right hip musculature to keep her balanced over the artificial leg. Caroline could bend the knee and hip joints of the prosthesis to walk or sit in a chair by shifting her weight to change the pull of gravity. She was too light to be able to use a spring hip, however, so was not able to sit on the floor while using her prosthesis. Her prosthesis also did not have a swivel knee that would have allowed her to rotate the knee to sit on the floor in a ring sitting position.

After a few weeks of intensive work, Caroline and her parents went back home. Knowing that PTs at home were not familiar

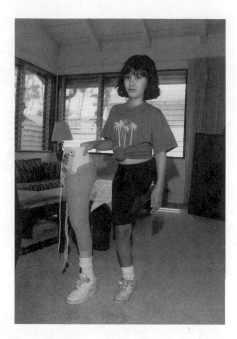

Figure 12-3 Caroline demonstrates how she puts on her prosthesis.

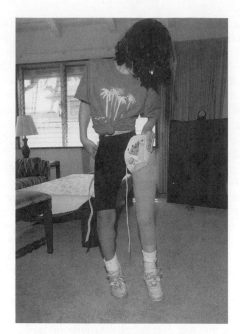

Figure 12-4

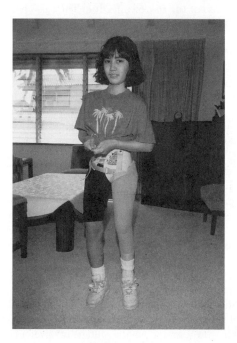

Figure 12-5

with her type of prosthesis, they brought home a video of Caroline using the device (Figures 12-3, 12-4, and 12-5).

Caroline missed more than half of her schooling for the rest of fifth grade and half of sixth grade because of the chemotherapy. She was too nauseated to eat while receiving chemotherapy and needed total parenteral nutrition (TPN) through an indwelling catheter in her chest. She developed a continuous nausea that was worse in the mornings and continued long after her chemotherapy ended. Her doctors were unable to find a cause for her illness, although it kept her out of school for large blocks of time during most of the year following her chemotherapy. Caroline and her mother found that when they adjusted her diet to include more fiber, it could control her upset stomach to some extent, although the nausea continues to this day. Sheila has learned to cook differently, and Caroline has become very sensitive to her own dietary needs. Caroline also takes medicine to control her nausea.

The school provided a tutor who worked with Caroline while she was in the hospital and at home. Her mother also qualified to be a home/hospital tutor so that she could help her daughter catch up during the summers when school services were not available. During Caroline's seventh grade year, Sheila was paid for the support she was giving Caroline. Caroline grew even closer to Lianne and her parents over the years that she struggled with feeling sick, and she fought to become more independent in her mobility and self-care skills.

Caroline's family needed to take some breaks, and Sheila took a job in a retail store in the evenings. By waiting on customers she felt a needed respite from her continuous role as caregiver and teacher, and she was able to bring a little money home. George became more involved in church activities. He was able to develop a social network outside the family for his own support.

Continued therapy services helped Caroline improve her strength and independence. It took her a long time to relearn how to do even very simple things such as going up and down stairs, balancing on the toilet, and picking up objects from the floor. The therapists from the school health services who provided services to her in school had not worked with many children who had amputations and had never worked with a child with a hemipelvectomy. They were honest about their lack of experience and worked hard with Caroline to identify her goals and help her work toward them. They were obviously unfamiliar with her prosthesis and gait training using the prosthesis. The video taken in New York of Caroline walking with her prosthesis was valuable as she struggled to walk with the help of her physical therapist and her mother.

Her parents had to readjust their thinking about her cancer and its treatment. They began to realize that the surgery and chemotherapy had far-reaching consequences for their daughter beyond just the cancer itself. Specifically, Caroline's organs were affected by chemotherapy causing secondary medical problems they had not anticipated including her nausea, diarrhea, and difficulty with eating. They joined a cancer support group and began to find that other families had similar experiences. George and Sheila became active in supporting a "Cancer Camp" for families and children with cancer, to encourage discussion and sharing among families. They were grateful for sponsors of the camp including the American Cancer Foundation and the Children's Cancer Foundation in their state. Caroline found these camps valuable as well.

Sheila and George found that they needed to make adaptations to their home for Caroline. Her bedroom was originally upstairs, and they moved it downstairs. Caroline could go up and down stairs using her crutches and the railing without too much difficulty after a while, but it took a significant amount of energy. When she found she had forgotten a book, her hairbrush, or another item upstairs, she had to make the trip up and down the stairs again. It became overwhelming to go up and down so many times. So her bedroom was moved into her mother's office downstairs. The office was moved into the space where the dining room used to be. It had to stay downstairs because Caroline needed to use the computer for her schoolwork. The dining room table was moved to one side of the living room. Sheila worried about where she was going to fit the Christmas tree! The bathroom remained upstairs, however. It was too expensive to put a new bathroom downstairs.

In the summer before eighth grade, Caroline found that her stump had shrunk more and that she needed a new prosthesis. The family went to New York for the third time to see the prosthetist. Luckily, space was available at the Ronald McDonald House for the three of them. A new prosthesis was made, and Caroline struggled to learn to use it before she returned home.

Because the prosthesis is intended to last for at least a few years, it has to be adjustable to accommodate for Caroline's growth and for normal shrinkage in her residual limb. For this reason, the metal shaft of the "femur" is extendable. In her new prosthesis Caroline was able to get an energy saving foot that returns energy gained during the stance phase of gait to the toe off phase. She still was not heavy enough for a spring hip, however, and did not get a swivel knee. Because of her small stature, she may never be able to use a spring hip. Because the manufacturer does not make pediatric sizes, the prosthesis' foot is bigger than Caroline's right foot. Sheila had to buy two pairs of shoes at a time for Caroline to accommodate this size difference. Caroline works hard to scuff up the shoe that the prosthesis wears so there will be equal wear. She feels conspicuous with a new white sneaker on one foot and an old scuffed one on the other. Her mother made a brocade cloth bag in which to keep the prosthesis and carry it from place to place. Caroline has a new video from New York to help her continue to improve her gait skills.

Back at School

When Caroline was able to return to school full time in eighth grade, it was difficult facing her classmates with her changed physical appearance. She had been seeing a psychologist for several months, which helped her deal with changing schools from elementary to intermediate, making new friends, and adjusting to being back at school full time. Caroline was comfortable with herself and her amputation, which helped her adjust. An oncology nurse and a child-life specialist from the hospital came to talk with her classmates and ease her transition back into school. Other challenges (e.g., access issues at the school and fatigue left over from the intensive chemotherapy) were hard to separate from the social issues and complicated Caroline's return to school.

The intermediate school where she moved for seventh and eighth grades is less accessible than her elementary school had been. It is on two levels and is quite spread out with some hills between the buildings. Caroline continues to receive services from special education for adaptations including the use of a locked elevator to go up to her second floor classes. Unfortunately, the key to the elevator is never given to students, so Caroline has to wait for an aide with a key each time she wants to go upstairs. She was frequently late to class because the aide became busy and was late to help her with the elevator. This was deeply frustrating. After she complained, all her classes were moved to the first level so the elevator was no longer a problem. Caroline felt that this solution was short sighted. Other students with mobility impairments still struggled with the elevator. As a result, she became very active in school government, especially relating to issues affecting students with disabilities.

Caroline is doing well in her classes in eighth grade and was on the Honor Roll last semester. She continues at the intermediate school and is taking English, social studies, math, and basic practical arts (home economics and shop) as core classes. As electives she is taking Japanese language and media production classes, where she is learning how to use a video camera and edit tape. Caroline continues to receive help from special education. She and her mother participated in Caroline's IEP meeting in the fall of eighth grade, along with her PT, the adaptive physical education teacher, several key subject teachers, and the school principal. (See Box 12-1 for a sample of integrated IEP goals for Caroline.) This meeting was a good opportunity for Caroline to explain to her eighth grade teachers about her disability and her need for adaptations in class. One accommodation the school has made is giving her an extra set of textbooks to keep at home and a secure locker to store her books at school. With two sets of books, she does not need to carry so much in her backpack.

This year Caroline does not feel the need to continue with her adapted physical education, although it was offered. She continues to get consultation from a physical therapist as needed to help with her strength and mobility skills in school. She does not wear her prosthesis in school yet since she cannot wear it for an entire school day; she does not feel comfortable taking it off in school, where there is no place to store it. One problem with wearing her prosthesis for extended periods is that she needs to take it off to use the bathroom. This is because she would need to remove the stretch fabric shorts she wears to protect her residual limb and the prosthesis comes close to her urethra, making cleaning it difficult. She plans to work with the school therapist closely when she is ready to begin wearing her prosthesis in school.

BOX 12-1   Sample Individual Education Program Goals for Caroline

1. Caroline will walk up a 12-foot-long ramp on campus using her prosthesis without using the railing.
2. Caroline will walk across campus using her prosthesis on a level surface at a consistent pace for 3 minutes.
3. Caroline will descend a full flight of stairs using an alternating step pattern while wearing her prosthesis.
4. Caroline will walk between buildings A and C on campus (100 feet) in 5 minutes.

Accommodations for Caroline in the individualized education program include the following:
1. Caroline will sit in the front of the class to accommodate for her hearing impairment.
2. Caroline will sit in a chair instead of the floor when students are sitting on the floor.

BOX 12-2   Physical Therapy Evaluation Summary: Caroline

Social and Medical History
Addressed in the Case Study.

Range of Motion
Upper extremities are both within normal limits, as are her right knee and ankle.
Right hip:

Hip flexion	100 degrees with pain in groin at end range
Hip internal rotation	30 degrees
Hip external rotation	25 degrees
Hip abduction	50 degrees
Hip extension	10 degrees

Spine is straight with normal ranges.

Posture
Caroline compensates for her lack of a left lower extremity by shifting her weight to the right in standing and sitting.

Muscle Strength, Tone, and Bulk

Hip flexion	4/5
Hip abduction	4/5
Hip extension	4 − 5
Hip internal rotation	4 − 5
Hip external rotation	4 − 5

Muscle bulk is on the low side of normal in her trunk, arms, and right lower extremity. Caroline has a small stature with a slight body type.

Reflexes and Developmental Reactions
Caroline has good balance reactions in sitting. She has learned to compensate for her amputation by using her arms and right leg more to compensate for balance challenges. In standing, she has fair/good balance on her right leg when not using her prosthesis, which is limited by weakness in her trunk and right leg muscles. When using the prosthesis, she has fair/good balance, although she is still learning how to shift her weight to compensate for balance challenges in stance and while moving.

Gait
Caroline uses either axillary or forearm crutches when walking without her prosthesis. She uses a swing-to gait with a normal walking speed. When using her left leg prosthesis, she walks with the following gait compensations: right hip hiking, decreased stance time on the left leg, and inconsistent/decreased alternate arm swing. Her endurance is only fair; she is able to walk only 100 feet at a normal pace before needing to rest or slow down. She can ascend or descend one step using her prosthesis without requiring a railing, but for more steps, requires a railing for an alternate gait pattern. She can walk up or down a short ramp, but finds it very challenging, and prefers to use a railing. She can walk on uneven surfaces such as grass or gravel with less confidence in her gait than when on flat surfaces.

Functional Skills
Caroline is independent in most mobility skills including walking with crutches and with her prosthesis up and down stairs and ramps and over uneven surfaces for short distances, but distance is limited by poor endurance and poorly developed balance skills. She can get up and down from the floor without her prosthesis or upper extremity support. She can hop on her right leg and can go up on her right toes briefly.

Adaptive Equipment
- Left full leg prosthesis with hip, knee, and ankle joints
- Bilateral axillary and forearm crutches

Activities of Daily Living
Caroline's self-care skills are generally age appropriate except for poor endurance and difficulties with mobility as described above.

Assessment/Summary
Caroline is a bright, motivated adolescent struggling with recurrent nausea as a consequence of her chemotherapy. She has decreased endurance and strength, with resulting limitations in her mobility skills. She has been experiencing right hip pain with slight decreases in right hip mobility and strength, which are probably musculoskeletal in origin from the stress of using her prosthesis. Specifically, she has tightness in her right tensor fasciae latae and iliotibial band with weakness in her gluteus medius muscle, which are responsive to tender point stretching, myofacial release techniques, and strengthening and coordination exercises. She is motivated to learn to use her prosthetic limb efficiently and follows through on treatment suggestions and exercises at home as she is medically able. She has a supportive family.

> **BOX 12-3** Home Exercises for Caroline
>
> Do all these exercise progressions at least once daily.
>
> ### Strengthening
>
> 1. Lie on your stomach and lift your leg off the mat. You may want to stabilize yourself by moving your arms out to your sides. Move your leg parallel to the floor out from your body, then back to midline again. Hold it up in the air for at least a count of 5. Repeat 5 to 10 times.
> 2. Lie on your back on a firm surface with your foot on the floor and your knee bent. Tuck your head forward and lift your head and shoulders off the mat so that your shoulder blades come off the surface. Hold for a count of 5. Repeat 5 to 10 times.
> 3. While sitting, have another person sit facing you and grasp your upper arms. The other person moves forward, backward, to the side, and in circular motions, moving you with them. The person can vary speed and direction. You give an opposing force. This challenges your balance and develops strength in your trunk muscles.
> 4. Lie on your back and slowly raise your leg straight up in the air until it is at about a 30-degree angle to the floor. Hold it for a count of 5. Bring it down slowly. Repeat 5 to 10 times.
>
> ### Flexibility
>
> 5. While sitting in a long sitting position (leg out straight in front of you), pull your toes back toward your body and lean your body gently toward your leg. You should feel a pull behind your thigh and in your calf. Stretch as far as you can.
>
> Hold it for a count of 5. Then stretch a little further and hold for another count of 5. Relax slowly. Repeat this 5 to 10 times.
> 6. Lie on your left side at the edge of a firm surface that is above the floor (table, firm bed). Gently let your right leg dangle down over the edge of the surface until you feel a stretch at the side of your thigh and hip. Make sure that your leg is turned a little inward (toes pointing in) and that your body is not rolling forward or backward. Hold the stretch for a count of 5. Repeat 5 to10 times.
> 7. When ascending stairs using crutches and a railing, put the toes of your foot on the edge of a step and let your body weight push downward through your heel. You should feel a stretch at the back of your calf. Hold for a count of 5. Stretch a little further, and hold for another count of 5. Repeat 5 to 10 times. You can also do this stretch with your foot on the floor and your body leaning forward using crutches or a wall for stability.
>
> ### General
>
> 8. Join a swim or other exercise class for general fitness. If you can find a friend (or relative) to do this with you, you may be more motivated to continue. If you need help adapting the exercises or activities for your specific needs, ask your physical therapist.
> 9. Walk when you have the opportunity rather than riding.
> 10. Take the stairs rather than the elevator if you have a choice.

Caroline has been receiving physical therapy services for several months outside of school from a therapist who specializes in orthopedic disorders. She has been experiencing pain in her right hip, especially after she walks with the prosthesis, and is not sure what is causing it. Medical test results were negative for more cancer, much to her relief, and the treatment focus has been on musculoskeletal causes. Her new PT, Barbara, performed an evaluation (Box 12-2) and determined that Caroline has some tightness of the iliotibial band and tensor fasciae latae (TFL) of her right hip, with weakness in her gluteus medius muscle. When walking with her prosthesis, Caroline tends to compensate for her weak right gluteus medius muscle by using her TFL and hip flexors, therefore, internally rotating her hip. The resulting tightness is probably what causes her pain. Barbara is working with Caroline weekly on stretching of her TFL and hip flexors, strengthening of her gluteus medius muscle, and gait training using her prosthesis (Figure 12-6). During gait training, they are focusing on alternating Caroline's arm swing while walking with the prosthesis. (Box 12-3 for home activities to support Caroline's physical therapy program.)

Sheila is busy after school driving Caroline to her school government meetings, youth orchestra practices and performances, and physical therapy appointments. On weekend evenings, when Sheila works, Caroline's sister sometimes takes her out to shop or to the movies. Lianne is in college now and is quite busy away from home most of the time, so the girls enjoy spending what time they can together. Sometimes they talk about Caroline's fu-

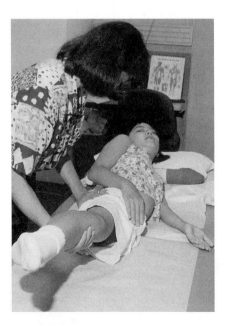

Figure 12-6 Caroline works with her physical therapist on strengthening activities for her right hip musculature.

ture. Her goals include going to college and having a career and a family. Although many things are difficult for her, she does not see any barriers that she cannot overcome. When she plants her foot firmly, she is as stable as anyone else!

Seeing a sick child wrenches our hearts like nothing else can. Working with a child who is in pain or feeling ill brings out the nurturing instincts in even the most callous among us. It does not seem fair that children should have to undergo illness when they have barely started living. But children do get sick, and some of them are very sick with diseases that can cause death or temporary or permanent disability.

One of the wonderful things about children is that they usually try their best and want to play and interact if they are feeling up to it. Physical therapy can help the sick child maintain or regain strength, endurance, and motor skills that allow them to play. Using play, the therapy provider can help the child have fun while working toward functional skills that may help the child go home from the hospital or participate in activities that bring them out of the world of illness and into the world of peers.

This chapter focuses on medical problems of childhood. The causes of medical problems are varied, and the outcomes are varied; but children with most of the disorders discussed in this chapter have frequent or prolonged contact with physicians and hospitals. Cardiopulmonary disorders include respiratory disorders such as asthma and cystic fibrosis (CF) and cardiac disorders such as congenital heart defects. Infectious disorders such as meningitis, infantile botulism, and Guillain-Barré syndrome (GBS) can cause acute and chronic problems with development. Childhood cancers vary in their type and prognosis, but all are traumatic to children and families and cause severe illness. Other medical disorders discussed in this chapter include seizure disorders, hemophilia, and sickle cell anemia (SCA).

The Case Study of Caroline, a teenager recovering from cancer, points out the unique role that physical therapy can play in the recovery and rehabilitation of children with severe illness. Caroline's cancer and her recovery from it has had a profound effect on her childhood. Caroline's resiliency, and that of her family, testifies to the resiliency in all of us.

The Applications section on medical technology (p. 415) helps the therapy provider be aware of and familiar with low- and high-technology medical interventions. Knowing what to do in case of accidental removal of tubes or lines, how to deal with beeping monitors, and when to call for help can encourage the physical therapist assistant (PTA) to be more comfortable working with children who need these medical appliances.

Children who are sick sometimes die. The special section on death and dying helps each of us explore our feelings regarding working with children who are terminally ill and dealing with the death of children we have come to know. As much as we would like to avoid it, death is a reality of life. Children who are terminally ill can be a source of great strength and joy, as well as a source of great pain to those around them. This section helps the PTA learn to be honest about feelings so that he or she can be a true support to the child and family with a significant illness.

Respiratory Disorders of Childhood

Respiration is a central function of the human body. Diseases that interfere with the transfer of gasses to nourish cells and take away waste not only interfere with school, family life, and peer relations but can cause a child to have little energy for even basic self-care tasks. Asthma is the most common chronic respiratory illness in children, and cystic fibrosis is the most common genetic disorder among whites. Both of these diseases have implications for exercise and pulmonary hygiene that concern physical therapy.

Asthma

Asthma is the only treatable chronic condition in the Western world that is increasing in prevalence (Sly, 1988). It also is killing more children than ever before (Weiss & Wagener, 1990). Physical therapy providers may encounter children with asthma in group exercise classes, children with neuromotor disabilities with whom they work may have asthma, or therapy providers may work directly with the child with asthma to help improve strength or endurance or to design an exercise program.

Prevalence and cause. It is estimated that between 5% and 10% of all children have asthma. The symptoms and severity may vary, but all these children have reversible airway disease. The airways of a child with asthma are hypersensitive to irritants including infection, cold temperatures, differences in humidity, exercise, irritants such as tobacco smoke or pollution, and allergens. Table 12-1 outlines some of the most common triggers and irritants for childhood asthma. Some children may have a stronger reaction to some stimuli than others. For instance, in a particular child asthma may be induced by exposure to dust mites or cockroach waste but not by animal dander or cold weather. Other children are affected by all these stimuli. Emotional arousal may also contribute to an

TABLE 12-1   Triggers or Irritants for Childhood Asthma

Trigger or irritant	Examples
Exercise	Running, team sports; swimming is the least asthma-provoking form of exercise.
Infections	Respiratory infections (bacterial and viral), colds, sinus infections
Allergies	Outdoor allergens (pollens, molds); indoor allergens (house dust, feathers, molds, pets); foods (milk, soy, eggs)
Irritants	Cigarette smoke, air pollution, strong odors, aerosol sprays, paint fumes
Weather	Cold air, weather allowing proliferation of molds or pollens
Emotions	Emotional responses triggering deep breathing such as laughing, crying, yelling, anger, frustration, anxiety

asthma attack. The anxiety caused by having an attack can promote hyperventilation and increase the severity of the symptoms. Many children are afraid of dying (Yoos & McMullen, 1996).

A genetic component to asthma has been identified. Approximately 75% to 80% of children with asthma have significant allergies as well. It is felt that children with asthma have a genetic propensity for the disease with environmental influences actually causing the asthma. It is not known why asthma has been significantly increasing in recent decades; theories range between increased air pollution over time to underreporting or underdiagnosing of asthma in the past. The percentage of children dying from asthma is also increasing significantly, although the perception is that better control of the disease has led to improved outcomes (Budetti & Weiss, 1993).

More boys than girls have asthma in younger ages; but as children grow, these percentages even out. Over half of children have their first asthma attack by the time they are 3 years old, and most children have had their first attack by the time they are 10 years old. More children of black ethnicity have asthma than those who are white. More children in urban areas have asthma than those in rural areas, and more children in Western areas of the United States have asthma than those living in Eastern areas (Gergen, Mullaly, & Evans, 1988).

Children who have had bronchopulmonary dysplasia or other respiratory problems in infancy are more likely to develop asthma. Children with extremely low birth weights are also more likely to develop this chronic disease than their peers.

Clinical features. Asthma is defined as a chronic reversible airway obstruction or narrowing of the airways that leads to air trapping and subsequent impairment of gas exchange. Asthma attacks or events may occur only a few times per year in response to easily identifiable stimuli or may occur much more frequently with triggers difficult to determine. Three events occur that impair the child's ability to breathe: (1) muscles that control airway diameter contract, causing decreased airway diameter; (2) the

mucous membranes become inflamed and swell, causing a further decrease in airway diameter; and (3) mucus production increases, causing blockages of some airway passages (Figure 12-7).

A child who has frequent coughing, frequent respiratory infections, coughing after exercise or crying, coughing at night, chest tightness, shortness of breath, irritability, or wheezing should be suspected of having asthma. Wheezing is caused by decreased diameter of the airways. It is not the most common symptom, but is the most easily identifiable, and consists of continuous high-pitched or hissing sounds with breathing. Wheezing sounds may be louder on expiration than on inspiration.

Asthma varies in its intensity, between different children and between attacks in the same child. If a child remains lying down with respiratory distress, he or she is probably having only a mild attack. A moderately or severely affected child chooses to sit upright or stand during an attack, possibly leaning forward with hunched shoulders. The most effective measures of the severity of an attack include pulmonary function tests such as peak expiratory flow rate (PEFR) or forced vital capacity. These measurements are taken using equipment specific to the task including spirometers or flow meters. Clinically, the PTA can determine the severity of an attack by observing the child's respiratory rate, level of alertness, ability to speak, use of accessory muscles to breathe, and skin color. Table 12-2 outlines parameters for these observations.

Eighty percent of children with asthma are affected by exercise, so monitoring children during athletic activities is prudent. Older children are able to monitor themselves to some extent. The PTA may be in a position to assist children with exercise-induced asthma (EIA) when asthma attacks are just beginning. The following section outlines how to most effectively intervene or support a child with asthma.

Asthma affects children differently, but most children experience many days lost from school and frequent trips to the emergency room with some subsequent hospitalizations (Figure 12-8).

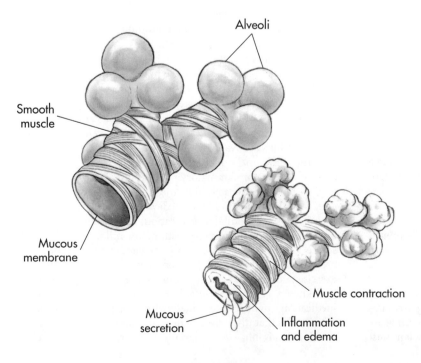

Alveoli

Smooth muscle

Mucous membrane

Mucous secretion

Muscle contraction

Inflammation and edema

Figure 12-7 Three events occur during an asthma attack. Contraction of muscles controlling airway diameter, swelling of mucous membranes, and an increased production of mucus.

TABLE 12-2   Clinical Estimation of Severity for Children With Asthma Attacks

	Respiratory rate	Level of alertness	Ability to speak	Accessory muscle use	Psychological state	Skin color
Mild	Normal to 30% higher than normal*	Alert	Speaks clearly in full sentences	Mild use of intercostal muscles	Normal to mildly anxious	Normal
Moderate	30% to 50% higher than normal	Alert	Speaks in phrases or short sentences	Moderate use of intercostal muscles, chest hyperinflation, use of sternocleidomastoid and neck muscles	Moderately anxious	Normal to pale
Severe	More than 50% higher than normal	May have decreased alertness	Speaks in single words or short phrases	Clear retractions, use of all accessory muscles, nasal flaring, chest hyperinflation	Severely anxious	Pale, may have some blueness (cyanosis) around mouth and nail beds

*Normal respiratory rates range for children with younger children having higher rates. A rule of thumb in breaths per minute follows:
Infants up to 1 yr: 30-35
Toddlers 1-4 yr: 23-29
School age 5-11 yr: 19-22
Adolescent 12 yr+: 16-18

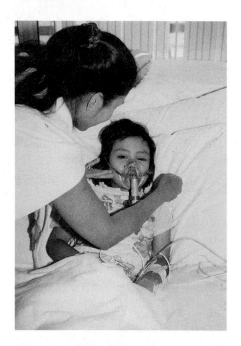

Figure 12-8 This 5-year-old child is hospitalized with an asthma attack. She is having a respiratory treatment, breathing medication directly into her lungs.

Social experiences and academic skill acquisition may be limited by school absences related to the disease, and parents may find themselves being overly protective of their children who have asthma.

Intervention. The most important intervention for the child with asthma is controlling the disease. This is a long-term approach based on prevention, rather than addressing each acute episode as a separate incident. The family and physician must work together to find the most effective method for controlling a particular child's disease. Controlling the disease involves the following:

- Avoidance of trigger factors
- Prophylactic medication
- Allergy injections when indicated
- A team approach with education for the child and family

Avoidance of trigger factors. Trigger factors must be identified, and the treatment or prevention approach is different depending on the specific factors involved with each child. For example, if a child is allergic to molds, dust, or pets, an effective approach is to minimize these substances in the home through regular cleaning, avoidance of carpets, finding pets a new home, use of dust barriers, and control of humidity to minimize mold. If the child is allergic to outside allergens, practices such as not having the child mow the lawn, staying inside when pollen levels are high, and air-conditioning the home might be effective. As children grow older, they learn to recognize trigger factors for themselves and learn to take steps to avoid them.

Medications. Medications are available that can significantly reduce the number and severity of asthma episodes. Four types of medications are available to help with asthma control:

- Inhaled bronchodilator medications
- Inhaled antiinflammatory medications
- Systemic corticosteroid medications
- Systemic bronchodilator medications

Inhaled bronchodilator medications are the most effective at opening airways narrowed by asthma for mild, moderate, and severe asthma. When used before exercise, this medication can prevent EIA. Children with EIA can participate normally in most exercise with proper premedication. Some Olympic athletes are well-known asthmatics, notably Florence Griffith Joyner. This medication can be taken via metered-dose inhalers (small hand-held bottles that dispense one dose at a time) or in a nebulized solution that is inhaled during a breathing treatment. Young children do not always use the inhaler properly, causing a decrease in the effectiveness of the medication. A spacer, a plastic tube between the child and the inhaler, helps deliver the correct dose in the correct manner and increases the effectiveness of this method of delivery. Although this medication is effective, overuse can cause a delay in evaluating severe asthma and a worsening of the asthma.

Inhaled antiinflammatory medications such as corticosteroids are taken consistently for children with moderate to severe disease to provide beneficial effects, which build up over days and weeks. Taking the medication inconsistently can cause a decrease in the effectiveness. Side effects of this medication include oral infections such as thrush.

Systemic bronchodilator medications such as theophylline can help prevent nighttime attacks of asthma or control of daily symptoms. Side effects are more common with the systemic medication. Systemic corticosteroid medications can help control chronic severe asthma or reverse severe episodes of asthma. Side effects can be severe, so the use of these medications is reserved only for those cases that cannot be controlled by other medications.

Allergy injections. Most children with asthma have significant allergies. Injections that help the child decrease sensitivity to allergens can be effective to treat the asthma as well. Some controversy exists as to whether these shots are effective for severe cases of asthma and which cases they might help the most. Whether the shots are more effective early in the course of asthma rather than later is also being debated (Sigman & Mazer, 1996).

A team approach. When parents and older children are involved as important members of the management team, control of the disease can be improved. With education, parents can monitor certain pulmonary functions at home and better understand when the child needs emergency medical care. In addition to managing the acute phases of the disease, parents can take an active role in preventing acute episodes through monitoring the environment, activities, and exercise of the child (Szczepanski et al., 1996).

Role of physical therapy. Maintenance of health is especially important for a child with a chronic disease like asthma. In addition to avoiding situations in which the child is exposed to respiratory infections, the child should take steps to actively promote health. An exercise program has been shown to improve the health of children with asthma without adversely affecting the disease itself (Fink, Kaye, Blau, & Spitzer, 1993). Once the child learns to control EIA, he or she can participate fully in sports.

The PT or PTA may be involved in adapting or implementing an exercise program for the child with asthma or creating a program to gradually build a level of fitness. Children who come to physical therapy for neurodevelopmental or orthopedic problems may also have asthma, which should be considered when designing a program for them.

Cystic Fibrosis

Incidence and cause. Cystic fibrosis (CF) is a genetic defect affecting 1 in 2000 to 3000 white children. Significantly lower incidences are found in Hispanic children and black children, and even lower incidences are found in Asian children. It is inherited in an autosomal recessive pattern, meaning both parents must carry the defective gene to pass it to their offspring. In 1989 a discovery was made of a defect in the long arm of chromosome 7 leading to a defect in the production of CF transmembrane regulator (CFTR). This protein affects the exocrine (mucus-producing) glands, and the defect produces problems in multiple systems throughout the body, most notably in the respiratory tract, gastrointestinal tract, reproductive tract, and in the sweat glands of the skin. It used to be called the "salty kiss disease," reminiscent of mothers who complained that they noticed salt on their children's skin when kissing them.

The life expectancy of a person with CF in the United States has increased significantly in the past 50 years, from about 6 years of age in the 1950s to well into the 40s for children born in the 1990s (Collins, 1992). Increasing knowledge of the disease process and advances in therapeutic treatment including antibiotics have contributed to this increase in life expectancy.

Clinical features. Because the disease affects mucus-producing glands, the respiratory tract is a key problem site. Thickened mucus results in poor ciliary action, stagnant mucus, and constant infections. Infections increase throughout life with multiple resistance built up to antibiotics and trauma to the structures of the respiratory tract, causing erosion and fibrosis of the lung tissues over time. The child with CF has a persistent productive cough, a barrel-shaped chest, and later on, clubbed fingers and toes from hypoxia.

Thick secretions block pancreatic ducts, leading not only to progressive fibrosis of the pancreas but also lack of appropriate enzymes in the intestinal tract to break down and absorb nutrients. Therefore stools are abnormally large with too much fat and protein; and absorption of nutrients is disturbed, leading to failure to thrive, easy bruising, and anemia. Rectal prolapse can be a major problem from the large stools, as are intestinal obstructions and impacted feces. Children with CF tend to be small and thin with little fat and have difficulty gaining weight.

Problems with exocrine production lead to deficiencies in saliva production with resultant mouth sores. Liver cirrhosis can occur from blocked liver ducts. A classic sign of CF is excessive amounts of chloride and sodium on the skin from faulty sweat glands. The child is at risk for dehydration and for abnormal electrolyte balance in the blood, especially during hot weather or times of excessive sweating.

Intervention. Greater knowledge of the mechanisms of the defects in CF is prompting greater efforts to address the roots of the problems, but unfortunately, many of these interventions are not yet fully developed or proven. Treatments involving gene replacement therapy, alteration of chloride channels, and thinning of hyperviscous mucus with various agents are being developed. Management of the pulmonary and gastrointestinal problems to reduce the negative effects of the disease has increased the life span of affected individuals and continues to be the mainstay of treatment.

Antibiotics to treat the multiple infections of the respiratory tract have been effective in decreasing the number and severity of infections. Chest physical therapy to expel thick secretions is a daily part of the life of a child with CF. Expulsion of the secretions can help to avoid infections and can increase the area of lungs available for gas exchange. The Applications section in Chapter 11 discusses postural drainage, percussion, vibration, and breathing exercises, the backbone of chest physical therapy.

Pulmonary complications of CF are usually the cause of death. For individuals in the later stages of the disease, transplantation of the lungs can improve function and increase the life span. Double lung transplantations are done for individuals with CF so that original lung tissue does not contaminate new lung tissue with infection.

Attention to nutrition through adequate diet, oral supplements, and intravenous or nasogastic supplementation during acute exacerbations can help the child with CF gain weight and grow. Provision of extra pancreatic enzymes helps the child absorb more nutrients through the intestinal tract (Green, Buchanan, & Weaver, 1995).

Exercise may be difficult because of frequent illness and poor respiratory capacity. Children with CF have increased energy requirements even at rest and even in the absence of respiratory disease (Shepherd et al., 1988). Because of the difficulty in getting adequate nutrition, fat stores for energy and muscle bulk may be depleted or absent. Some efforts are being made with recombinant growth hormone treatment to promote physical strength and endurance in children with CF. The goal is to help the children be more active to improve their respiratory status (Wong, 1995). Electrolyte balance, especially sodium and chloride, is important to watch during exercise because of the potential for more sweating than usual and the tendency to excrete large amounts of these electrolytes through the sweat glands. Encouraging the child to drink electrolyte replacement fluids with high sodium and chloride content may be helpful during exercise.

An exercise program that allows for a gradual increase in performance demand and a controlled environment should be designed for children with CF. Avoidance of trauma, overexertion, and careful monitoring of a child's respiratory status during exercise helps ensure safety and positive results. Stationary bicycle, walking or light running on a treadmill, or swimming are excellent activities. Attention to making the activity fun through setting goals, documenting progress on a chart, creating fantasy "journeys," or setting up mild competition between children or between the therapy provider and the child can encourage greater consistency with the exercise program. Ongoing pulmonary function tests are the best method of assessing a child's pulmonary status over time and can indicate an early decrease in respiratory function from infection or other causes. Attention to pulmonary hygiene before and after exercise through assisted coughing, percussion and drainage, or inhalant treatments can maximize the benefits of the exercise.

Heart Disease in Children

Congenital heart disease (CHD) is a common occurrence in the United States and throughout the world. Children whose hearts do not work well frequently develop respiratory problems, as well as decreased strength and endurance. These can lead to delays in developmental skills. Physical therapy may be involved to encourage strength, endurance, and developmental skills in children who have extended hospital stays to prepare for or recover from heart surgery. Although the trend is toward early complete repair of congenital heart defects in infancy, several surgeries may be required to repair multiple defects. The physical therapy provider may see the child throughout childhood in school, as an outpatient, or as an acute inpatient.

 Ask a nurse. The nurse is an endless well of information regarding medical issues and social issues about a particular hospitalized child. She or he is a valuable resource for therapists.

Children may also have acquired heart disease. The child's healthy heart is affected through infection, autoimmune responses, environmental effects, and familial tendencies. In this section we focus on congenital heart defects because they are more common. Principles of treatment are similar between congenital and acquired defects.

Incidence and Cause

The incidence of CHD is about 8 to 10 per 1000 live births (Hoffman, 1995; Montafna et al., 1996). Many more infants with CHD associated with chromosomal abnormalities die in utero as either miscarriages or stillbirths. Genetic defects are one cause of CHD. Although genetic defects other than chromosomal abnormalities are thought to cause CHD, specific genes have not yet been identified, and factors such as low incidences of heart disease within individual families of children with CHD (leading to an explanation other than genetic) have yet to be explained. Other causes of CHD include exposure to teratogens such as infectious agents. Most researchers subscribe to a multifactorial mechanism of causation, which includes single genes, teratogens, and chance (Bristow, 1995). Over 90% of CHD has no identifiable cause. Some prenatal factors are correlated with a higher incidence of CHD including maternal rubella during pregnancy, maternal alcoholism, maternal age over 40 years, and maternal insulin-dependent diabetes (Wong, 1995).

Anatomy of the Healthy Heart

The heart can be thought of as a wonderfully efficient double pump (Figure 12-9). Deoxygenated blood from the body is brought to the right atrium of the heart via the inferior and superior venae cavae. The blood is pumped into the right ventricle, the first efficient pumping station of the heart. Blood is vigorously pumped from the right ventricle through the pulmonary artery to the lungs where gas exchange takes place. Pressures are low in the right side of the heart because relatively little pressure is needed to circulate the blood through the lungs. In the lungs the carbon dioxide waste products in the blood are exchanged for fresh oxygen. To get distributed to the tissues where oxygen is needed, the blood must return to the left atrium of the heart by way of the pulmonary veins. The blood is then delivered to the second pumping station, the left ventricle, which pumps it through the aorta and out to the various tissues of the body. The pressure needed to pump blood to the entire body is significantly higher than that needed to pump blood to the lungs. Therefore pressure on the left side of the heart is much higher than that on the right side. All these events occur simultaneously and in a consistent rhythm that is carefully modulated by electrical impulses in the heart itself.

Fetal circulation is different than postnatal circulation (Figure 12-10). Because the blood is oxygenated through the placenta, the lungs are not essential to fetal circulation. Several anatomical

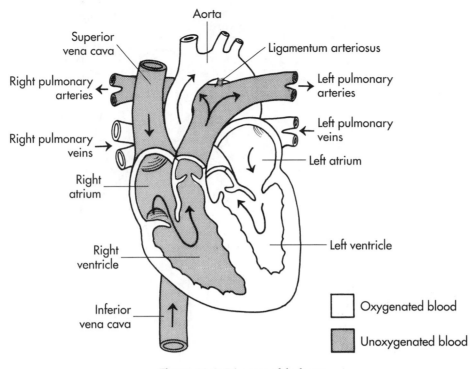

Figure 12-9 Diagram of the heart.

differences between a fetus and an infant exist to promote efficiency in fetal circulation. In the fetus the umbilical vein carries oxygenated blood to the liver from the placenta. Here the vein divides, with some blood going into the liver circulation and the rest of the blood going to the fetal heart via the inferior vena cava. Deoxygenated blood from lower body tissues is returned to the heart by the inferior vena cava, joining the oxygenated blood from the placenta. Once in the heart, this blood passes directly from the right to the left atrium via the foramen ovale, an opening between the two chambers. Oxygenated blood then goes into the left ventricle to get pumped into the aorta to go to the brain and other tissues. Deoxygenated blood from the upper body returns to the heart via the superior vena cava and also enters the right atrium. This blood passes through to the right ventricle and is pumped to the pulmonary artery where some of it goes to the developing fetal lungs. The majority, however, is shunted via the ductus arteriosus to the descending aorta and brought back to the placenta via the umbilical arteries for more oxygen.

Any abnormalities in the anatomy of the heart, including persistence of fetal structures, can cause significant disruption in the ability of the infant's lungs to function and of the tissues to obtain oxygenated blood.

Clinical Features

Two main categories of CHD are traditionally recognized: those that result in cyanosis and those that do not, called cyanotic and acyanotic cardiac lesions. Cyanosis is characterized by a bluish color of highly vascularized tissues such as nail beds and lips resulting from poor oxygen saturation of the hemoglobin in the blood. A number of different abnormalities can lead to each of

these conditions and are discussed below. Although CHD can be divided into cyanotic and acyanotic categories, in actuality, symptoms accompanying cardiac defects often have elements of both. Some children may have several heart defects at the same time, causing multiple problems. Understanding the effects of a child's heart defects is necessary to understand the consequences of activity and exercise for the child during physical therapy.

Acyanotic heart defects. All CHDs are characterized by compromised circulation of blood to the tissues. Acyanotic defects are those in which blood is adequately saturated with oxygen but may be poorly distributed to the body.

Defects in this category can cause too much blood to go to the lungs, resulting in congestive heart failure. The resulting damage and congestion of the heart and lungs causes inefficient pumping of oxygenated blood to the rest of the body. Symptoms include pulmonary hypertension, respiratory distress, diaphoresis (inappropriate sweating), and fatigability. Tachycardia, weakness, restlessness, decreased blood pressure, and cool extremities also may be seen. Fast breathing, coughing, wheezing, pale or blue lips and nail beds, and flaring nostrils are also common symptoms. Difficulty with feeding because of poor endurance and resultant poor weight gain are common signs in infants. Developmental delays result from poor tolerance to activity.

The most common defect, affecting almost one third of children with CHD is the ventricular septal defect (VSD), an opening between the right and left ventricles. Normally, all the oxygenated blood in the left ventricle would be pumped out the aorta to the body; but with an opening between the ventricles in children with a VSD, higher pressures in the left ventricle cause blood to flow into the right ventricle. There the blood joins unoxygenated blood and is pumped into the pulmonary artery to go back to the lungs. The result is that too much blood goes to

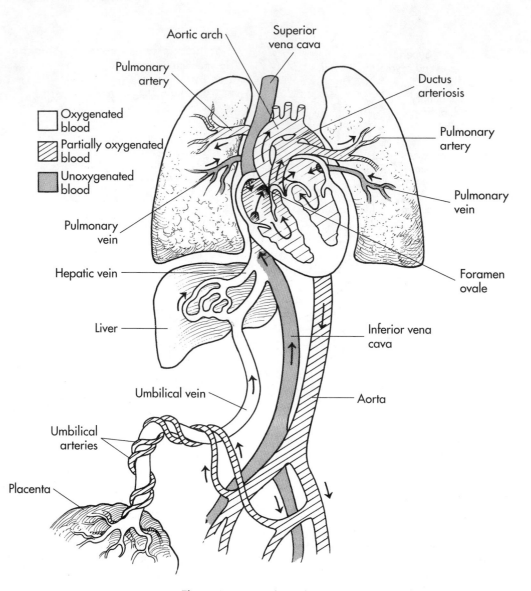

Figure 12-10 Fetal circulation.

the lungs. Damage to delicate lung tissues from too much pressure and subsequent lung congestion can result. VSD is seen in children with Down syndrome or fetal alcohol syndrome, among others. Surgery is usually required to place a synthetic patch over the opening; the procedure is done earlier in children with larger defects to try to limit the negative effects on growth and development.

Patent ductus arteriosus (PDA) (also discussed in Chapter 11) is a failure of the fetal shunt between the pulmonary artery and the descending aorta to close. It occurs in about 8% of congenital heart defects. In the infant, blood is shunted from the aorta to join the blood in the pulmonary artery and travels into the lungs, causing congestion. This defect is seen commonly in children with prematurity, Down syndrome, or rubella syndrome. The treatment of choice is indomethacin, a drug that can result in closure of the PDA, or surgery in cases where the drug is ineffective.

About 7% of children with congenital heart defects have an atrial septal defect (ASD), a hole in the septum between the atria. Blood is shunted from the left atrium to the right (instead of to the left ventricle and through the aorta to the body), passing from the right atrium to the right ventricle and to the pulmonary artery to the lungs. This defect is seen in many syndromes, notably Down syndrome and fetal alcohol syndrome. Problems from this disorder are not usually as severe as some other CHDs, and the heart is usually surgically repaired when the child is between 6 months and 2 years old.

Other disorders can also lead to congestive heart failure and include narrowing of the pathways in which the blood moves away from the heart, sometimes known as obstructive defects. Some of the symptoms relating to these defects include those of congestive heart failure. Other symptoms may include a heart murmur, high blood pressure, or differences in blood pressure and pulses between the upper and lower extremities. Coarctation of the aorta (7% of CHD) involves a narrowing of the descending aorta. Aortic stenosis (3% of CHD) involves a narrowing at the entrance to the aorta. Pulmonary stenosis (8% of CHD) involves a narrowing at the entrance to the pulmonary artery. Any of these conditions can cause blood to back up into the heart and lungs. Surgical repair is always required if function is affected.

Other treatments that may be used with children in congestive heart failure include diuretics, drugs used to decrease the fluid levels in the body through urinary excretion. Digitalis may be used to increase the contractility of the heart resulting in decreased edema, decreased heart size, and increased cardiac output. A class of drugs called angiotensin-converting enzyme inhibitors make it easier for the heart to pump by dilating blood vessels in the kidneys and lungs and lowering blood pressure. Balloon angioplasty is sometimes used as a less invasive intervention to dilate valves or blood vessels in obstructive defects.

Cyanotic heart defects. Several heart defects can cause poor oxygen saturation, including those that shunt unoxygenated blood to the tissues. Defects in this category are significantly less common than acyanotic defects. Symptoms can include cyanosis, a pale or bluish color of the lips, nail beds, and other normally pink tissues. Cyanosis can occur in acute episodes that may follow crying or feeding when the infant's oxygen requirements exceed the supply. For older children, clubbing of the fingers, poor growth, or possible tachycardia or dyspnea may be seen as a result of chronic hypoxia. Children with these defects are at risk for strokes, brain abscess, and seizures. Exercise and activity are severely curtailed because of low oxygen supplies. Children are at risk for significant developmental delays because of illness and decreased activity.

The most common of the cyanotic defects is tetralogy of Fallot (TOF), a constellation of four different defects that occur together in about 4% of children with CHD. The child with TOF has a VSD, pulmonary stenosis, an overriding aorta (the aorta overrides the ventricular septum, increasing the likelihood of unoxygenated blood being pumped through it to the tissues), and right ventricular hypertrophy (because the right ventricle has to work harder than normal). Blood flow and oxygenation may be assisted with a shunt between the subclavian artery and pulmonary arteries using a Blalock-Taussig or modified Blalock-Taussig shunt, until the child is large enough and strong enough to undergo a complete repair. The surgical repair is usually done in the first year of life and involves repairing the VSD and widening the pulmonary stenosis.

Tricuspid atresia, a failure of the valve between the right atrium and ventricle to form, is the second most common cyanotic defect and occurs in over 3% of children with CHD. In children with this defect, oxygenated and unoxygenated blood mix in the left side of the heart through an ASD and proceeds to the pulmonary artery through a VSD. Complicated surgeries done in steps to create shunts between systemic arterial blood and the pulmonary artery can help to increase blood flow to the lungs but does not correct the defects. An advanced procedure called the modified Fontan procedure connects the right atrium to the pulmonary artery in an attempt to get greater flow of unoxygenated blood to the lungs. Children with this cardiac defect never have normal cardiac anatomy and long-term survival is not known.

Hypoplastic left heart syndrome occurs in 3% of children with CHD. The left ventricle is poorly formed, and is not functional in pumping oxygenated blood to the tissues. A persistence of the ductus arteriosus between the aorta and the pulmonary artery helps to mix oxygenated and unoxygenated blood to go to the tissues. Surgical procedures done in stages can improve the heart function, but some believe that transplantation is the best option. Prognosis is not good for these children, and some surgeons advocate no treatment at all.

Less than 3% of children with CHD have transposition of the great arteries, where the aorta and the pulmonary arteries have switched positions. Oxygenated blood is pumped to the lungs, and unoxygenated blood is pumped to the tissues of the body. Septal defects allow the blood to mix so that oxygenated blood can be transported to the body, and unoxygenated blood can be transported to the lungs. Several surgical procedures are done to change the flow of blood, including an arterial switch procedure where the major arteries are surgically moved to their originally intended positions.

Physical Therapy Intervention

Because of the sometimes severe lack of oxygen to the tissues for a child with CHD, physical therapy intervention may be limited to parent teaching about positioning and handling during infancy. The child may gain more strength and endurance with growth or with surgical procedures, allowing greater handling and intervention as the child grows older. Facilitation of normal developmental skills is generally the focus of therapy, especially those skills that allow the child to participate in age-appropriate activities. For the young child, tolerating handling for a few minutes may be an initial goal; where sitting without support, standing, and walking may be later goals. Use of age-appropriate toys and activities can help engage young children. Modeling activities for parents or nursing staff and directly teaching others to carry on the activities can help ensure that activities are carried on when the therapy provider is not present.

Observation of the child's color, respiratory rate, level of sweating, affect, fatigue, and level of irritability are essential to avoid overstressing the child with CHD. Frequent rests during the therapy session can help the child work or play for longer periods of time. Knowing when to end the therapy session to allow the child deeper rest is important. If the child is hospitalized, parents or nurses will be able to help the PTA read the child's signs. At home, the parent will be the primary caregiver and should be relied on to give this type of support.

Supplementary oxygen may be used routinely at home or in the hospital or may be available to help the child during increased activity such as therapy sessions. The hospitalized child may require mechanical ventilation, may require suctioning, and may use an oxygen saturation monitor (see Applications section in this chapter). The PTA working with a child with CHD must be familiar with the operation of this equipment and its use. Suc-

> If a pulse oxymeter alarm is sounding and you want to get an accurate readout of the child's oxygen saturation, put your fingers gently over the tape holding the sensor to keep it close to the skin. This allows the machine to read the oxygen saturation.

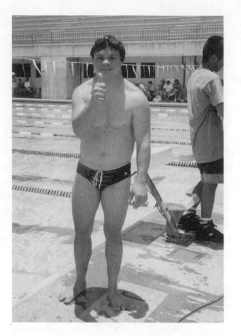

Figure 12-11 This young man with Down syndrome recently underwent cardiac surgery to correct a ventricular septal defect. He loves to swim and regularly participates in the Special Olympics.

tioning will likely be done by the nurse or parent rather than the therapy provider, depending on the circumstances and level of training.

Children with repaired cardiac defects can develop exercise endurance and strength, allowing them to participate in vigorous activity (Figure 12-11). The physical therapy provider may work with the child through several childhood and early adult surgeries, helping maintain a positive attitude toward exercise, as well as learning specific exercise skills.

Acquired/Infectious Neurological Disorders of Childhood

The well infant or child may acquire a disease of bacterial, viral, or other origin that causes temporary or permanent disability. Several of these are discussed in this section including meningitis, encephalitis, GBS, and infantile botulism. Children who have contracted these diseases generally need rehabilitation to recover their premorbid skills or to develop functional skills after brain damage has occurred.

Meningitis and Encephalitis

Meningitis is an inflammation of the meninges or covering of the brain or spinal cord. It is a serious illness that can lead to brain damage in previously healthy children. Encephalitis is an infection of the brain caused by a virus. Both diseases can cause serious brain injury and are common causes of acquired cerebral palsy.

Incidence and cause. Two major causes of meningitis are bacteria and viruses. Bacterial meningitis is not only the most common but is usually the most serious. It affects between 35 and 50 people per 100,000 in the United States (Jackson & Saunders, 1993). Children from infancy to 5 years of age account for 90% of the cases of bacterial meningitis, with the most common ages being between 6 months and 2 years.

The most common forms of bacteria to cause meningitis include meningococcus, *Haemophilus influenzae* type b (HiB), and pneumococcus. A vaccine is currently available against HiB but not against the other forms. Most of these bacteria live harmlessly in the back of the mouth and throat and cannot be avoided. They must, however, infect the meninges to cause meningitis. This usually occurs via a primary infection in the nose, throat, or skin infecting the blood with organisms that then travel to the meninges. For this reason, meningitis frequently follows a respiratory illness.

Aseptic meningitis and encephalitis are less common than bacterial meningitis and can be caused by a wide variety of organisms, most commonly viruses. Causes include viral sources such as mumps, poliovirus, herpes simplex, hepatitis, and human immunodeficiency virus (HIV). Illness may occur after infection from measles, rubella, or smallpox. Bacterial causes include tuberculosis, syphilis, and partially treated bacterial meningitis. Other causes include amebic causes, drug reactions, and reactions to vaccines. Aseptic meningitis and encephalitis commonly affect children with leukemia. Encephalitis may be caused by mosquito-borne viruses and therefore frequently arises during warm weather.

Clinical features. Initial symptoms of bacterial meningitis include fever, nuchal rigidity (stiff neck), vomiting, and malaise (general aching). In a child younger than 2 years old, symptoms might be slightly different, including fever, vomiting, seizures, poor feeding, a bulging fontanelle (opening between the plates of the skull), and irritability. A young child's neck may be supple rather than stiff.

A child with aseptic meningitis or encephalitis may have a gradual or abrupt onset of illness. Headache, fever, malaise, sore throat, abdominal pain, vomiting, chest pain, back and leg pain, or sensitivity to light may be present. Aseptic meningitis cannot be treated except symptomatically and usually resolves in 7 to 10 days. Meningitis caused by tuberculosis may be more serious and could result in hydrocephalus because of discharge blocking the route of cerebral spinal fluid in the ventricles.

Because encephalitis is frequently associated with childhood diseases such as rubella and mumps, its incidence has greatly diminished with the advent of good vaccination programs against these diseases. Encephalitis can mimic aseptic meningitis and be fairly mild and benign; however, it can also be a life-threatening illness, leaving children with severe disabilities. Mosquitoes and ticks carrying viruses that can lead to encephalitis are active during summer months, so this disease arises more frequently in the summer in temperate climates and all year round in tropical and subtropical climates. Symptoms include headache, fever, malaise, dizziness, apathy, neck stiffness, nausea, vomiting, ataxia, tremors, hyperactivity, and speech difficulties (Wong, 1995). Symptoms of more severe illness include stupor, seizures, disorientation, spasticity, and coma. Cranial nerve palsies may occur, leading to blindness or deafness.

Intervention. Bacterial meningitis is very dangerous and is treated as an emergency situation. A lumbar puncture is taken to determine the presence of bacteria and to define what type of bacteria to treat. Treatment with antibiotics is started immediately intravenously. The child is monitored in the hospital for more severe manifestations of the disease and to make sure that the he or she responds to the antibiotics. Aseptic meningitis is not usually treated except symptomatically.

Severe forms of encephalitis are also an emergency. A lumbar puncture may detect the virus or organism causing the inflammation, but intravenous treatment with acyclovir, an agent that fights viral infections, is started immediately. Medical interventions to control seizures, counteract swelling in the brain caused by the inflammation, and ensure adequate hydration and nutrition can help to minimize any neurological damage from the disease.

Children who have meningitis at younger ages, especially in the first months of life, have a greater chance of having residual problems. The infecting organism is also a factor in the outcome; children with infection from HiB have a worse outcome than children with infections from other organisms. Sixty-five percent of children with HiB bacterial meningitis recover completely. Thirty-five percent of children with HiB infections have residual problems from the disease, which may include hearing impairments (10%), language disorders or delays (15% to 34%), visual impairments (2% to 4%), motor impairments (3% to 7%), seizures (8%), and mental retardation (10%) (Jackson & Saunders, 1993). Vaccination against HiB is now available and is hoped to decrease the rate of disability from the disease.

Up to 60% of children with encephalitis have residual problems of headache and fatigue; with more severe problems of behavior changes, impaired motor function, mental retardation, or seizures (Jackson & Saunders, 1993).

Physical therapy is rarely involved in the acute phase of treatment of the child with meningitis or encephalitis but may become involved as the child reaches the recovery phase and functional motor deficits become apparent. Intervention is very similar to that of children with cerebral palsy, and the reader is referred to Chapter 7 for interventions for different types of motor problems related to cerebral palsy. Each child with motor deficits from meningitis or encephalitis looks different, depending on the pattern of infection, the amount and areas of the brain damaged, associated deficits such as hearing or vision impairments, and the age of the child.

Guillain-Barré Syndrome

Sometimes called acute polyneuropathy, acute polyradiculitis, infectious or acute idiopathic polyneuropathy, Landry's ascending paralysis, or acute segmentally demyelinating polyradiculoneuropathy, Guillain-Barré syndrome (GBS) is a devastating but reversible disease that causes progressive paralysis resulting from demyelination of the peripheral neurons (Figure 12-12). Children become progressively weaker, sometimes needing mechanical ventilation to help them breathe, and then get progressively stronger again as the peripheral nerves remyelinate. Demyelination occurs over the peripheral nerves, nerve roots, and cranial nerves. In severe cases some axons in the spinal cord are also affected. Most children recover completely but may take months or years to regain lost strength and function. Some children have permanent disability from residual weakness, especially in distal muscle groups.

Incidence and cause. This relatively rare disease can affect individuals of all ages but is becoming increasingly more common in children. GBS generally is seen in children between the

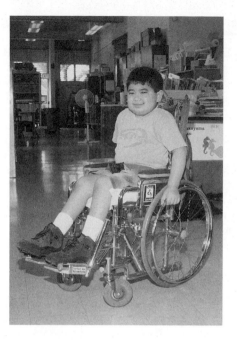

Figure 12-12 Clinton was diagnosed with Guillain-Barré syndrome 11 months ago. He continues to use a wheelchair for most of his mobility needs at school.

ages of 4 and 10, although younger and older children can also be affected. Although the cause is not known, in most cases the disease occurs about 1 to 3 weeks after a minor infection, immunization, or surgical procedure. It is thought to have an autoimmune basis.

Clinical features. The child with GBS may complain of weakness, fatigue, and sensory abnormalities such as paresthesias or areas of anesthesia. The legs generally are affected before the arms, and the paralysis progresses up the spinal cord. Motor symptoms are generally worse than sensory symptoms. The onset of symptoms is rapid and progressive; this progression is considered a medical emergency because the child may lose respiratory function without warning.

The extent of paralysis varies between children, and some have involvement of lower extremities and trunk muscles only. About 30% of children, however, progress to a full paralysis within days, including respiratory muscles, requiring mechanical ventilation. About 5% of children die during the acute phase, and about 10% to 20% of children who recover have residual neurologic impairment. Five percent to 10% suffer a relapse after beginning recovery. Clinton, described in Box 12-4, demonstrates a severe case of GBS with at least one relapse.

Usually within a few weeks or months, a gradual return of motor function begins as the nerves remyelinate. Sensory hypersensitivity may continue for months and may be a limiting factor in the recovery. Some children cannot bear weight or allow anything to touch their feet because of sensory hypersensitivity. A gradual return of strength and function allows the child to be discharged from the hospital and continue rehabilitation from home as an outpatient. Some children require months or years of rehabilitation as they gradually gain more function. Others have a gentler course and may fully recover within a few months.

Intervention. Medical intervention focuses on the mainte-

BOX 12-4   Clinton, A Boy Recovering From Guillain-Barré Syndrome

Clinton is the only child of his single mother. They have a close relationship, and his mother is very involved in all aspects of Clinton's life. He was 6 years old when he complained of dizziness and being unable to walk while in school one day. He also was vomiting and had a headache. He was taken to the hospital where his symptoms rapidly progressed. Three days later, he was completely paralyzed and required a ventilator to help him breathe. Physical therapy immediately became involved with Clinton to help him maintain his range of motion and prevent joint contractures while he was paralyzed. Resting ankle splints helped him prevent severe contracture of his plantar flexor muscles. Two months later, Clinton had improved enough that the ventilator and endotracheal tube could be removed, and he was moved from the intensive care unit to the regular pediatrics floor. He suffered a relapse within a few weeks and went back to the intensive care unit for 2 more weeks. He suffered from severe depression during his hospital stay, which required treatment. He finally went home almost 5 months after his initial illness, with considerable residual weakness. Because of difficulty with malnourishment while Clinton was in the hospital, a gastrostomy button was placed. The button was not removed, since it would be needed if Clinton has another relapse. The button allowed nutritional supplementation at night and administration of nighttime medications after he went home.

Problems after he went home included the following:

- Limitations in range of motion in ankle dorsiflexion and hip extension bilaterally
- Absent or trace muscle strength in his ankle dorsiflexors and plantar flexors bilaterally
- Poor strength in his hip extensors bilaterally
- Good strength in his hip abductors, adductors, and knee flexors bilaterally
- Weak normal strength in knee extensors bilaterally
- Continued hypersensitivity to touch and pressure in his feet and legs

Clinton was not walking independently and refused to bear weight through his legs because of hypersensitivity on the plantar surface of his feet. During the next few months he agreed to bear weight with shoes on and learned to walk while holding first both hands and then one hand of an adult (Figure 12-13). He learned to roll, come to sitting, move between sitting and quadruped, and pull himself up to stand using a modified half-kneel position. Although he now walks while pushing his wheelchair, he has independent mobility propelling his wheelchair around his home and school. His gait is characterized by genu recurvatum (back knee) bilaterally, foot drag, no heel-to-toe motion, decreased stride length, and dependence on upper extremity support for balance and to assist weight bearing. Gait is limited by continued contractures in both ankles, continued hypersensitivity of his feet, and poor endurance.

Medical insurance has refused to pay for dynamic ankle foot orthoses or for physical therapy treatments as an outpatient in the local pediatric hospital. Clinton gets physical therapy from Cheryl, a PTA, in school twice per week. He is in a regular second grade classroom. Cheryl works closely with his mother and teacher to support his gross motor skills when she is not with him. In his physical therapy sessions, Cheryl helps Clinton work on improving his strength and functional skills such as moving between the floor and his wheelchair (Figure 12-14), improving his strength and endurance while walking, climbing stairs, and ensuring that his equipment needs are met. The school loans him the wheelchair he is using, and Cheryl has tried an adapted tricycle and other equipment with Clinton. Although he is cooperative for the most part, Clinton is embarrassed to be seen doing his physical therapy activities and refuses to ride the tricycle because peers might see him. He is aware of his altered appearance (weight gain, round face) caused by the steroid medications he is taking and is self-conscious with strangers.

---

nance of body functions such as respiration, nutrition, and elimination. Attention to the child's respirations and cough can indicate whether the intercostal muscles are becoming too weak to support independent respiration. Insertion of an endotracheal tube and use of a mechanical ventilator are some of the most intrusive lifesaving supports. Intravenous or nasogastric feeding, use of diapers or catheters to manage elimination, and positioning to prevent skin breakdown are some basic nursing interventions.

Physical therapy can assist with prevention of contractures and maintenance of comfort through provision of daily range of motion, resting ankle splints, and helping with positioning while the child is acutely ill. Protection of the hypersensitive feet and legs from the touch of the bedcovers can be achieved through a framework to hold the sheets and blankets over the feet.

As recovery begins, activities to help the child sit up, stand, reach for toys, and develop independent movement skills can be initiated. Awareness of the tactile hypersensitivity that almost always accompanies this disease is important to maintain the confidence of the child and family. Allowing the child to make

choices of activities or influence timing of activities can help the child feel more in control and take more responsibility for his or her rehabilitation.

Helping the child communicate while intubated and while very weak can be a challenge. Creative methods include modified switches attached to communication boards, visual scanning devices, and manual communication boards using a yes/no method of choice. The parent or primary caregiver should be involved with the primary nurse, the speech-language pathologist, PT, and any other team members regularly involved with the child in creating and deciding on a communication method. A workable method of communication can help to counter the stress of hospitalization and decreasing function, which can lead to depression.

As the child readies to leave the hospital and return home and to school, communication with therapists in the community settings is essential. Services should be in place before the child needs them. Medical rehabilitation is generally not in the purview of school health services (see Applications section, Chapter 5), but therapists in the school are able to support the

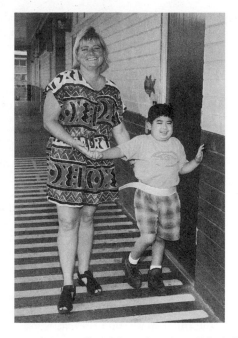

Figure 12-13 Clinton walks while trailing the wall for balance and holding Cheryl's hand for support.

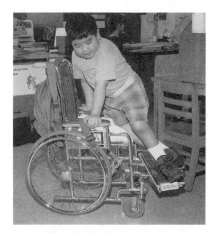

Figure 12-14 Clinton demonstrates how he gets into his wheelchair.

child so that he or she can benefit from the educational setting. The actual level of involvement of school therapists varies according to specific policies in each state and school district.

Infantile Botulism

The symptoms of botulism, a neuromuscular disease, can be very similar to those of GBS: progressive weakness and paralysis, with a wide range of effects. The course of the disease may be affected by the cause, the age of the child, and the child's susceptibility to the disease.

Incidence and cause. Botulism is a disease seen mostly in adults. The classic form with which most people are familiar is caused by ingesting foods that have been contaminated with botulism spores. Home canned foods that have been improperly

sterilized are the most common source of this illness. Parents still warn children not to eat food from cans that have swollen because of the proliferation of botulism spores and the resultant production of toxin in the food.

A second form of botulism is that caused by contaminated wounds. Botulism spores can infect a wound causing symptoms 1 to 2 weeks after exposure. It is most often found in wounds sustained in open areas or farms.

The most common form of botulism in children is infantile botulism, caused by ingestion of spores that then multiply in the gastrointestinal tract, causing toxins to be produced inside the body. Spores are found in honey and in lesser amounts in light or dark corn syrup. They can also be found in the air in rural areas. Sweeteners may be put on nipples to get infants to eat or mixed with foods by well-meaning caregivers who are unaware of the risks. Infants from rural areas may have no history of being given sweeteners and may have ingested spores from the air. Infants with a history of decreased bowel movements may have a greater likelihood of getting the disease because the decreased elimination allows spores to grow in the intestinal tract.

Clinical features. This disease is most commonly seen in very young infants of 2 to 3 months. Constipation may be an early sign of the disease; in some infants, constipation is the only symptom. Other infants have a decrease in spontaneous movements with generalized weakness. Poor feeding, a weak cry, and a decrease or absence of deep tendon reflexes are other symptoms that may occur. Progressive paralysis leading to failure of spontaneous respiration can lead to a medical emergency and death if the infant is not supported by mechanical ventilation. The infant may need ventilatory and nutritional support for weeks or months as the disease takes its course. Most infants recover completely, but a few may have residual weakness or paralysis.

Intervention. Older children and adults can receive botulinum antitoxin made from horse serum to combat the disease. This intervention has not been shown to be useful in infants and young children, and the dangers of reaction to the serum far outweigh the usefulness of this treatment in young children. Medical support for respiration and nutrition are the most important interventions as the disease runs its course. Children with severe disease may have a tracheotomy performed to allow greater ease in ventilation. A nasogastric tube may be placed for nutritional support; for children with a longer course, a gastrostomy tube may be placed to provide nutrition directly to the stomach.

Physical therapy intervention is important to address the child's musculoskeletal and developmental needs during the long acute hospitalization. Early intervention for positioning to avoid contractures is essential. Passive range of motion to maintain joint integrity and range while the child has little or no active movement can also be useful. If the family is able to spend time with the child, teaching them these basic skills can give them a concrete role at the bedside and ensure that optimal positioning and passive range occurs even when the nursing staff are busy. The child fatigues easily with active motion because the toxins affect the ability of the nerve endings to release acetylcholine, dimishing nerve conduction to the muscles.

As the child gains strength, feedings may be resumed. Attention to the length of time it takes an infant to nipple a feeding and quality of sucking and swallowing is important because muscle weakness can result in aspiration, which can lead to further illness.

Developmental gross motor skills including head control, rolling, propping on arms in the prone position, coming to the sitting position, and supported standing can be facilitated to promote normal sensory experience and help the child develop age-appropriate skills. Fine motor skills of grasp and release, transfer of toys from one hand to another, finger feeding, and reaching can also be supported through play with toys, food, and other objects. The cranial nerves may be affected by the disease, causing diploplia (double vision), ptosis (closed eyelids), and facial paralysis; however, sensory input including mirrors, toys with high contrasting colors, sounds such as from children's music tapes, and conversation should be emphasized to encourage normal developmental stimulation. The child's musculoskeletal system has been affected by the disease, but the intellectual function remains intact. The child continues to need stimulation to foster developmental skills, especially in a hospital environment.

The child with botulism poisoning may recover adequate respiratory and oral-motor function but require continued physical therapy intervention as an outpatient to promote optimal gross motor skills. Given enough time, most children recover completely.

Childhood Cancers

Cancers in children have been increasing over past decades, but the rate of recovery has also been increasing as more effective medical interventions are found. Childhood cancers have been increasing 1% to 2% per year in the past two decades, especially cancers of the brain, bone, and blood. These trends have been especially marked for children younger than 2 years of age (Gurney et al., 1996). The rate of survival from many childhood cancers has also increased dramatically throughout the world. Mortality from childhood cancers has decreased from 8.3 per 100,000 to 3.6 per 100,000 from 1950 through 1986 (Fernback & Vietti, 1991). The survival from childhood leukemia has risen from 20% of children diagnosed in the 1960s to almost 80% in the 1990s. This increase in survival well outweighs the increase in incidence.

> Let parents and family members take the lead when the subject of death or the terminal nature of a disease arises. Be open to their need to talk about it. Listen.

The types of cancer to affect children are different from adult cancers. Whereas adult cancers affect the lungs, colon, breast, prostate, and pancreas, children get cancers of the blood, brain, bone, and lymphatic system, as well as tumors of the muscles, kidneys, and nervous system. Each is characterized by an uncontrolled proliferation of cells, and this proliferation causes different symptoms in the different cancers. Cancers in children are more active than those in adults; 80% of children have cancer already spread to distant body sites on diagnosis, whereas this is true for only 20% of adults. Cancer is the most potent killer disease of childhood and kills more children than any other cause except injury.

Because more children are being diagnosed with cancer and more children are living longer with cancer, physical therapy is more likely to be needed. Interventions from physical therapy range according to the type of cancer and the age of the child but include helping a child improve general strength and endurance, controlling pain in acute cases, and providing rehabilitation for amputation or other surgical intervention. Children may be seen acutely in the hospital, as an outpatient, or may be followed at school for long-term physical therapy needs.

Incidence and Cause

The cause of most childhood cancers is unknown. This is opposed to the strong relationship between lifestyle and environmental exposures such as cigarette smoking, sun exposure, and chemical exposures including asbestos that can lead to many adult cancers. Some relationship has been established between a viral component and some cancers, including the human T-cell leukemia-lymphoma virus (HTLV), and the Epstein-Barr virus with some leukemias and lymphomas in adults, leading to speculation about a possible viral link in children.

Risk factors have been identified for some cancers in children. Exposure to ionizing radiation has been shown to lead to cancer in adults and children. It is thought that exposing pregnant women to radiation may predispose the fetus to cancer. Some drugs containing radioisotopes and immunosuppressive agents can increase the risks of a child developing cancer. Maternal exposure to diethylstilbestrol (DES), a drug once used to prevent miscarriage during pregnancy, has been shown to significantly increase the female offspring's risk for vaginal cancers during adolescence and young adulthood. This drug is no longer being prescribed for this purpose, and most daughters of mothers who took the drug are now in middle adulthood.

Exposure to electromagnetic radiation through power lines is suspected of having a small relationship to the development of childhood cancers, as is exposure to some pesticides and some parental occupational exposures, although definitive studies have not yet been done (Zahm & Devesa, 1995).

A genetic component to childhood cancers is strongly suspected. Some cancers occur more frequently in siblings, especially twins. Patterns of inheritance can be identified for some pediatric tumors, especially eye, brain, and kidney tumors. Children with some chromosomal abnormalities have a higher incidence of some cancers. For example, children with Down syndrome are 15 times more likely to develop leukemia than children who do not have Down syndrome.

About 8000 children are diagnosed with cancer each year in the United States (Zahm & Devesa, 1995). The incidence is about 141 per 1,000,000 white children for all pediatric cancers, but this figure changes according to the specific cancer (Zahm & Devesa, 1995). Black children have a slightly higher incidence, and boys are slightly more susceptible than girls to most cancers. Table 12-3 lists the percentages of different types of pediatric cancers.

Clinical Features

In general, cancers are made up of abnormal cells that have a rapid growth rate and lose the orderly function of nearby cells. These proliferating cells impair the function of the organ or system they are invading. They are able to metastasize or spread to distant sites of the body via the blood or lymph systems or

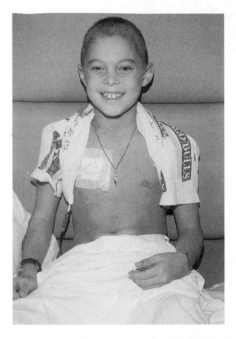

Figure 12-15 John, who has acute lymphoid leukemia, is receiving red blood cells through an indwelling catheter in his chest to treat anemia.

TABLE 12-3	Types of Pediatric Cancers

Type	Total pediatric cancers (%)
Leukemia	39
Brain and nervous system cancers	22
Lymphomas (cancers of the lymph system)	10
Kidney	6
Bone	6
Soft tissue (muscle)	5
Other	12
Total	100

through mechanical disruption such as through a needle biopsy. Cancer cells compete with healthy tissue for nutrients and space, killing normal cells. The cancer cells invade adjacent tissues, making it impossible for normal cells to perform their functions. Solid tumors expand, compressing nearby tissues and causing more cell death and functional damage. Different cancers have different properties. The principal cancers of childhood are described below.

Leukemia. The most common childhood cancer, leukemia, is a cancer of the tissues of the body that make blood cells, including the bone marrow and the lymph system. Vascular tissues of the body are the most severely affected, especially the spleen and the liver. Leukemia most commonly affects children between 2 and 6 years of age but can affect younger or older children as well (Figure 12-15).

Two forms of leukemia include acute lymphoid leukemia (ALL) and acute myelogenous leukemia (AML). ALL has its origins in the lymph cells and is the most common type of child-

hood leukemia, affecting almost 80% to 90% of all children with leukemia. Subtypes of ALL, L_1, L_2, and L_3 are based on the structure of the leukemic cells. Eighty-four percent of children with ALL have subtype L_1, which has the best prognosis (Wong, 1995). AML has its origins in bone marrow. It affects between 10% and 20% of all children with leukemia.

The onset of leukemia may be sudden or gradual. A child may feel tired with a decreased appetite and continued fever after a minor illness like a cold or may feel gradually more tired over a course of weeks. Symptoms including increased bruising or bleeding, bone and joint pain, and fatigue may mimic mononucleosis or arthritis.

These symptoms are similar for all types of leukemia and arise from the suppression of normal bone marrow function. Abnormal cells form in the bone marrow and create white blood cells that do not perform their proper functions. The abnormal cells crowd out the normal cells, causing the body to be lacking in normal white blood cells, red blood cells, and platelets. Absence of normal white blood cells leads to increased infections, absence of platelets causes increased bleeding, and absence of normal red blood cells leads to anemia. Eventually, the abnormal cells weaken the bone, causing bone and joint pain and fractures. When the periosteum is invaded, the pain can become severe. Related symptoms include pallor, fever, and anorexia or absence of appetite.

Other organ systems are also affected by the leukemic cells. The spleen, liver, and lymph glands can become enlarged. Central nervous system (CNS) involvement can occur, although new medications are decreasing this complication. Leukemic infiltration of the meninges leads to interference of the flow of cerebral spinal fluid and resulting increase in intracranial pressure. This can lead to neck and back pain, vomiting, irritability, lethargy, and finally, coma. Proliferation of abnormal cells can cause other normal body cells throughout the body to become starved for nutrition. General muscle wasting and weight loss are common symptoms in children who have survived active leukemia for a period of time. Invasion of other body tissues including the testes, ovaries, kidneys, prostate, gastrointestinal tract, and lungs are also common in long-term survivors.

Interventions range from chemotherapeutic drugs, CNS irradiation, or bone marrow transplants, depending on the symptoms of the child and the type of leukemia. Most children with leukemia are treated at regional medical centers that participate in large scale therapeutic protocols through coordinating national treatment groups such as the Children's Cancer Group or the Pediatric Oncology Group (Ross, Severson, Pollock, & Robison, 1996). Treatment protocols are developed and implemented across the country and are constantly being revised based on results. A large national database for treatment protocols and results is therefore available. This national, and in some cases, world-wide coordination of pediatric cancer treatment is probably the reason for the huge advances in treatment success.

Brain and nervous system cancers. Cancers of the brain and nervous system are the next largest group of pediatric cancers beside leukemia and are the most common type of solid tumors in children. Brain and nervous system tumors are differentiated by the type of tissue involved and by their location. Table 12-4 outlines the most common types of tumors in the CNS and peripheral nervous system and their signs and symptoms.

Treatment for these tumors is usually surgical resection and

TABLE 12-4　Types of Nervous System Tumors in Children

Type of tumor	Symptoms	Prognosis	Treatment
Astrocytoma Affects almost half of children with brain tumors; two major types			
Cerebellar: About 10%-20% of childhood CNS tumors	Ataxia, clumsiness, awkward gait, vomiting, headache, irritability, personality changes, fatigue, anorexia	70%-90% cure rate	Surgery
Supratentorial: About 35% of childhood CNS tumors	Visual disturbances, seizures, headache, vomiting, irritability, personality changes, fatigue, anorexia	75%-85% cure rate for low grade, lower for high grade	Surgery, radiation, chemotherapy
Medulloblastoma Affects about 15% of children with CNS tumors; usually occurs in the cerebellum	Ataxia, headache, vomiting, irritability, personality changes, fatigue, anorexia	50% cure rate; highest for low grade, lower for high grade	Surgery, irradiation
Brain Stem Glioma Affects about 15% of children with CNS tumors	Cranial nerve dysfunction, gait disturbances	Poor	Irradiation
Ependymoma Affects 5%-10% of children with CNS tumors	Seizures, ataxia, clumsiness, hemiparesis, hydrocephalus in infants, headache, vomiting, irritability, personality changes, fatigue, anorexia	50% cure rate	Surgery, irradiation
Craniopharyngioma Affects 6%-9% of children with CNS tumors	Visual disturbances, headache, vomiting, endocrine disturbances	Benign tumor	Surgery, irradiation if needed
Neuroblastoma Arises in the sympathetic nervous system with common sites being adrenal glands or paraspinal ganglions; occurs in young children	Pain, abdominal mass, persistent diarrhea, bone pain, pallor, weakness, irritability, anorexia, weight loss	75% for children younger than 1 year of age, 50% for children older than 1 year of age; in some children, the tumor spontaneously regresses	Surgery, chemotherapy, irradiation if needed

CNS, Central nervous system.

may include chemotherapy and/or irradiation if the entire tumor is not able to be removed surgically. The location of the tumor indicates the functional deficits a child may experience from the effects of the tumor or treatment for the tumor.

Neuroblastoma is a particularly difficult type of cancer to diagnose because it generally begins early in life. Sites of the tumor may vary considerably. The tumor has frequently metastasized before diagnosis and has many sites with diverse resultant problems. This type of cancer has a poor prognosis and is particularly difficult for parents and families.

Lymphoma. Two types of cancers of the lymphatic system include Hodgkin's disease (HD), and non-Hodgkin's lymphoma (NHL). NHL is more common in younger children, but HD becomes more common in adolescence, with an incidence ap-

proaching that of leukemia. Both diseases are more common in boys than girls. HD is characterized by swelling of peripheral lymph nodes, with metastases to sites outside the lymph system including bone marrow, spleen, liver, lungs, and mediastinum. NHL most frequently involves the abdomen and mediastinum. Cancer cells in NHL are more undifferentiated and the disease is usually more diffuse than HD, with children between the ages of 7 and 11 most commonly affected. An intensive treatment protocol for both HD and NHL includes chemotherapy and irradiation. Children in the early stages of the disease can be cured, and about 50% of children in later stages recover.

Wilms' tumor. Also called nephroblastoma, Wilms' tumor of the kidney is the most common solid tumor seen in the abdomen. It is seen more frequently in young children, and peak

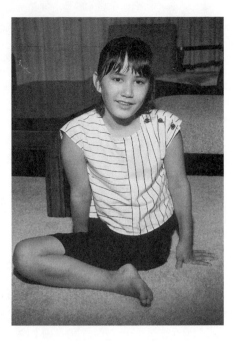

Figure 12-16 Losing a limb can be a devastating consequence of osteosarcoma in adolescents.

incidence is 3 years of age. Wilms' tumor has a definite genetic inheritance pattern with an increased incidence in identical twins and siblings. This tumor is associated with congenital deformities including genitourinary deformities and aniridia (absence of iris in the eye). Other associated but less common deformities include microcephaly and mental and growth retardation. A swelling or mass in the abdomen is the most common presenting symptom. Treatment includes surgery and chemotherapy with or without irradiation.

Bone cancers. Osteosarcoma is the most common bone cancer in children and peaks between 10 and 25 years of age (Figure 12-16). Most tumors occur in the epiphyses of the long bones, with more than half occurring in the femur, especially the distal portion. Other bones involved with this type of tumor can include the tibia, humerus, phalanges, jaw, and pelvis. Initial symptoms may include pain, swelling, or pathological fracture.

Treatment is somewhat controversial with some physicians advocating radical surgery, amputating the limb with at least 3 inches of bone proximal to the tumor to prevent reoccurrence. Others recommend limb salvage procedures where a wide margin of unaffected tissue around the tumor is resected with prosthetic replacement of resected bones and joints. Children with distal femoral involvement could undergo a rotationplasty where the distal femur and proximal tibia are removed and the lower leg is rotated 180 degrees so the ankle can serve as a knee joint. In this way, a child can use a below-knee prosthesis with the additional function that would provide. Chemotherapy is used as an adjunct to surgery to ensure the tumor is completely gone.

Ewing's sarcoma is another type of bone cancer common in children in the same age range, peaking from 10 to 25 years of age. This cancer arises in the marrow-producing portion, the shaft, of long bones and may also be seen in the ribs, pelvis, scapula, or skull. Ewing's sarcoma is not usually addressed surgically, and a combination of irradiation and chemotherapy is

the most common treatment modality. Irradiation may affect the epiphyses of the bone, producing deformity and slow growth that will be with the child for the rest of his or her life. The limb, however, will be spared.

Soft tissue tumors. Soft tissue tumors can occur in muscles, tendons, bursae, and fascia. They may also occur in fibrous tissue, connective tissue, or lymphatic or vascular tissue. The most common type of soft tissue tumor is rhabdomyosarcoma, a tumor of striated muscle tissue, which can be found anywhere in the body. This tumor may appear in a child of any age but is more common in children younger than 5 years old. The most common sites include the head and neck, especially the orbits of the eyes. Clinical symptoms vary according to the site but can include earache, runny nose, or an abdominal mass. The tumors are fast growing with frequent metastases and require vigorous intervention. Combined chemotherapy and irradiation with surgery as a less frequently used option are treatments of choice. If the disease is caught early, up to 90% or 100% of children may be cured. For children in later stages, especially when metastatic disease is present at the time of diagnosis, the prognosis is less favorable with less than 50% being cured.

Medical Interventions

As described in the preceding section, different cancers respond better to different interventions; however, the primary types of intervention include some combination of irradiation and/or chemotherapy to shrink the tumor and surgery to remove the tumor. Other interventions include bone marrow transplantation and immunotherapy.

Irradiation. Irradiation is the targeting of cancer cells by high-energy electromagnetic emissions to disrupt the DNA of the cell and result in the shrinkage or death of the tumor. The child is usually treated daily in a radiology facility for several weeks. The amount of radiation is limited by the tolerance of surrounding tissues to the modality.

Chemotherapy. Chemotherapy consists of administering a variety of toxic drugs in combination to attack a particular form of cancer. Drug trials have demonstrated that drugs in combinations are more effective in addressing cancerous cells while minimizing toxic side effects and minimizing the build up of resistance by cancer cells. Some drugs are able to be administered continuously in higher doses using syringe pumps to avoid the higher toxicity when they are administered intermittently.

Surgery. The goals of surgery are usually to biopsy a tumor or to resect the tumor as completely as possible. The trend is to use a combination of chemotherapy and irradiation to support the surgery and do less radical surgeries. An example is using limb sparing procedures when possible for children with osteosarcoma rather than complete amputations.

Bone marrow transplantation. Bone marrow transplantations are used for children with leukemia who are not responding well to traditional chemotherapy. Children with AML usually do not respond as well to chemotherapy than those with ALL and may need a bone marrow transplantation at the first remission. Those with ALL are usually coaxed through at least two remissions before the bone marrow transplantation is attempted. Children have a 50% chance of recovering from a bone marrow transplantation.

TABLE 12-5 Cancer Interventions and Residual Effects

Intervention	Types of cancer	Side effects/residual effects
Surgery	Brain and nervous system tumors Lymphomas (HD, NHL) Kidney Bone (osteosarcoma) Soft tissue tumors	Amputation/limb deficiency Poor wound healing Infection Poor body image
Irradiation	Leukemia (some CNS prophylaxis) Brain and nervous system tumors Lymphomas (HD, NHL) Kidney Bone (Ewing's sarcoma) Soft tissue tumors	Impairment of intellectual function Impairment of motor function Delayed or deficient growth Hormonal dysfunction Decreased fertility or sterility Skeletal deformities including scoliosis, leg length discrepancy, skull and facial disfigurement Osteoporosis Pathological fractures Dental caries Postirradiation somnolence can develop 5-8 wk after CNS irradiation and last for 4-15 days (fever, nausea, vomiting, anorexia)
Chemotherapy	Leukemia Brain and nervous system tumors Lymphomas (HD, NHL) Kidney Bone Soft tissue tumors	Infection Bleeding Anemia Nausea, vomiting Anorexia Mucosal ulceration Severe constipation Foot drop, weakness, and numbing of the extremities Jaw pain Alopecia (hair loss) Hemorrhagic cystitis
Immunotherapy	Leukemia	Similar as for chemotherapy
Bone marrow transplantation	Leukemia	Infection Skin breakdown Delayed wound healing Death

CNS, Central nervous system; *HD,* Hodgkin's disease; *NHL,* non-Hodgkin's lymphoma.

The procedure for the transplantation includes three phases. In the first, drugs and irradiation are administered to kill all existing bone marrow cells and the disease that exists in them, as well as to immunosuppress the child for the greatest chance of success at accepting the new bone marrow. New bone marrow is provided from a histocompatible donor through blood transfusions in the second phase. The third phase involves supporting the child in medical isolation as the new bone marrow implants and begins to grow new bone marrow cells. The child is kept in strict isolation during this period of time, with administration of blood transfusions and antibiotics to minimize the risk of infection. Infection, rejection of the new bone marrow, and illnesses such as interstitial pneumonia are some of the greatest risks leading to death.

Each of these interventions has significant side effects that can impact the life of a child and family (Table 12-5). A therapy provider should be aware of these side or residual effects and also aware of the long-term effects of interventions for childhood cancer.

Physical Therapy Intervention

The child with weakness and poor endurance. The child with cancer may have weakness and decreased endurance during hospitalizations and chemotherapy treatments that can be addressed with physical therapy. During this acute phase of treatment, nausea, vomiting, and fatigue are common side effects of the drugs. Before the administration of the chemotherapy, the therapy provider could meet with the older child to design an exercise program for use during an extended hospitalization. An exercise bicycle, small trampoline, free weights, or other exercise aid may be supplied to the adolescent with instructions on how to use the equipment and a brief exercise program. The child can then use the equipment when he or she feels up to it and can call the therapy provider for assistance whenever needed.

The child who is facing surgery for amputation or a limb salvage procedure may need strengthening and general conditioning to prepare for surgery and maximize recovery after surgery. A written exercise protocol for the child to do at home under the supervision of parents or other adults may be all that is needed.

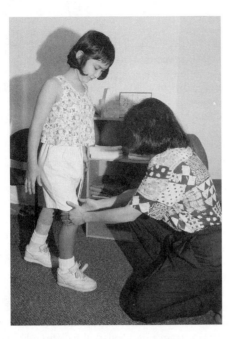

Figure 12-17 Caroline works with her physical therapist to improve her gait using the prosthesis.

To increase compliance with the program, a chart documenting progress should be an integral part of the plan, with a system of positive feedback when small goals are met. Many adolescents are devastated by the diagnosis of bone cancer and have difficulty complying with medical interventions, including an exercise program. A psychologist familiar with cancer and adolescents should be included in the team if possible to meet with the child and help develop a plan of recovery that is acceptable to all.

The child with weakness and contractures from chemotherapy and frequent hospitalizations. Young children receiving extended or repetitive chemotherapy may have neurological effects from the drugs, including foot drop, paresthesias, and weakness. Because of plantar flexion contractures and weakness, the child may lose the ability to walk. Splints to maintain ankle range of motion and bed mobility activities for parents or nursing staff to do with the child including passive range of motion and simple active movements integrated in a play activity may help prolong functional skills. The children with these problems are frequently those who are the most sick and those who are not responding well to treatment. The therapist should work with the team to ensure that only appropriate interventions are given and that the child and family's overall needs for nurturing and comfort are considered foremost.

Rehabilitation of the child with a surgical amputation. Rehabilitation for strengthening and range of motion of a residual limb in preparation for a prosthesis is generally complicated by repeated rounds of chemotherapy and long-term effects of the treatment regimen. Working closely with the team, including the family, can help the process of appropriate planning. Training to use the prosthesis may occur sporadically because of illnesses and chemotherapy (Figure 12-17). For more specific information about prostheses, see Chapter 5 and the Case Study in this chapter.

Other Medical Disorders of Childhood

Three other medical disorders of childhood are addressed in this chapter. Seizures are a problem that can occur either alone or in conjunction with other disorders. Because seizures are so common among children who receive physical therapy services, being familiar with not only the different types of seizures but also appropriate intervention is necessary for safety.

Hemophilia and sickle cell anemia are inherited disorders that can result in orthopedic impairments and medical problems. Understanding the cause of the orthopedic disorders can help PTs and PTAs plan and implement appropriate interventions for children with these disorders.

Seizures in Children

Seizures are usually brief episodes of unconsciousness, motor activity, sensory experiences, or inappropriate behavior caused by malfunctions of the brain's electrical system. Different types of seizures can look very different from one another. Seizures are associated with many childhood illnesses and disabilities, including cerebral palsy, fragile X syndrome, autism, traumatic brain injury, brain tumors, or fever, and frequently are associated with no other medical or developmental problem at all.

Incidence and cause. Epilepsy, a condition of chronic seizures, affects 1% of typically developing children (Zupanc, 1996). Isolated seizure activity such as that occurring with fevers is more common, occurring in up to 3% of children. Children with developmental disabilities including mental retardation and cerebral palsy have an overall 3% risk of chronic seizures (Nevo et al., 1995).

Seizures are caused by abnormalities in the structure or function of the brain. Some individuals have a lowered threshold to seizures, a trait that may run in some families. Transient seizures may be related to elevated temperature (fevers) or biochemical imbalances. Other causes of seizures include trauma to the brain tissue from birth trauma, traumatic brain injury, bleeding in the brain, brain cancer, or disease. Chemical imbalances of the blood and tissues can cause seizure activity as well.

Seizures can be classified as idiopathic, with no obvious cause, or symptomatic, related to a particular cause. Most idiopathic seizure activity begins in children between 2 and 14 years of age. In children younger than 2, developmental causes such as birth trauma or metabolic disease can usually be identified. Adults who begin seizure activity usually have an identifiable cause such as brain cancer, traumatic head injury, or other brain disease such as encephalitis.

Clinical features. Understanding the way seizures are described involves learning specific terminology related to seizures. Table 12-6 outlines classifications for seizures. Seizures can be classified as partial, general, or unclassified, depending on the outward manifestations of the seizure itself and the implied amount of abnormal brain activity contributing to the seizure. Partial seizures can be simple, with no loss of consciousness, or complex, involving a loss of consciousness. Simple partial seizures may involve motor symptoms such as jerking of one part of the body, which may spread to other parts, or may involve sensory symptoms including smells, visions, or feelings like fear or anger. Both sensory and motor symptoms may be present at the same time.

TABLE 12-6   Classification of Seizures

International classification of seizures	Older term(s) for classifying seizures	Manifestations of the seizure
Generalized seizure	Generalized seizure	Seizures that are generalized to the entire body; always involve a loss of consciousness
Tonic-clonic seizure	Grand mal seizure	Begin with a tonic contraction (stiffening) of the body, then change to clonic movements (jerking) of the body
Tonic seizure		Stiffening of the entire body
Clonic seizure	Minor motor seizure	Myoclonic jerks start and stop abruptly
Atonic seizure	Drop attacks	Sudden lack of muscle tone
Absence seizure	Petit mal seizure	Nonconvulsive seizure with a loss of consciousness; blinking, staring, or minor movements lasting a few seconds
Akinetic seizure		Lack of movement, "freezing" in place
Partial seizure	Focal seizure	Seizures not generalized to the entire body; a variety of sensory and/or motor symptoms may accompany this type of seizure
Simple partial seizure	Jacksonian seizure	No loss of consciousness or awareness
• With motor symptoms		Jerking may begin in one small part of the body, and spread to other parts; usually limited to one half of the body
• With sensory symptoms		Sensory aura may precede a motor seizure
Complex partial seizure	Psychomotor seizure Temporal lobe seizure	Loss of consciousness occurs during the seizure, either at the beginning or the end of the event; may develop from a simple partial seizure and/or develop into a generalized seizure; may include automatisms like lip smacking, staring, or laughing
Unclassified seizure		Seizures that do not fit into the above categories including some neonatal and febrile seizures

A complex partial seizure always involves a loss of awareness of surroundings and may include purposeless behavior, wandering, or total loss of consciousness. Sometimes bizarre behavior is associated with this type of seizure, such as opening the door of a moving car, running around the room knocking over furniture, or removing clothes in public. The child has an impairment of consciousness and is not aware of his or her actions. An aura, or sensory experience may be the initiating symptom of the seizure. A complex partial seizure may progress to other seizure activity including a generalized seizure. Older children may recognize an aura as the beginning of a seizure and take precautions.

Generalized seizures are characterized by the type of motor activity that accompanies the episode. The tonic-clonic seizure, formerly called a grand mal seizure, involves initial stiffening with loss of consciousness and subsequent jerking motions of the entire body. The seizure may last from a few seconds to several minutes, and in severe cases, even longer. The tonic-clonic seizure is the most common type of seizure, especially in children with developmental disabilities. Most tonic-clonic seizure activity is followed by a postdictal period of deep sleep, headache, muscle soreness, or focal motor or sensory phenomena. Children sometimes sleep for hours or a complete day after a major seizure.

Tonic seizures are characterized by stiffening of the muscles. Clonic seizures are characterized by repetitive jerking of the muscles. The jerking may start in one part of the body and generalize to the entire body. Atonic seizures are also called drop attacks because the individual loses all muscle activity or tone and falls to the floor. Akinetic seizures are characterized by lack of movement, and the person may freeze in place. Absence seizures are brief seizures characterized by an absence of convulsions. Blinking, staring, or minor automatic movements may accompany a loss of consciousness.

Children with cerebral palsy or mental retardation are at greater risk for developing seizures than the general population. Common types of seizures seen in this population include tonic-clonic, myoclonic, atypical absence seizures, and partial complex seizures. Some children have more than one type of seizure. Children with milder forms of mental retardation or cerebral palsy are more likely to have partial seizures; conversely, children with more severe mental retardation and cerebral palsy are more likely to have generalized seizures (Steffenburg, Hagberg, & Kyllerman, 1996.)

A critical condition when seizure activity continues for an indeterminate length of time is called status epilepticus. One seizure may follow another so rapidly that they appear to be one long seizure. In other cases, seizures follow one another at brief intervals. Sometimes hours or days may pass with no abatement of seizure activity. This condition is a medical emergency. Death or brain damage could result from lack of oxygen.

Intervention. Medical intervention includes careful diagnosis of the seizure activity. Some seizure activity is subtle or could be mistaken for behavior manifestations rather than abnormal brain activity. Assessing the cause of the seizures can help decide on the course of treatment. The PTA working with a child can help this process by documenting very carefully any seizure activity including the time and length of the seizure, behavior of the child, motor components of the seizure, and affect of the child after the seizure. Documenting environmental stimuli that may have contributed to the seizure such as flashing lights, noises, or activities can also be helpful.

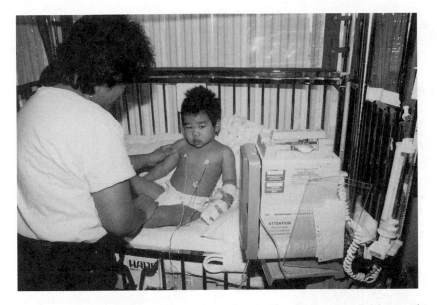

Figure 12-18 Kevin, a child with a chronic seizure disorder, has developmental delays, with no expressive language skills at 2 years of age.

Some partial seizures can simply be observed, with relevant data documented. For instance, a teacher may notice the child staring blankly one minute, and returning to work the next. A PTA may notice a child freeze briefly when participating in therapy. These episodes should be noted and brought to the attention of parents or caregivers.

If a seizure includes a motor component, more vigorous intervention needs to occur. The child should be protected from harm by moving furniture to allow space to move, providing a pillow or soft clothing under the head, and loosening any restrictive clothing. The child should be rolled onto his or her side to minimize the risk of aspiration. Nothing should be inserted into the child's mouth. Someone should stay with the child for reassurance once he or she regains consciousness. If seizures are a regular occurrence in the child's life, the teacher or school nurse should be able to assess whether or not medical intervention is necessary. At a minimum, details about the seizure should be written to the parent or guardian. If seizures are not a normal occurrence for this child or if the seizure lasts longer than usual, medical intervention should be obtained by calling the parent, the child's physician, or by calling an ambulance.

Medications to control seizure activity are usually administered initially in high doses and subsequently titrated over time to the lowest dose that is effective at controlling the seizures. Most neurologists prefer to control seizures with only one drug; but if an effective drug cannot be identified, combinations of drugs may be used (Morton & Pellock, 1996). Different drugs have varying side effects, but all cause some drowsiness or lethargy. Children may have difficulty learning or behavioral challenges because of the medications. This side effect can be severe in many children, with significant improvement in their ability to attend and learn when they are weaned off the drugs. Hyperplasia of the gums is common in children who take phenytoin (Dilantin) and may result in bleeding or mouth tenderness. Other side effects of seizure medications may include a skin rash, nystagmus, anemia, dysarthria, nausea, dizziness, and ataxia.

Children with a seizure disorder may have developmental delays either related to their underlying condition such as cerebral palsy or traumatic brain injury or related to the seizure disorder itself (Figure 12-18). A team approach to address the child's needs usually includes physical therapy if the child is demonstrating motor delays. Because the medical management of the seizures is directed by the child's response to the medication, excellent communication between therapists, teachers, parents, and physicians is essential. Getting to know the child's common pattern of seizures can help the therapy provider recognize a seizure. Parents or teachers who know the child well can inform the PTA of the proper procedures to follow.

A physical therapy provider may see a child with an acute seizure episode in the hospital or for outpatient therapy related to an acute loss of function. Usually, however, the child with seizures is followed in an infant development program or at school for chronic delays in development or motor deficits related to brain damage (Figure 12-19)

The Child With Hemophilia

Although a genetic disorder, hemophilia is included in this chapter because its effects are more orthopedic from the physical therapy standpoint, than developmental. The PT or PTA is more likely to see the child with hemophilia in an acute care or an outpatient setting than for long-term therapy in school or at home.

Hemophilia is an X-linked genetically transmitted disorder leading to a deficiency of clotting factors in the blood. The two major types of hemophilia include hemophilia A, which is a deficiency of factor VIII, and hemophilia B, which is a deficiency of factor IX. More than 80% of hemophiliac children have hemophilia A, the more common type. The clinical manifestations of both disorders are similar, although treatments differ because of the different clotting factors needing to be replaced.

Etiology and incidence. Because hemophilia is an X-linked disease, almost all the affected children are boys. A few girls who

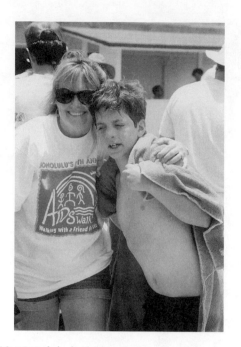

Figure 12-19 Luke's disabilities first appeared as seizure activity when he was an infant. Seizures are still a common experience for him.

have an affected father and a carrier mother may exhibit the disease. Some girls who are carriers may exhibit mild symptoms of the disease. Hemophilia affects approximately 1 in 10,000 children.

Clinical features. Three levels of severity have been identified based on the level of clotting factor in the blood. Children with mild disease have between 5% and 25% of normal clotting factor in their blood. They are at risk for bleeding from moderate to severe trauma or surgery but will not usually have problems resulting from mild trauma such as that resulting from falls or general sports participation, excluding contact sports like boxing or football.

Children with moderate disease have between 1% and 5% of clotting factor in their blood. They are at risk for excessive bleeding from mild to moderate trauma and will have some bleeding into their joints but will seldom have spontaneous bleeding. Playing contact sports is not a good idea for these children, but they may participate in swimming, jogging, and gentle team sports like golf.

Children with severe disease have less than 1% of clotting factor in their blood. They are at risk for bleeding from even very mild trauma and may have spontaneous bleeding into their joints, muscles, or other areas of the body for no apparent reason. More than 60% of children with hemophilia have this severe form of the disease.

Bleeding into joints is the most common manifestation of the disease and will occur in all children with moderate and severe hemophilia. Recurrent bleeding can lead to chronic inflammation and joint changes including damage to and loss of articular cartilage. The most common joints to be affected include the knee, elbow, and ankle. The degree and type of disability resulting from bleeding into the joints is directly related to the severity of the disease and consequently the number and severity of the bleeding episodes.

Disability resulting from hemarthrosis (bleeding into joints) can include joint contracture, weakness of surrounding muscles, and functional disturbances of gait or other functional skills.

Bleeding may also occur in other parts of the body. Parents are counseled to put lightweight helmets on toddlers with moderate to severe disease as they learn to walk to prevent severe bleeding from mild head trauma.

Children who received clotting factor replacement therapy before 1985 are at risk for becoming HIV positive. After 1985, blood has been routinely screened for HIV. It is estimated that 70% of children in this category are infected with HIV (Brown, Schultz, & Gragg, 1995). These children are now entering adolescence and must make choices about responsible and irresponsible sexual activity. The prognosis for many children who are HIV positive is improving with the advent of new drug therapies (see Chapter 10), but the issues of growing older with HIV have yet to be explored thoroughly.

A more common side effect of factor replacement therapy is contracting hepatitis from contaminated blood. Hepatitis B affects 80% of children with severe hemophilia. The recent widespread use of hepatitis B vaccine may decrease the incidence of this complication. Other blood-borne pathogens may not have yet been identified or may be less serious, but children with multiple infusions of factor replacements are at high risk for blood-borne diseases because of the number of donors to whom they are exposed.

Mayes et al. (1996) suggest that children with hemophilia may be more often enrolled in gifted programs than children without hemophilia but also had higher proportions of attention-deficit hyperactivity disorder (ADHD) and learning disabilities. It is certain that children with chronic illnesses like hemophilia have a different experience of childhood than their peers.

Intervention. During the past 20 years, management of hemophilia has changed to allow a much improved outlook. Emphasis is on preventing bleeding episodes that can threaten function or life before they happen, rather than simply treating them after they occur. Intravenous factor replacement therapy is the most effective means of preventing excessive bleeding and usually is given in the early phases of bleeding to decrease its severity. Home therapy is now practiced throughout the country where children can receive factor replacement at home. About 10% to 15% of children with hemophilia A develop antibodies against factor VIII. These children can be treated with large doses of factor replacement for acute episodes but are at much greater risk for bleeding because of ineffective responses to factor therapy. They do not usually benefit from prophylactic therapy and may need to take even more precautions to prevent injury. Elective surgery is not an option for them.

Children with hemarthrosis usually need to immobilize the joint and stay off the limb until the swelling and pain are reduced. Splinting, taping, or in a few cases casting may be used for immobilization. The least restrictive form of immobilization is usually the best because allowing some joint movement can help speed recovery. Conversely, immobilizing a joint for too long can lead to stiffness and contracture. The therapist may be involved in fabricating appropriate splints to protect joints after bleeding or after surgery.

The child may need to use crutches for mobility. Once the limb can be moved, the child can receive therapy. Passive range of motion is contraindicated for a child with hemophilia because of the risk of unintentionally injuring the joint. Active range of motion, however, is encouraged to maintain mobility and strength. Pool or water activities can serve multiple purposes of active ranging and strengthening, and be fun for a child.

Muscles surrounding a frequently injured joint usually become weak and need rehabilitation to regain strength and function. Care should be taken to design exercises that are age-appropriate and fun and do not stress the joint. Jumping on a trampoline, for example, may not be appropriate for a child recovering from bleeding in the knee. Jumping in the swimming pool, however, may provide the same benefit while protecting the joint.

Surgical intervention to reduce joint pain, decrease episodes of bleeding, and improve function includes synovectomies. Hypertrophied synovial membrane is removed through open surgery or arthroscopy to allow more normal joint function. The most common joints for this procedure are the knee and elbow. When the child is older, more invasive surgery may be needed to alleviate pain and preserve joint function. Joint replacements (especially the hip), joint fusion, and osteotomies may be helpful with severe joint destruction.

The importance of regular exercise to both treat and prevent joint injury is being recognized. Habits of regular exercise should be started at an early age in all children, but especially in children with hemophilia. Regular swimming, golf, light jogging, table tennis, or other exercise that does not overly stress joints may provide some protective factor against joint bleeding (Buzzard, 1996). Children should be encouraged to be active throughout their lives. Intramural sports can be allowed for children with mild or moderate disease with prophylactic factor replacement before the participation. For children with acute bleeding or severe disease, prophylactic factor replacement may be necessary before participating in physical therapy.

Role of the PTA. The PTA may follow the child with hemophilia as an outpatient in a clinic or hospital setting. Therapy goals usually include strengthening, decreasing contractures, and improving functional skills such as walking. Most children recover from acute bleeding and do not need assistive devices such as crutches or a wheelchair for the long term. Preventing bleeding while enhancing strength and range of motion is sometimes a difficult balance. It is important to take the child's cues seriously. Sometimes a vague feeling of stiffness or pain indicates early bleeding.

The Child With Sickle Cell Anemia

Incidence and cause. Sickle cell anemia (SCA) is a hereditary disease and is one of a series of related diseases that have abnormal variants of hemoglobin formation. SCA affects about 3% of black people in the United States.

It is thought that the sickle cell trait protects against malaria, and therefore genetic selection over the generations has caused it to be more common in those living in tropical areas where mosquitoes carry malaria. In fact, almost 40% of black Africans carry the trait. In the United States about 8% to 13% of black Americans carry the trait. It is found in a few white Americans as well, primarily in people from the Mediterranean region.

Persons who carry the trait generally are well, although may have minor health disturbances related to the sickle cell trait. Some abnormalities of hemoglobin are present but not enough to cause significant health impairment such as anemia. When two parents who both carry the sickle cell trait have children, each offspring has a 25% chance of developing SCA, a 50% chance of carrying the trait and therefore possibly passing it on to his or her offspring; and a 25% chance of having normal hemoglobin.

Persons with SCA can live into the fifth decade or longer, although many die earlier. Causes of death include infection, pulmonary emboli, renal failure, or occlusion of a blood vessel supplying vital tissues such as the brain or heart. Management of the disease has improved over the past few decades so that life expectancy for individuals with SCA is significantly longer than in the past. Issues of living with a chronic disease have gained more importance as more individuals survive longer with the disease.

Clinical features. Persons who inherit SCA have significant health impairment caused by abnormally shaped red blood cells. Figure 12-20 outlines some of the most common sites of pain or disease caused by SCA. The genetic substitution of one amino acid for another in the 574 amino acids of the hemoglobin chain causes the red blood cell to take a sickle shape. It becomes stiff and inflexible. Because of these qualities, the sickled cell cannot pass through small capillaries and may clump together, blocking small blood vessels and causing hypoxia to the tissues. The sickle cell is fragile and less tolerant of the mechanics of circulation, breaking down faster than a normal red blood cell. Anemia results when too few red blood cells carry oxygen to the tissues. Jaundice results when the products of too much red blood cell destruction cannot be metabolized fast enough.

Children with SCA have multiple problems. Because of persistent anemia and resultant lack of oxygen to the muscles and other tissues, children with SCA are tired most of the time. This persistent anemia can cause a decrease of oxygen to vital tissues and can result in heart failure if severe enough.

The primary problem causing pain and tissue destruction is the vasoocclusive nature of the disease. Sickled cells can occlude small blood vessels anywhere in the body. Organs that are particularly sensitive include those with heavy blood supply such as the spleen, liver, kidney, and bone. These organs may demonstrate enlargement, tissue necrosis, and scarring. The spleen may be enlarged during childhood, but by adulthood the spleen is so fibrotic it is barely palpable. The liver, an organ important in blood purification, can become enlarged and tender resulting from back up of blood. Kidney failure may result from tissue death. Bones become osteoporotic and skeletal deformities may occur including spinal lordosis or kyphosis.

Acute infections, especially viral, can precipitate aplastic crisis when the red blood cell production in the bone marrow is slowed. Severe anemia can result.

Painful exacerbations, usually caused by occlusion of blood vessels can include hand-foot syndrome. This painful swelling and tenderness of the hands and feet in young children is due to infarction of the short tubular bones of the hands and feet and usually resolves in a few weeks. Chest syndrome is characterized by chest pain, cough, fever, and anemia and is related to occlusions in lung tissue. Strokes or miniinfarctions of brain tissue result from occlusions in brain tissue and can lead to significant neurological damage. Up to 25% of children with SCA experience identified strokes (Childs, 1995), and those who experience one have a 60% probability of experiencing multiple strokes.

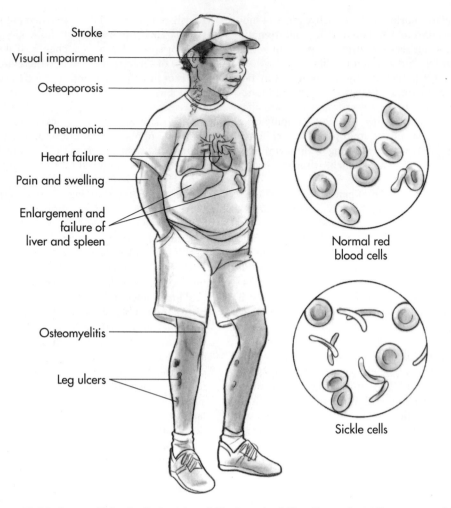

Figure 12-20   Some red blood cells form in a sickle shape in sickle cell anemia. Different parts of the body may be affected by the disorder.

More children have what are termed "silent strokes," where brain damage can be seen after death on autopsy but may not produce clinical symptoms. Children may experience pain in joints, long bones, and ulcers of the skin, all caused by sickled cells occluding blood vessels.

Sequestration, or a pooling of blood, can occur in the spleen, either acutely or chronically. The result can include severe shock from a decreased blood volume circulating to the other organs and possibly death. Children younger than 5 years of age are most susceptible to the acute form of this problem.

Infection is a significant threat to children with SCA. In addition to causing aplastic crisis, infection can be overwhelming because of defective splenic function and resultant inability to fight the infection. Children younger than 5 are at most risk for dying from the disease, most often from overwhelming infection. Crises become less frequent as children grow older, but critical episodes can cause disability and death at any age. Adolescents usually have delayed physical and sexual maturity, although most catch up to peers eventually. Many individuals with SCA can live with this chronic disease in adulthood, although the average life of a child with SCA is shortened significantly compared with peers without the disease.

Intervention.   Treatment is not available to remediate the underlying disease of sickled cells; however, supportive and preventive practices can provide greater comfort and less permanent disability to individuals with SCA. Early prophylactic treatment of young children with penicillin has proven to reduce the incidence of infection and resultant mortality. As pain is a major complaint, the use of analgesics including narcotics can provide some relief. Medical support for splenic sequestration and subsequent anemia has increased the survival rate from these complications. Prophylactic transfusions to treat anemia and decrease the number of abnormal red blood cells in circulation can help children function better. Treatment with some chemotherapy agents including hydroxyurea has shown some promise in reducing the incidence of painful crises and improving hemoglobin content. Bone marrow transplantations are being explored as a possible cure for SCA; but the mortality with this procedure is high, and the difficulty of matching individuals with donors presents significant problems.

A physical therapy provider may see a child who has sustained either orthopedic or neurologic damage from SCA. A child with leg ulcers may be seen for debridement to improve healing. A child with osteoporosis may sustain a fracture and need treatment for mobility training or strengthening. A child with brain injury from stroke will need physical therapy as part of a team effort to help learn appropriate developmental and functional skills. Therapy may be scheduled around blood transfusions so the child has more energy. Being aware of the child's pain level and tolerance, manifestations of pain crises, and the side effects of medical treatments can help the therapy provider design and implement appropriate therapeutic activities. Strategies for therapy vary considerably depending on the age of the child and the injury or disability that the child sustains.

APPLICATIONS

Medical Equipment for the Physical Therapist Assistant

CLARK E. RATLIFFE

PTAs encounter many different types of medical equipment in the course of providing treatments to children. Because physical therapy often involves moving a child, care must be exercised so that necessary equipment does not become dislodged or broken. The purpose of each piece of equipment and how it works should be understood. It is important to know what equipment can and cannot be removed during treatment and why. Additionally, knowledge of how to move equipment and what to do if something becomes dislodged or disconnected is necessary. A good practice to adopt when first working with a child is to carefully follow each line and wire from the child to the device to which it is attached. Learning the function of each wire and tube can help a therapy provider feel more secure and address problems or emergencies with confidence.

Feeding Equipment

Many children have problems that make oral feeding difficult or impossible. For instance, a child who is chronically dependent on a ventilator is not able to take food orally because of the risk of aspiration. Sometimes children remain unable to feed orally even after they are no longer ventilator dependent because they have no experience of oral gratification with food. While they are learning to eat, they may not be able to take enough nutrition orally and require supplementation with tube feedings. Children who are unconscious need to be fed either intravenously or through a tube.

Nasogastric Tube

As its name implies, the nasogastric (NG) tube is passed through the nasopharynx, through the esophagus, and into the stomach (Figure 12-21). The tube is either clear or a white opaque color and is usually anchored by tape near the nose. This tube can be used to either instill food into the stomach or drain gastric contents. When the NG tube is draining gastric contents, it is attached to a collection canister that may, in turn, be attached to a suction source providing intermittent suction. Draining gastric secretions is necessary for children who have a bowel obstruction or whose intestinal motility has been diminished after surgery. It is important not to disconnect the NG tube from the collection canister for long periods during procedures because the stomach continues to produce secretions that need to be emptied.

When the NG tube is used for feeding and/or administering medication, it is attached to a pump that delivers formula and/or medication either continuously or intermittently. Knowledge of the feeding schedule is important to schedule physical therapy sessions. If the child is fed bolus feedings (large amounts at one time similar to our eating a meal all at once), periods of activity should be scheduled before the feeding so that the child is not moving around vigorously with a full stomach. If the stomach is full, an increased risk of emesis leads to the possibility of aspiration.

Nasogastric tube dislodgment. If the NG tube becomes accidentally dislodged, it is not a medical emergency. In the hospital the nurse should be informed immediately if the NG tube is being used for gastric drainage; otherwise, it is usually fine to wait until the activity is finished. In the home or clinic environments it is probably best to let the family know what happened right away.

The NG tube usually must be reinserted. If the child is at home, parents may prefer to have reinsertion done at a doctors office or clinic rather than attempting to do it themselves at home. Insertion is quite unpleasant for the child and therefore usually difficult for a parent.

Gastrostomy Tube or Button

The gastrostomy (G) tube is used in children who need to be fed via a tube over an extended period of time. An NG tube passing

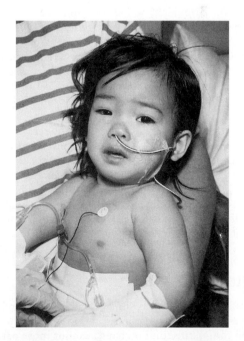

Figure 12-21 The nasogastric tube goes through the nasopharynx and into the stomach to provide nutrition and medications.

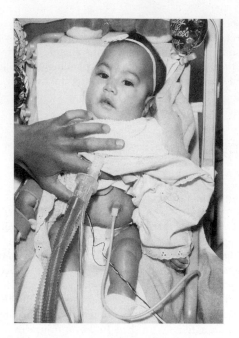

Figure 12-22 Christene uses a feeding tube attached to her gastrostomy button for all her feedings.

through the nose may damage the nares and the delicate tissues of the nasal septum over time. Therefore for children who need it, a tube or a receptacle for a tube is surgically implanted through the abdominal wall directly into the stomach.

A rubber catheter, called a Foley catheter, has a balloon on one end that can be inflated with saline solution. The tube is passed through the new opening into the stomach. Once there, the balloon is inflated to prevent the catheter from coming back out. The tube should be taped to the skin to prevent accidentally pulling it out. Any pulling should stress the tape rather than the inflated balloon in the stomach. The end of the tube should be secured to the skin or clothing for the same reason.

Gastrostomy tube dislodgment. If the G tube is accidentally dislodged, determination should be made if the stomach and abdominal wall are torn or injured. If so, surgical repair may be necessary. Usually, however, these tubes become dislodged because the balloon in the Foley catheter leaks saline and deflates, allowing it to slide through the opening. The remedy is for the nurse or parent to simply and painlessly insert a new catheter.

The gastrostomy "button" is a small receptacle for a feeding tube. When the feeding tube is not in use, it can be removed and the hole in the abdomen closed with a cap. The button is much less obtrusive than a G tube. Dislodging it is nearly impossible. Most children who need long-term tube feeding are fitted with these "buttons" (Figure 12-22).

Monitors

Many different kinds of monitors are encountered in both the hospital and home care environments. Monitors in the hospital are more complicated and perhaps monitor more parameters than those encountered in the home, but often the general concepts and reasons for monitoring are the same. Anyone interact-

ing with a child as a medical professional should have at least a basic understanding of why each machine is needed and what to do if an alarm is sounded or the connections become dislodged. It is also important to know which machines can be disconnected for treatments and how to move or change the connections to the child.

Cardiorespiratory Monitor

The cardiorespiratory (CR) monitor is one of the most commonly seen pieces of equipment in the hospital setting. Its purpose is to monitor the rate and quality of each heartbeat and respiration. In the hospital setting these monitors usually have an oscilloscope type of screen on which is displayed a tracing of the heart's electrical activity (ECG) and the respiratory pattern. The heart and respiratory rates are displayed as well. A paper strip may be spit out of the monitor when it alarms to provide a hard copy of the event that caused the alarm.

In the home setting CR monitors are much simpler and do not have CR tracings. They typically count the heart and/or respiratory rate and alarm when the child's rates are outside set parameters.

Alarms. Before alarms can be addressed, the reason a particular monitor is being used should be understood. The monitor may be used to monitor the heart rate, respiratory rate, or both. The reasons that the child needs monitoring are important. The child may have sleep apnea, for example, or may have a congenital heart defect. The child in the hospital may have medical problems that do not directly affect the heart or lungs but put the child at risk for respiratory or cardiac failure. For instance, a child with a head injury may have brain swelling that can compress the centers that control heart or respiratory rates. High doses of antiseizure medication may also affect the respiratory rate. It is important to take the time to find out why any monitor is being used.

Alarm parameters should be clear. Alarm settings should make sense when the purpose of the monitor is known. Alarms are typically set at a level that is about 5 beats above and below the child's usual heart or respiratory rate. For a child who has sleep apnea, however, the lower levels only need to be set.

When working with a child with sleep apnea, the monitor may be disconnected during the therapy session. It is important to reconnect it when the therapy is finished.

If a CR monitor alarm sounds, it is important to find out why and do something about it. Always go first to the child, not the machine. After determining that the child is all right, go to the machine to assess why the alarm went off.

Artifact. When an alarm sounds, if an infant is kicking and gleefully batting at a mobile, it is clear that there is not a problem with low heart or respiratory rate. The monitor may show disorganized squiggles. Because the infant is moving around, the leads are being disturbed. The monitor is interpreting the kicking and batting motions as an abnormal heart rate. This is called "artifact." A nurse or parent may initially help to determine if an alarm is due to artifact, but it soon becomes clear that when the tracing is very haphazard, yet the child appears fine, artifact is the likely cause.

Lead disconnection. If the child appears fine and a monitor screen displays a tracing that is completely flat, it is usually because a monitor lead has become disconnected. A lead is a wire that is adhered to the skin and is attached to the monitor. Through these wires the electrical flow from the heart is monitored. These wires are always color coded, indicating where they should be placed on the chest. The colors are black, white, and either red or green. The white lead goes on the upper right portion of the chest. This can be remembered because "white" and "right" rhyme. The next one is easy to remember because black is the opposite color of white and therefore goes on the opposite side of the chest. The remaining lead, either green or red, goes under the rib cage straight down from the black lead. Sometimes the leads are placed on the child's chest and sometimes on the child's back. Both work just as well. Sometimes it is a good idea to place the leads on the back to get them out of the way of curious hands.

Home Apnea Monitor

The home apnea monitor is very simple in its function because it simply measures the length of time between breaths and alarms if the child does not take a breath in a reasonable space of time (apnea). Usually there is no cardiac monitoring function attached to this monitor. A home apnea monitor is used for infants that may be at risk for sudden infant death syndrome (SIDS) because of a seizure disorder, prematurity, respiratory infection, or other reasons. The child may have had a previous near SIDS incident of unknown cause.

Alarms. The monitor is usually attached by means of a flexible strap that is wrapped around the infant's lower chest. Sensors in this strap detect each respiration. Usually the alarm in these monitors are expressed in terms of seconds of apnea rather than respirations per minute. The monitoring strap can usually be removed during a therapy session. Be sure to check with the parents before removing it and to learn how to reattach the strap. The positioning of this strap is important to avoid false alarms. Each child is different, and the parents are usually the best source of information on strap positioning.

Pulse Oxymeter

The pulse oxymeter monitors the percent of the hemoglobin in the blood that is saturated with oxygen (Figure 12-23). This function indicates how effectively the lungs are doing their job. In a normal person the hemoglobin should be 95% to 100% saturated.

Hemoglobin saturation is measured by assessing the color of a light passed through the skin, veins, and arteries. A small light source is on one side of the measuring device, and a receiver is on the other. These two parts usually are contained in a small piece of tape that can be wrapped around a finger or toe so that the light source is on one side and the receiver on the other. The device is easily recognized on the child because of an orange glow seen through the tape, with a wire running from the tape to a monitor.

Alarm. For the pulse oxymeter to read oxygen saturation accurately, it must sense a pulse through the finger or toe around which the probe is placed. Movement sometimes makes this difficult, and a low reading is obtained. When a child is moving around, there are frequent false alarms. The heart rate that is displayed on the pulse oxymeter monitor can be compared to the rate displayed by the CR monitor to assess whether the pulse

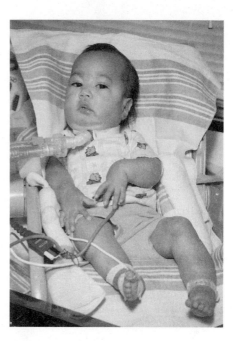

Figure 12-23 Notice the pulse oxymeter sensor wrapped around Christene's right toe. She also has a gastrostomy tube and monitor leads coming from under her shirt. Christene is supported by a ventilator attached to her tracheostomy.

oxymeter is giving a false reading. The pulse oxymeter is designed so that it never gives a false high reading. Therefore if you see a reading above 95%, the child is fine. If the child does not have a CR monitor, the child's pulse can be palpated to see if the machine is picking up each heartbeat.

When working with a child using an oxygen saturation monitor, the therapy provider know what actions to take if the saturation goes below 95%. The child may be stressed from the physical therapy treatment, causing oxygen saturation to go down. Giving the child a break may help. Additional oxygen may be needed and can be provided either by turning up the oxygen the child is already receiving or turning on a ready oxygen source. It is important to be prepared and ready before an emergency occurs. Whenever possible, anticipate rather than react, and prepare rather than scramble. Know where the oxygen source is and how to administer it.

Intravenous Devices

Intravenous Lines

When a child needs fluids and medication delivered intravenously, a catheter is introduced into a vein (Figure 12-24). The veins used could be located almost anywhere. Feet and hands are the most common locations, but it is not unusual to see intravenous lines (IVs) placed in an infant's scalp veins. In children who may need longer term IV therapy, catheters may be placed into larger veins such as the subclavian vein under the clavicle. These central lines feed directly into the heart. In pediatrics all IVs are precious and delicate and need to be carefully guarded against being accidentally dislodged. Because of the small diameter of a child's veins and the child's inability to hold still during

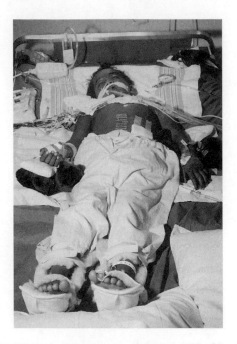

Figure 12-24 In the intensive care unit, this child with a head injury has an intravenous line in his left wrist and an arterial line in his right radial artery. The lines running from the right side of his neck are central lines. He also has an endotracheal tube—going into his mouth and trachea—to which a ventilator is attached.

insertion, starting IVs on children is difficult and often traumatic for the child. Therefore be careful.

Intravenous pump and alarms. It is the standard of care to use an IV pump on all pediatric patients who have running IVs. This pump usually is able to detect an IV that has infiltrated (no longer is discharging its contents into a vein but into the tissues surrounding a vein), has air in the line, or is out of solution. Different brands of pumps have various alarms, but it is important not to ignore any IV alarm. If an IV alarm is sounding, find someone who can deal with it properly by assessing what the alarm is communicating. Simply turning off the alarm is not good enough. Because of the small lumen only a few minutes with no fluid running through a line may cause it to clot.

In the event you are seeing a child with a running IV who is not on a pump but has a gravity feed IV, the drip chamber of the IV can indicate the rate of flow. This small reservoir into which IV fluid is slowly dripping is in the IV. Look at this drip rate and get a sense for how fast it is flowing. If during the course of the treatment session the flow stops or is dripping considerably faster, get assistance.

Arterial Lines

The arterial line (art line) is only encountered in the intensive care setting in critically ill children who need intensive medical intervention to survive. This line is threaded into a small peripheral artery such as the radial or pedal arteries. It is then attached to a transducer for the purpose of measuring blood pressure continuously. The art line is also used to sample arterial blood to test respiratory gas content as a measure of respiratory function. The PTA is usually not involved with these children

until they are out of intensive care and no longer have an art line. There may be exceptions to this, however.

Arterial line dislodgment. Because art lines are on the arterial or "high-pressure" side of the circulatory system, special care must be taken to not dislodge them. If they become disconnected or pulled out, the ensuing bleeding can be forceful and profuse. If this happens, immediately put pressure on the site and call for help.

Oxygen Equipment

Numerous pieces of equipment can provide oxygen to a child. The type that is used depends on what percentage of oxygen the child needs. Most children in the hospital who are receiving oxygen will have their oxygen saturation continually monitored (see discussion of pulse oxymeter, p. 417). Outside the hospital setting, the oxygen saturation may not be monitored because the child's oxygen need will be stable and known. In either case it is important to find out how well a child tolerates activity and a lowered oxygen supply. It is not unusual, for instance, for an oxygen mask to become dislodged during a physical therapy activity. It is important to know how carefully to guard against this eventuality.

Mask

A good way to deliver high concentrations of oxygen is with a mask. Different types of masks deliver different amounts of oxygen. For instance, the Venturi type of mask typically has a small attachment that is placed between the mask and the oxygen source. This attachment can be adjusted to provide oxygen levels between 27% and 35%. The important thing to remember about this type of mask is that sufficient liters per minute of oxygen must flow through the Venturi valve for the oxygen delivered to the patient to remain constant.

Another type is called a rebreather mask. This can be recognized by the bag that is attached to the bottom of the mask. The purpose of this bag is to collect oxygen between each breath so that on inhalation a greater volume of oxygen is available. With any mask the child breathes all the oxygen-rich gas in the mask first, then pulls in room air for the remainder of the inhalation. This mixing of room air lowers the possible percentage of oxygen that the child actually breathes. While a rebreather mask is theoretically able to provide nearly 100% oxygen, in practice children are rarely able to receive much more than about 75%.

Masks have significant problems. Most oxygen masks are easily dislodged. Many children in the 2- to 6-year-old range feel claustrophobic with the mask on their face. If they are having trouble breathing, they will not tolerate something over their nose and mouth. As children get into the school-aged years, they are more likely to do what is asked of them and keep the mask in place. Finally, a mask is not a good option for an infant because of difficulty of fit and an infant's difficulty in cooperating.

Nasal Cannula

A nasal cannula is a small tube that delivers oxygen directly to the nose (Figure 12-25). This method works very well for children of any age as long as only low concentrations of oxygen are needed. Delivering concentrations of oxygen of more than about

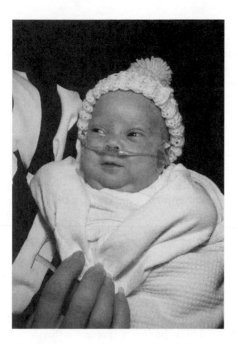

Figure 12-25 This premature infant is receiving oxygen via a nasal cannula.

25% by nasal cannula is difficult. The cannula can be taped directly to the child's cheeks and will stay in place quite well. Some hospitals use sticky-backed loop material stuck directly on the child's cheeks. This lasts longer than tape and is very effective at holding a cannula that has the hook portion of the hook and loop dyad in place. Older children can hook the cannula over their ears to hold it in place. Children may find it uncomfortable to have much more than 2 L/min of oxygen flowing into the nose. Although the oxygen is always humidified before delivery to the child, at high flow rates it still can be very drying to the delicate mucous membranes.

Tents and Hoods

To reliably provide a high concentration of oxygen to an active infant, it may be necessary to create an oxygen-rich environment for the infant's whole head or body. An oxygen tent is a clear plastic covering that is placed over the entire crib. The "tent" can be filled with enough humidified oxygen to achieve concentrations up to 100%. The humidity can also be controlled. Children with respiratory infections such as croup, which is often treated in part with humidification because it is soothing to sore bronchioles, may especially benefit from an oxygen tent. Oxygen can be administered in other controlled environments similar to a tent, such as Isolette.

Although the tent can provide high concentrations of oxygen to an active child, there are disadvantages. With the whole crib covered by the tent, it is not possible to get to the child without allowing oxygen to escape, thus lowering the concentration in the tent. Usually another source of supplemental oxygen is provided directly across the child's face at this time. Obviously, an infant needs to be touched and held and changed and fed in addition to any physical therapy treatments, all of which require lowering the oxygen concentration during the activity. Once the

tent is sealed again, oxygen concentration can take a long time to rise to desired levels because of the large volume of air in the tent. The child must be watched closely during this period to ensure adequate oxygenation.

An oxygen hood is another alternative for the smaller infant. This small hood fits over the infant's head with a semicircular opening for the neck. The hood is similar to the oxygen tent in that it provides an enclosed area where the oxygen and humidity can be controlled. Because it is smaller, the infant's body can be moved for diaper changing or exercise without losing oxygen. Another advantage over the tent is that the ambient air can be brought up to a given level of oxygen concentration faster. Disadvantages are that an active infant would soon roll out of the hood.

Blow-by Oxygen

An oxygen delivery system may become disconnected during a physical therapy session. If the child does not tolerate an absence of oxygen, some form of supplemental oxygen must be readily available. Blow-by oxygen is administered through a flexible tube attached to an oxygen source. The delivery end may be attached to a mask, or it may be an open tube. It can be moved near the child's face to blow humidified oxygen across the child's nose and mouth. When working with a child who has oxygen needs, this supplemental source should always be readily available in case of need. Blow-by oxygen can avert an emergency by delivering a high concentration of oxygen quickly.

Bagging and Suctioning

For children who are not able to breathe on their own, some form of mechanical ventilation is used. The PTA is not expected to operate these machines but is responsible for making sure a child using a ventilator is adequately oxygenated during therapy activities. Mechanical ventilators deliver oxygen and tidal volume (breaths) to children through either an endotracheal tube or a tracheostomy.

Endotracheal tubes. An endotracheal (ET) tube is a clear plastic tube that is passed through either the nose or mouth into the trachea for the purpose of delivering oxygen and ventilatory assistance (see Figure 12-24). Most children who have these tubes in place are dependent on this ventilatory assistance and may experience general respiratory failure within minutes of an accidental removal of the tube (extubation). For this reason, these children are encountered only in the intensive care environment.

"Bagging" is manual provision of ventilation for a child. The bag is a device that inflates with oxygen (usually 100%) and can be fitted over the ET tube or a tracheostomy. It can also be attached to a tightly fitting mask that is used in case the ET tube comes out. There are two types of bags. One is a floppy bag called an anesthesia type bag. This bag is flow dependent in that it requires oxygen flow to inflate. The second type of bag is more commonly used and is called an Ambu bag. The Ambu bag is stiffer and has resilience, which makes it self-inflating. It is not necessary to have any flow of gas into this bag to provide ventilation. Learn which type your patient has and how to use each.

If during the course of a therapy session a child becomes accidentally extubated, perform the following actions immediately and in this order:

1. Call for help. Say "Extubation! Help!"

2. While calling for help get the bag and the mask and put them together. You should have already looked to see where everything is located when you first arrived at the bedside.
3. Make sure oxygen is flowing to the bag.
4. In an intensive care unit there will be plenty of help at the bedside by this time. A nurse or physician will remove the tube the rest of the way if necessary, place the mask over the nose and mouth of the child, and begin delivering breaths.
5. The child's oxygen saturation, heart rate, breath sounds, and color will be constantly checked while preparing for reintubation.
6. Finally, think carefully and honestly about what happened. What led to the extubation, and how can it be prevented in the future? Of course you will feel terrible, but do not let this stop your learning from the experience. An incident report will need to be completed in most medical centers. Your supervisor and intensive care unit staff can help with this report.

Tracheostomy. An ET tube would cause tracheal erosion if left in place for an extended period of time. A tracheostomy ("trach") is used for children whose need for ventilatory support is chronic and therefore long term. Children who have significant difficulty handling secretions or those with chronic respiratory difficulties may also use a tracheostomy, although they may not need ventilatory support. A short, curved tube is placed into the trachea via a hole (ostomy) cut through the front of the neck. For children the one piece plastic tube does not have an inner cannula. Tracheostomies are much more secure than ET tubes and less likely to become dislodged. They are tied around the child's neck. Children with tracheostomies are likely to be in the home or nonacute care settings rather than a hospital setting.

A few weeks after the ostomy has healed, the hole in the trachea tends to stay open if the cannula is removed. This makes rapid and easy replacement much more likely should it become dislodged. It is a common practice to keep two extra cannulas at the bedside in case of accidental dislodgment or blockage. One is usually the size the child currently has in place and the other is one size smaller. The immediate availability of the smaller cannula increases the chances of successfully replacing it in an emergency.

In case of an accidental dislodgment of the cannula, the following should be done:

1. Call for help. Say "Trach came out. Help!"
2. Get the bag and mask and make sure oxygen is flowing. Do not put the mask on the bag. While doing this observe whether the child is breathing through the ostomy. If the answer is yes, go to number 3. If the answer is no, go to number 5.
3. Cut the tie holding the old cannula if necessary, and put it back into the ostomy. If the child seems to be breathing easily through the ostomy, you may have time to get the new cannula from the bedside.
4. Attach the bag to the cannula and give a few breaths if necessary.
5. If the child is not breathing through the ostomy, attach the mask to the bag and place over the nose and mouth.
6. Give a breath and observe for chest wall movement. The ostomy will likely need to be covered with your finger to prevent air escaping.

Being able to handle a cannula dislodgment is much less stressful if you have replaced one before. Parents are trained to replace the cannula every month or so. You may want to watch this process if a child you are working with has a tracheostomy.

Suctioning. When children have a tube in their trachea and are unable to breathe on their own, they are often unable to clear their secretions by coughing. If a patient coughs up mucus into an ET tube, there is every likelihood that the mucus will be pushed back by the machine during the next breath delivered. A child in this situation needs to have secretions suctioned out (Figure 12-26). Any therapy provider must be comfortable using suctioning equipment. Most institutions teach their particular technique and give guidelines as to who is able to perform suctioning. Usually the nursing and respiratory therapy staff perform suctioning for children who are intubated. A broader range of care providers like nurses' aides and PTAs, however, may perform suctioning for a child with a tracheostomy once trained.

Suctioning of an ET tube is a sterile procedure. Suctioning kits that include all the necessary equipment such as gloves, sterile water, and a suction catheter should be at the bedside. The catheter is threaded down the ET tube until it gets to the first bifurcation of the bronchiole tree. Suction is then applied and the catheter slowly removed, sucking up mucus as it goes.

Suctioning of a tracheostomy is a little different. If a child with a tracheostomy does not require a mechanical ventilator, the child may be able to cough up mucus into the trach itself. In this case all that is necessary is to remove it from the trach. Generally, this is a clean rather than sterile procedure, and the suction catheter is passed only the length of the trach. This is called shallow rather than deep suctioning. Nursing staff or parents can train the physical therapy staff to provide this service to a child.

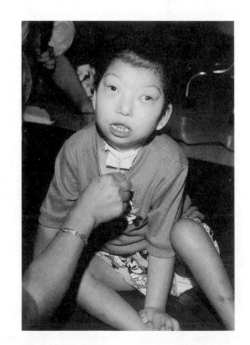

Figure 12-26 Secretions are being suctioned through Nicole's tracheostomy.

Death and Dying—Celebrating Life

KAREN J. TESSIER

Kendra is an infant with whom you are working. She suffered severe anoxia from birth trauma, and her mother died soon after the delivery. She is being cared for by her father and grandmother.

Ryan has a progressive neuromuscular disorder, and has been using a wheelchair for mobility. He is now 16, and has been growing noticeably weaker in the last few months.

Jennifer is 8. She was seriously injured in a car crash that killed her father and brother. She and her mom are trying to put their lives back together.

You have been treating Jason, 12, who has a brain tumor. Today when you go to visit, you find out that he died over the weekend.

Mindy got the HIV virus from her mother at birth. She is now 4 and has full-blown acquired immunodeficiency syndrome (AIDS). Her mother is also in the last stages of AIDS.

Paul, 3, was badly burned in a fire at his home. His grandmother, who lived in the same house and cared for the children while their parents were at work, died in the fire.

So many stories, each one so different, yet all with a common thread. Each one of these children and their families are dealing with death and grief. You, as a provider of care to these children, are also affected. You have your own feelings to sort out and experience, *and* you have an opportunity to help support these children and their families.

Morse and Perry (1990) studied children who had near-death experiences. They found that most parents and caregivers avoided talking with the child about dying. They limited their interactions to brief encounters and pretended everything was "okay," even to the point of lying to the child. This was their method of coping with their own discomfort about the subject.

Death in our society is often denied and ignored. We pretend that it does not exist so that we do not have to face our feelings of fear and dread that it will take us or someone we love. Yet it is just this denial that makes death so much harder to handle when it does occur, and the reality is that we all face it sooner or later.

The death of a child is especially hard for most people. Children are not supposed to die and certainly not before their parents. It is not the natural order of things. Being with a child who has to cope with the death of a loved one is also something that we never want to face. Death is "too awful," and we protect our children from awful things.

While many people grow to adulthood without experiencing the death of someone close to them, the reality is that many children do suffer a loss. In a school district of 6000, at least three children die each year, and 20% of all students lose a parent to death during their school years (Wolfelt, 1983).

Believe it or not, there is good news in all of this. We can learn how to support those who are dying or are bereaved, and we can grow in the process. For a child, an experience with death can be an opportunity to learn about life and living, as well as death and dying. Death does not have to be awful, and the opportunity to be with someone who is facing it can be a rich and rewarding experience. Very seldom do most of us have the chance to really make a difference in someone's life and to absolutely know that what we did helped someone to get through an especially hard time in their life. Because we were there and were willing to take

a risk to reach out in spite of our discomfort, we were able to help someone be less alone.

A mother whose child died after a long illness stated, "The only thing, when the chips are down, that really matters is kindness. . . . I know you have to turn it off . . . so you can carry on . . . but please don't stifle your compassion or your kindness" (Sahler, 1978). What we need to learn is how to express the kindness so that it becomes part of our professional skills.

While some people have a gift for knowing and doing the "right" thing, most of us have to learn. Having some knowledge as a guide helps us to support the bereaved person rather than add to their pain. This section provides you with information that can help you in working with death and dying.

To effectively help others cope with grief, we must give ourselves permission to feel and express our own grief. If it is denied or ignored, the incongruity between our feelings and our actions is obvious and gets in the way of the relationship. We also need to understand what this death means to those others who are affected by it.

The Child's Response to Death

It is important to have an understanding of a child's concept of death to know how to work with a dying child or one who has lost a loved one.

We can learn a lot about the way children view death by lis-

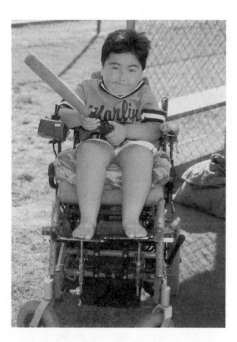

Figure 12-27 Rik has a progressive neuromuscular disease. He is healthy now, but his family wrestles with the fact that he will likely suffer from respiratory complications as his respiratory muscles get weaker. Rik loves baseball, Ninja stars, and video movies. He lives every moment to the fullest, as do most children.

tening to them. Grief is not about what is in our minds or our ability to understand but what is in our hearts and what we feel. "Any child mature enough to love is mature enough to grieve" (Wolfelt, 1983). Even a very young child is affected by a loss, although the outward expression of that experience may be difficult to notice, especially by someone who either does not know the child well or is so consumed by their own grief that they cannot see beyond it. Sometimes we are so caught up in our own reaction to the loss that we forget that the child is also experiencing grief.

Wolfelt (1983) believes that a child's ability to cope with a death depends on several factors, including the following: (1) the relationship with the person who has died (what the death means to the child), (2) the nature and circumstances of the death, (3) the child's personality, (4) previous experiences with death, (5) chronological and developmental age, (6) availability and type of support, (7) behavior and attitudes of significant adults.

Concepts of Death

Many studies have been done on children's understanding and perception of death by age levels. Interestingly, there is quite a bit of variability among these studies, perhaps because of where and when they were conducted and the circumstances of the children's lives at the time. For instance, children in Hungary who saw many people killed during wartime could be expected to view death differently than children in a safe environment in the United States 30 years later.

Despite the differences, there were common findings about the way the majority of children viewed death as they matured from infancy to adolescence. These are summarized in Table 12-7. An awareness of the child's developmental level helps you understand the possible reactions that may occur and lets you respond more appropriately to support the child.

Remember, the behaviors listed in Table 12-7 are useful only as guidelines and each child shows variations in perceptions and responses to death based on his or her own life experiences and

family values. Religion can play a major part in the child's response if it is important in the family's life. Past experience with death also affects the response.

There are also differences based on the death experience itself. A sudden and unexpected death is perceived differently from the anticipated death of someone who has had a long and painful illness. Those who have a family member dying or who are dying themselves undergo anticipatory grief, which is the process studied by Elisabeth Kübler-Ross. She worked with the dying, and the stages she described elucidate the process that the dying person goes through: from denial, anger, bargaining, and depression to acceptance.

Phases/Stages of Grief

Other theorists have defined the process of mourning or grief. Bowlby and Parkes describe four common phases among which those in grief move (Limbo & Wheeler, 1986). Table 12-8 delineates the duration and characteristics of each of these phases (Davidson, 1984; Heath & Gensch, 1994).

It is important to know that one does not move along a linear path through these phases. Those who are grieving go back and forth among them and may even experience all of them at once. The process can be described as coming in waves or moving along a spiral. Ideally, the general movement is forward, and yet there are many slides backward along the path.

Wolfelt (1983) identifies 13 dimensions of grief typically exhibited by children. These can be compared to the grief phases listed above. As caregivers recognize these dimensions, they can use behaviors that support the child in the healing process.

The initial response is often referred to as shock or denial or disbelief or numbness. This is temporary and usually short lived. It is important to be supportive and caring and not to force the child to accept more than he or she is ready to handle.

A difficult dimension for many adults is what appears to be lack of feelings. This is actually part of the above response and is a

TABLE 12-7 Children's Perception and Response to Death by Age Level

Age	Concepts	Behaviors
Birth-3 years	No actual concept of death Awareness of separation Fear of abandonment	May be fussy, cry for parent, especially mother, inconsolable Responds to nurturing from other caring person
3-5 years	Death is temporary, reversible Magical thinking Dead have biological functions Degrees of death	Grieves in "short bursts" Continues play and other normal activities most of time Asks when dead person will "wake up"
5-9 years	Death happens to others Death is final Death associated with punishment and mutilation	Plays involves rituals, morbid talk, jokes about death Can respond to logical explanation Influenced by others Feels some guilt
10-12 years	Death is final and inevitable More adult perception	Feels more guilt Asks many questions May exhibit bad behavior to hide fear
Adolescence	Death in relation to natural order of things Search for meaning and values related to death	Denial of death, especially their own Takes risks (defy death)

normal protective behavior for the child. The caregiver should be aware that this response is natural and not punish the child for it.

Children and adults in grief often experience physiological changes. These can include tiredness, lack of energy, difficulty sleeping or excessive sleep, lack of appetite or excessive appetite, tightness in the throat, shortness of breath, general nervousness, trembling, headaches, stomach pain, weakness, and skin rashes. In addition, someone who had a physical disorder before the death tends to become worse afterward. Another response of the child may be to identify with the feelings or symptoms of the person who died. The adult should be understanding of these physical changes and help the child to see them as a temporary response to grief.

A normal response for a child to the stress of loss is regression, or a return to an earlier developmental stage where the child felt safe and protected. Behaviors may include refusal to go out to play, asking to be rocked or nursed, or to sleep with the parent. The child may cling, ask to have things done that he or she is capable of doing independently, or talk "baby talk." Other behaviors may be refusing to go to school, demanding extra at-

TABLE 12-8 Phases of Bereavement

Phase	Duration	Characteristics
Shock and numbness	Most intense first 2 weeks	Short attention span
		Concentration difficult
		Impaired decision making
		Stunned, disbelief
		Resistant to stimuli
		Functioning impeded
		Denial
		Time confusion
		Failure to accept reality
Searching and yearning	Dominant 2 weeks to 4 months	Sensitive to stimuli
		Anger, guilt
		Dreams
		Restless or impatient
		Irritable
		Weight gain or loss
		Problems with sleep
		Preoccupation with deceased
		Resentment, bitterness
		Time confusion
		Palpitations, sighing
		Weakness, headaches
		Testing what is real
Disorientation	Dominant 5 to 9 months	"Going crazy"
		Social withdrawal
		Disorganized, forgetful
		Aware of reality
		Depressed
		Guilt
		Insomnia
		Anorexia
		Weight gain or loss
		Sadness
		Exhaustion
		Difficulty concentrating
		Feeling ill
		Lack of energy
Reorganization	Dominant 18 to 24 months	Sense of release
		Renewed energy
		Decision making easier
		Eating and sleeping back to normal
		Able to laugh and smile again
		Increased awareness of own well-being
		Again look toward future

tention, or a breakdown in peer relationships. The helping adult needs to be understanding and supportive while this is in the early stages. If the regressive behavior continues, either the child's emotional needs are not being met or the behavior is being encouraged to meet the needs of the parent.

An opposite response to regression is the big man or big woman syndrome. The child is attempting to grow up quickly and become the man or woman of the house, perhaps to replace a dead parent. This response should be sensitively discouraged. It is important that children be allowed to develop normally rather than rush through or skip stages.

A response that may occur suddenly and without warning is disorganization and panic. This is a common reaction for people as they fight against the reality of the death. They may have experienced a memory, either good or bad, or conversely have lost all memories of the person who died. Either way, this is a scary and painful experience. They may have bad dreams, be restless, irritable, or unable to concentrate. They may cry at odd times or be unable to eat or sleep. This reaction peaks at 1 to 6 months after the death of a significant loved one. The grieving person needs the physical presence and contact of a loving support person. Crying and talking should be encouraged. This helps to move through the grief.

An upsetting response to witness is explosive emotions. These can include anger and rage and are often a mask for feelings of pain, helplessness, frustration, and hurt. This can be a means of psychological survival and is a natural part of grief. We need to accept these feelings without judgment and reassure the grieving person that they will pass.

Some children express their grief by acting-out behaviors such as fighting, defying authority, running away from home, or even rebelling against everything. It is important that the adult understand the underlying factors behind this behavior. The children may need affection or security and reassurance that they are still loved.

Another common response is fear. Children worry that they will die or someone else close to them will. They are afraid to love again because they may lose again. The child needs reassurance, loving support, and acceptance.

For children and for adults, guilt and self-blame are common reactions after loss. They may believe that something they did (wishes, feelings, thoughts) caused the death, and they fear verbalizing this. It is important to provide opportunities for the bereaved to talk openly about the person who died and to show warmth and acceptance.

A less obvious emotion may be relief. This is natural after a long illness, and yet survivors may feel guilty about this feeling. It is important that they be given a chance to talk about it.

Perhaps the most difficult dimension is that described as loss or emptiness or sadness. This typically occurs 6 to 10 months after the loss. The person may show any of the following: a lack of interest in self and others, change of appetite and sleeping patterns, prolonged withdrawal, nervousness, inability to experience pleasure, or low self-esteem. They may feel totally alone and empty. They may be discouraged by the time it is taking to work through their grief. Dealing with grief may be the hardest work anyone ever has to do, and it cannot be rushed or avoided. It is important that the bereaved person complete this grief work. One way to help is to encourage the child to talk, draw, write, or play. The adult can also model other acceptable and therapeutic ways of expressing feelings.

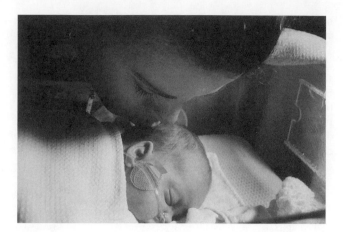

Figure 12-28 This infant was born very prematurely at 26 weeks of gestation. Her parents are getting ready to take her home from the hospital now, after the wild roller-coaster ride of her early life near death.

The final dimension of grief is reconciliation. This is when a person emerges from the grief. *Reconciliation* is a more appropriate term than *resolution* or *recovery*. There is no "getting over it" or "returning to normal" after the death of a loved one. The survivor is forever changed by the grief and loss.

Reconciliation is not an event but a process. It does not happen all at once and is often a very slow and painful process. There is no specific timetable in which this happens, and each person's way of getting there is unique. Moving *toward* grief rather than away from it is important in reaching reconciliation. Changes that may be noted during the reconciliation process include a return to previous eating and sleeping patterns, a renewed sense of energy and well-being, a sense of release from the person who has died, increased ability to think and make decisions, the ability to enjoy activities, a recognition of the reality and finality of the death, the establishment of new and healthy relationships, and the discovery of the ability to cope successfully with the loss resulting from the death.

We must recognize that grief is complex and varies from person to person. People should not be protected from grief; rather we can encourage them to not be ashamed of grief or to hide from it. It is essential that as helpers we be open and honest if we wish to help the bereaved through this process.

How Can I Help?

As a caregiver who has developed a relationship with the child and family, you are in a unique position to help in a grief situation. Whether you are treating a child who is dying, a child who has lost someone close, or are providing comfort to an adult whose child has died, you can learn to do and say helpful rather than hurtful things.

First, however, you need to know yourself and how you are reacting to this loss. If it is so devastating to you that you are having a hard time coping, you will be of minimal help to others. You need to accept that this is okay and take care of yourself. Your sharing this grief with others close to it will be a comfort in itself. Leave it to others to provide more active support. Table 12-9 pro-

Level	Relationship	Contact
	TABLE 12-9 Suggested Level of Contact by Relationship	
1	Close family and friends	Be physically present immediately and continue intermittently throughout grieving period. Assist in talking openly about the loss and give ongoing support.
2	Other family and friends	Call from time to time and send personal handwritten notes. Openly acknowledge what has happened. Help with maintenance needs if necessary.
3	Acquaintances	Send handwritten note. Make contribution to relevant charity, if appropriate, and ask that it be acknowledged to family.

vides some guidelines for the level of contact appropriate in a loss situation (Lord, 1988).

Practical Support

Some of the most helpful things to do after a death are practical ones. A list of suggestions follows for what family and friends might do. There may be something in the list that is appropriate for you, as an involved health care professional, as well.

- Bring food, especially something that can be frozen or saved.
- Run errands.
- Help with other children.
- Clean house.
- Help with transportation.
- Shop for family.
- Help address thank you notes.
- Send a note.
- Give a journal or diary for them to write in.
- Write reminiscences about the child and send to family, especially on the birthday or anniversary date. This is especially appreciated from classmates of a child who has died and can be helpful for those children as a way of dealing with their feelings of loss.
- Attend the funeral.
- Help with phone calls.
- Help in planning the funeral or memorial service.

Empathetic Listening

Listening is crucial in comforting others. One of the best things to do for someone who is grieving, whether after a death or in anticipation of one, is to listen. The person needs to talk and to have someone there who will really hear, with no judgment or need to "fix" anything.

What grieving people want is to be allowed to talk about what they are going through when they want to and to have all their feelings accepted. No one can make others hurry through their pain, and as much as we may want to, we cannot make them feel better. All we can do is let them know that we care and are willing to share in the suffering. Attempts to prematurely lift people out of their pain can be resented and rejected; they do not *want* to feel better at first. It is also not helpful to talk trivia or to keep the conversation light so they do not think about the pain in their life. Accepting the reality and sharing honest, open communication means much more than acting like nothing happened.

What Not to Say

The comments that people say to someone who is grieving are meant to help the person "feel better." Many of them do the opposite. Reactions to these comments include anger, bitterness, withdrawal, denial, frustration, loneliness, disbelief, and depression. The following are examples of hurtful comments:

- Everything's going to be okay. (How do you know that? Maybe they won't be okay.)
- It was God's will. (You can't speak for God.)
- You have an angel in heaven. (They would rather have their angel here on earth with them.)
- You're young, you can have other children. (Maybe they can't.)
- At least you have other children. (That doesn't make this loss any easier to bear.)
- It was for the best. (Not for you to decide.)
- It could have been worse. (What could be worse than their child dying?)
- You're looking great! (When they aren't.)
- You're so strong. (They may be barely holding themselves together.)
- Are you feeling better yet? (Makes it seem like they should be.)
- Don't be sad. Don't cry. Don't worry. Don't dwell on it. I can't believe you're saying that. You shouldn't feel. . . . (Denies their right to their feelings.)
- You'll get over it. (Maybe they won't.)
- Get over it. Just put it behind you. You need to move on. Forget about it. Get on with your life. It can't be that bad. (Diminishes the loss and their feelings.)
- I know how you feel. (No one knows how someone else feels.)
- You'll be a better person now that this happened. (They'd rather have their child than be a "better person.")
- If you need anything, call me. (They won't.)
- We'll take care of everything for you. (You can't, nor should you.)
- You can't bring the child back. (They know that, and they still want to.)
- Feeling like that won't help. (It's still okay for them to feel like that for now.)
- Let's not talk about that. (You're cutting off communication because of your own discomfort.)

Helpful Things to Say

The simplest things to say are the most helpful and comforting. This is indeed a case of "less is more." The following are examples of things to say:

- I'm sorry.
- I can't even imagine how you must be feeling.
- This must be so hard for you.
- What can I do for you right now?
- I'm here. I want to listen.
- I wish there was something I could do.
- I'd give anything to be able to make it better for you, and I know I can't. Just know that I am here for you.
- How are you feeling today? (Better than "How are you?")
- I was thinking of you and wondering what kind of day you were having.
- Do you feel like talking about it? (Respect the answer.)
- It's okay to cry in front of me.
- Tell me about . . .
- You'll never forget . . .
- What is it like without . . .
- How are you coping?
- What is it like when . . .
- It seems to me like you feel . . .
- I had a child (or a parent) who died, too (if this is so).
- Nothing (silence).

Things to Do

A list of some helpful things to do follows:
- Cry with them if it comes naturally. Don't cry more than they do. They don't need to be comforting you.
- Offer to be with them. *Ask* them if they want company. If the answer is yes, arrange for a time to be alone with them so they can talk. It may not be comfortable for them to do this at work or in public places. They may be trying very hard to maintain control.
- Be comfortable with silences and crying.
- Be willing to hear the story over and over. They need to keep talking about it.
- Ask open-ended questions.
- Reminisce about the "good times" and your memories of the person who died.
- Use the person's name.
- Use their words at first. "Death" may be too hard for them to hear or say at first.
- Encourage them to cry and sigh (both release tension and anxiety).
- Encourage expressions of anger that are not destructive.
- If you have had a loss, share your own experience briefly if they ask about it, then refocus on them.

Advice on Self-Care

An essential message for the caregiver is to remember to take care of yourself. It is easy to get caught up in "doing for others" and neglect yourself and your needs. You will not be any good for someone else or for yourself if you get overworked, overtired, or overstressed. Those in the health care and helping professions are often the worst about taking care of themselves. A conscious effort needs to be made to include self-care in our lives. Keep in mind that you cannot be a rescuer; you cannot save them from this. You can offer support, but individuals must go through their own grief process. You cannot do it for them.

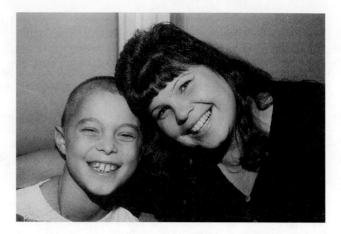

Figure 12-29 John, a 9-year-old boy with leukemia, has a close relationship with his mother. Both of them have to consider the possibility of his death from the disease. They enjoy each moment with each other.

It is important to maintain your own circle of emotionally healthy friends and spend time with them. Do things for yourself that are enjoyable and energizing. Stay healthy. Eat properly, rest, and exercise.

Process your own feelings. Remember not to tell yourself "You shouldn't feel. . . ." However you feel is what is. Accept it and go from there. If you do or say the "wrong" thing, apologize, then drop it. You did the best you could.

If the grief or death you are experiencing is of someone with whom you work or for whom you provide care, recognize that you cannot turn off your feelings about it when you go home. It may help to develop a ritual or activity for yourself to help address your feelings. This can include talking over your feelings with a sympathetic listener; collecting a special rock, shell, or flower for each person who dies and keeping it with others in a special place; including the person in your prayers; or taking a walk in memory of the person who dies.

Most of all, believe that your efforts have made a difference, even if they are not acknowledged. The person who is grieving may barely be able to get through each day; there is no energy or clarity of focus left over to be aware of others and their needs. You can be sure, however, that they know you were there for them when they needed someone most and they will always remember you in a special way.

EXERCISES

1. The world of acute care can be overwhelming if you are not familiar with it. Volunteer at a local hospital that serves children to get a sense of what a hospital is like. You do not have to volunteer in the physical therapy department (although this would be great experience) to get a sense of what the experience of hospitalization is like for children. You could volunteer to play with children in the playroom, to carry messages between floors, or to deliver flowers.
2. Invite your classmates who have experienced any acute care procedures and equipment (oxygen mask, nasal cannula, CR

monitor, NG tube, pulse oxymeter, etc.) to describe the experience for the class if they are willing.

3. In a safe environment explore your own feelings about death and dying. You may want to write about your feelings in a journal, discuss them with family or close friends, or with a few classmates. Describe any experiences you may have had when someone close to you died or was very ill. Can you identify stages of grief that you experienced or are experiencing? Think about how your own experiences or lack of experiences regarding death in your own life might influence your interactions with children and families who are experiencing death or loss.

● ▬▬▬ QUESTIONS TO PONDER ▬▬▬ ●

1. Hospitals are an institution that provide much needed services. Some children grow up in this environment if they need more medical care than their families or community settings can provide. Christene (see Figure 12-23), for example, has spent her entire life in the hospital and is dependent on medical technology. Children like Christene cost millions of dollars of taxpayers' money to support in this expensive environment. What can be done to provide care to them in a more natural setting that costs less? Is it appropriate to try to move them out of hospitals?

2. It is now possible to do more medical procedures at home than ever before. Children with IVs, trachs, and ventilator dependence can be supported at home through parent training and visiting nursing support. Is it fair to expect parents to operate medical equipment like ventilators and carry out medical procedures like suctioning? How far should we go in encouraging medical procedures to be done at home?

3. Death is a subject that is not talked about much in our society. Can you identify some of the cultural values related to death? How do these values dictate societal practices related to death? Should we be trying to change values about death? Why or why not?

Annotated Bibliography

Batshaw, M. L., & Perret, Y. M. (1992). *Children with disabilities: A medical primer (3rd ed.).* Baltimore, MD: Brookes.

Written by a physician and a social worker, this book is a complete and easily accessible text on medical and social issues associated with common disabilities of childhood. Chapters address specific diagnoses including Down syndrome, prematurity, cerebral palsy, and traumatic brain injury, as well as functional issues including feeding, nutrition, and medical dependence on technology. The authors make complex medical information understandable. This text is on my bookshelf, and I refer to it frequently, both as a teaching tool and as a reference.

Berkow, R. (1992). *The Merck manual (16th ed.).* Rahway, NJ: Merck Research Laboratories.

This manual is a steadfast standby, where information about almost all medical conditions can be found, including etiology, signs and symptoms, diagnosis, prognosis, and treatment. The information is presented in a rather dry, technical manner, but most of its information is up to date. Because it is an academic text, it does not give the flavor of a child's or family's experience with a disease or condition and tends to skew the reader toward impersonal objectivity. It is a wonderful resource for factual information, however. This book is a good one to have on the shelf as a basic reference text for medical disorders.

References

Bristow, J. (1995). The search for genetic mechanisms of congenital heart disease. *Cellular and Molecular Biology Research, 41,* 307-319.

Brown, L. K., Schultz, J. R., & Gragg, R. A. (1995). HIV-infected adolescents with hemophilia: Adaptation and coping: The Hemophilia Behavioral Intervention Evaluation Project. *Pediatrics, 96,* 459-463.

Budetti, P., & Weiss, K. B. (1993). Asthma care in the U.S. *Medical Care, Supplement, 3*(MS1), 1.

Buzzard, B. M. (1996). Sports and hemophilia: Antagonist or protagonist. *Clinical Orthopedics, 328,* 25-30.

Childs, J. W. (1995). Sickle cell disease: The clinical manifestations. *Journal of the American Osteopathic Association, 95,* 593-598.

Collins, F. (1992). Cystic fibrosis: Molecular biology and therapeutic implications. *Science, 256,* 774-779.

Davidson, G. W. (1984). *Understanding mourning.* Minneapolis: Augsburg.

Fernback, D. J., & Vietti, T. J. (1991). General aspects of childhood cancer. In D. J. Fernback & T. J. Vietti (Eds.), *Clinical pediatric oncology (4th ed.).* St. Louis, MO: Mosby.

Fink, G., Kaye, C., Blau, H., & Spitzer, S. A. (1993). Assessment of exercise capacity in asthmatic children with various degrees of activity. *Pediatric Pulmonology, 15,* 41-43.

Gergen, P. F., Mullaly, D. I., & Evans, R. (1988). National survey of prevalence of asthma among children in the US, 1976-1980. *Pediatrics, 81,* 1-7.

Green, M. R., Buchanan, E., & Weaver, L. T. (1995). Nutritional management of the infant with cystic fibrosis. *Archives of Disease in Childhood, 72,* 452-456.

Gurney, J. G., Davis, S., Severson, R. K., Fang, J. Y., Ross, J. A., & Robison, L. L. (1996). Trends in cancer incidence among children in the U. S. *Cancer, 78,* 532-541.

Heath, L. S., & Gensch, B. K. (Eds.). (1994). *RTS counselor training manual.* LaCrosse, WI: RTS National Office.

Hoffman, J. I. (1995). Incidence of congenital heart disease: II: Prenatal incidence. *Pediatric Cardiology, 16,* 155-165.

Jackson, D. B., & Saunders, R. B. (1993). *Child health nursing.* Philadelphia, PA: Lippincott.

Limbo, R. K., & Wheeler, S. R. (1986). *When a baby dies.* LaCrosse, WI: Resolve Through Sharing, LaCrosse Lutheran Hospital/Gundersen Clinic, Ltd.

Lord, J. H. (1988). *Beyond sympathy.* Ventura, CA: Pathfinder Publishing.

Mayes, S. D., Handford, H. A., Schaefer, J. H., Scogno, C. A., Neagley, S. R., Michael-Good, L., & Pelco, L. E. (1996). The relationship of HIV status, type of coagulation disorder, and school absenteeism to cognition, educational performance, mood, and behavior of boys with hemophilia. *Journal of Genetics and Psychology, 157,* 137-151.

Montafna, E., Khoury, M. J., Cragan, J. D., Sharma, S., Dhar, P., & Fyfe, D. (1996). Trends and outcomes after prenatal diagnosis of congenital cardiac malformations by fetal echocardiography in a well defined birth population, Atlanta, Georgia, 1990-1994. *Journal of the American College of Cardiology, 28,* 1805-1809.

Morse, M., & Perry, P. (1990). *Closer to the light.* New York: Ivy Books.

Morton, L. D., & Pellock, J. M. (1996). Diagnosis and treatment of epilepsy in children and adolescents. *Drugs, 51,* 399-414.

Nevo, Y., Shinnar, S., Samuel, E., Kramer, U., Leitner, Y., Fatal, A., Kutai, M., & Harel, S. (1995). Unprovoked seizures and developmental disabilities: Clinical characteristics of children referred to a child development center. *Pediatric Neurology, 13,* 235-241.

Ross, J. S., Severson, R. K., Pollock, B. H., & Robison, L. L. (1996). Childhood cancer in the United States: A geographical analysis of cases from the Pediatric Cooperative Clinical Trials groups. *Cancer, 77,* 201-207.

Sahler, O. J. Z. (1978). *The child and death.* St. Louis, MO: Mosby.

Shepherd, R. W., Holt, T. L., Vasques-Velasquez, L., Coward, W. A., Prentice, A., & Lucas, A. (1988). Increased energy expenditure in young children with cystic fibrosis. *Lancet, 1,:* 1300-1303.

Sigman, K., & Mazer, B. (1996). Immunotherapy for childhood asthma: Is there a rationale for its use? *Annals Allergy Asthma Immunology, 76,* 299-305.

Sly, R. M. (1988). Mortality for asthma, 1979-1984. *Journal of Allergies and Clinical Immunology, 82,* 705-717.

Steffenburg, U., Hagberg, G., & Kyllerman, M. (1996). Characteristics of seizures in a population-based series of mentally retarded children with active epilepsy. *Epilepsia, 37,* 850-856.

Szczepanski, R., Gebert, N., Hfummelink, R., Kfonning, J., Schmidt, S., Runde, B., & Wahn, U. (1996). Outcome of structured asthma education in childhood and adolescence. *Pneumologie, 50,* 544-548.

Weiss, K. B., Wagener, D. K. (1990). Changing patterns of asthma mortality: Identifying target populations at high risk. *Journal of the American Medical Association, 264,* 1683-1687.

Wolfelt, A. (1983). *Helping children cope with grief.* Muncie, IN: Accelerated Development.

Wong, D. L. (1995). *Whaley and Wong's nursing care of infants and children,* (5th ed.). St. Louis: Mosby.

Yoos, H. L., & McMullen, A. (1996). Illness narratives of children with asthma. *Pediatric Nursing, 22*(4), 285-290.

Zahm, S. H., & Devesa, S. S. (1995). Childhood cancer: Overview of incidence trends and environmental carcinogens. *Environmental Health Perspectives, 103* (6), 177-184.

Zupanc, M. L. (1996). Update on epilepsy in pediatric patients. *Mayo Clinic Procedures, 71,* 899-916.

Glossary

abduction Moving away from the midline of the body.

accessible Able to be accessed, entered, or used by persons with disabilities. This may include having a ramp or elevator for wheelchairs, a large bathroom stall to allow wheelchairs, telephone communications for the deaf, or Braille markings for the blind.

acetabulum Cuplike cavity in the side of the pelvis where the head of the femur articulates with the pelvis, forming the hip joint.

acute Sharp or severe. An acute disease has a rapid onset and a short course.

ADA Americans with Disabilities Act. Passed by the United States Congress and signed into law in 1990, this Act guarantees many equal rights for persons with disabilities.

adaptive equipment Equipment that has been adapted for the use of a person with a disability to assist with posture, positioning, mobility, or performance of functional tasks. Examples of adaptive equipment include a wheelchair, grab bars, and a switch-activated cassette player.

adaptive skills Skills to assist a person in coping with the demands and opportunities of daily life such as communication, self-care, social interaction, community use, self-direction, health and safety, academics, leisure, and work.

adduction Moving toward the midline of the body.

adhesion Condition that occurs when discrete body tissues bind together.

amniocentesis Prenatal procedure where a small amount of amniotic fluid is extracted from the amniotic sac using a needle. The purpose of the procedure usually is to examine the fluid for genetic material to assess the genetic health of the fetus.

amputation To cut off, usually a limb or body part. Amputation can occur traumatically through injury or surgically.

analgesic Medication or intervention that reduces pain such as aspirin or heat.

ankylosis Stiffening or fusion of a joint.

anorexia nervosa Disorder characterized by unreasonable fear of becoming obese and consisting of a distorted self-image, severe weight loss, and physiological changes related to excessively low body fat. The disease is most often seen in young women.

anoxia Absence of oxygen.

antalgic Painful. Usually referring to an antalgic gait where pain in the hip causes a person to lean over the painful hip during the stance phase of gait.

anterior Toward the front.

apex Highest point. The apex is the highest point on the convexity of a curve such as in scoliosis.

Apgar score System of assessing the general condition of a newborn baby. The Apgar score assesses the infant's heart rate, respiratory effort, muscle tone, reflex irritability, and color.

apnea Absence of breathing.

approximation Pressure through a joint. A therapeutic technique designed to stimulate postural tone and give proprioceptive feedback through a joint.

apraxia Loss of the ability to perform coordinated movements.

APTA American Physical Therapy Association. The national professional organization, made up of physical therapists and physical therapist assistants, that advocates for their interests to the legislature and the public.

arthralgia Joint pain.

arthritis Inflammation of a joint.

arthrodesis Joint fusion.

ASL American sign language.

asphyxia Condition where the body has too little oxygen and too much carbon dioxide, leading to loss of consciousness or death.

aspirate To breathe liquid or solid material into the lungs.

assessment Ministeps included in the evaluation process such as the use of specific measurement tools and their interpretation. Assessment also means the ongoing evaluation of a child's progress or the outcome of therapeutic intervention.

assistive technology Any tool or item that increases, maintains, or improves functional capabilities of individuals with disabilities in diverse areas including seating, mobility, learning, self-care, and recreation.

astigmatism Blurry vision caused by an unequal curvature of the cornea, preventing light rays from converging on a single point.

ataxia Loss of the ability to coordinate muscular movement, characterized by a wide base of support, tremors, and poor coordination. For example, drunkenness causes ataxia.

ATNR Asymmetrical tonic neck reflex. A normal infant reflex present up to 6 months of age with a stimulus of turning the head to the side and a response of flexion of the arm and leg on the scalp side of the head and extension of the arm and leg on the face side of the head.

atrophy Reduction in the size of an organ or muscle because of weakness or disuse.

augmentative communication Methods or devices to enhance communication. These may include a manual communication board, speech synthesis, or computer generated language.

autonomic dysreflexia Disinhibition of the sympathetic nervous system which can occur in people with spinal cord injuries above T6. Some signs and symptoms include headache, nausea, bradycardia, and hypertension. This condition can be life threatening if not controlled.

avulse To separate or pull away.

axilla Armpit.

babbling Language that includes long strings of repeated sounds.

barotrauma Trauma caused by excessive pressure.

bilateral On both sides.

bilirubin Breakdown product of red blood cells. Excessive bilirubin can cause jaundice.

biomechanics Study of the effects of forces such as muscle pull and gravity on the musculoskeletal system.

bradycardia Abnormally slow heart rate.

bulimia Eating disorder common among young women that is characterized by binge eating sometimes followed by purging or purposeful vomiting. Severe diets, excessive fasting, and other methods of rebounding from binge eating can also occur. Severe health problems can result from poor nutrition.

cardiac Relating to the heart.

carpal Referring to the small bones in the wrist.

cataract Opacity or thickness of the lens of the eye causing an impairment in vision.

caudal Having to do with the tail. In the direction of the tail.

cephalic Having to do with the head. In the direction of the head.

cervical Relating to the neck.

choreoathetoid Involuntary, unpredictable small movements of the distal parts of the extremities.

chorionic villi sampling Prenatal procedure where a small amount of chorionic villi from the placenta is sampled and examined for genetic material to assess the genetic health of the fetus.

chromosome Strand of hereditary material in the nucleus of plant and animal cells. The chromosomes carry the genes and are the carriers of the hereditary information that specify all aspects of the organism.

chronic Lasting for a long time or having frequent recurrences. Diseases such as lupus, arthritis, and multiple sclerosis are chronic diseases.

clavicle Collarbone. The bone crossing the upper chest that connects to the sternum on one end and the shoulder on the other end.

cleft palate Incomplete fusion of the palate during embryonic development, causing an opening or fissure.

clonus Repetitive contraction and relaxation of muscle resulting from a disinhibition of the normal stretch reflex. For example, in a person with a spinal cord injury or cerebral palsy, characteristic repetitive "jumping" of a leg when the foot is supported is caused by clonus at the ankle.

clubfoot Deformity of the foot and ankle characterized by adduction of the forefoot, varus position of the hindfoot, and equinus at the ankle. In lay terms the forefoot is curved inward in relation to the heel, the heel is bent inward in relation to the leg, and the ankle is fixed in plantar flexion with the toes pointed down.

cocontraction Contraction of muscles at the same time. Usually refers to contraction of muscles around a joint to provide joint stability.

collagen Fibrous protein. A component of bone, skin, and other connective tissue.

coma Prolonged state of unnatural unconsciousness, usually relating to a head injury, poisoning, or other injury or disease.

commode chair Positioning equipment used for personal care. The commode chair can be used over a regular toilet for toileting, in a shower for showering, or can be used with a removable bowl for toileting.

congenital Acquired at birth or during uterine development from hereditary or environmental influences.

consultation To meet with one or more team members to discuss issues related to a child's needs.

contracture Chronic or permanent tightening of soft tissues, causing decreased range of motion at a particular joint.

costovertebral Referring to joints between the ribs and the vertebrae of the spine.

COTA Certified Occupational Therapy Assistant. The COTA usually has an associate degree from an accredited COTA educational program. The COTA is qualified to carry out an occupational therapy intervention program under the supervision of an occupational therapist.

cranial nerve Any of 12 pairs of nerves that arise from the brain stem and exit the brain through openings in the skull. These nerves innervate diverse structures and functions, including eye and facial muscles, swallowing, and hearing.

cruise Walking while holding on to furniture. A child cruises before walking independently.

crutch-walking Ambulating with the assistance of crutches.

cultural competence Also known as cultural sensitivity, cultural competence includes understanding of one's own culture, knowledge of other cultures and traditions, willingness to use this information in interacting with others, and the ability to take cultural differences into account when interacting with others.

cyanosis Bluish color of the mucous membranes and skin, especially around the nail beds and lips, resulting from inadequate oxygenation of the tissues.

cytotoxic Relating to a toxic (causing injury or death) effect on cells.

debridement Removal of dead or dying tissue and foreign matter from a wound.

decerebrate Positioning after a brain lesion that is characterized by extension of all extremities.

decorticate Positioning after a brain lesion that is characterized by flexion of the arms and extension of the legs.

decubitus ulcer Ulceration or breakdown of the integrity of the skin, usually caused by excessive pressure in partially or completely insensate skin or caused by long periods in bed coupled with poor nutritional status.

deformity Abnormality in the shape or size of tissues because of disease, abnormal mechanical forces, genetic disorder, or malformation.

deinstitutionalization The process of moving individuals who have lived in institutions into community residential settings.

developmental Relating to the sequences of skill development in a child.

developmental age Child has been tested or observed to perform developmental skills similarly to other children of this age, no matter what the chronological age of the child.

developmental delay Differences in developmental skills where a child's skills (e.g., walking or talking) are not as developed as chronologically age-equivalent peers.

diaphoresis Inappropriate sweating.

diplegia Paralysis or spasticity of the legs and trunk, with the arms involved to a lesser extent.

disinhibition Loss of inhibition. When referring to muscle innervation, this term implies a central nervous system injury blocking normal inhibition of muscle contraction. The result is excessive muscle contraction, or spasticity.

dislocation Condition in which one bone completely slides out of the enclosing joint.

distal Away from the midline of the body. For example, the hand is more distal than the shoulder.

dorsiflexion Bending the joint toward the dorsal surface (back of the hand, top of the foot).

dorsum Back. The dorsum of the hand is the back of the hand; the dorsum of the foot is the top (back) of the foot.

durable medical equipment (DME) Medical equipment financed by medical insurance that is anticipated to last for several years before needing replacement. For example, a walker, a wheelchair, and a hospital bed.

dysarthria Abnormal or impaired verbal articulation, including slurred speech.

dysfunction Abnormal or impaired function.

dysgenesis Abnormal or defective development of an organ, particularly the testes or ovaries.

dyslexia Disability involving difficulty in reading and comprehending written words.

dysmorphia Abnormal form, shape, or structure.

dysplasia Abnormal development or growth of body tissues.

dyspnea Difficulty breathing.

dyspraxia Inability to organize and select speech.

dysrhythmia Abnormal rhythm, usually of the pattern of cardiac contractions or brain wave patterns.

dystonia Abnormal muscle or skin tone.

early intervention Referring to services provided to children between the ages of birth and 2 years who have developmental delays or are at risk for having developmental delays.

echolalia Immediate repetition of words or phrases spoken by someone else. Echolalia my preclude or impede the initiation of purposeful speech.

eclampsia Condition during pregnancy, or during or after childbirth, involving seizures and loss of consciousness that constitutes a medical emergency.

edema Swelling, usually in and of bodily tissues.

EHA Education of All Handicapped Children Act. See PL 94-142.

electrolytes Essential ions or electrically charged particles in the blood such as sodium, potassium, or chloride. These particles adjust the flow of water across a cell membrane.

embryo Developing infant in the first 8 weeks of gestation.

encephalopathy Any disease of the brain.

endfeel Subjective feeling in a joint at the end of range. Endfeel may be hard, soft, bouncy, empty (painful), or squishy, among others.

environmental Relating to the environment and environmental contexts such as school, home, schoolbus, bathtub, or backyard.

environmental assessment Evaluation of the child's skills and needs in the different environmental contexts of his or her life.

environmental intervention Intervention performed at the specific times and in the places where the skill or function is to be used.

epidural Outside or over the dura level of membranous tissue surrounding the brain and spinal cord.

epiphysiodesis Surgical fusion of a growth plate.

epiphysis Cartilaginous growth plate in the end of long bones. The epiphysis fuses on skeletal maturity.

equilibrium Balance.

equilibrium reactions Adjustments for changes of the body's orientation in space such as righting the head and trunk against gravity when tilted.

equinovarus Foot deformity characterized by ankle plantar flexion and inversion. (Toes pointed down with the bottom of the foot facing inward.)

equinus Plantar flexion at the ankle (toes pointed down).

eschar Thick necrotic tissue that inhibits wound healing. It is found in deep partial thickness and full thickness burn wounds, and usually must be removed to allow healing.

etiology Cause or origin, usually of a disease of medical problem.

evaluation Total process of measuring a child's abilities and drawing conclusions, which result in a final report.

eversion To turn the foot so that the inner aspect of the foot faces caudally.

extension Straightening. Increasing the angle of a joint.

external rotation Rotating the joint so that the limb (leg or arm) turns away from the midline of the body. Usually pertaining to the hip and shoulder.

extrapyramidal tracts Referring to the extrapyramidal tracts of neurons in the brain, damage to which causes athetosis or ataxia. Extrapyramidal tracts control postural muscles.

exudate Substance that has oozed or been discharged, usually from a wound.

fabricate To make, construct, or create.

facilitate To make something easier. A therapy provider facilitates posture and movement for a child with disabilities to help the child learn to move more efficiently.

facilitated communication Technique for helping nonverbal persons communicate that involves physically facilitating the typing of a message on a typewriter, communication board, or augmentative communication device, simply by holding the individual's hand, arm, or sleeve.

failure to thrive Deceleration from previous growth pattern, or growth consistently below the 5th percentile for age in height and weight.

family-centered In this model of service delivery, the family directs the services and supports for the child. The model reflects the understanding that the family is with the child for life and should have the key role in directing interventions.

femur Bone between the pelvis and the knee, the thighbone.

fetus Developing infant after the first 8 weeks of gestation and before delivery.

fibula Smaller lower leg bone between the knee and the ankle, on the outside of the leg.

fine motor Having to do with small muscles that control small movements such as those involved with handwriting, picking up small objects, and some handicrafts.

flaccid Absence of muscle tone, floppy or limp.

flexion Bending. When the angle of a joint decreases.

footplate Plate conforming to the foot used as a base for molding or casting an orthosis for foot and ankle positioning.

forefoot Front part of the foot, including the metatarsals and phalanges.

functional Related to a function or use, useful. For example, putting colored shaped blocks into a shape sorter toy may not be a functional task for an adult with mental retardation, but putting appropriate coins into a vending machine leads to getting a drink or food.

fusiform Shape that is characterized by being fatter in the middle than on the ends.

gait Pattern of movement associated with upright mobility (walking or running).

Galant Also known as the trunk incurvation reflex, the stimulus for the Galant reflex is pressure along the spine of an infant up to 2 months of age, causing lateral flexion of the spine toward the side of the stimulus.

gavage Tube feeding through the nose or mouth.

gene Building block of the chromosome, the genetic material of the cells. Each gene determines specific characteristics in an organism.

genetic Relating to genetics or genes. Usually related to characteristics inherited in genetic material.

goal Usually used in the context of a "long-term goal." A skill or measuring point for treatment that can usually be attained in 3 months to 1 year. For example, Bob's long-term goal is to run as fast as the other boys during kickball.

groin Anterior and inner surface of the legs where they meet the pelvis. The groin area often includes the genitalia.

gross motor Having to do with large muscles that control posture and large movements including standing and walking.

growth plate See epiphysis.

handicap Barrier or property of the environment that results in a person with a disability being excluded from participation in an event in which others without disabilities can participate. For example, the lack of a wheelchair ramp was a handicap to Joan who wanted to go into the restaurant.

handling Using placement of hands on a child's body to control abnormal muscle tone and facilitate posture, functional skills, or movement patterns.

hematoma Localized swelling caused by bleeding into tissues.

hemianopsia Loss of vision in half the visual field because of central neurologic deficit.

hemiplegia Paralysis or spasticity in half the body, usually involving one arm and one leg on the same side.

hernia One type of tissue protruding through another tissue that usually bounds or contains it. For example, an inguinal hernia is a protrusion of the bowel through the abdominal muscle in the inguinal region. Brain tissue can herniate through the foramen magnum, a hole is the base of the skull where the spinal cord passes.

hindfoot Back part of the foot, including the calcaneus and the talus bones.

home care Services provided in the home to help a person with an illness or disability to maintain or improve health and functional skills. Services may include nursing, physical therapy, occupational therapy, or speech-language pathology.

humerus Bone in the upper arm between the shoulder and the elbow.

hydrocephalus Build up of the fluid in the ventricles of the brain caused by an interference with the normal flow of cerebrospinal fluid around the brain and spinal cord.

hyperactivity Behavior affected by activity levels above the range of normal including difficulty remaining seated, constant fidgeting with hands or feet, and inability to focus attention for long periods.

hypertonicity High muscle tone. Characterized by resistance to passive movement and by involuntary movements (spasms).

hypertrophic Enlargement or overgrowth of tissue or organ as a response to abnormal stimulation or abnormal response to normal stimulation.

hyperventilation Abnormally fast breathing causing too much carbon dioxide to be removed from the blood with resultant physiologic changes of falling blood pressure, tingling in the hands and feet, and sometimes fainting.

hypoplasia Underdevelopment, usually of a bone or organ.

hypothermia Abnormally low body temperature.

hypotonicity Low muscle tone. Characterized by lack of resistance to passive movement, poor definition of muscles, hypermobility of joints and sometimes decreased strength and endurance.

hypoxygenation *See* Hypoxia.

hypoxia Insufficient oxygenation of the blood or tissues.

IDEA Individuals with Disabilities Education Act. See PL 105-17.

idiopathic Relating to a disease with no known cause.

IEP Individual education program (also known as individualized educational plan). This plan is created for children 3 years of age and older by an interdisciplinary team that includes family members to guide educational and related services for the child during each school year.

IFSP Individual family support plan (also known as individualized family service plan). This plan is written for all children younger than 3 years of age who are receiving early intervention services. It is created by a team of service providers including family members and reflects the needs of the family.

inclusion To include means to take in as a member. Inclusion refers to the educational practice of teaching children with disabilities in a regular education classroom with support but as full members of the class. This concept can be expanded to include community settings as well.

inguinal Relating to the inguinal canal in the groin.

inhibit To suppress or restrain. A therapy provider inhibits abnormal movements and postures for a child with disabilities to help the child learn to move more efficiently on his or her own.

integrated To bring diverse parts together. When physical therapy services are provided in the same environments and during the same activities as educational, recreational, and other services, they are said to be integrated.

intensive care Services provided in an acute care hospital to preserve life or health that involve very close medical supervision and usually technological support.

interdisciplinary When two or more disciplines work together to plan, assess, or intervene, team members are working in an interdisciplinary manner.

internal rotation Rotating the joint so that the limb (leg or arm) turns toward the body. Usually pertaining to the hip or shoulder.

interstitial Relating to or affecting the spaces between cells or tissues.

intervention To enter into the affairs of another. To provide treatment or consultation that may change the direction or outcome otherwise predetermined.

intrinsic muscles Muscles situated entirely within the body part on which they act. Usually referring to the small muscles of the hands and feet.

inversion To turn the foot so that the outer aspect of the foot faces caudally.

ischemia Decrease or cessation of blood flow to a discrete area, usually causing tissue death.

isokinetic Exercises where a muscle contraction against variable resistance results in a movement of the limb at a constant speed.

isometric Exercises where a muscle contraction against resistance results in the muscle length remaining the same.

jaundice Yellow cast to the skin and tissues caused by difficulty excreting high concentrations of bilirubin, a breakdown product of red blood cells. This condition is common in newborns, and can become dangerous if the bilirubin concentrations are too high.

keloid Overgrowth of scar tissue, usually red, raised, and fibrous.

keyboard Set of keys or buttons allowing one to enter data.

kinesiology Study of the mechanics of human movement, especially the actions of the muscles.

kinesthesia Sense that detects body position, movement, and weight.

kyphoscoliosis Severely abnormal spinal curve with excessive forward and lateral flexion of the spine. Most kyphoscoliotic curves also have abnormal rotation of the spine.

kyphosis Excessive forward curvature or flexion of the spine manifesting in a concave deformity, which usually occurs in the thoracic region.

last Shape of the sole of the foot.

lateral Away from the midline of the body. The scapulae are lateral to the spine.

laxity State of being slack or loose.

ligament Band or sheet of fibrous tissue that attaches one bone to another.

linear In one plane, flat. Usually referring to a seating system that is flat rather than curved or contoured.

longitudinal Lying lengthwise; along the length.

lordosis Excessive extension of the spine manifesting in a convex deformity. It usually occurs in areas where there is typically spinal extension such as the lumbar or cervical levels.

lumbar Area of the back between the ribs and the pelvis.

mainstream To include a student with disabilities into a class or specific activity in which typically developing peers are participating.

malaise Bodily discomfort including ache and fatigue such as that accompanying a flu.

manual muscle test Objective method of measuring strength. Six grades are usually assessed including normal (grade 5), good (grade 4), fair (grade 3), poor (grade 2), trace (grade 1), and absent strength (grade 0).

MAPS McGill action planning system. A method for long-term planning and visioning for the future of a person, especially a person with a disability.

medial Toward the midline of the body. The spine is medial to the scapulae.

Medicaid Program financed jointly by the federal government and individual states that provides medical services for people that can not afford to pay. Because medical expenses can be very high for people with disabilities, many are covered under this program.

medically fragile State of having a chronic disease or disability requiring medical support such as suctioning, tube feeding, or respiratory treatments. The medically fragile person is at risk for becoming seriously ill within a short time if medical supports are withdrawn or if exposed to people and the diseases they carry in the general population.

Medicare A federal program under the United States Social Security Administration that provides for medical care for people older than 65 years and people with disabilities.

medulla Inner core of long bones where bone marrow is formed.

medulla oblongata Lowermost portion of the brain that controls primary functions such as respiration and temperature regulation.

microcephaly Abnormally small head size, below the 5th percentile.

midline Imaginary line down the center of the body, running from the head to the feet.

mobility base Base with wheels, usually to a seating or positioning system (e.g., the wheels and frame of a wheelchair or a stroller).

modalities Therapeutic methods or agents that involve a physical intervention. Physical therapy modalities include ultrasound, massage, electrotherapy, and hydrotherapy, among others.

motor Involving or relating to movement of the muscles.

motor control Involving control of the muscles and resultant movement of the limbs and trunk.

motor planning Planning and coordinating movements of the arms, legs, head, and trunk in the right sequence and force to achieve a motor goal.

multimedia Combined use of several different media such as graphics, text, music, and video, especially for the purposes of education or entertainment. Many computer programs boast of being multimedia programs.

muscle tone Resistance to passive movement of a muscle. A person with muscle tone outside the normal range is said to have hypotonicity (low tone) or hypertonicity (high tone).

musculoskeletal Relating to the muscles and bones.

mutation Sudden change in the genetic structure of a cell where a new character or trait is manifested.

myalgia Muscle pain.

myelin White fatty substance forming a sheath around some nerve fibers. Nerve impulses travel significantly faster in myelinated fibers than unmyelinated fibers.

myofacial release System of therapeutic intervention designed to release tightened muscle and other soft tissues through deep massage and manipulation.

myopia Nearsightedness. Objects far away appear blurred.

NDT Neurodevelopmental treatment. This method of intervention for people with neuromuscular disabilities, including cerebral palsy, traumatic brain injury, and strokes, emphasizes normal postural reactions in the learning and relearning of motor skills.

necrosis Death or disintegration of tissues caused by interruption in the blood supply from disease or injury.

neonatal Relating to newborns.

neurological Relating to the nervous system including the brain, spinal cord, and peripheral nerves.

neurotransmitter Chemical substance that transmits nerve impulses from one neuron to another.

NICU Neonatal intensive care unit.

nystagmus Rapid, involuntary side-to-side motion of the eyeball.

obtunded Dull or deadened, usually referring to a person's level of awareness or consciousness.

occiput Posterior portion of the head or skull.

opisthotonic Describing an abnormal posture that has strong muscle tone pulling the trunk and neck into hyperextension and all four limbs into extension. This posture cannot be relaxed easily.

orthopedic Relating to the musculoskeletal system including bones, muscles, joints, tendons, and ligaments.

orthostatic hypotension Low blood pressure caused by a sudden upright position such as standing or sitting upright.

orthotic External support for one or more joints.

orthotist Professional trained to fabricate, fit, and adapt orthotics.

ossification To calcify and change to bony tissue.

osteoporosis Condition of decreased bone density, leading to brittle bones and an increased risk for fractures.

osteotomy Surgical procedure removing a portion of bone.

ostomy Surgical construction of an artificial opening such as a gastrostomy (opening to the stomach), iliostomy (opening to the ilium), colostomy (opening to the colon), or tracheostomy (opening to the trachea). The opening is usually used to introduce vital elements such as nutrition or oxygen or to allow excretions to be eliminated.

palmar Relating to the palm of the hand.

palmar grasp Neonatal reflex with a stimulus of pressure in the palm of the hand and a response of flexion of the fingers. This reflex is seen in typically developing children up to 4 months of age.

paralysis Loss of ability to move one or more body parts, usually as a result of damage to nerves innervating muscles that provide movement.

paraplegia Complete paralysis of the lower half of the body, usually as a result of spinal cord injury. The injury can be as high as the first thoracic level.

patella Kneecap.

pediatric Relating to infants and children.

pelvic belt Belt used to maintain the position of the pelvis in an optimal position during seating. This belt may also be used for safety to prevent someone falling out of a chair.

percutaneous Through the skin.

pericardium Membranous sac that encloses the heart and major blood vessels coming from the heart.

perinatal Relating to the period of time around childbirth.

perineum Area of the body between the genitals and the anus.

periosteum Double layer of fibrous connective tissue that surrounds and nourishes bone.

peritoneum Membrane lining the walls of the abdominal cavity.

phalanges Individual bones in each segment of the fingers and toes.

phenylketonuria Genetic disorder where phenylalanine cannot be metabolized and builds up, causing brain damage and mental retardation. If the condition is recognized early in the child's life, intake of foods containing phenylalanine can be limited and disability can therefore be limited.

phocomelia Term indicating the lack of formation of the proximal portion of a limb. The distal portion (hand or foot) usually extends directly from the trunk (shoulder or hip).

physiological flexion Flexion of the arms and legs characteristic of a typical newborn.

physiology Biological study of the functions of living organisms. Human physiology includes the mechanisms of body function such as respiration and digestion.

physiotherapist Physical therapist. This term is used outside of the United States.

PL 94-142 Education of All Handicapped Children Act (EHA). This Act was passed in 1975 and was the first legislation mandating a free and appropriate education for all children regardless of disability.

PL 99-456 The Education of the Handicapped Act Amendments of 1986 extended the earlier legislation of PL 94-142 to serve children younger than 6 years including infants, toddlers, and preschoolers and their families.

PL 105-17 Individuals with Disabilities Education Act (IDEA). The Act was passed in 1997 and reauthorized the earlier legislation of EHA (1975) and its amendments in 1986, as well as the earlier version of IDEA in 1991.

planar In one plane, flat. Usually referring to a seating system that is flat rather than curved or contoured.

plantar Relating to the plantar surface, or bottom, of the foot.

plantar flexion Pertaining to the ankle. Bending the joint toward the plantar surface of the foot, or pointing the toes downward.

plantar grasp Neonatal reflex with a stimulus of pressure at the base of the toes and a response of flexion of the toes. This reflex is seen in typically developing children up to 9 months of age.

plateau Stable period with little change in condition.

plinth Raised, padded, usually narrow table used to support a patient during medical intervention.

pneumothorax Accumulation of gas in the pleural (lung) cavity, usually as a result of injury or disease to the lung tissue.

PNF Proprioceptive neuromuscular facilitation. This approach to physical rehabilitation emphasizes diagonal patterns of muscle use to regain functional strength and motor control.

positioning Assisting a child to obtain and maintain a functional position using adaptive equipment, the therapist's body, or other supports.

posterior Toward the back.

postural reactions Righting, equilibrium, and protective responses that not only protect the developing infant but lead to greater variety of movements and skills.

posture Alignment of body parts in relationship to each other and to the environment.

Practice Act Act of law that governs the professional practice of a set of individuals (for example, physical therapists or physicians).

premature Delivery of a fetus before 37 weeks of gestation.

primitive reflexes Reflexes that appear in infancy and are integrated into normal movement patterns as the infant develops during the first 6 months of life.

prognosis Prediction of the probable course and outcome of a disease or injury.

pronate To turn the forearm so that the palm faces a caudal or posterior direction. To turn the foot so that the inner aspect of the foot faces caudally.

prone Lying with the face or front downward.

prone stander Equipment used to promote weight bearing through the legs. A person is positioned on the stander, leaning slightly forward with support through the anterior trunk. A mobile stander allows the user to propel the device either by turning the large wheels or through a motorized feature.

proprioception Perception of movement and orientation of body parts in relation to each other and in space. Nerve receptors in the joints and muscles feed information to the brain to perceive movement and orientation.

prosthesis Artificial device used to replace a missing body part. For example, prostheses for missing limbs.

prosthetist Professional trained to fabricate, fit, and adapt prostheses, especially for missing limbs.

protective responses Protective responses help the infant learn to protect from falls and bear weight through arms and legs to prepare for more upright positions and mobility.

protraction To extend or protrude. Usually used in the context of holding or moving one body part anterior or in front of other body parts such as protracting the shoulders.

proximal Toward the midline of the body. For example, the shoulder is more proximal than the hand.

pseudohypertrophy Deceptive enlargement. Usually referring to enlargement of the calf muscles of a child with Duchenne's muscular dystrophy caused by fat deposits rather than muscle strengthening.

PTA Physical therapist assistant. This person usually has an associate degree from an accredited PTA educational program and has licensing requirements in most states. The PTA is qualified to carry out a physical therapy intervention program under the supervision of a physical therapist.

pull-out Therapists working with children in educational environments may use a pull-out model of therapy, where a child is pulled out of class to participate in therapy, then reintroduced to the class after the therapy session.

pulmonary Relating to the lungs.

pyramidal tracts Referring to pyramidal tracts of neurons in the brain, damage to which causes spasticity. The pyramidal tracts control voluntary muscles.

quadriparesis Weakness or partial paralysis of the body from the neck down, including all four limbs. This term is sometimes used to describe a person who has cerebral palsy involving all four extremities but who has some functional skills.

quadriplegia Paralysis of the body from the neck down, including all four limbs.

radiograph Film image produced by passage of x-rays through the body.

radius Forearm bone on the thumb side, between the elbow and the wrist.

range of motion Full excursion of a joint from one extreme to the other. Sometimes used as a verb, meaning to move someone's joints through their available range.

reciprocal To move in an alternating pattern. A reciprocal gait is one where one leg moves and then the other reciprocates, following the same pattern of movement.

referral Request for services, usually from a physician or agency.

reflex Involuntary response to a stimulus.

rehabilitation Therapy or education designed to restore previous functional levels. Rehabilitation is usually undertaken after a disease or injury has reduced a person's functional skill level.

retraction To draw back or in. Usually used in the context of holding a limb or portion of the body in a posterior plane to the rest of the body such as retracting the hip or shoulder.

retrolental fibroplasia Also called retinopathy of prematurity, where, high levels of oxygen stimulate abnormal growth of the blood vessels in the premature retina causing visual impairment.

rheumatic Relating to a pathological condition of the muscles, tendons, joints, bones, or nerves resulting in stiffness, pain; and discomfort.

rhizotomy Surgical severance of a nerve root.

righting responses Keeping the head and body oriented to each other and to gravity.

rigidity Involuntary increased muscle tone throughout the body with little voluntary movement and a high risk for developing contractures.

role release Transferring knowledge or skills traditionally accorded to one discipline to persons from other disciplines to benefit a child. Thus a teacher may be taught to carry out gait training for a child, or a parent may adjust a splint under specific circumstances.

sagittal Longitudinal plane running from front to back on the body that divides the body into two sections.

scan To move a finely focused beam of light across a paper to transmit its image into a computer.
Method of communication whereby a person scans a selection of choices and then chooses one using a switch or a physical communication.

scoliosis Lateral curvature to the spine with or without a rotational component.

screening Quick test with only a few items to assess whether a child is functioning at the same level as peers.

seating Custom postural support designed to allow the individual a functional seated position to facilitate mobility, learning, recreation, self-help skills, or comfort.

seating system Combination of supports allowing an individual to sit upright, usually placed on a mobility base.

Section 504 Refers to Section 504 of the Rehabilitation Act of 1973. If a disability does not affect educational performance and therefore students do not qualify for special education, they may qualify for physical therapy services and civil rights protections under this section.

seizure Brief episode of unconsciousness, motor activity, sensory experience, or inappropriate behavior caused by a malfunction of the brain's electrical system.

sensory Having to do with the sensory system such as touch, taste, movement in space, sight, or sound.

sensory defensiveness Excessive aversion to most forms of sensory stimulation including touch.

serial casts Process of stretching soft tissues through constant stretch produced by casting and recasting a joint at progressively greater angles.

shunt Flexible plastic tubing system running under the skin from the ventricles of the brain to either the peritoneum or the atrium of the heart of an individual with hydrocephalus to drain excess spinal fluid and prevent brain damage.

SIB Self-injurious behaviors, also known as self-abusive behaviors. Behaviors that cause physical harm to the self, such as head banging, slapping, or biting the self.

sidelyer Device to position a child on his or her side. It usually has an L shape, with the child lying on his or her side on one wing of the L and resting his or her back against the other. Straps secure the child in place.

SIDS Sudden infant death syndrome.

SMH Severely multiply handicapped.

SMI Severely multiply impaired.

software Programs, routines, and languages that direct a computer to perform certain functions.

somatosensory Relating to sensory stimulation of the body.

spastic Referring to muscles that have abnormal innervation and increased resistance to passive movement. The muscles may react strongly to any stimulus with jerky movements or strong contractions that pull the extremity into flexion or extension.

spica cast Cast designed to keep one or both hips aligned during healing of bone or soft tissue injury or surgery. The cast usually extends from the nipple line to the knees or ankles on at least one side. A cut out is made around the perineum for elimination.

spirometer Instrument for measuring the volume of air entering or leaving the lungs.

splinting Use of a splint or orthotic to maintain joint alignment over a period of time.

static Not moving.

stereotypical behavior Repetitive and apparently purposeless behaviors such as hand flapping or finger flicking.

stimulate To rouse to greater activity or action.

STNR Symmetrical tonic neck reflex. The stimulus for this reflex is flexion or extension of the neck. When the neck is in flexion, flexion is seen in the arms and extension in the legs; when the neck is in extension, extension is seen in the arms and flexion in the legs.

strabismus Disorder of the muscles of the eye, causing abnormal alignment. Both eyes may turn in, out, or only one eye may deviate.

subcutaneous Under the skin.

subdural Under the dura level of membranous tissue surrounding the brain and spinal cord.

subluxation Condition in which one bone partially slides out of the enclosing joint. A partial dislocation.

suckling Early pattern of feeding that involves mouth closure, tongue pressure on the nipple, and tongue shortening and broadening to strip milk from the nipple.

supinate To turn the forearm so that the palm faces anterior or in the direction of the head. To turn the foot so that the outer aspect of the foot faces caudally.

supine Lying with the face or front upward.

supine stander *See* tilt table.

switch Device used to break or open an electrical circuit. Different types of switches help people with disabilities access electrical devices including battery-powered toys, household appliances, and computers.

sympathetic nervous system Part of the autonomic nervous system that speeds up the heart rate, contracts blood vessels, and reduces gastric secretions, among other functions, in response to danger or excitement.

syndrome Group of symptoms or conditions that characterize a disease or genetic abnormality.

synovectomy Surgical removal of the synovial membranes, the lining of joints, tendon sheaths, and bursae.

systemic Affecting the entire body.

tachycardia Abnormally fast heart rate.

tactile Relating to the sense of touch.

tardive dyskinesia Serious side effect of neuroleptic drugs that typically occurs after long periods (years) of treatment and includes facial grimaces and unusual movements of the body and hands.

task analysis Breaking down a task into its component parts to more easily teach the task.

temperament Characteristic behaviors and ways of reacting to environmental influences.

temporomandibular joint (TMJ) Joint between the temporal bone of the skull and the mandible (lower jaw). It is located just in front of the ear.

tendon Band of dense fibrous tissue that attaches a muscle to a bone.

teratogen Agent that causes malformation of an embryo or fetus.

therapeutic exercise Exercise designed to have a therapeutic effect, that of promoting improved health or improved functional skills.

thoracic Area of the trunk between the diaphragm and the neck.

thrombosis Formation, development, or presence of a fibrous clot in a blood vessel.

tibia Larger lower leg bone on the inside of the leg, between the knee and the ankle.

tilt table Equipment used to promote weight bearing through the legs. A horizontal table that can be either electrically or mechanically cranked to a vertical or semivertical position after a person has been positioned on the table with feet flat against a shelf and the person secured with straps for safety.

tilt-in-space Postural support system with the ability to change orientation in space while maintaining a set angle between the seat and the back.

tinnitus Sound heard in one or both ears without an external source. The sound is described as buzzing, ringing, or whistling.

TLR Tonic labyrinthine reflex. The stimulus for this reflex is the position of the head with a supine position resulting in extension of the trunk and extremities and a prone position resulting in flexion of the trunk and extremities.

tongue thrust Forceful protrusion of the tongue beyond the lower lip that makes eating and swallowing difficult.

torsion Twisting.

trackball Method of providing input to a computer using a movable ball rolling in place on a stable base.

trailing Method of mobility for persons who are blind where one hand is "trailed" on a wall to assess position in the environment.

transdisciplinary Working closely with others from different disciplines across disciplinary boundaries to carry out comprehensive services to individuals with disabilities and their families.

transfer To move from one place to another. In physical therapy this term usually implies moving from one type of adaptive equipment such as a wheelchair to another such as a bed or mat table.

transition Moving from one form of service delivery to another, usually associated with age milestones. For example, moving from an infant development program to school-based services or from school to a vocational setting.

transverse Lying across, crosswise.

trauma Serious injury to tissues usually caused by external forces.

Trendelenburg Drop in the non–weight-bearing side of the pelvis during stance. This is usually caused by weakness in the gluteus medius muscle on the opposite (weight-bearing) side.

ulna Forearm bone on the pinkie side, between the elbow and the wrist.

ultrasound Modality using ultrasonic waves to direct deep heat into soft tissues. This modality is also used diagnostically by trained technicians to visualize internal body structures.

unilateral On one side.

valgus Joint position characterized by the portion of the limb distal to the joint moving away from the midline of the body.

varus Joint position characterized by the portion of the limb distal to the joint moving toward the midline of the body.

vascular Pertaining to the blood vessels.

ventilator Mechanical device that delivers oxygen and tidal volume (breaths) to children who need assistance to breathe through either an endotracheal tube or a tracheostomy.

ventricle Cavity in the interior of the brain. Four ventricles in the brain produce cerebrospinal fluid that is circulated throughout the central nervous system.

vertebra One of the 24 independent small bones contributing to the spinal column.

vestibular Pertaining to balance. The vestibular system is situated in the middle ear.

volar Front. The volar surface of the hand is the palm; the volar surface of the foot is the plantar surface.

webspace Space between the thumb and the first finger or between the fingers or toes usually composed of a web-like tissue.

weight bearing Taking weight through the long axis of long bones. Weight bearing may be passive in passive standing or active when muscles control balance or gait activities.

Index